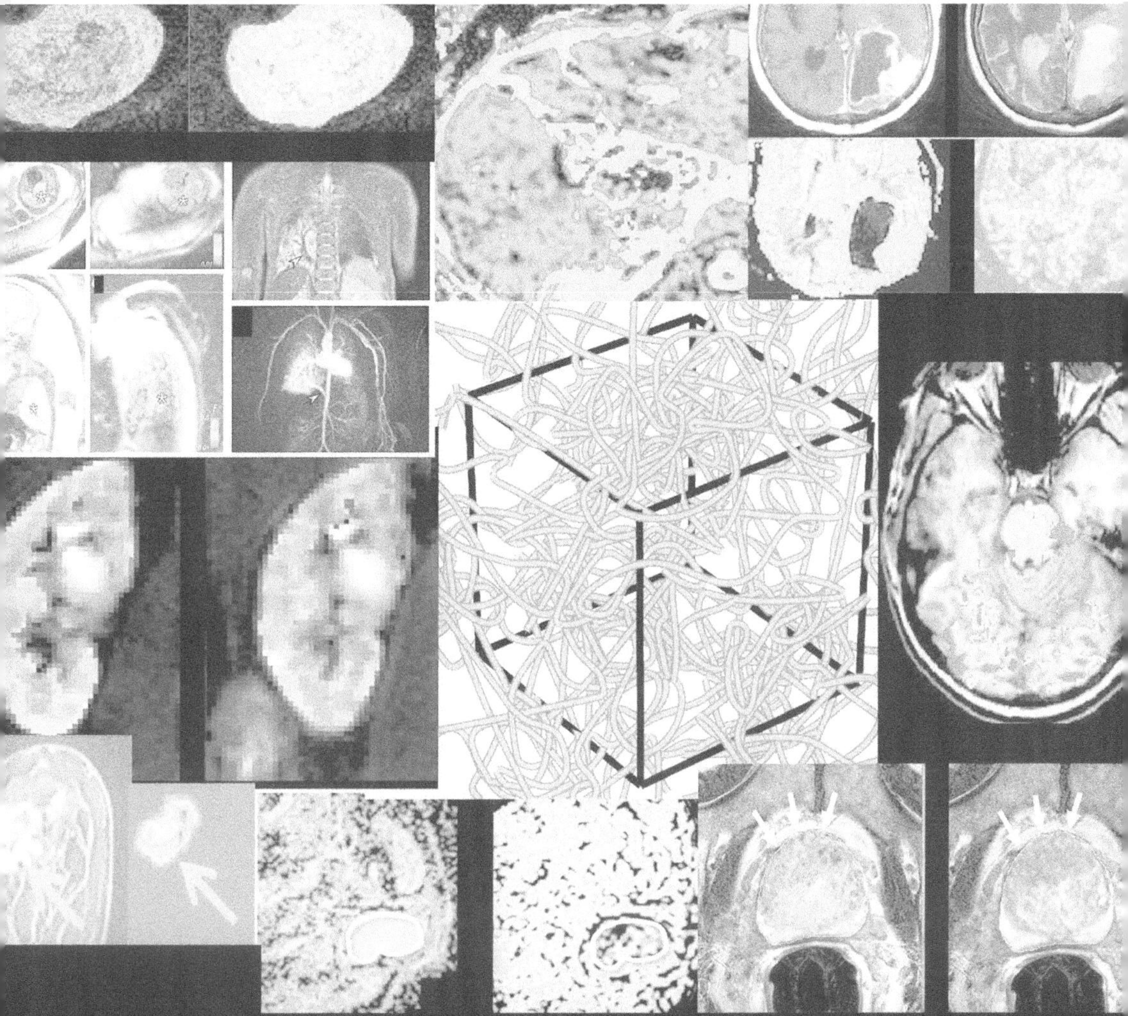

Intravoxel Incoherent Motion (IVIM) MRI

Intravoxel Incoherent Motion (IVIM) MRI

Principles and Applications

edited by
Denis Le Bihan | Mami Iima
Christian Federau | Eric E. Sigmund

PAN STANFORD PUBLISHING

Published by

Pan Stanford Publishing Pte. Ltd.
Penthouse Level, Suntec Tower 3
8 Temasek Boulevard
Singapore 038988

Email: editorial@panstanford.com
Web: www.panstanford.com

British Library Cataloguing-in-Publication Data
A catalogue record for this book is available from the British Library.

Intravoxel Incoherent Motion (IVIM) MRI: Principles and Applications

ISBN 978-981-4800-19-8 (Hardcover)
ISBN 978-0-429-42727-5 (eBook)

To the memory of our friend and colleague,

Alain Rahmouni, M.D., Ph.D.

who passed away during the preparation of this book.

*We all continue to miss this outstanding clinician and scientist,
who made significant contributions to the field of radiology
and was a fervent supporter of IVIM MRI.*

Contents

Foreword

Herbert Y. Kressel, MD

Miriam H. Stoneman Professor of Radiology, Radiologist in Chief Emeritus
Beth Israel Deaconess Medical Center, Harvard Medical School, Boston, MA

The clinical introduction of magnetic resonance imaging (MRI) heralded the beginning of a new era in medical imaging. Radiologists immediately recognized the remarkable image contrast and the multiplanar capabilities and quickly realized that imaging features could now be routinely identified on MRI images that could not be seen with X-ray, nuclear medicine, or ultrasound-based imaging techniques. Most importantly, contrast in MRI images was fundamentally multiparametric and based primarily on the T1 and T2 relaxation times and proton density. It was recognized that molecular diffusion and flow were also potentially available as MRI contrast determinants, but initially these could not be easily harnessed in imaging. The repetition time (TR) and the echo time (TE) were varied to configure the earliest MRI spin-echo pulse sequences in order to increase the weighting of one of the contrast determinants and decrease the importance of the other two to image contrast.

However, despite the clear clinical value of MRI imaging afforded by the early imaging techniques and the remarkable increase in sensitivity to disease afforded by the improved contrast resolution and multiplanar imaging, it became apparent that there was variability in the relaxation times in lesions of patients with the same disease and overlap in the relaxation times in patients with a number of different disease states. As a result, there was considerable interest among investigators in developing additional imaging approaches to harness the other potential image contrast determinants, including diffusion and flow.

In 1986, Denis Le Bihan and colleagues, in France, published the first of two papers that would eventually profoundly reshape the approach to MRI imaging [1]. They noted that in fluids, molecular

Brownian motion is responsible for molecular diffusion and that gradient application in MR imaging causes some signal intensity diminution due to an induced phase shift that is dependent on the gradient intensity, the diffusion coefficient of the tissue or substance imaged, and the measurement time. They went on to explain that the overall diffusion in tissues was related to what they termed "intravoxel incoherent motion (IVIM)" in tissue. The overall diffusion was multifactorial and related to tissue perfusion, including the capillary geometry and capillary blood flow velocity, as well as the intracellular restricted diffusion and free water diffusion. They further proposed a method to image and determine the relative contributions of this intravoxel incoherent motion by varying the strength, duration, and timing of gradient applications during image acquisition. They termed this method "IVIM imaging."

Their initial reports demonstrated that, using their approach, they could reproducibly determine the apparent diffusion coefficient (ADC) and in a few selected examples of human imaging, show an increase in the ADC in a cystic lesion in the brain, as well as a decrease in the ADC in a low-grade astrocytoma. This work was followed in 1988 by a larger, albeit still preliminary, study, in which they explained in more detail the mathematical basis for the model of IVIM they proposed and further demonstrated how to separate and determine the alterations in signal due to perfusion from those more related to "pure diffusion" [2]. In this study, they suggested that altered perfusion to tumor vascularity, as well as edema related to cerebral ischemia, may be identified on IVIM imaging.

While interest in diffusion imaging grew, there was initially a great deal of skepticism about IVIM. Or, as Dr. Le Bihan described in 2008, "diffusion . . . perfusion . . . confusion" [3]. This skepticism was largely the result of existing instrument limitations, due to available magnetic field strength, which limited signal-to-noise ratios, particularly in lower-field-strength systems, and limitations due to available gradient strength and stability. Thus, early imaging attempts at diffusion imaging and IVIM, particularly outside the brain, frequently suffered from motion degradation and poor image quality. Moreover, it was not possible to get adequate image quality at the longer *b* values needed to optimally separate the perfusion from restricted diffusion in tissue. In this case, the model proposed by Le Bihan and colleagues was better than the MRI units available to implement and utilize this technique, which had resulted in disappointing initial results when these techniques were tried. Happily, as machine performance improved, results improved, and the range of clinical applications for diffusion-related techniques grew rapidly. In addition, the advent of echo-planar techniques and parallel imaging, which sped up image acquisition, made inclusion of these techniques in routine clinical imaging exams quite feasible.

While diffusion-related clinical applications were initially established in the brain, particularly in the evaluation of acute and chronic stroke, more recently we have seen a dramatic growth in interest in and utilization of diffusion IVIM imaging elsewhere in the body [4–8]. The growth in clinical applications has been most pronounced in a wide range of oncologic applications in the head and neck, prostate, liver, kidney, and breast [9–19]. IVIM techniques have demonstrated value in diagnosis and staging and in determining response to therapy. Moreover, as further improvements in MRI hardware and software have been introduced that make it feasible to obtain images at higher *b* values than previously, it has increased interest in imaging based on non-Gaussian (kurtosis) diffusion imaging, which is sensitive to tissue and cellular heterogeneity commonly seen in malignancies [19–21].

The current volume, *Intravoxel Incoherent Motion (IVIM) MRI: Principles and Applications,* edited by leading experts Denis Le Bihan, Mami Iima, Christian Federau, and Eric E. Sigmund, with contributions from leading clinical investigators from around the world, begins with a clear yet concise description of IVIM and related diffusion techniques. Then follow chapters on the full range of neuro-IVIM and body-IVIM applications, as well as the next frontiers for IVIM imaging. This work is a welcome addition to our understanding of this burgeoning area of investigation and growing clinical applications.

References

1. Le Bihan D, Breton E, Lallemand D, Grenier P, Cabanis E, Laval-Jeantet M. MR imaging of intravoxel incoherent motions: application to diffusion and perfusion in neurologic disorders. *Radiology* 1986, 161(2), 401–407.

2. Le Bihan D, Breton E, Lallemand D, Grenier P, Cabanis E, Laval-Jeantet M. MR imaging of intravoxel incoherent motions: application to diffusion and perfusion in neurologic disorders. *Radiology* 1986, 161(2), 401–407.
3. Le Bihan D. Intravoxel incoherent motion perfusion MR imaging: a wake-up call. *Radiology* 2008, 249(3), 748–752.
4. Moseley ME, Cohen Y, Mintorovitch J, et al. Early detection of regional cerebral ischemia in cats: comparison of diffusion- and T2-weighted MRI and spectroscopy. *Magn. Reson. Med.* 1990, 14(2), 330–346.
5. Schlaug G, Siewert B, Benfield A, Edelman RR, Warach S. Time course of the apparent diffusion coefficient (ADC) abnormality in human stroke. *Neurology* 1997, 49(1), 113–119.
6. Lövblad KO, Baird AE, Schlaug G, et al. Ischemic lesion volumes in acute stroke by diffusion-weighted magnetic resonance imaging correlate with clinical outcome. *Ann. Neurol.* 1997, 42(2), 164–170.
7. González RG, Schaefer PW, Buonanno FS, et al. Diffusion-weighted MR imaging: diagnostic accuracy in patients imaged within 6 hours of stroke symptom onset. *Radiology* 1999, 210(1), 155–162.
8. Sugahara T, Korogi Y, Kochi M, et al. Usefulness of diffusion-weighted MRI with echo-planar technique in the evaluation of cellularity in gliomas. *J. Magn. Reson. Imaging.*, 1999, 9(1), 53–60.
9. Padhani AR, Koh DM, Collins DJ. Whole-body diffusion-weighted MR imaging in cancer: current status and research directions. *Radiology* 2011, 261(3), 700–718.
10. Thoeny HC, De Keyzer F, King AD. Diffusion-weighted MR imaging in the head and neck. *Radiology* 2012, 263(1), 19–32.
11. Sumi M, Nakamura T. Head and neck tumours: combined MRI assessment based on IVIM and TIC analyses for the differentiation of tumors of different histological types. *Eur. Radiol.* 2014, 24(1), 223–231.
12. Luciani A, Vignaud A, Cavet M, et al. Liver cirrhosis: intravoxel incoherent motion MR imaging—pilot study. *Radiology* 2008, 249(3), 891–899.
13. Turkbey B, Shah VP, Pang Y, et al. Is apparent diffusion coefficient associated with clinical risk scores for prostate cancers that are visible on 3-T MR images? *Radiology* 2011, 258(2), 488–495.
14. Patel J, Sigmund EE, Rusinek H, Oei M, Babb JS, Taouli B. Diagnosis of cirrhosis with intravoxel incoherent motion diffusion MRI and dynamic contrast-enhanced MRI alone and in combination: preliminary experience. *J. Magn. Reson. Imaging.* 2010, 31(3), 589–600.

15. Koh DM, Scurr E, Collins DJ, et al. Colorectal hepatic metastases: quantitative measurements using single-shot echo-planar diffusion-weighted MR imaging. *Eur. Radiol.* 2006, 16(9), 1898–1905.
16. Chandarana H, Kang SK, Wong S, et al. Diffusion-weighted intravoxel incoherent motion imaging of renal tumors with histopathologic correlation. *Invest. Radiol.* 2012, 7(12), 688–696.
17. Turkbey B, Shah VP, Pang Y, et al. Is apparent diffusion coefficient associated with clinical risk scores for prostate cancers that are visible on 3-T MR images? *Radiology* 2011, 258(2), 488–495.
18. Guo Y, Cai YQ, Cai ZL, et al. Differentiation of clinically benign and malignant breast lesions using diffusion-weighted imaging. *J. Magn. Reson. Imaging* 2002, 16(2), 172–178.
19. Rosenkrantz AB, Sigmund EE, Johnson G, et al. Prostate cancer: feasibility and preliminary experience of a diffusional kurtosis model for detection and assessment of aggressiveness of peripheral zone cancer. *Radiology* 2012, 264(1), 126–135.
20. Filli L, Wurnig M, Nanz D, Luechinger R, Kenkel D, Boss A. Whole-body diffusion kurtosis imaging: initial experience on non-Gaussian diffusion in various organs. *Invest. Radiol.* 2014, 49(12), 773–778.
21. Iima M, Yano K, Kataoka M, et al. Quantitative non-Gaussian diffusion and intravoxel incoherent motion magnetic resonance imaging: differentiation of malignant and benign breast lesions. *Invest. Radiol* 2015; 50(4), 205–211.

Preface

The intravoxel incoherent motion magnetic resonance imaging (IVIM MRI) concept was introduced in the mid-1980s together with diffusion MRI as it was immediately realized that MRI diffusion measurements could also be sensitive to blood microcirculation in capillary vessels. While diffusion is a physical phenomenon which had been known for more than a century (although its "molecular" origin was shown only in 1905 by Einstein), the idea that blood microcirculation could be seen as a pseudodiffusion phenomenon, due to the pseudorandom organization of capillary vessels in space, was coming out of the blue. Not so surprisingly, the concept was not well understood and received at the time, although the original *Radiology* article was accompanied by a laudatory editorial article by Thomas Dixon. Diffusion MRI was also seen as obscure. Diffusion MRI took off when Moseley et al. showed (indeed, using the IVIM MRI method to evaluate perfusion in a cat stroke model) that water diffusion dropped at the early stages of brain ischemia. However, it took much longer for IVIM MRI to be recognized as a potential perfusion imaging method. Because of the IVIM concept, diffusion MRI has been associated for many years with perfusion imaging, and therefore the many diffusion/perfusion sessions at meetings and workshops, or even book chapters, or journal key words, although they refer to completely different phenomena, both physically and biologically. However, the unexpected association of "diffusion" and "perfusion" was a little bit puzzling at the beginning for some, who at some point did not hesitate to display such aphorisms as "diffusion, perfusion, … confusion," printed on T-shirts worn by them at the first SMRM-sponsored workshop on diffusion/perfusion MRI, organized in Bethesda in 1989. In their defence, perfusion-driven IVIM effects were sometimes elusive and not clearly visible given the low signal level achievable at the time and the occurrence of severe motion artefacts before the advent of echo-planar imaging (EPI). It is fair to say that diffusion and IVIM MRI entered the clinical application field when EPI became available on clinical MRI systems (as well as systems operating at 1.5 T). IVIM MRI has also been the first imaging method providing images and measures of tissue perfusion completely noninvasively, without the use of tracers or contrast agents, well before the advent of arterial spin labeling (ASL). This also has been seen as a provocative step and challenged by R. M. Henkelman in his article "Does IVIM measure classical perfusion?" IVIM MRI has survived and been refined by this history and has gradually made its way to the clinical MRI world. Today, the seminal IVIM article, (*Radiology*, 1986, 3500 citations) has become the 5th most-cited article of all time in the field of radiology (just after the Hounsfield article introducing CT), and the *Radiology* (1988) article on perfusion IVIM MRI the 18th most cited article (2500 citations). Thanks to the tremendous technical improvement of MRI scanners, perfusion-driven IVIM MRI has become available for clinical applications, with great potential in oncology, as a non-contrast imaging modality. Therefore, we thought it was a good time to summarize all the currently available knowledge, either methodological or clinical, on perfusion IVIM MRI, in a book to help clinicians, researchers, and students alike to use and further advance and improve the method and concept. To our welcome surprise, we discovered that IVIM MRI was even more widely used than we realized, even to assess the placenta or foetal lungs, a completely unexpected outcome in the 1980s. Indeed, the approach has sufficiently grown in both depth of contrast and breadth of application beyond its original concept that it became a challenge for us to select topics to highlight in a limited number of chapters. If the book modestly contributes to the further development of IVIM MRI and to its expansion in the clinical world, we will feel greatly rewarded.

The successful realization of this book is directly the reflection of the committed efforts of our many contributors and the extended hours given by them. We are deeply indebted for their kind willingness to give their best in their efforts to contribute their chapters despite their already busy schedules. We profoundly thank our families for the long hours they have given up so that this book could be written and edited. We cannot overstate our appreciation for their continuous love and devotion. We also extend our gratitude to our support staff. Finally, successful completion of this project can also be attributed to the competent and motivational efforts of the staff of Pan Stanford Publishing, especially Jenny Rompas, Stanford Chong, Sarabjeet Garcha, and Shivani Sharma.

Denis Le Bihan
Mami Iima
Christian Federau
Eric E. Sigmund

Autumn 2018

Section I

INTRODUCTION TO IVIM MRI

Chapter 1

Introduction to IVIM MRI

Denis Le Bihan
NeuroSpin/Joliot/CEA Saclay, Bat 145,
91191 Gif-sur-Yvette, France
denis.lebihan@gmail.com

Intravoxel incoherent motion magnetic resonance imaging (IVIM MRI) allows both tissue microstructure (from molecular diffusion) and tissue microcirculation (perfusion) to be investigated at once. Besides brain and head tumors perfusion-driven IVIM MRI is currently being investigated to assess malignant lesions in the liver, the prostate, or the breast or evaluate tissue function in the kidney or even the placenta or the fetus. Indeed, IVIM MRI is experiencing a remarkable revival for applications throughout the body. The first reason is certainly that vast progress has been made in MRI scanner hardware and sequence developments, satisfying the signal-to-noise-ratio-hungry IVIM method. The second reason is that diffusion MRI has become a pillar of clinical MRI, part of many protocols, so that one may get IVIM/perfusion images "for free," together with the diffusion images, without the need for additional scanning time. Perfusion imaging, as permitted by IVIM MRI, gives valuable

Intravoxel Incoherent Motion (IVIM) MRI: Principles and Applications
Edited by Denis Le Bihan, Mami Iima, Christian Federau, and Eric E. Sigmund

ISBN 978-981-4800-19-8 (Hardcover), 978-0-429-42727-5 (eBook)
www.panstanford.com

information on neoangiogenesis or microvascular heterogeneity, as well as on treatment efficacy of chemo- or radiotherapy, and especially the effectiveness of antiangiogenic drugs or vascular targeting agents. The third reason is that IVIM MRI does not involve contrast agents, serving as an interesting alternative to perfusion MRI in some patients with contraindications for contrast agents, such as patients with renal failure at risk for nephrogenic systemic fibrosis (NSF). Recently, an accumulation of gadolinium deposits in the brain or other organs in patients who have received multiple injections of contrast agents has been demonstrated [1, 2]. The IVIM method, thus, appears particularly appealing for patients requiring multiple MRI scans, as well as for children or pregnant patients. This section will introduce the IVIM concept. In Section II of this book other perfusion MRI methods will be presented. Section III will provide a detailed overview of the many potential clinical applications (neuro, body, and musculoskeletal) of perfusion-driven IVIM MRI that are currently under evaluation. Finally, Section IV will address methodological issues and look at further developments.

1.1 The IVIM Concept

"IVIM refers to translational movements which within a given voxel and during the measurement time present a distribution of speeds in orientation and/or amplitude" [3–5]. The concept was introduced in 1986, together with the foundation of diffusion MRI [3], as it was realized that the flow of blood in capillaries (perfusion) would mimic a diffusion process and impact diffusion MRI measurements. However, perfusion and diffusion effects can be disentangled in diffusion MRI, leading to separate maps and measurements of molecular diffusion and perfusion [4]. Diffusion and blood microcirculation are two completely different physical phenomena, taking place at very different spatial and temporal scales, but because both can be addressed with IVIM MRI, they have been associated for many years in the MRI and radiology communities where "diffusion and perfusion MRI" often appear as session titles or journal keywords.

1.1.1 Molecular Diffusion

Molecular diffusion is just one type of IVIM. Due to their thermal energy all molecules move, colliding against each other. Each collision results in a change in the motion direction of each molecule, and the overall process is well described by a random walk, as first realized by Einstein. For liquid water the average of *individual* molecular displacement between two "collisions," l, in 3D space, is in the 10th of a nanometer range while mean "velocity" (a concept more valid for a gas phase than a liquid phase), $\mathbf{v}$, is around 100 m/s, which correspond to a diffusion coefficient, D, around 10^{-9} m^2/s based on Einstein equation ($D = l\mathbf{v}/6$) [6]. Diffusion refers to the random movement of individual molecules, but on a statistical basis, taking into account billions of molecules, each one diffusing on its own, this movement translates into an overall probability displacement along one spatial direction that obeys a Gaussian distribution. For water at body temperature the average diffusion distance is 17 μm during a time interval of 50 ms, a perfect scale to explore the microstructure of biological tissues in vivo (Fig. 1.1).

1.1.2 Perfusion-Driven Pseudodiffusion

Apparent motion randomness for perfusion results from the geometry of the vessel network where blood circulates, under the hypothesis that the microvascular network can be modeled by a series of straight segments randomly oriented in space and uniformly distributed over 4π within each voxel in the 3D space. Here, randomness thus results from the *collective* motion of blood water molecules in the network, flowing from one capillary segment to the next, in addition to the individual diffusion movement of blood water molecules. This collective movement has been described as a pseudodiffusion process where the average displacement, l, would now correspond to the mean capillary segment length and the mean velocity, $\mathbf{v}$, would be that of blood in the vessels (Fig. 1.1) [4]. Using Einstein's diffusion equation for pseudodiffusion one gets a value for the pseudodiffusion coefficient, $D^* = l\mathbf{v}/6$, which is around 10^{-8} m^2/s, taking l as 100 μm and $\mathbf{v}$ as 1 mm/s. It is really fortunate that D^* is close enough to D for it to be possible to make diffusion MRI sensitive to both diffusion and blood microcirculation, both resulting, separately, in a monoexponential decay of the MRI signal with the b value (see below). But the blood microcirculation component decays 10 times faster, which allows the two independent phenomena to be separated. Interestingly, the value for D^* is found to be similar across other species that have been scanned, which is not completely surprising as small animals have shorter capillary segments but higher flow velocities [7].

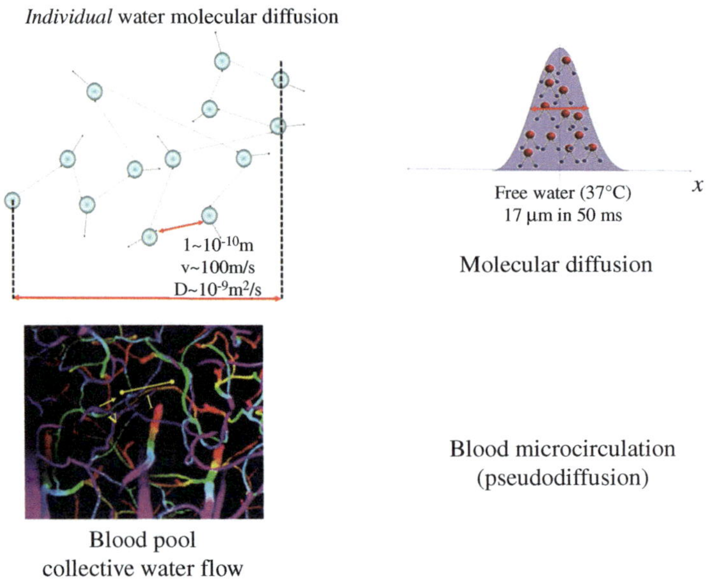

Figure 1.1 Molecular diffusion and blood pseudodiffusion. Molecular diffusion (top) is a random process at the individual molecular level. According to Einstein's equation, the diffusion-driven distribution of molecular displacements is a Gaussian distribution of molecular displacement (free diffusion). Pseudodiffusion (bottom) for blood flow (BF) results from the collective water flow in the randomly orientated capillary segments.

1.1.3 Other Sources of IVIM

By definition IVIM does not specifically refer to diffusion and blood microcirculation, and other sources of IVIM are possible. Some examples are given at the end of this chapter, especially in the domain of virtual elastography, but the chapters of this book will exclusively focus on perfusion-driven IVIM.

1.2 IVIM MRI

1.2.1 IVIM Contribution to the MRI Signal

The random displacement of individual molecules results in a signal attenuation in the presence of magnetic-field-encoding gradient pulses. This attenuation increases with the diffusion coefficient and the degree of sensitization to diffusion of the MRI pulse sequence (so-called b value, which depends on the gradient pulse shapes, duration, and separation times; see Refs. [3, 4]). With free (Gaussian) molecular diffusion the overall MRI signal attenuation, $S(b)/S(0)$, follows a monoexponential decay [3]:

$$S(b)/S(0) = \exp(-bD), \tag{1.1}$$

where $S(b)$ and $S(0)$ are the MRI signal intensities at a given b value and $b = 0$, respectively. In the presence of blood microcirculation, the overall MRI signal attenuation, $S(b)/S(0)$, becomes the sum of two exponentials (biexponential decay), one for tissue diffusion and one for the blood compartment (assuming water exchange between blood and tissues is negligible during the encoding time, a hypothesis which has not yet been deeply investigated):

$$S(b)/S(0) = f_{\mathrm{IVIM}} \exp[-b(D^*+D_{\mathrm{b}})] + (1-f_{\mathrm{IVIM}}) \exp(-bD), \tag{1.2}$$

where f_{IVIM} is the flowing blood fraction (sometimes also called f_{p}, or even simply f), D^* is the pseudodiffusion coefficient ascribed to blood random microcirculation, D is the water diffusion coefficient in the tissue, and D_{b} is the water diffusion coefficient in blood (as diffusion of individual water molecules also occurs in blood). Because the fraction of the flowing blood is usually small (a few percent) compared to the overall tissue water content, the perfusion-driven IVIM signature appears more as a deviation as small b values of the tissue diffusion–driven monoexponential signal decay (Fig. 1.2).

1.2.2 Extracting Diffusion and Perfusion Parameters

When both diffusion and flowing blood effects are present the apparent diffusion coefficient, ADC [3], calculated from signals $S(b)$ and $S(0)$ as $\ln[S(b)/S(0)]/b$ is higher than D. This difference is mostly seen when using small b values. As f_{IVIM} is usually small, one has ADC

$\approx D + f_{\text{IVIM}}/b$, and f_{IVIM} simply appears as the (negative) intercept of the diffusion component of the signal decay in log plots with b values (Fig. 1.3) [4].

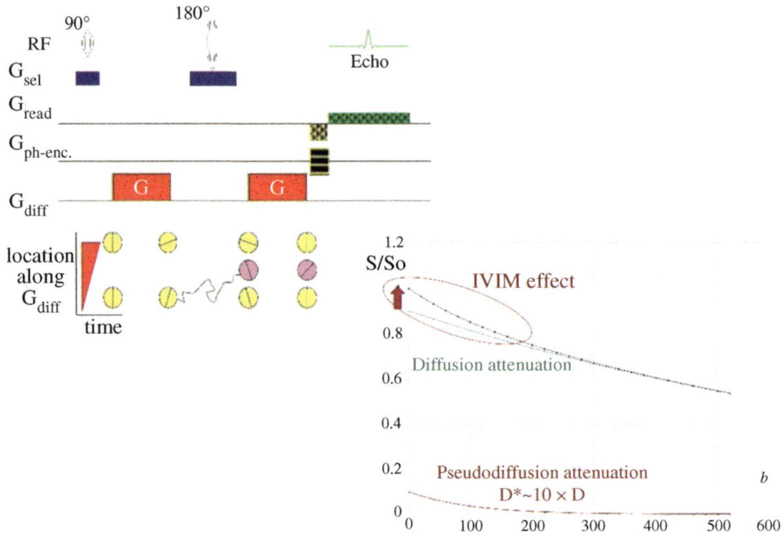

Figure 1.2 Effects of diffusion and pseudodiffusion on the MRI signal. Random water displacements (either from individual molecular motion or from collective water incoherent flow at the voxel level) result in an exponential decay of the signal amplitude with the degree of field gradient encoding (*b* value). The tissue diffusion and BF component contribute separately to the signal, resulting in a biexponential shape. However, as *D**>>*D* the IVIM (BF) effect appears as a deviation of the tissue diffusion signal decay at low *b* values.

On the basis of this observation, the first perfusion-driven IVIM measurements were obtained just by using three b values (0, 100, and 200 s/mm^2, the highest achievable value with the hardware available at that time) [4] (Fig. 1.3). The three b values scheme used at the beginning of IVIM MRI has gained popularity recently although with the larger gradient strengths available, as this approach minimizes acquisition times. The IVIM concept was first validated in a dedicated phantom (Fig. 6 in Ref. [4]) and in a small series of patients with tumors [4]. Phantoms mimicking both perfusion and tissue diffusion are tricky to make. We used calibrated sephadex beads, inside which water could diffuse and between which a flow of water was maintained, mimicking random flow in capillaries.

The IVIM concept was further confirmed by other groups in normal subjects and animal models [8–11].

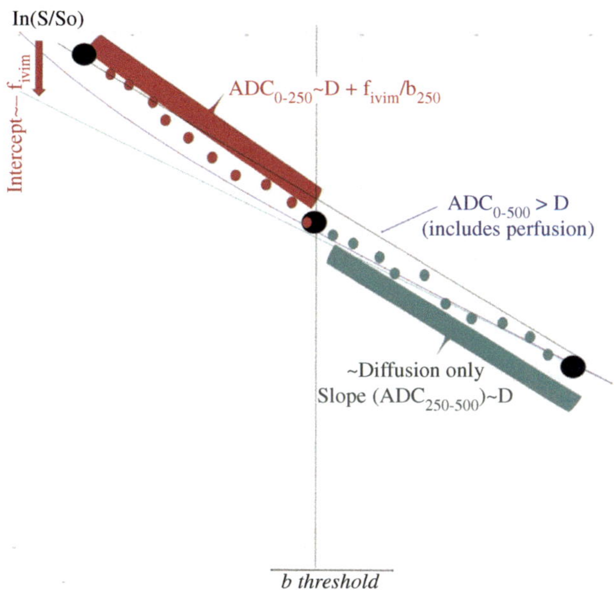

Figure 1.3 Strategies to process IVIM/diffusion data sets. Above a given threshold (which depends on the tissue IVIM/diffusion intrinsic parameters) for the *b* values only tissue diffusion contributes to the signal decay. The ADC obtained with *b* values higher than this threshold (e.g., $ADC_{250-500}$) is the tissue diffusion coefficient, *D*. At lower *b* values (e.g., ADC_{0-250}) the ADC includes the BF component. Hence, the flowing blood fraction (f_{IVIM}, which is the intercept of the tissue diffusion decay curve) can be obtained from those two ADC values, making only three *b* values in total. Alternately, one may prefer fitting the overall signal attenuation curve with an IVIM/diffusion model. To reduce the effect of noise, one often performs fitting in two steps, first estimating diffusion from high *b* value signals, then subtracting the tissue diffusion component from the overall signal to estimate the IVIM parameters.

IVIM really entered the clinical world when echo-planar imaging (EPI) became available, as a signal acquired at multiple and higher *b* values could be obtained free of motion artifacts [12], allowing the first clinical validation of IVIM perfusion MRI in a series of patients with liver lesions [13]. If one considers that IVIM effects are completely negligible for *b* values above 250 mm^2/s (see below) the slope of the signal attenuation between $b = 250$ and, say,

500 s/mm^2 is, according to Eq. 1.2, just the tissue diffusion coefficient D: $ADC_{250-500} \approx D$, while $ADC_{0-250} \approx D + f_{IVIM}/250$. The perfusion fraction would then come as $250 \times (ADC_{0-250} - ADC_{250-500})$, where the ADC is defined as:

$$ADC_{bi\text{-}bj} = \ln[S(b_i)/S(b_j)]/(b_j - b_i) \tag{1.3}$$

However, D^* cannot be estimated with this simplistic approach. Furthermore, parameter estimates could be noisy unless one acquires multiple signals at those three b values and average them out. Then, the total acquisition time increases, and considering three repeated acquisitions for each of the $3b$ values, becomes identical to the acquisition of signals at 15 different b values. With so many acquired signals at hand one may rather consider fitting those signals with the IVIM/diffusion model. Equation 1.2 can be rewritten more generally as:

$$S(b) = S_{0IVIM}F_{IVIM}(b) + S_{0diff}F_{diff}(b) \tag{1.4}$$

Here S_{0diff} and S_{0IVIM} are the fractions of pure diffusion and IVIM components to the overall signal, respectively, with $S_{0diff} = S(0)(1 - f_{IVIM})$ and $S_{0IVIM} = S(0)f_{IVIM}$. $F_{diff}(b)$ and $F_{IVIM}(b)$ are, respectively, the diffusion and perfusion-related IVIM signal attenuation as a function of diffusion weighting (b value). It should be noted here that tissue and blood contribute to $S(0)$ with different T_2 and T_1 weightings, which means that f_{IVIM} values might be misestimated, depending on the echo time (TE), and the field strength $\mathbf{B}_0$, as well as the tissue voxel content (e.g., local blood oxygen level), an issue when comparing literature results (see also Chapter 19 about this issue). With the pseudodiffusion model introduced above, the expression for $F_{IVIM}(b)$ is simply:

$$F_{IVIM}(b) = \exp[-b(D_b + D^*)] \tag{1.5}$$

However, other models can be used, such as the "sinc" model introduced later in this chapter or in more detail in Chapter 19.

As for the diffusion component, with the common monoexponential model one has, as in Eq. 1.1:

$$F_{diff}(b) = \exp(-bD), \tag{1.6}$$

where D is the diffusion coefficient of water in the tissue. Here also, other models are now being used, especially when using high b values, as the monoexponential model assumes diffusion is

Gaussian (free), which is far from the case in biological tissues and an important source of errors in the estimation of IVIM parameters (see below).

With a dataset comprising signals acquired at multiple b values one may get estimates of $S(0)$, f_{IVIM}, D^*—usually D_b is included in D^* but might be estimated [14]—and D by fitting the signal with Eq. 1.2 or 1.4. However, the fitting process is known to be sensitive to noise (and then to local minima) and may lead to erroneous or inaccurate parameter estimates if the number of acquired signals is not very large compared to the number of parameters to estimate. Considering that the IVIM component become negligible at some point when b increases (as D^* is much higher than D), a popular, elegant, and more robust approach is to split the signal in two parts and switch to a two-step fitting process, first fitting the experimental data for high b values (above 200–600 s/mm^2) with the diffusion model for $F_{\text{diff}}(b)$ and then fitting the residual signal after removing the diffusion component at low b values [15] with the IVIM model $F_{\text{IVIM}}(b)$.

For this two-step approach, one needs to determine the threshold b value that separates the pure diffusion part and the IVIM/diffusion mixed part. Unfortunately, there is no generic response, as this threshold value depends highly on the parameters one has to estimate, f_{IVIM}, D^*, and D. In the normal brain f_{IVIM} is less than 5% and D is around 0.001 mm^2/s, so the IVIM component accounts for less than 0.3% of the signal for $b > 200$ s/mm^2. In body tissues, however, f_{IVIM} values as high as 20% are not uncommon while D may be on the order of 0.002 mm^2/s, so the IVIM component at $b = 400$ s/mm^2 may still be around a few percent and higher threshold b values might be required. Hence, the b value threshold should be chosen according to the expected level of perfusion (low in the brain, higher in the body) and, of course, the overall signal-to-noise ratio (SNR) of the data.

In summary, there is no consensus, yet, on the best processing approach of IVIM data. There is extensive literature investigating the pros and cons of fitting algorithms, simultaneous or multistep [16, 17], as well as other methods, such as the Bayesian algorithm [18–21] or even an adaptive thresholding approach [20]. Those approaches will be reviewed in detail in Section IV of this book.

1.3 Pitfalls to Consider for an Accurate Estimation of Perfusion-Driven IVIM Parameters

1.3.1 Non-Gaussian Tissue Diffusion

An accurate estimation of the IVIM parameters first requires proper handling of the diffusion component within the IVIM/diffusion MRI signals that account generally for more than 90% of the total signal at low *b* values. Although the ADC concept has been (and still is) extremely useful, it does not provide a precise estimate of the diffusion-sensitive MRI signal decay. Because the diffusion process in tissues is not Gaussian and the semi log plot of the signal decay, F_{diff}, in biological tissues is not straight (as assumed intrinsically by the ADC and Eq. 1.6) but exhibits a curvature [22] (Fig. 1.4). In the presence of non-Gaussian diffusion, the use of Eq. 1.6 to fit the diffusion component of the signal above the *b* value threshold will introduce a significant bias to the estimated perfusion parameters: Fitting the curved diffusion signal attenuation with a straight line (in log plots) according to Eq. 1.6 results in an artifactual IVIM effect, as acquired data points at low *b* values will automatically appear above the fitted diffusion signal decay (Fig. 1.4). The perfusion fraction, f_{IVIM}, will, thus, be *overestimated*. Furthermore, the shape of the residual signal decay at low *b* values will appear close to an exponential, mimicking Eq. 1.5, which would be misleading (D^* values would be overestimated as well).

Several models have been proposed to empirically handle this non-Gaussian behavior, such as the polynomial or kurtosis model [23] (also called diffusion kurtosis imaging, DKI [24]), the biexponential model [25, 26], the statistical model [27], the stretched exponential model [28], and others [29, 30], with various degrees of success, depending on the context and the tissues under examination. With the kurtosis model one has:

$$F_{\text{diff}} \approx \exp[-b\text{ADC}_0 + (b \cdot \text{ADC}_0)^2 K/6] \quad (1.7)$$

Here ADC_0 is the virtual ADC that would be obtained when *b* approaches 0 (free, Gaussian diffusion). The dimensionless coefficient *K* (kurtosis) characterizes the degree of deviation of the signal behavior from a monoexponential decay ($K = 0$ when the diffusion-driven molecular displacements obey a Gaussian law), a marker of the heterogeneity of the diffusion environment. Hence, Eq. 1.2 now changes to:

$$S(b)/S(0) = f_{\text{IVIM}} \exp[-b(D_{\text{b}} + D^*) + (1 - f_{\text{IVIM}}) \exp[-b \cdot \text{ADC}_0 + (b \cdot \text{ADC}_0)^2 K/6] \quad (1.8)$$

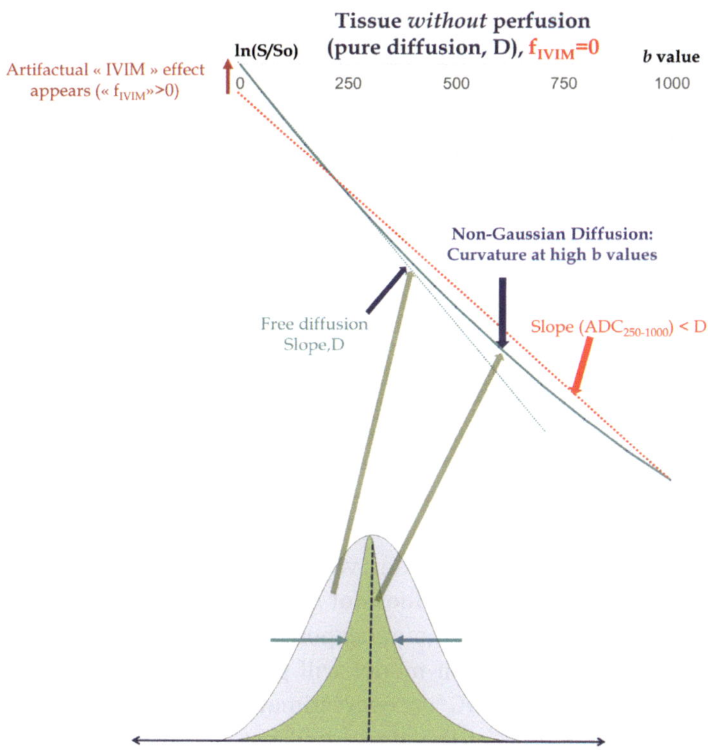

Figure 1.4 Non-Gaussian diffusion. Failing to take into account non-Gaussian diffusion effects might lead to erroneous f_{IVIM} and D^* parameter estimates (overestimation), as shown here in a simulated tissue model without perfusion. Non-Gaussian diffusion that becomes visible at high *b* values originates from the interaction of water-diffusing molecules with obstacles, such as cell membranes, and results in a curvature of the signal attenuation. Modeling the tissue diffusion component with a monoexponential model underestimates genuine diffusion (ADC < *D*) when the signal at high *b* values is included, which, in turn, creates an artifactual IVIM effect (left). Non-Gaussian diffusion must be properly handled using adequate models, such as the kurtosis model or other models, to avoid such erroneous IVIM effects.

On the other hand, ignoring the IVIM component at low *b* values will lead to an overestimation of kurtosis value when fitting signals with Eq. 1.8 in a single step. More generally, one should be aware that the kurtosis model is only one possible model to handle non-Gaussian diffusion in $F_{\text{diff}}(b)$, which implicitly means that it is not a perfect model. The kurtosis model is known to fail at very high *b* values or when the kurtosis parameter is high (a practical limit is that the triple product ADCo·K·b must be smaller than 3). In short, any imperfection in fitting the diffusion part of the signal (at high *b* values) will lead to artifactual IVIM effects (at low *b* values) and a misestimation (generally an overestimation) of IVIM parameters. This is an important point to keep in mind, although it might sound counterintuitive.

1.3.2 Rician Noise

A particular source of systematic error in diffusion and perfusion parameter estimation results from the non-Gaussian nature of the noise in magnitude reconstructed images, resulting in a systematic shift from a noise-free signal [31, 32]. This source of error is particularly prominent at high *b* values for which the SNR becomes low. The main effect of such noise is that it may mimic a curvature in the diffusion signal attenuation plot (Fig. 1.5) and a "kurtosis" effect: At high *b* values, when SNR becomes low, the signal reaches a "noise floor" and does not get to 0. The signal attenuation appears curved, even for monoexponential diffusion, and fitting signals with any diffusion model will give erroneous values (e.g., underestimation of ADC or overestimation of kurtosis). As the diffusion component of the signal will not be estimated properly, the perfusion component, which is very sensitive to such errors, will, in turn, be affected, with an *underestimation* of f_{IVIM}, which can even become "negative." It is thus particularly important to correct for this noise bias all IVIM MRI data, especially when using high *b* values for the diffusion component. Unfortunately, the retrieval of true signal values from noise-corrupted data is far from simple, both theoretically and practically [32, 33]. Furthermore, with the use of phased-array coils instead of single coils, the noise structure becomes even more complex (noncentral chi square distribution) [34–37], and nonstationary with parallel imaging methods, because of the correlation between receiving channels and the under sampling of k-space. Noise correction becomes more problematic, often requiring a large amount of repeated measurements or long computation times.

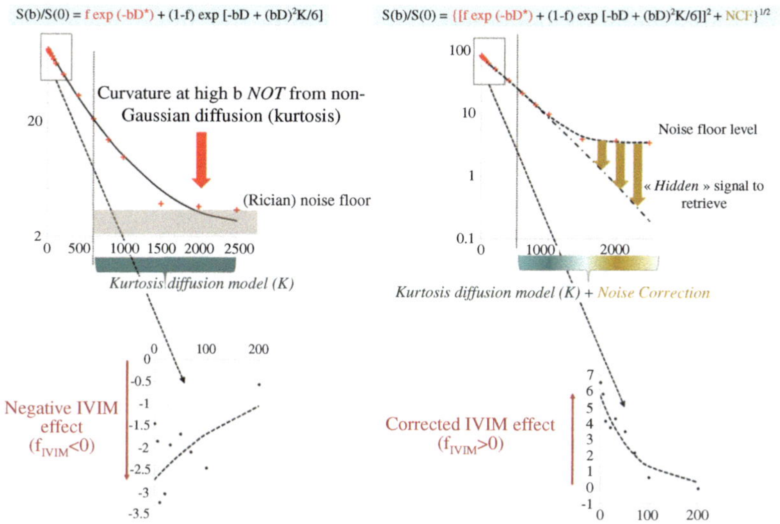

Figure 1.5 Effect of Rician noise of IVIM parameters estimates. At high b values the signal becomes low and may reach the Rician noise floor (the mean of which is not 0), resulting in a curvature of the signal decay, not to be confused with the curvature produced by non-Gaussian diffusion. Failing to remove the noise contribution to the signal amplitude leads to an overestimation of non-Gaussian diffusion (e.g., K parameter), which in turn results in an underestimation of f_{IVIM} (the IVIM residual part of the signal may even become negative, as shown in the lower left graph of this example). After noise correction is properly applied (using the noise correction factor, NCF, parameter) the curvature is much reduced and the signal decay becomes close to a straight line; K becomes close to 0 in this example, and ADC_0 decreases. The estimated signal at low b values (insert and bottom right) remains higher than the measured signal, and the estimated f_{IVIM} value is positive, as expected.

We recently introduced a simplified procedure where a noise correction factor (NCF) is experimentally obtained through a phantom calibration process relying on the diffusion MRI signal property itself [15]. The NCF is a parameter that characterizes the "intrinsic" noise contribution from the image acquisition setup (depending on the coils, the MRI sequence parameters, etc., but assuming little difference between phantom and in vivo noise features). If noise correction is not applied one finds a high *K* value and a very high ADC_0 value (Fig. 1.5). Such erroneous parameter estimates would result, in turn, in an estimated signal lower than the measured signal at low *b* values, which would mimic a nonperfused tissue (f_{IVIM} could even become negative, a physical impossibility).

Importantly, although non-Gaussian diffusion and noise effects affect signals acquired at high *b* values, the impact is seen at low *b* values, as IVIM effects are small. A proper estimation of diffusion and IVIM parameters, as shown in Figs. 1.4 and 1.5 [15], might require the inclusion of high *b* value signals, not only the signal acquired at moderate *b* values (less than 1000 s/mm^2), as often found in the literature.

1.3.3 Erratic Signals

Spin-echo signals are formed when 90° and 180° radiofrequency pulses are used sequentially. Unfortunately, if those pulses are not perfectly calibrated, spurious signals are generated, such as free induction decay signals following imperfect 180° pulses or stimulated echoes considering the multiple pulses used for multislice acquisitions. Those signals add up to the spin-echo signals but do not share the IVIM/diffusion encoding of the main spin-echo signals, leading to errors when fitting the overall signals with the IVIM/diffusion model. Pulse imperfections are unavoidable, resulting from inhomogeneities in the B1 field generated by coils, poor shimming, or errors in the determination of resonance frequencies. Generally, those unwanted signals are suppressed with the use of the so-called crusher or spoiler gradient pulses placed on each side of the 180° pulses or after each slice readout signal. Those spoiler pulses, however, obviously act as IVIM/diffusion encoding gradients and must be taken into account when calculating *b* values, which is clearly unfavorable for IVIM, as the "*b* = 0 value" is never reachable in the presence of spoiler gradients (or else gradient pulses used for MRI spatial encoding). Obviously, the lowest achievable *b* values highly depend on each vendor MRI hardware and software item or component. Values as high as 10–15 or even around 50 s/mm^2 are not uncommon, as instabilities in gradient amplifiers may also render low *b* values unreliable. Conversely, gradient pulses used for diffusion encoding act as spoiler pulses, which means that signals acquired with sufficient diffusion encoding are immune from artifacts created by those unwanted signals, while signals at low *b* values carrying the perfusion IVIM information are not.

1.4 Perfusion-Driven IVIM MRI and "Classical" Perfusion

1.4.1 IVIM MRI Reflects Capillary Network Architecture and Blood Flow

The IVIM exponential model used for Eqs. 1.2 and 1.5 assumes that flowing blood water changes directions (capillary segments) many times in randomly oriented capillaries (at the voxel level) during the diffusion encoding time, mimicking a collective random walk ("pseudodiffusion") (Fig. 1.1). Overall, there is an empirical consensus that this monoexponential IVIM model is appropriate to fit data for clinical application studies, as IVIM/diffusion encoding times remain long given the limited capacity of clinical systems' gradient hardware. However, this model might not be accurate when the encoding time becomes short, the blood velocity is slow, or capillary segments are long. In those conditions blood may remain in single, straight capillary segments during the entire encoding time. If those segments are, nonetheless, randomly oriented over 4π in 3D space the signal attenuation can be modeled as a sinc function [4, 5] (Fig. 1.6):

$$F_{\mathrm{IVIM}}(c) = \exp(-bD_{\mathrm{b}})\,\mathrm{sinc}\,(cv), \tag{1.9}$$

where *c* is another pulse gradient factor, similar to the *b* factor [in the case of a pure pulsed-gradient spin-echo sequence with two pulses of length δ separated by a time interval Δ one has $c = (b\Delta)^{1/2}$ when $\delta << \Delta$]. Within this regime, one may also define a pseudodiffusion coefficient, D^*, by calculating the Taylor expansion limited to the first orders of $f_{\mathrm{IVIM}}(c)$, as $D^* = v^2c^2/(6b)$ [5]. An important consequence of this model is that while D^* still depends on the capillary blood velocity, it does not depend on the capillary segment length, *l*, as spins never get to probe the entire capillary segments. Noticeably, this sinc behavior has never been reported experimentally, even at short diffusion times. One possible explanation might lie in spatial or temporal variation of the capillary velocity in the voxel. It can be shown that when blood velocities, *v*, follow a Gaussian distribution in the capillary network, or when BF changes direction at least three times during the encoding time, $F_{\text{IVIM}}(c)$ becomes exponential anyway [35] (Fig. 1.6) (see Chapter 19).

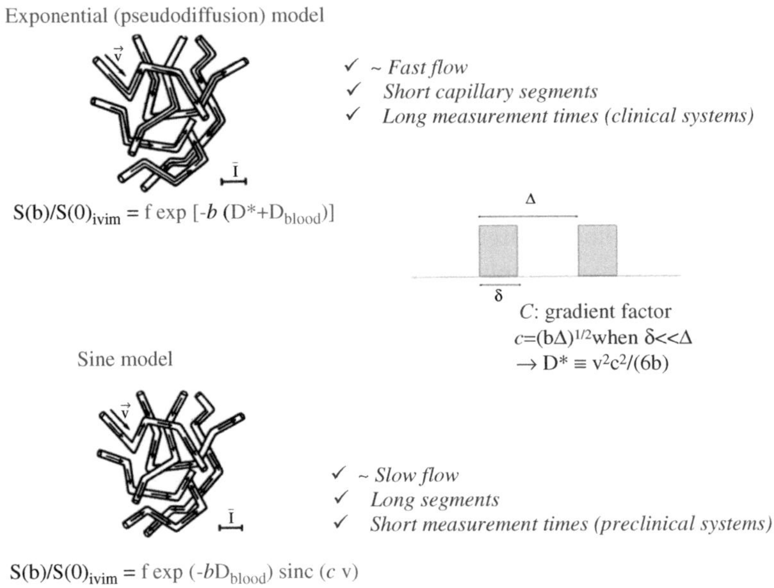

Figure 1.6 IVIM blood flow models. The exponential pseudodiffusion model (top) assumes blood changes direction (capillary segment) several times during the encoding time. This condition is met when flow is fast enough, capillary segments are not too long, and the encoding time is long enough to accommodate those direction changes. In the opposite case, where no change in direction occurs, the IVIM signal can be modeled by a sinc function if capillary segments are randomly oriented (bottom).

Other models have been proposed to handle intermediate regimens between the monoexponential and sinc IVIM models, taking into account the existence of several vessel functional pools. For instance, Kennan et al. [38] have introduced a model based on a velocity autocorrelation function. Arguing that the Gaussian phase approximation assumed by Kennan et al. is invalid in some cases, Wetscherek et al. [39] introduced another model based on normalized phase distributions. These two models assume that only flow in capillaries contributes to the IVIM signal. Noticing some disagreement between experimental data and the standard monoexponential model, other authors have suggested models that take into account not only capillaries but all types of vessels [40, 41]. Those models will be analyzed in detail in Chapter 19.

1.4.2 Link with Tracer-Perfusion Methods

An important issue is to establish whether and how a bridge can be established between the IVIM parameters, f_{IVIM} and D^*, and those that have been used with classical perfusion measurements [42–44], on the basis of the delivery of tracers, as with positron emission tomography (PET) or single-photon emission computed tomography (SPECT) or other MRI methods used to estimate tissue perfusion (arterial spin labeling [ASL] and contrast-enhanced MRI; please refer to Chapter 2). Classical perfusion parameters are, for instance, the blood volume (BV), the BF, and the mean transit time (MTT).

It has been shown that, under some hypotheses, one has [44]:

$$f_{\text{IVIM}} = \text{BV}/f_{\text{w}}, \tag{1.10}$$

$$\text{MTT} = L/\mathbf{v} = Ll/6D^*, \tag{1.11}$$

and

$$\text{BF} = (6f_{\text{w}}/Ll)\, f_{\text{IVIM}} D^*, \tag{1.12}$$

where f_{w} is the MRI-visible water content fraction and L is the total capillary length (from artery to vein). As shown from Eq. 1.11 the element bridging the classical perfusion and IVIM parameters is the capillary network geometry, and more especially two specific lengths characterizing this network: the capillary segment length and the total capillary length. Those quantities are constant for a given tissue, so relative perfusion or BF can potentially be estimated from the product $D^* \cdot f_{\text{IVIM}}$. Furthermore, the MTT could also be evaluated (at least in a relative manner) from D^* without the need to estimate an arterial "input function," which is not a trivial parameter to estimate, and without the confusion of the inclusion of the transit time of blood in the large feeding vessels.

In any case, there is still the need for a deeper insight into the IVIM concept to fully exploit the benefit of the IVIM-based perfusion imaging in the clinical setting, as will be shown in the chapters of Sections III and IV of this book. The flowing blood fraction, f_{IVIM}, appears correlated with vessel density [45, 46], and recent studies have shown a correlation between f_{IVIM} and cerebral blood volume (CBV) derived from dynamic susceptibility contrast (DSC) MRI in gliomas [47, 48] or dynamic contrast–enhanced (DCE)-derived parameters in renal tumors [49], head and neck tumors [50], or breast tumors [51]. But other studies failed to observe such a correlation [52]. One also has to keep in mind that IVIM imaging has a differential sensitivity to vessel sizes, according to the range of b values that are used, but is sensitive to all randomly flowing blood in each voxel. Direct comparison with other methods, such as ASL, is not straightforward, as ASL monitors only the transit of blood that has been labeled outside of the voxels, while IVIM reflects all randomly flowing blood in each voxel. Chapter 2 will summarize the concepts used with non-IVIM perfusion MRI methods, a very important step to understand the conditions when correlation between the results obtained by either approach is expected or not expected.

1.5 Non-perfusion-Driven IVIM MRI

IVIM MRI is sensitive to any fluid flow, not only blood, as long as there is an intravoxel distribution. In the brain cerebrospinal fluid (CSF) flow is clearly visible on IVIM images [3], and IVIM MRI has been proposed as a CSF flow mapping approach. On the other hand, this sensitivity might also appear as a confound when evaluating perfusion in the brain cortex if it is included as a partial volume effect. CSF suppression techniques may alleviate this pitfall. In other organs, such as the kidneys, IVIM MRI may be used to investigate vascular and tubular flow, although they may be difficult to disentangle [53]. Active transport resulting from glandular secretion (breast ducts, salivary glands, and pancreas) may also be explored in addition to microcapillary perfusion.

Apart from random capillaries BF may also experience incoherent intravoxel dephasing in larger vessels, considering that laminar flow (or even more turbulent flow) leads to a distribution of velocities within the vessel lumen and to an IVIM signal attenuation, which could be much larger than the perfusion-driven IVIM effect. This feature can be successfully exploited to identify vessels containing voxels and generate IVIM 3D angiograms without the need for contrast agents (Fig. 1.7A).

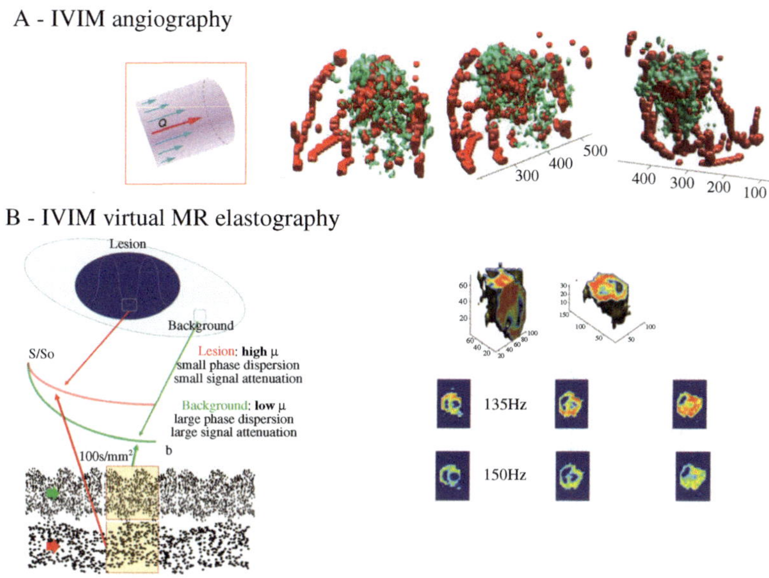

Figure 1.7 Other IVIM MRI applications. (Top) The spatial distribution of blood velocities in vessels also results in an IVIM effect that can be used to identify voxels containing blood vessels and produce IVIM-based angiograms (here in a normal breast) without the need for contrast agents. (Bottom) Mechanical vibrations used for MR elastography also induce phase distributions in each tissue voxel and an IVIM effect when considering the amplitude of the signal. This IVIM effect will be larger in normal tissues than in lesions, presenting higher elasticity values, and IVIM MRI could be used, potentially, to estimate those elasticity values. Conversely, if those elasticity values are known (they can be directly derived from diffusion maps, without the need for using mechanical vibrations) virtual IVIM elastographic images can be generated, producing a new kind of contrast that would depend on the combinations of vibration frequencies or amplitudes, as shown here in a breast tumor.

Another emerging field of application is IVIM/diffusion virtual magnetic resonance elastography (dMRE). With standard MRE, propagating shear waves through tissues lead to microscopic tissue displacements, resulting in phase shifts in the presence of magnetic gradient pulses, which can be exploited to estimate tissue shear stiffness. For instance, the degree of liver fibrosis could be derived from elasticity measurements [54]. Recently, it has been suggested that tissue shear stiffness (in kPa) could be directly obtained from diffusion MRI without the need to use any mechanical vibration device [55]. This is possible due to a striking relationship that has been revealed, at least in the liver, between tissue elasticity and tissue water diffusion. This correlation might not be surprising as both relate, although in a different way, to tissue microstructure, but it still remains to be investigated. On the other hand, mechanically induced phase shifts induced by standard MRE are spatially distributed and result in a phase dispersion in each voxel and an amplitude signal attenuation, that is an IVIM effect [56]. The degree of attenuation in those IVIM images would depend on the tissue elasticity and on the choice of acquisition parameters (mainly IVIM b value, vibration frequency, and amplitude of the propagating shear waves), creating a new kind of contrast to highlight lesions that are most often associated with a high stiffness. This elasticity-driven IVIM approach, using standard MRE, is challenging, though, as the wave amplitude dampens very quickly when waves penetrate tissues. However, this elasticity-driven IVIM contrast can be emulated *virtually* once the tissue elasticity is known—information that can be obtained directly from diffusion MRI without using any mechanical vibration [55]. This new elasticity-driven IVIM contrast can be emulated for any range of virtual vibration frequencies and amplitudes not limited by MRE or MRI hardware capacity, acting as a sort of postprocessing filter and revealing tissue details not readily visible with MRE or diffusion MRI (Fig. 1.7).

1.6 Conclusion

While the main source of IVIM remains molecular diffusion, which is now extensively used in research and clinical practice, providing exquisite and unique information on tissue microstructure completely noninvasively ("virtual biopsy" concept), other types of IVIM, especially blood microcirculation in the capillary network (perfusion), have a great potential for clinical applications, especially in oncology. IVIM-based perfusion MRI can provide information on tissue microcirculation and BF in addition to information on tissue microstructure from diffusion MRI using the same MRI sequence and without the need for contrast agents, as will be reviewed in the chapters of Section III. Work remains to fully characterize and model the effects of BF at different spatial and temporal scales on the overall IVIM signal. Optimization of IVIM/diffusion data processing pipelines requires attention, given the small range of the flowing BV in most tissues. Especially non-Gaussian diffusion behavior and Rician noise might significantly impact IVIM parameters estimation if not properly accounted for, although such effects are visible mainly in data acquired at high *b* values. Those technical considerations will be the object of Section IV in this book.

References

1. Kanda T, Ishii K, Kawaguchi H, Kitajima K, Takenaka D. High signal intensity in the dentate nucleus and globus pallidus on unenhanced T1-weighted MR images: relationship with increasing cumulative dose of a gadolinium-based contrast material. *Radiology* 270: 834–841, 2014.
2. Kanda T, Osawa M, Oba H, Toyoda K, Kotoku J, Haruyama T et al. High signal intensity in dentate nucleus on unenhanced T1-weighted MR images: association with linear versus macrocyclic gadolinium chelate administration. *Radiology* 275: 803–809, 2015.
3. Le Bihan D, Breton E, Lallemand D, Grenier P, Cabanis E, Laval Jeantet M. MR imaging of intravoxel incoherent motions: application to diffusion and perfusion in neurologic disorders. *Radiology* 161: 401–407, 1986.
4. Le Bihan D, Breton E, Lallemand D, Aubin ML, Vignaud J, Laval-Jeantet M. Separation of diffusion and perfusion in intravoxel incoherent motion MR imaging. *Radiology* 168: 497–505, 1988.
5. Le Bihan D. Magnetic resonance imaging of perfusion. *Magn. Reson. Med.* 14: 283–292, 1990.
6. Einstein A. *Investigations on the Theory of Brownian Motion.* Furthe R, Cowper AD, Eds. New York: Dover, 1956.
7. Pavlik C, Rackl A, Bing RJ. Quantitativecapillary topography and blood flow in the cerebral cortex of cats: an in-vivo microscopic study. *Brain Res.* 208: 35–58, 1981.
8. Powers TA, Lorenz CH, Holburn GE, Price RR. Renal artery stenosis: in vivo perfusion MR imaging. *Radiology* **178**(2): 543–8, 1991.
9. Morvan D. In vivo measurement of diffusion and pseudo-diffusion in skeletal muscle at rest and after exercise. *Magn. Reson. Imaging.* 13: 193–199, 1995.
10. Pickens DR III, Jolgren DL, Lorenz CH, Creasy JL, Price RR. Magnetic resonance perfusion/diffusion imaging of the excised dog kidney. *Invest. Radiol.* 27: 287–292, 1992.

11. Neil JJ, Bosch CS, Ackerman JJ. An evaluation of the sensitivity of the intravoxel incoherent motion (IVIM) method of blood flow measurement to changes in cerebral blood flow. *Magn. Reson. Med.* 32: 60–65, 1994.
12. Turner R, Le Bihan D, Maier J, Vavrek R, Hedges LK, Pekar J. Echo-planar imaging of intravoxel incoherent motions. *Radiology* 177: 407–414, 1990.
13. Yamada I, Aung W, Himeno Y, Nakagawa T, Shibuya H. Diffusion coefficients in abdominal organs and hepatic lesions: evaluation with intravoxel incoherent motion echo- planar MR imaging. *Radiology* 210: 617–623, 1999.
14. Funck C, Laun FB, Wetscherek A. Characterization of the diffusion coefficient of blood. *Magn. Reson. Med.* Sep 23, 2017. doi: 10.1002/mrm.26919. [Epub ahead of print] PubMed PMID: 28940621.
15. Iima M, Yano K, Kataoka M, Umehana M, Murata K, Kanao S et al. Quantitative non-Gaussian diffusion and intravoxel incoherent motion magnetic resonance imaging: differentiation of malignant and benign breast lesions. *Invest. Radiol.* 50: 205–211, 2015.
16. Lemke A, Stieltjes B, Schad LR, Laun FB. Toward an optimal distribution of b values for intravoxel incoherent motion imaging. *Magn. Reson. Imaging* 29: 766–776, 2011.
17. Barbieri S, Donati OF, Froehlich JM, Thoeny HC. Impact of the calculation algorithm on biexponential fitting of diffusion-weighted MRI in upper abdominal organs. *Magn. Reson. Med.* 75(5):2175–84, 2016.
18. While PT. A comparative simulation study of bayesian fitting approaches to intravoxel incoherent motion modeling in diffusion-weighted MRI. *Magn. Reson. Med.* 78(6):2373–2387, 2017.
19. Orton MR, Collins DJ, Koh DM, Leach MO. Improved intravoxel incoherent motion analysis of diffusion weighted imaging by data driven Bayesian modeling. *Magn. Reson. Med.* 71(1):411–20, 2014.
20. Wurnig MC, Donati OF, Ulbrich E, Filli L, Kenkel D, Thoeny HC, et al. Systematic analysis of the intravoxel incoherent motion threshold separating perfusion and diffusion effects: Proposal of a standardized algorithm. *Magn. Reson. Med.* 74(5):1414–22, 2015.
21. Spinner GR, von Deuster C, Tezcan KC, Stoeck CT, Kozerke S. Bayesian intravoxel incoherent motion parameter mapping in the human heart. *J. Cardiovasc. Magn. Reson.* 6;19(1):85, 2017.
22. Iima M, Le Bihan D. Clinical intravoxel incoherent motion and diffusion MR imaging: past, present, and future. *Radiology* 278: 13–32, 2016.

23. Chabert S, Meca C, Le Bihan D. Relevance of the information about the diffusion distribution in vivo given by kurtosis in q-space imaging. *Proceedings of the 12th Annual Meeting of ISMRM, Kyoto, Japan.* 2004;1238.

24. Jensen JH, Helpern JA, Ramani A, Lu H, Kaczynski K. Diffusional kurtosis imaging: the quantification of non-gaussian water diffusion by means of magnetic resonance imaging. *Magn. Reson. Med.* 53(6):1432–1440, 2005.

25. Niendorf T, Dijkhuizen RM, Norris DG, van Lookeren Campagne M, Nicolay K. Biexponential diffusion attenuation in various states of brain tissue: Implications for diffusion-weighted imaging. *Magn. Reson. Med.*, **36**: 847–857, 1996.

26. Mulkern RV, Haker SJ, Maier SE. On high b diffusion imaging in the human brain: ruminations and experimental insights. *Magn. Reson. Imaging* 27(8):1151–1162, 2009.

27. Yablonskiy DA, Bretthorst GL, Ackerman JJ. Statistical model for diffusion attenuated MR signal. *Magn. Reson. Med.* 50(4):664–669, 2003.

28. Bennett KM, Schmainda KM, Bennett RT, Rowe DB, Lu H, Hyde JS. Characterization of continuously distributed cortical water diffusion rates with a stretched-exponential model. *Magn. Reson. Med.* 50(4):727–734, 2003.

29. Hall MG, Barrick TR. From diffusion-weighted MRI to anomalous diffusion imaging. *Magn. Reson. Med.* 59(3):447–455, 2008.

30. Zhou XJ, Gao Q, Abdullah O, Magin RL. Studies of anomalous diffusion in the human brain using fractional order calculus. *Magn. Reson. Med.* 63(3): 562–569, 2010.

31. Henkelman RM. Measurement of signal intensities in the presence of noise in MR images. *Med. Phys.* 12: 232–233, 1985.

32. Gudbjartsson H, Patz S. The Rician distribution of noisy MRI data. *Magn. Reson. Med.*. 34: 910–914, 1995.

33. Sijbers J, Den Dekker AJ, Scheunders P, et al. Maximum-likelihood estimation of Rician distribution parameters. *IEEE Trans. Med. Imaging* 17: 357–361, 1998.

34. Brion V, Poupon C, Riff O, et al. Parallel MRI noise correction: an extension of the LMMSE to non central χ distributions. *Medical Image Computing and Computer-Assisted Intervention–MICCAI*, Springer; 2011: 226–233, 2011.

35. Constantinides CD, Atalar E, McVeigh ER. Signal-to-noise measurements in magnitude images from NMR phased arrays. *Magn. Reson. Med.* 38: 852–857, 1997.

36. Aja-Fernández S, Tristán-Vega A, Hoge WS. Statistical noise analysis in GRAPPA using a parametrized noncentral chi approximation model. *Magn. Reson. Med.* 65: 1195–1206, 2011.

37. André ED, Grinberg F, Farrher E, et al. Influence of noise correction on intra-and inter-subject variability of quantitative metrics in diffusion kurtosis imaging. *PLOS One* 9:e94531, 2014.

38. Kennan RP, Gao JH, Zhong J, Gore JC. A general model of microcirculatory blood flow effects in gradient sensitized MRI. *Med. Phys.* 21: 539–545, 1994.

39. Wetscherek A, Stieltjes B, Laun FB. Flow-compensated intravoxel incoherent motion diffusion imaging. *Magn. Reson. Med.* 74: 410–419, 2015.

40. Constantinides CD, Atalar E, McVeigh ER. Signal-to-noise measurements in magnitude images from NMR phased arrays, *Magn. Reson. Med.* **38**: 852–857, 1997.

41. Aja-Fernández S, Tristán-Vega A, Hoge WS. Statistical noise analysis in GRAPPA using a parametrized noncentral Chi approximation model, *Magn. Reson. Med.* **65**: 1195–206, 2011. https://doi.org/10.1002/mrm.22701

42. Zierler K. Indicator dilution methods for measuring blood flow, volume, and other properties of biological systems: a brief history and memoir. *Ann. Biomed. Eng.* **28**: 836–848, 2000.

43. Henkelman RM. Does IVIM measure classical perfusion? *MRM* 16: 470–475, 1990.

44. Le Bihan D, Turner R. The capillary network: a link between IVIM and classical perfusion. *Magn. Reson. Med.* 27: 171–178, 1992.

45. Iima M, Reynaud O, Tsurugizawa T, et al. Characterization of glioma microcirculation and tissue features using intravoxel incoherent motion magnetic resonance imaging in a rat brain model. *Invest. Radiol.* 49(7):485–490, 2014.

46. Lee HJ, Rha SY, Chung YE, et al. Tumor perfusion-related parameter of diffusion-weighted magnetic resonance imaging: Correlation with histological microvessel density. *Magn. Reson. Med.* 71(4):1554–1558, 2014.

47. Federau C, Meuli R, O'Brien K, Maeder P, Hagmann P. Perfusion measurement in brain gliomas with intravoxel incoherent motion MRI. *AJNR Am. J. Neuroradiol.* 35(2):256–262, 2014.

48. Kim HS, Suh CH, Kim N, Choi CG, Kim SJ. Histogram analysis of intravoxel incoherent motion for differentiating recurrent tumor from treatment effect in patients with glioblastoma: initial clinical experience. *AJNR Am. J. Neuroradiol.* 35(3):490–497, 2014.

49. Chandarana H, Kang SK, Wong S, et al. Diffusion-weighted intravoxel incoherent motion imaging of renal tumors with histopathologic correlation. *Invest. Radiol.* 47(12):688–696, 2012.

50. Fujima N, Yoshida D, Sakashita T, et al. Intravoxel incoherent motion diffusion-weighted imaging in head and neck squamous cell carcinoma: assessment of perfusion-related parameters compared to dynamic contrast-enhanced MRI. *Magn. Reson. Imaging* 32(10):1206–1213, 2014.

51. Liu et al. Intravoxel incoherent motion MR imaging for breast lesions: comparison and correlation with pharmacokinetic evaluation from dynamic contrast-enhanced MR imaging. *Eur. Radiol.*, 26(11): 3888–3898, 2016.

52. Bisdas S, Braun C, Skardelly M, Schittenhelm J, Teo TH, Thng CH, et al. Correlative assessment of tumor microcirculation using contrast-enhanced perfusion MRI and intravoxel incoherent motion diffusion-weighted MRI: is there a link between them? *NMR Biomed.* 27(10):1184–1191, 2014.

53. Notohamiprodjo M, Chandarana H, Mikheev A, et al. Combined intravoxel incoherent motion and diffusion tensor imaging of renal diffusion and flow anisotropy. *Magn. Reson. Med.* 73(4):1526–1532, 2015.

54. Morisaka H, Motosugi U, Ichikawa S, Nakazawa T, Kondo T, Funayama S, et al. Magnetic resonance elastography is as accurate as liver biopsy for liver fibrosis staging. *J. Magn. Reson. Imaging.* Oct 14, 2017. doi:10.1002/jmri.25868. [Epub ahead of print].

55. Le Bihan D, Ichikawa S, Motosugu U. Diffusion and Intravoxel Incoherent Motion (IVIM) MRI based virtual elastography: A hypothesis generating study in the liver. *Radiology* 285(2):609–619, 2017.

56. Glaser KJ, Felmlee JP, Manduca A, Ehman RL. Shear stiffness estimation using intravoxel phase dispersion in magnetic resonance elastography. *Magn. Reson. Med.* 50: 1256–1265, 2003.

Section II

Other MRI Approaches to Perfusion Imaging

Chapter 2

Other MRI Approaches to Perfusion Imaging (ASL, DSC, DCE)

Emmanuel L. Barbier, Sylvie Grand, Alexandre Krainik, and Jan M. Warnking
Grenoble Institut des Neurosciences, Univ. Grenoble Alpes, Inserm, CHU Grenoble Alpes, Grenoble, F-38000, France
emmanuel.barbier@univ-grenoble-alpes.fr

2.1 The Perfusion Parameters: The Microvascular Network and Physiological Principles

Perfusion characterizes the microvascular network. The “micro” scale refers here to the size of the capillary diameter: about 6 μm. From an in vivo imaging point of view, this scale is far below the voxel size (about 1000 μm). Therefore, each voxel of a perfusion map contains hundreds or even thousands of microvessels. The perfusion value associated with that voxel is generally a mean value across these numerous microvessels. Obtaining quantitative values is not always easy and not always useful, from a clinical point of view. Often,

Intravoxel Incoherent Motion (IVIM) MRI: Principles and Applications
Edited by Denis Le Bihan, Mami Iima, Christian Federau, and Eric E. Sigmund

ISBN 978-981-4800-19-8 (Hardcover), 978-0-429-42727-5 (eBook)
www.panstanford.com

relative index values are derived. The available perfusion estimates primarily depend on the choice of acquisition method. In most cases, several parameter maps may be derived from one acquisition. A list of examples is shown in Table 2.1.

Table 2.1 Main perfusion-related parameters that can be monitored with MRI perfusion techniques

Parameter Name	Abbreviation	Unit	Technique
Blood flow	F	mL/100 g/min.	ASL, DSC, DCE
Blood volume fraction	BVf	mL/100 g	DSC, DCE
Mean transit time	MTT	s	DSC
Time of maximum of the residue function	T_{max}	s	DSC
Permeability	K_{trans}	mL/100 g/min.	DCE
Vessel size index	VSI	µm	DSC, steady-state
Vessel density	VD	Vessels/mm^2	DSC, steady-state
Tissue oxygen saturation	StO_2	%	Quantitative BOLD

2.2 Perfusion Tracers

To estimate perfusion parameters, imaging techniques generally rely on tracers. A perfusion tracer is a molecule introduced in the blood stream in small quantities and that does not perturb perfusion. For practical reasons, all clinical tracers are plasmatic. Indeed, labeling erythrocytes is a complex procedure not adapted to a routine clinical setting.

We will first introduce how tracers may be used to quantify perfusion parameters, from a biophysical point of view, without considering the imaging part. Then, we will consider how imaging tracers, also called contrast agents (CAs), impact the magnetic resonance imaging (MRI) signal and how MRI can be turned into perfusion MRI.

Injection mode: To avoid any increase in arterial pressure, tracers are injected into the venous system. Then, the left heart distributes the tracer into the arterial system at a physiological pressure. In addition, tracers are generally flushed with saline to ensure that the tracer reaches a large vein (i.e., the vena cava) as a bolus (<5 s).

At the organ level: From a biophysical point of view, tracers are either diffusible or nondiffusible. In other words, during the imaging sequence (or imaging session), a tracer either extravasates or remains intravascular. This depends on the organ of interest. The same tracer may be diffusible for a particular organ and nondiffusible for another (e.g., a gadolinium chelate is diffusible in the skin but not in the brain). The behavior of the tracer depends on its size (the hydrodynamic diameter), its charge, its lipophilicity, etc. The extravasation may be passive (e.g., driven by the concentration gradient between intra- and extravascular spaces) or active (e.g., active transport by vesicles) or a combination of both. In the healthy brain, capillaries are impermeable to MRICAs in almost every region [1], unless the blood–brain barrier is altered. From a biophysical point of view, a diffusible tracer is generally modeled as a tracer that passively crosses the vessel wall at a rate characteristic of the vessel wall permeability and then freely diffuses into the extravascular space.

In blood: The temporal evolution of the tracer concentration in the feeding arteries of the organ of interest is called the arterial input function (AIF). Evaluating the AIF is the most challenging part in perfusion studies. Following the intravenous injection, the left heart distributes the tracer into the arterial system and every organ sees a "first pass" of the tracer. The evolution of the tracer concentration in the draining veins of the organ of interest is called the venous output function (VOF). The interorgan difference in tracer circulation time (approximately 15 to 40 s) [2] and in blood volume is such that a second pass can be visible in some organs (such as the brain) before the tracer concentration becomes homogeneous across the entire vascular system.

Finally, the tracer concentration in blood decays. The exact mechanisms of tracer excretion depend on the tracer and are outside the scope of this chapter. Pharmaceutical companies may provide an estimate of the plasmatic half-lives for tracers for various species, including humans [3].

2.3 Biophysical Modeling of Nondiffusible Tracers

Considering an organ and a nondiffusible CA for that organ, there are two main strategies to obtain perfusion-related parameters: a dynamic approach and a steady-state approach.

2.3.1 Dynamic Approach

This approach, used in dynamic susceptibility contrast (DSC) MRI or in perfusion CT, was proposed by Hering as the "indicator dilution method" in 1824 [4]. Considering the tracer concentration over time in arterial blood, $\mathrm{AIF}(t)$, and in a particular voxel, $C_{\mathrm{voxel}}(t)$, and assuming a bolus injection, no extravasation of tracer, and no tracer recirculation, the blood volume fraction (BVf), may be computed as:

$$\mathrm{BVf} = \frac{\int_0^{\infty} C_{\mathrm{voxel}}(\tau)d\tau}{\int_0^{\infty} \mathrm{AIF}(\tau)d\tau} \tag{2.1}$$

Eq. 2.1 shows that the area under the concentration time curve of each voxel is proportional to voxel BVf. For flow, F, the following relationship holds:

$$C_{\mathrm{voxel}}(t) = F \cdot \mathrm{AIF}(t) \otimes R(t), \tag{2.2}$$

where $R(t)$ is the residue function. Following the arrival of an infinitely short dose of tracer, the residue function is the remaining fraction of that dose of tracer in the voxel at time t. This function decays from 1 (at $t = 0$, all the tracer is in the voxel) to 0 (at long t values, all the tracer has left the voxel). Deconvolving $C_{\mathrm{voxel}}(t)$ by $\mathrm{AIF}(t)$ yields the function $F{\cdot}R(t)$. The deconvolution is very sensitive to noise and has to be made insensitive to the tracer arrival delay [5]. In theory, the value of this function at $t = 0$ provides an estimate of F since $R(0) = 1$. In practice, there is a delay between the AIF and the tracer concentration time course in the voxel, which may be characterized by the time of the maximum of $R(t)$, called $T_{\max}$ [6].

A last important principle is the central volume theorem, established by Meier and Zierler [7]. Under the assumptions described above, blood volume, blood flow (F), and mean transit time (MTT) are related:

$$\text{MTT} = \text{BVf}/F, \tag{2.3}$$

Assuming that the microvascular network inside the voxel has one input and one output, MTT is the mean time taken by the CA to travel along the possible microvascular pathways between the input and the output.

2.3.2 Steady-State Approach

In this approach, measurements are performed before and after the injection of a CA, once the CA concentration in blood may be considered homogeneous and stable for the acquisition duration. The ratio between the blood and the voxel CA concentrations is the voxel BVf, assuming the CA remains purely intravascular. The required stability in the intravascular CA concentration limits the scope of usable CAs.

The steady-state and dynamic approaches may be coupled: The data obtained at beginning and at the end of the dynamic acquisition may be used to perform a steady-state analysis of BVf. As the steady-state analysis does not depend on an AIF, the BVf estimate can be used to refine the dynamic analysis, such as in the book end approach [8].

2.4 Biophysical Modeling of Diffusible Tracers

We now consider an organ and a diffusible CA—an exogenous tracer such as a gadolinium chelate or simply intravascular water. Three physiological situations may be considered [9]:

- The flow-limited situation, in which the permeability is high compared to the flow. The flow is thus the limiting factor to the arrival of the tracer into the tissue. This case is the one considered if water is used as a tracer, such as in arterial spin labeling (ASL).
- The permeability-limited situation, where the flow maintains an almost constant concentration of the tracer across the vascular system in the voxel and a small fraction of the tracer extravasates.
- The mixed situation, where both flow and permeability limit the arrival of the tracer to the tissue. This case is the one

generally considered in dynamic contrast–enhanced (DCE) MRI.

From a formal point of view, these situations may be described by the extraction fraction, E, that is, the fraction of tracer within blood that enters the tissue compartment:

$$E = 1 - \exp(-PS/F), \tag{2.4}$$

where P is the permeability of the vessel wall (in cm·s^{-1}) and S is the surface of the vessel wall (in cm^2). The permeability-surface product PS is thus a flux of tracer through the vessel wall, like F is the flux of blood through the vessels. As tracers are generally plasmatic, there is a hematocrit factor between the blood and the plasmatic concentrations of the CA.

To measure perfusion parameters, there is again a dynamic approach and a steady-state approach.

The dynamic approach, used in DCE MRI, relies on a pharmacokinetic modeling of the tracer distribution inside the voxel. As for nondiffusible tracers, we will consider that AIF(t) describes how a tracer enters into a voxel over time. After its extravasation, the tracer is distributed only in the extravascular and extracellular space (EES) [9]. Assuming that the diffusion through the vessel wall is driven by the concentration gradient across that wall, and assuming that the voxel may be modeled as two compartments, the blood and the EES, one has:

$$C_{\text{voxel}}(t) = \text{BVf} \cdot \text{AIF}(t) + v_{\text{e}} \cdot k_{\text{pe}} \int_0^{\infty} \text{AIF}(\tau) \exp\left[-k_{\text{ep}}(t-\tau)\right] d\tau, \tag{2.5}$$

where k_{pe} and k_{ep} represent the forward and reverse rate constants of CA exchange between blood and EES. This equation is known as the extended Kety model [9]. The product $v_{\text{e}} \cdot k_{\text{pe}}$ is called K_{trans} in literature and is used as a reporter of permeability. Other models exist [10–12]. For example, assuming that the tracer does not return from tissue to blood during the measurement, Eq. 2.5 may be simplified. On the basis of this approach, Patlak et al. proposed a graphical analysis to derive the vessel wall permeability [13]. Conversely, more complex models that account for blood flow in the vascular compartment have also been proposed [14, 15], such as:

$$\frac{dC_{\text{microv}}(t)}{dt} = \frac{F}{\text{BVf}} \cdot [\text{AIF}(t) - \text{VOF}(t)] - \frac{PS}{\text{BVf}} [C_{\text{microv}}(t) - dC_{\text{EES}}(t)], \tag{2.6}$$

and
$$\frac{dC_{\text{EES}}(t)}{dt} = \frac{PS}{v_{\text{EES}}} [C_{\text{microv}}(t) - dC_{\text{EES}}(t)], \tag{2.7}$$

where C_{microv} and C_{EES} represent the tracer concentration in the microvasculature of the voxel and in the EES space, respectively, and v_{EES} represents the EES volume.

In the flow-limited situation, an equilibrium between CA concentrations in intra- and extravascular spaces is often assumed, such that the venous concentration may be obtained from the voxel concentration, using the coefficient of partition for the considered tracer (i.e., the ratio of plasma and tissue tracer solubilities) [16]:

$$\frac{dC_{\text{voxel}}(t)}{dt} = F \cdot [\text{AIF}(t) - \text{VOF}(t)]. \tag{2.8}$$

This is the case of ASL, which uses labeled water as the CA, where in addition the decay of label due to longitudinal relaxation needs to be considered (see Section 2.6). ASL allows quantifying blood flow, as well as arrival or transit times.

For the steady-state approach, images are obtained before and at a time point after tracer injection, when the intravascular concentration may be considered stable for the acquisition duration. It can be used to qualitatively evaluate permeability to a gadolinium chelate.

An alternative to the use of models is to simply define metrics of the signal change, such as the area under the curve of signal change, following CA injection. This phenomenological approach is more robust to noise and model fit failure than model-based approaches and obviates the need for an AIF [17].

2.5 Exogenous Tracers: DSC, Steady-State Approaches, and DCE

2.5.1 Impact of Exogenous Tracers on the MR Signal

Most exogenous tracers are detected indirectly in MRI via their impact on the water proton signal. There are two simultaneous effects: the susceptibility effect and the relaxivity effect. For a given acquisition strategy, usually one or the other of these effects is predominant and CA concentration can be derived from the magnetic resonance (MR) signals. Perfusion parameters are then calculated from that concentration on the basis of the appropriate tracer kinetic model. Difficulties arise when both of these effects have a significant impact on the signal but only one is modeled.

The relaxivity effect is an acceleration of the relaxation of the longitudinal and transverse magnetization components of water. The longitudinal relaxation time, T_1, and the CA concentration (noted as [CA]) are linked through:

$$T_1 = \frac{1}{T_{10}} + r_1 \cdot [\mathrm{CA}], \tag{2.9}$$

where T_{10} is T_1 in absence of a CA and r_1 is the relaxivity of the CA [18]. The same relation holds for tissue transverse relaxation time, T_2. The r_1 and r_2 relaxivities of a CA depend on the biochemical environment, on the temperature, and on the magnetic field.

The susceptibility effect is a perturbation of the magnetic field around the CA. Every CA particle becomes magnetized when placed within the magnetic field, depending on the magnetic susceptibility of the CA. As exogenous MRI CAs are either paramagnetic or superparamagnetic, they all have a positive magnetic susceptibility, that is, their magnetization locally increases the magnetic field in which they are placed. If the CA concentrations are heterogeneous inside a voxel due to a difference between intra- and extravascular concentrations, the CA-induced perturbations of the magnetic field broaden the distribution of resonance frequencies within the voxel. This yields a faster apparent transverse relaxation, that is, a CA in a voxel shortens its T_2*.

In the case of a nondiffusible CA, the vessels containing a CA may be seen as perturbations of the magnetic field. Assuming that vessels can be modeled by cylinders, several authors [19–23] contributed to a model of the intravascular susceptibility effect on the MR signal, as reviewed in Ref. [24]. Interestingly, as shown in Ref. [25], there is a dependence on the microvessel diameters of ΔR_2. For ΔR_2^*, the dependence exists as well but only for microvessel diameters smaller than the physiological ones. ΔR_2^* is directly proportional to

BVf. Assuming a small BVf (i.e., BVf < 15%), the changes in relaxation rates, ΔR_2^* and ΔR_2 are:

$$\Delta R_2^* = \frac{4\pi}{3} \cdot \gamma \cdot \Delta\chi \cdot B_0 \cdot \mathrm{BVf} \tag{2.10}$$

and

$$\Delta R_2 = 0.909 \cdot \mathrm{D}^{1/3} \cdot \mathrm{BVf}^{1/3} \cdot \mathrm{VSI}^{-2/3} \cdot (\Delta R_2^*)^{2/3}, \tag{2.11}$$

where γ is the gyromagnetic ratio ($\mathrm{Hz \cdot T^{-1}}$), $\Delta\chi$ (dimensionless) is the increase in the intravascular magnetic susceptibility due to the CA, and B_0 is the flux density of the main magnetic field (**T**), D is the apparent diffusion coefficient for water, and VSI stands for vessel size index (a metric representing the distribution of microvessel diameters inside the voxel). $\Delta\chi$ depends on the blood CA concentration of paramagnetic agents and on both CA concentration and magnetic field of superparamagnetic agents. As deoxyhemoglobin is paramagnetic and therefore plays the role of a CA, these equations also apply to the blood-oxygenation-level-dependent (BOLD) contrast. It has been shown that quantitative maps of microvascular blood oxygen saturation (also called tissue oxygen saturation) may be obtained on the basis of these equations [26–30].

2.5.2 Dynamic Susceptibility Contrast MRI

In DSC MRI, an exogenous nondiffusible tracer is injected as a bolus while the signal change in the organ of interest is dynamically imaged. The vast majority of clinical protocols use the susceptibility effect: the gadolinium chelate is paramagnetic, and its compartmentalization inside the microvessels induces strong susceptibility effects, mostly observed with gradient echo (GE) contrast (Fig. 2.1). As long as the CA remains intravascular, intravascular relaxivity effects are limited to blood plasma and thus negligible. Water exchange between intra- and extravascular compartments can, however, amplify these intravascular relaxivity effects. DSC is mainly applied to map brain perfusion and rarely in other organs. The requirement for a high temporal resolution limits the spatial resolution.

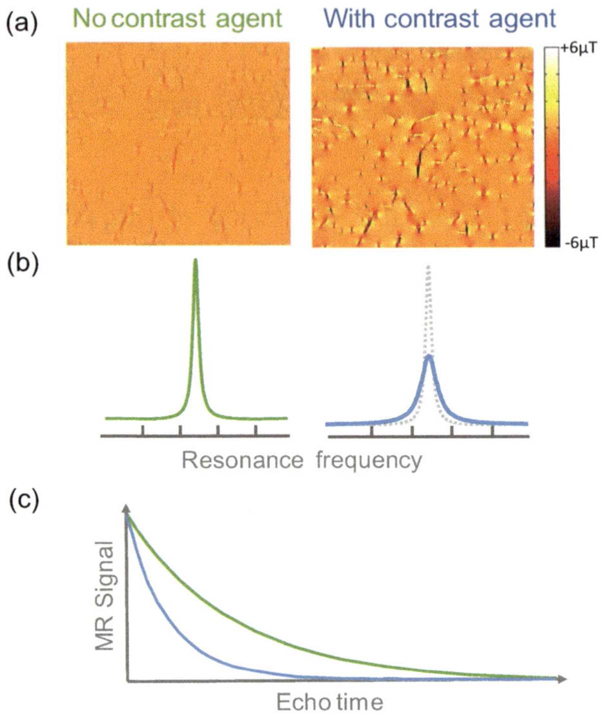

Figure 2.1 Impact of an intravascular contrast agent of the gradient echo signal via susceptibility effects. (a) Simulation of the magnetic field distribution in a voxel containing capillaries. In the absence of a paramagnetic contrast agent, the difference between intra- and extravascular magnetic field depends on oxygen saturation (deoxyhemoglobin is paramagnetic). (b) Schematic of the distribution of resonance frequencies without and with an intravascular paramagnetic contrast agent. (c) The intravascular contrast agent accelerates the gradient echo signal decay.

From literature, it is obvious that there is no consensus on the recommended acquisition and processing approach [31, 32]. A detailed paper by Willats and Calamante published in 2013 reviews all the steps to perform a robust DSC experiment [33]. For clinicians, recommendations have been provided by the acute stroke imaging roadmap group [34, 35] and by the American Society of Functional Neuroradiology [36]. We will not go into the details of all the parameters here but will focus on the main steps that require some discussion, based on recent publications:

Acquisition

- Prepare a strategy to account for CA extravasation due to blood–brain barrier leakage. One strategy is the use of postprocessing schemes [37, 38]. Another strategy is the injection of a preload of the CA (a quarter to a full dose): the extravasated CA reduces the tissue T_1 such that the longitudinal relaxation becomes almost complete during each repetition time (TR). Thereby, the second injection (the DSC bolus of CA) yields almost no further T_1 effects. Yet another strategy is the use of double-echo acquisitions [39]. This way, the apparent transverse relaxation may be estimated independently of changes in longitudinal relaxation. Overall, the last two schemes are reported as the most efficient [40, 41].
- At 1.5 T or 3.0 T, use a sequence with a TR no higher than 1.5 s to obtain sufficient temporal resolution to be able to perform deconvolution. A multiecho acquisition can also be used to improve AIF determination, by automatically identifying and removing voxels exhibiting truncation artifacts [42], a recurrent issue.
- Acquire many baseline points to obtain a robust baseline (e.g., 30 s of baseline).
- Acquire data to cover the entire bolus passage and avoid truncation errors, especially in the case of major flow reduction, such as in a stroke (~120 s).

Data processing

- Use preprocessing to assess data quality, correct for patient motion, filter in the space and time dimensions, correct for CA extravasation, and remove macrovessel artifacts.
- Convert the signal change $S(t)$ to $\Delta R_2^*(t) = -1/\mathrm{TE} \cdot \ln[S(t)/S_0]$, where TE is the echo time and S_0 the baseline signal.
- Detect the AIF. This is usually done using magnitude images, but phase images [43] or complex images [44] are of interest. Indeed, the relation between tracer concentration and phase is linear for large BVf values, while the relation between magnitude signal and tracer concentration is not. Several

algorithms have been described to automatically detect the AIF (early and narrow concentration time curves) [45]. As the area under the AIF should be similar to the area under the VOF, the VOF may be used to correct the AIF [46]. Indeed, the AIF may be corrupted by partial volume, signal saturation, and limited temporal resolution, while the VOF is less sensitive to these factors.

- Perform the deconvolution. While deconvolution is recommended in most studies, a few papers claim that summary parameters normalized to normal tissue may have advantages over deconvolution in terms of lower noise and AIF sensitivity [47].

Regarding postprocessing software, numerous tools are available: the main manufacturers propose a tool directly at the console, some academic tools are available through the web page of the perfusion study group of the International Society for Magnetic Resonance in Medicine, and some private companies propose their own solutions. There are a few comparisons across software solutions [48–50], but there is no consensus on the best postprocessing pipeline to perform.

Despite the variety of protocols, DSC yields very reproducible results. When repeating a DSC exam five days after the first one using the same scanner and the same region of interest for normalization, both gradient echo (GE) and spin echo (SE) DSC were highly repeatable [51]. Normalized parameters were more repeatable than the ones obtained using AIF deconvolution.

Most DSC protocols rely on GE signals due to their high signal change during bolus passage. SE signals may also be of interest, as SE signals are more sensitive to microvascular changes than to macrovascular changes [24, 52]. One can also acquire both GE and SE using a modified sequence to produce VSI or vessel density maps [53–58]. With the availability of multiband acquisitions and compressed sense, whole-brain coverage with multiple echoes may be achieved during bolus passage. This is clearly an opportunity to gather more information. Finally, new strategies have been proposed to derive from DSC data information related to oxygenation [59] and capillary transit time heterogeneity [60, 61], a surrogate marker of tissue oxygenation. These new approaches enhance the informative potential of DSC MRI (Fig. 2.2).

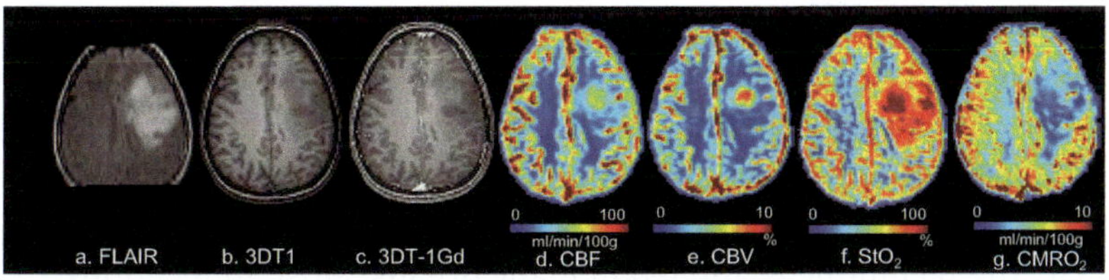

Figure 2.2 Typical MRI images and maps obtained for a patient bearing a glioblastoma. (a) FLAIR image, on which the tumor is well depicted. (b, c) 3D-T1w image, before and after injection of a Gd chelate. (d) CBF map, (e) cerebral blood volume (CBV) map, (f) StO_2 map, and (g) $CMRO_2$ map. CBF and CBV were obtained using dynamic susceptibility contrast (DSC) MRI. StO_2 and $CMRO_2$ were obtained using a quantitative BOLD approach (unpublished data from Grenoble Institut des Neurosciences/CHU Grenoble Alpes).

2.5.3 Steady-State Susceptibility MRI

The steady-state approach, based on exogenous nondiffusible tracers like DSC, does not allow the mapping of dynamic parameters, such as flow or transit time. However, it has the advantage of providing more acquisition time, thus increasing spatial resolution. ACA with a stable concentration during the measurement time is required. Iron oxide particles fulfill the requirements but are currently not authorized as CAs in humans. Some off-label research projects have, however, been conducted. Thereby, using either T_2* or T_1 contrast, high-resolution BVf maps were obtained [62–64].

GE DSC and T_1-based-steady-state MRI may be combined. This approach, called the bookend technique [65, 66], uses the steady-state cerebral blood-volume (CBV) measurement to rescale the DSC-derived parameters.

Steady-state susceptibility MRI may also be used to map VSI, microvessel density, or microvascular oxygenation [23, 27]. More recently, a strategy to combine steady-state susceptibility MRI and MR fingerprinting, termed "MR vascular fingerprinting" [67, 68], has been proposed. This approach relies on a dictionary of simulated MR signals to analyze microvascular MRI protocols. It provides BVf, VSI, and tissue oxygen saturation maps. Steady-state MRI and multiecho DSC MRI provide similar estimates of BVf and VSI [56].

2.5.4 Dynamic Contrast–Enhanced MRI

The DCE injection protocol is similar to that of DSC, but here the kinetics of the extravasation of the CA are modeled. The vast majority of clinical protocols rely on the T_1 relaxivity effect: the extravasation of a gadolinium chelate may enhance the signal by a factor of 3 (Fig. 2.3). Since DCE accounts for tracer extravasation, as opposed to DSC, the technique is applied in many organs. Most applications are focused on cancer to assess tumor angiogenesis and the response to the tumor to therapy.

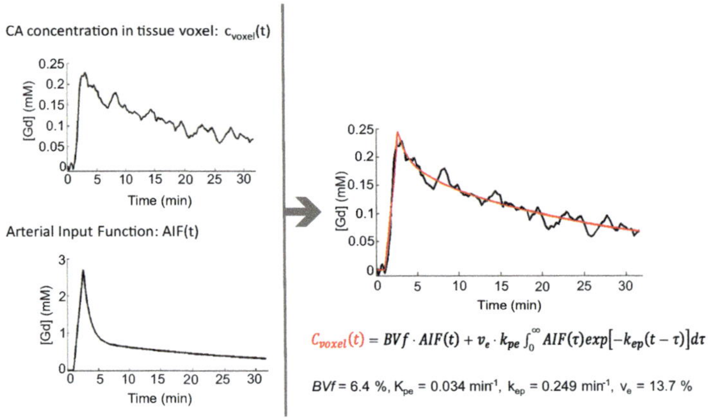

Figure 2.3 Example of measured $C_{\text{voxel}}(t)$, a reference AIF(t), and the fit (in red) of Eq. 2.5 to the data.

A steady-state version of this approach is the subtraction between two T_1-weighted images, one acquired before and the other after the CA injection. This approach can highlight clearly areas with leaky vascular walls. Using adequate calibration, it can be used to derive surrogate markers of vessel wall permeability. In the heart, quantitative T_1 maps are subtracted to assess extracellular volume [69].

For the dynamic version of the protocol, the choice of the imaging sequence used may depend on the type of analysis performed. To map flow, a high temporal resolution is required in order to estimate the AIF. For the extended Tofts model, a lower temporal resolution is sufficient. In either case, the acquisition duration is longer than that of DSC: the tracer needs time to extravasate. As acquisition parameters vary across organs, it is advised to search for optimal protocols per organ.

Similar to DSC, the determination of an AIF is challenging in DCE MRI. Several strategies have been proposed, such as using a reference tissue [70], the complex MRI signal [44], or the phase of the signal [71, 72]. Using the latter approach, it has been shown that DCE MRI and DCE-CT yield similar K_{trans} values in prostate cancer [72]. Even though DCE MRI takes extravasation of the CA into account, a low dose of the CA may be injected prior to the DCE experiment to monitor the AIF more accurately [73].

The situation of postprocessing tools is similar to that of DSC. Some academic tools are available through the web page of the perfusion study group of the International Society for Magnetic Resonance in Medicine, and some private companies propose their own solutions.

In the clinic, studies rely on the use of small gadolinium chelates, the only approved clinical CAs. There is, however, some potential in using tracers with different hydrodynamic diameters. In a rat model of glioma, gadolinium chelates of two different sizes reveal differential enhancement after radiation therapy and antiangiogenic therapies [74], presumably because of microfenestrations of different sizes [75]. Following blood–brain barrier opening using focused ultrasound microbubbles and using a CA with a different hydrodynamic diameter, Marty et al. showed that the closing of the blood–brain barrier is progressive [76]. Even large iron oxide particles with a hydrodynamic diameter of about 25 μm may extravasate in tumors [77].

To obtain more characteristics of tissue perfusion, there is an interest in performing combined protocols. The CA distribution can be monitored using multiecho sequences [39, 78]. The same CA can be injected twice and its effect monitored using different sequences. In the case of diffusible tracers, the first injection can be used to perform DCE MRI and at the same time act as a preload for the second injection, which can be monitored by DSC. Another strategy is to inject iron oxide particles to map BVf and VSI and then inject a diffusible tracer to monitor permeability [79, 80].

2.6 Endogenous Tracer: Arterial Spin Labeling

ASL is a technique to measure blood flow using arterial water as an endogenous tracer by saturating or inverting its magnetization upstream of the microvascular network of the tissue of interest [81]. Water diffuses largely unhindered across vessel walls in all organs, including the brain. Thus, after delivery of the bolus of labeled water to the tissue, reduced tissue magnetization can be observed using gradient-echo or spin-echo acquisitions. The duration of the bolus is usually on the order of seconds, and the label decays with the local longitudinal relaxation time. Given the rates of perfusion in most tissues, only a small fraction of the total water in each voxel is replaced by magnetically labeled water prior to signal acquisition. ASL relies on subtraction of images without (control image) and with prior labeling of arterial water (label image) to remove the contribution from static tissue spins in the MR signal. This difference signal is commonly referred to as the ASL signal. Assuming fixed bolus duration and complete delivery of labeled spins to the tissue prior to imaging, the ASL signal is proportional to the local blood flow [82, 83].

The fact that ASL requires signal subtraction where only a small fraction of water molecules contribute to the final signal renders the technique sensitive to subtraction errors. The magnetic label is created using "label" radio frequency (RF) pulses designed to saturate or invert arterial spins but which may also perturb the magnetization of static tissue spins due to off-resonance effects, such as magnetization transfer (MT). The control image is thus generally acquired after similar "control" RF pulses [81], designed to leave the magnetization of arterial water unperturbed while reproducing these off-resonance effects on static spins, either within a single imaging slice or over multiple slices, depending on the label technique.

The small subtraction signal in ASL for measurements of F, on the order of a few percent of the static tissue signal, also limits the signal-to-noise ratio (SNR) of this technique, which usually requires repeated acquisitions and signal averaging to produce maps of diagnostic quality. Typically, about 30 averages are required for cerebral blood flow (CBF) mapping. At the same time, the noninvasive and short-lived nature of the bolus enables rapid repetition of measurements and thus dynamic studies of blood flow with a temporal resolution of seconds, information which is not accessible with exogenous CAs.

2.6.1 ASL MRI Sequences

Many ASL sequences exist [84–86], primarily differing in the ways the blood is labeled and the control experiment is performed. This section aims to give a brief overview of the main features of common ASL sequences. Three ways of selectively labeling arterial water are commonly distinguished: pulsed labeling, continuous labeling, and velocity-selective labeling.

Pulsed ASL (PASL) applies a short, spatially selective, inversion pulse to a large region, including a portion of the feeding arteries [87, 88]. The duration of the bolus of labeled water depends on the length of the arterial segments within this region and on blood flow velocities in the arteries. To obtain the well-defined bolus duration required for the quantification of F, saturation pulses are usually used to truncate the bolus after a given time [89].

Continuous ASL (CASL) [90] or *pseudocontinuous ASL (pCASL)* [91] employs long, continuous or rapidly repeated, RF pulses targeted to a slice upstream of the organ of interest in the presence of a magnetic field gradient, leading to continuous flow-driven inversion of water spins traveling in arterial blood across this slice. The bolus duration is defined by the duration of RF transmission. Due to the long RF pulses, CASL and especially pCASL lead to a significantly higher specific absorption rate (SAR) than PASL. Undesired MT effects are most pronounced in CASL; PASL requires much lower RF power, and pCASL employs a stronger slice-select gradient during RF pulses, leading to a frequency offset that can be large with respect to the macromolecular spectrum. For applications targeting the brain, both the SAR and the MT effects can be effectively mitigated by the use of specialized labeling RF coils located at the neck to target the carotid arteries [92], at the cost of significantly increased experimental complexity.

Velocity-selective ASL (vs-ASL) selects arterial spins on the basis of their flow velocity, not their location in vessels outside the organ of interest. vs-ASL is able to label spins much closer to the tissues they perfuse, significantly reducing transit times [93–95].

A significant improvement in the SNR based on velocity-selective inversion, instead of the more common saturation of spins in this technique, has been demonstrated recently [96]. The duration of the bolus of labeled spins is usually not controlled explicitly in vs-ASL, and a bolus lasting from the label pulse to the image acquisition is assumed.

The most important sequence parameters for ASL preparation are the post label delay (PLD, commonly termed inversion time, TI, in the context of PASL and vs-ASL), the label duration in CASL and pCASL, the spatial label width in PASL, and the cutoff velocity of the label in vs-ASL. These parameters are of importance for the quantification of F from the ASL signal and need to be chosen according to the physiology of the organ considered and the hypotheses of the signal model used.

The SNR limitations inherent in ASL are mitigated mainly by three strategies: signal averaging through repeated acquisitions, suppression of the background signal from static spins through presaturation and repeated inversion pulses during label and PLD [97], and optimization of the readout module through fast low-resolution acquisitions, preferably with 3D encoding [98].

Since the adoption of pCASL as an accepted standard sequence for CBF mapping, this has become the workhorse sequence in many applications. However, the flexibility of ASL, its noninvasive nature, and the short lifetime of the label have enabled its use to obtain additional information beyond baseline F. Acquisitions performed at multiple PLDs (termed multi-TI acquisitions for PASL) allow extracting additional information about the kinetics of the arterial transit [99, 100], most notably the bolus arrival time, simultaneously providing robustness to variations in this parameter for the assessment of F [101]. Time-encoded pCASL provides a particularly efficient way of obtaining the same information, by dynamically switching between label and control conditions according to a Hadamard scheme during the ASL labeling, making use of the multiple repetitions required for signal averaging to gain additional temporal resolution with little to no penalty in SNR and acquisition time [102].

2.6.2 Analyzing the ASL Signal

At the simplest level, subtracting images acquired in the label condition from those acquired in the control condition allows localizing labeled spins in the imaged region. Depending on the delay between generation of the label and image acquisition relative to arterial transit times, these spins are located within large vessels, or they have reached the microvascular network or extravascular space. Accordingly, acquisitions at a short PLD are useful for angiography, while acquisitions at a long PLD allow assessing tissue perfusion [103].

In most cases, the PLD used and the spatial distribution of the ASL signal are the only sources of information available to interpret the ASL signal as either vascular or tissular. Accordingly, if F is to be assessed on the basis of ASL images measured at a single PLD, a PLD exceeding expected bolus arrival times throughout the organ is chosen during data acquisition. For the measurement of the CBF, the recommended values for PLD vary between 1500 ms in children and 2000 ms in neonates, older healthy subjects, and patients [104]. Such recommendations do not exist outside the brain.

Even for a long PLD, hyperintense vascular signals are seen in the presence of vascular disease. These signals should be interpreted as a marker of delayed arrival times, not local hyperperfusion, and spatial signal variation has been shown to be a surrogate for the measurement of arterial transit times [105]. Conversely, ASL hypointense signals downstream of vessels with a delayed transit are not necessarily a marker of hypoperfusion. Sensitivity to transit delays is considered an advantage or disadvantage of ASL compared to other perfusion imaging techniques, depending on the perspective.

Assuming complete delivery of labeled blood to the tissue prior to decay of the label, ASL permits absolute quantification of F maps. The vast majority of the literature focuses on human CBF measurements. In this context, the most common model considers a single spin compartment inside the perfused voxel, equivalent to flow-limited distribution of the labeled water [83, 90]. Given that the label relaxes with a T_1, which at common field strengths is significantly shorter in the human brain than vascular transit times from the arteriolar to the venular compartment, the venous outflow of labeled spins is neglected. The currently recommended analysis procedure for clinical F mapping via ASL is based on the simplifying assumption that the label relaxes with blood T_1 throughout the duration between labeling and signal acquisition. F can then be calculated for CASL or pCASL according to

$$F = \frac{\lambda \cdot (\mathrm{SI}_{\mathrm{control}} - \mathrm{SI}_{\mathrm{label}}) e^{\frac{\mathrm{PLD}}{T_{1b}}}}{2 \cdot \alpha \cdot T_{1b} \cdot \mathrm{SI}_{\mathrm{PD}} \left(1 - e^{-\frac{\tau}{T_{1b}}}\right)}, \tag{2.12}$$

and for PASL according to

$$F = \frac{\lambda \cdot (\mathrm{SI}_{\mathrm{control}} - \mathrm{SI}_{\mathrm{label}}) e^{\frac{\mathrm{TI}}{T_{1b}}}}{2 \cdot \alpha \cdot \mathrm{TI}_1 \cdot \mathrm{SI}_{\mathrm{PD}}}, \tag{2.13}$$

where λ is the blood–brain partition coefficient of water (0.9 mL/g [106]); SI stands for the MR signal intensities for control condition, label condition, and proton-density (PD) weighted images; PLD and TI denote the delay between the (end of) labeling and imaging in CASL and PASL, respectively; τ and TI_1 denote the duration of the bolus in CASL and PASL, respectively; $T_{1\mathrm{b}}$ is blood T_1; and α is the inversion efficiency of the label RF pulse.

Absolute quantification of tissue blood flow requires a reference signal $\mathrm{SI}_{\mathrm{PD}}$, obtained directly from a separately acquired proton-density-weighted image or calculated from the control signal intensity by correcting for incomplete T_1 relaxation, given the sequence parameters and a measured or assumed tissue T_1 value. The inversion efficiency α is frequently assumed to be known from literature (0.85 for pCASL [91] and 0.98 for PASL [107]). While this is a robust assumption for PASL, the flow-driven adiabatic inversion in CASL and pCASL depends on flow velocity and may thus be prone to variability due to pulsatility of flow and intersubject variations, especially in the presence of vascular disease. In addition, pCASL is sensitive to off-resonance ($\mathbf{B_0}$) effects. At a very high magnetic field, optimization of the interpulse phase increment in the pCASL pulse train and measurement of inversion efficiency in individual subjects is recommended [108].

Multi-PLD and time-encoded ASL approaches rely on more complex data processing, based on fitting models of the ASL signal evolution [109–111] or based on a model-free approach relying on deconvolution with an AIF similar to DSC MRI [100]. Two-compartment models can take advantage of multi-PLD data to account for different relaxation times between the intra- and extravascular compartments inside the voxel and a finite vascular permeability to water [112].

2.6.3 Applications of ASL

ASL is mainly employed to measure CBF in humans. It is now considered a mature technique for this application, thanks to an effort by the research and clinical communities to establish a consensus on the acquisition and analysis methods [104], followed by implementation of these methods by all major MRI vendors and multicentric methodological trials [113]. Perfusion measurements in tissues with longer transit times and lower perfusion than cerebral gray matter remain challenging but not impossible [114].

ASL can also be used to measure F in the kidney [115] and heart [116] due to the high blood flow in these organs, provided cardiac and respiratory motion is controlled using appropriate gating techniques. Proofs of concept for applications in other organs, such as retina [117] and lung [118], exist. ASL for limb muscles has a very low SNR for perfusion measurements at baseline blood flow. In this case, ASL is applied during hyperemia, induced either by cuff-occlusion reperfusion or by exercise [119]. While ASL was initially demonstrated in rodents, the vast majority of the subsequent work on the development of the technique was performed in humans. These technical advances are now progressively transferred back to small-animal imaging as well [108, 120–123].

If spatial selectivity within the label plane is added to the labeling scheme, groups of arteries or individual arteries can be targeted to obtain perfusion territory maps [124–126]. For ASL angiography, a time-resolved signal readout can be employed, enabling "4D" vessel-selective ASL angiography [127].

Signal readouts sensitive to a specific MR contrast may add information about the environment of the labeled spins in ASL. For example, the difference in T_2 between blood and tissue spins enables observation of the extravasation of labeled spins by combining T_2 relaxometry with a multi-PLD ASL sequence, either globally [128] or spatially resolved [129]. Inversely, ASL combined with a short PLD may be used as a magnetization preparation to specifically target vascular spins. Since blood oxygenation has an impact on T_2, ASL targeted to the venous blood, followed by T_2 relaxometry, has been proposed to measure venous blood oxygenation, since ASL is insensitive to the T_2 of tissue and since label and tissue signals subtract out during ASL processing [130, 131].

Finally, the short-lived nature of the label enables dynamic studies of perfusion, which opens a broad field of clinical applications [132]. Despite the limited SNR of individual subtraction images, statistical analysis of ASL time series [133] allows producing maps of functional changes in perfusion in response to tasks [134], at the resting state to reconstruct functional connectivity [135], or in response to hypercapnia to assess cerebral vasoreactivity [136].

2.7 Conclusion

Perfusion is a complex physiological phenomenon best characterized by several parameters. Most of the perfusion imaging techniques described in this chapter allow access to several parameters, but the set of available parameters differs between techniques. The diversity of available techniques, each with a different technological maturity, does not stand in favor of a rapid clinical acceptance. Almost 30 years after the papers on perfusion imaging by the group at Massachusetts General Hospital [137], one can observe strong improvement in the quality and reliability of perfusion parameter maps. However, there are still unresolved issues.

Today, there is no consensus on the best processing pipeline to analyze contrast-injected perfusion MRI. Efforts are being made to overcome this by the Quantitative Imaging Biomarkers Alliance (QIBA, http://www.rsna.org/QIBA) of the Radiological Society of North America (RSNA) or the European Imaging Biomarkers Alliance (EIBALL, https://www.myesr.org/research/esr-research-committee) of the European Society of Radiology (ESR).

So far, absolute quantification has not been a radiological need. With the development of standardized protocols, with the potential of artificial intelligence for data reconstruction and data interpretation, the need for more quantitative or at least less variable data sets may arise. Less variability would facilitate comparisons between centers and between patients in space and in time. One could also possibly argue that artificial intelligence (AI) will find quality among noisy data, a success observed in the context of magnetic resonance fingerprinting. Whatever the radiological demand for quantification, one can surely predict the development of AI will lead to a rethink of the current acquisition and processing procedures.

References

1. Banks W. A. Characteristics of compounds that cross the blood-brain barrier. *BMC Neurol,* 9 Suppl 1, S3 (2009) doi:10.1186/1471-2377-9-S1-S3.
2. Bae K. T. Intravenous contrast medium administration and scan timing at CT: considerations and approaches. *Radiology* 256, 32–61 (2010). doi:10.1148/radiol.10090908.
3. Weinmann H. J., Laniado M., Mützel W. Pharmacokinetics of Gd-DTPA/Dimeglumine after intravenous injection into healthy volunteers. *Physiol. Chem. Phys. Med. NMR* 16, 167–172 (1984).
4. Zierler K. Indicator dilution methods for measuring blood flow, volume, and other properties of biological systems: a brief history and memoir. *Ann. Biomed. Eng.* 28, 836–848 (2000).
5. Wu O. et al. Tracer arrival timing-insensitive technique for estimating flow in MR perfusion-weighted imaging using singular value decomposition with a block-circulant deconvolution matrix. *Magn. Reson. Med.* 50, 164–174 (2003) doi:10.1002/mrm.10522.
6. Calamante F. et al. The physiological significance of the time-to-maximum, (Tmax) parameter in perfusion MRI. *Stroke* 41, 1169–1174 (2010) doi:10.1161/STROKEAHA.110.580670.
7. Meier P., Zierler K. L. On the theory of the indicator-dilution method for measurement of blood flow and volume. *J. Appl. Physiol.* 6, 731–744 (1954).
8. Sakaie K. E. et al. Method for improving the accuracy of quantitative cerebral perfusion imaging. *J. Magn. Reson. Imaging* 21, 512–519 (2005). doi:10.1002/jmri.20305.
9. Tofts P. S. et al. Estimating kinetic parameters from dynamic contrast-enhanced T(1)-weighted MRI of a diffusable tracer: standardized quantities and symbols. *J. Magn. Reson. Imaging* 10, 223–232 (1999).

10. Cuenod C. A., Balvay D. Perfusion and vascular permeability: basic concepts and measurement in DCE-CT and DCE-MRI. *Diagn. Interv. Imaging* 94, 1187–1204 (2013). doi:10.1016/j.diii.2013.10.010.

11. Khalifa F. et al. Models and methods for analyzing DCE-MRI: a review. *Med. Phys.* 41, 124301 (2014). doi:10.1118/1.4898202.

12. Sourbron S. P.,Buckley D. L. Classic models for dynamic contrast-enhanced MRI. *NMR Biomed.* 26, 1004–1027 (2013) doi:10.1002/nbm.2940.

13. Patlak C. S., Blasberg R. G.,Fenstermacher J. D. Graphical evaluation of blood-to-brain transfer constants from multiple-time uptake data. *J. Cereb. Blood Flow Metab.* 3, 1–7 (1983).

14. Brix G. et al. Quantitative assessment of tissue microcirculation by dynamic contrast-enhanced MR imaging. *Advances in MRI Contrast* 2, 68–77 (1994).

15. de Bazelaire C. et al. Comprehensive model for simultaneous MRI determination of perfusion and permeability using a blood-pool agent in rats rhabdomyosarcoma. *Eur. Radiol.* 15, 2497–2505 (2005).

16. Kety S. S. Measurement of local blood flow by the exchange of an inert, diffusible substance. *Methods Med.Res.* 8, 228–236 (1960).

17. Cheng H. L. Improved correlation to quantitative DCE-MRI pharmacokinetic parameters using a modified initial area under the uptake curve, (mIAUC) approach. *J. Magn. Reson. Imaging* 30, 864–872 (2009). doi:10.1002/jmri.21916.

18. Stanisz G. J., Henkelman R. M. Gd-DTPA relaxivity depends on macromolecular content. *Magn. Reson. Med.* 44, 665–667 (2000).

19. Kiselev V. G. On the theoretical basis of perfusion measurements by dynamic susceptibility contrast MRI. *Magn. Reson. Med.* 46, 1113–1122 (2001).

20. Kiselev V. G., Posse S. Analytical theory of susceptibility induced NMR signal dephasing in a cerebrovascular network. *Phys. Rev. Lett.* 81, 5696–5699 (1998).

21. Kiselev V. G., Posse S. Analytical model of susceptibility-induced MR signal dephasing: effect of diffusion in a microvascular network. *Magn. Reson. Med.* 41, 499–509 (1999).

22. Yablonskiy D. A., Haacke E. M. Theory of NMR signal behavior in magnetically inhomogeneous tissues : the static dephasing regime. *Magn. Reson. Med.* 32, 749–763 (1994).

23. Tropres I. et al. Vessel size imaging. *Magn. Reson. Med.* 45, 397–408 (2001).

24. Tropres I. et al. Imaging the microvessel caliber and density: Principles and applications of microvascular MRI. *Magn. Reson. Med.* 73, 325–341 (2015) doi:10.1002/mrm.25396.

25. Boxerman J. L., Hamberg L. M., Rosen B. R.,Weisskoff R. M. MR contrast due to intravascular magnetic susceptibility perturbations. *Magn. Reson. Med.* 34, 555–566 (1995).

26. An H., Lin W. Quantitative measurements of cerebral blood oxygen saturation using magnetic resonance imaging. *J. Cereb. Blood Flow Metab.* 20, 1225–1236 (2000) doi:10.1097/00004647-200008000-00008.

27. Christen T. et al. Tissue oxygen saturation mapping with magnetic resonance imaging. *J. Cereb. Blood Flow Metab.* 34, 1550–1557 (2014). doi:10.1038/jcbfm.2014.116.

28. Christen T. et al. Evaluation of a quantitative blood oxygenation level-dependent, (qBOLD) approach to map local blood oxygen saturation. *NMR Biomed.* 24, 393–403 (2011). doi:10.1002/nbm.1603.

29. He X., Yablonskiy D. A. Quantitative BOLD: mapping of human cerebral deoxygenated blood volume and oxygen extraction fraction: default state. *Magn. Reson. Med.* 57, 115–126 (2007). doi:10.1002/mrm.21108.

30. Yablonskiy D. A., Sukstanskii A. L.,He X. Blood oxygenation level-dependent, (BOLD)-based techniques for the quantification of brain hemodynamic and metabolic properties—theoretical models and experimental approaches. *NMR Biomed.* 26, 963–986 (2013). doi:10.1002/nbm.2839.

31. Dani K. A. et al. Systematic review of perfusion imaging with computed tomography and magnetic resonance in acute ischemic stroke: heterogeneity of acquisition and postprocessing parameters: a translational medicine research collaboration multicentre acute stroke imaging study. *Stroke* 43, 563–566 (2012). doi:10.1161/STROKEAHA.111.629923.

32. Boxerman J. L., Shiroishi M. S., Ellingson B. M., Pope W. B. Dynamic susceptibility contrast MR imaging in Glioma: review of current clinical practice. *Magn. Reson. Imaging. Clin. North Am.* 24, 649–670 (2016). doi:10.1016/j.mric.2016.06.005.

33. Willats L., Calamante F. The 39 steps: evading error and deciphering the secrets for accurate dynamic susceptibility contrast MRI. *NMR Biomed.* 26, 913–931 (2013). doi:10.1002/nbm.2833.

34. Wintermark M. et al. Acute stroke imaging research roadmap. *Stroke* 39, 1621–1628 (2008). doi:10.1161/STROKEAHA.107.512319.

35. Warach S. J. et al. Acute stroke imaging research roadmap III imaging selection and outcomes in acute stroke reperfusion clinical trials: consensus recommendations and further research priorities. *Stroke* 47, 1389–1398 (2016). doi:10.1161/STROKEAHA.115.012364.
36. Welker K. et al. ASFNR recommendations for clinical performance of MR dynamic susceptibility contrast perfusion imaging of the brain. *AJNR Am. J. Neuroradiol.* 36, E41-51 (2015). doi:10.3174/ajnr.A4341.
37. Leu K. et al. Improved leakage correction for single-Echo dynamic susceptibility contrast perfusion MRI estimates of relative cerebral blood volume in high-grade Gliomas by accounting for bidirectional contrast agent exchange. *AJNR Am. J. Neuroradiol.* 37, 1440–1446 (2016). doi:10.3174/ajnr.A4759.
38. Stokes A. M., Semmineh N., Quarles C. C. Validation of a T1 and T2* leakage correction method based on multiecho dynamic susceptibility contrast MRI using MION as a reference standard. *Magn. Reson. Med.* 76, 613–625 (2016). doi:10.1002/mrm.25906.
39. Barbier E. L. et al. A model of the dual effect of gadopentetate dimeglumine on dynamic brain MR images. *J. Magn. Reson. Imaging* 10, 242–253 (1999).
40. Paulson E. S., Schmainda K. M. Comparison of dynamic susceptibility-weighted contrast-enhanced MR methods: recommendations for measuring relative cerebral blood volume in brain tumors. *Radiology* 249, 601–613 (2008). doi:10.1148/radiol.2492071659.
41. Leu K., Boxerman J. L., Ellingson B. M. Effects of MRI protocol parameters, preload injection dose, fractionation strategies, and leakage correction algorithms on the fidelity of dynamic-susceptibility contrast MRI estimates of relative cerebral blood volume in Gliomas. *AJNR Am. J. Neuroradiol.*38, 478–484 (2017). doi:10.3174/ajnr.A5027.
42. Newton A. T., Pruthi S., Stokes A. M., Skinner J. T., Quarles C. C. Improving perfusion measurement in DSC-MR imaging with multiecho information for arterial input function determination. *AJNR Am. J. Neuroradiol.* 37, 1237–1243 (2016). doi:10.3174/ajnr.A4700.
43. Bleeker E. J., van Buchem M. A., Webb A. G.,van Osch M. J. Phase-based arterial input function measurements for dynamic susceptibility contrast MRI. *Magn. Reson. Med.* 64, 358–368 (2010). doi:10.1002/mrm.22420.
44. Simonis F. F., Sbrizzi A., Beld E., Lagendijk J. J.,van den Berg C. A. Improving the arterial input function in dynamic contrast enhanced MRI by fitting the signal in the complex plane. *Magn. Reson. Med.* 76, 1236–1245 (2016). doi:10.1002/mrm.26023.

45. Yin J., Yang J., Guo Q. Automatic determination of the arterial input function in dynamic susceptibility contrast MRI: comparison of different reproducible clustering algorithms. *Neuroradiology* 57, 535–543 (2015). doi:10.1007/s00234-015-1493-9.

46. Wirestam R., Lind E., Ahlgren A., Stahlberg F., Knutsson L. Dynamic susceptibility contrast perfusion MRI using phase-based venous output functions: comparison with pseudo-continuous arterial spin labelling and assessment of contrast agent concentration in large veins. *MAGMA Magn. Reson. Mater. Phys. Biol. Med.* 29, 823–831 (2016). doi:10.1007/s10334-016-0567-y.

47. Meijs M., Christensen S., Lansberg M. G., Albers G. W.,Calamante F. Analysis of perfusion MRI in stroke: To deconvolve, or not to deconvolve. *Magn. Reson. Med.* 76, 1282–1290 (2016). doi:10.1002/mrm.26024.

48. Korfiatis P. et al. Dynamic susceptibility contrast-MRI quantification software tool: Development and evaluation. *Tomography* 2, 448–456 (2016). doi:10.18383/j.tom.2016.00172.

49. Kelm Z. S. et al. Variability and accuracy of different software packages for dynamic susceptibility contrast magnetic resonance imaging for distinguishing glioblastoma progression from pseudoprogression. *J. Med. Imaging, (Bellingham)* 2, 026001 (2015). doi:10.1117/1.JMI.2.2.026001.

50. Conte G. M. et al. Reproducibility of dynamic contrast-enhanced MRI and dynamic susceptibility contrast MRI in the study of brain gliomas: a comparison of data obtained using different commercial software. *Radiol. Med.* 122, 294–302 (2017). doi:10.1007/s11547-016-0720-8.

51. Jafari-Khouzani K. et al. Repeatability of cerebral perfusion using dynamic susceptibility contrast MRI in glioblastoma patients. *Transl. Oncol.* 8, 137–146 (2015). doi:10.1016/j.tranon.2015.03.002.

52. Wong A. M., Yan F. X., Liu H. L. Comparison of three-dimensional pseudo-continuous arterial spin labeling perfusion imaging with gradient-echo and spin-echo dynamic susceptibility contrast MRI. *J. Magn. Reson. Imaging* 39, 427–433 (2014). doi:10.1002/jmri.24178.

53. Kellner E. et al. MR evaluation of vessel size imaging of human gliomas: Validation by histopathology. *J. Magn. Reson. Imaging* 42, 1117–1125 (2015). doi:10.1002/jmri.24864.

54. Kiselev V. G., Strecker R., Ziyeh S., Speck O., Hennig J. Vessel size imaging in humans. *Magn. Reson. Med.* 53, 553–563 (2005). doi:10.1002/mrm.20383.

55. Stokes A. M., Quarles C. C. A simplified spin and gradient echo approach for brain tumor perfusion imaging. *Magn. Reson. Med.* 75, 356–362 (2016). doi:10.1002/mrm.25591.
56. Pannetier N. et al. Vessel size index measurements in a rat model of glioma: comparison of the dynamic, (Gd) and steady-state, (iron-oxide) susceptibility contrast MRI approaches. *NMR Biomed.* 25, 218–226 (2012). doi:10.1002/nbm.1734.
57. Jensen J. H., Lu H., Inglese M. Microvessel density estimation in the human brain by means of dynamic contrast-enhanced echo-planar imaging. *Magn. Reson. Med.* 56, 1145–1150 (2006). doi:10.1002/mrm.21052.
58. Emblem K. E. et al. Vessel caliber—a potential MRI biomarker of tumour response in clinical trials. *Nat. Rev. Clin. Oncol.* 11, 566–584 (2014). doi:10.1038/nrclinonc.2014.126.
59. Gersing A. S. et al. Mapping of cerebral metabolic rate of oxygen using dynamic susceptibility contrast and blood oxygen level dependent MR imaging in acute ischemic stroke. *Neuroradiology* 57, 1253–1261 (2015). doi:10.1007/s00234-015-1592-7.
60. Eskildsen S. F. et al. Increased cortical capillary transit time heterogeneity in Alzheimer's disease: a DSC-MRI perfusion study. *Neurobiol. Aging* 50, 107–118 (2017). doi:10.1016/j.neurobiolaging.2016.11.004.
61. Mouridsen K., Hansen M. B., Ostergaard L., Jespersen S. N. Reliable estimation of capillary transit time distributions using DSC-MRI. *J. Cereb. Blood Flow Metab.* 34, 1511–1521 (2014). doi:10.1038/jcbfm.2014.111.
62. Christen T. et al. High-resolution cerebral blood volume imaging in humans using the blood pool contrast agent ferumoxytol. *Magn. Reson. Med.* 70, 705–710 (2013). doi:10.1002/mrm.24500.
63. Rivera-Rivera L. A. et al. Comparison of ferumoxytol-based cerebral blood volume estimates using quantitative R1 and R2* relaxometry. *Magn. Reson. Med.* (2017). doi:10.1002/mrm.26975.
64. Blondiaux E. et al. Evaluation of rat heart microvasculature with high-spatial-resolution susceptibility-weighted MR imaging. *Radiology* 269, 277–282 (2013). doi:10.1148/radiol.13122152.
65. D'Ortenzio R. M. et al. Comparison of quantitative cerebral blood flow measurements performed by bookend dynamic susceptibility contrast and arterial spin-labeling MRI in relapsing-remitting multiple sclerosis. *AJNR Am. J. Neuroradiol.* 37, 2265–2272 (2016). doi:10.3174/ajnr.A4939.

66. Lindgren E. et al. Absolute quantification of perfusion by dynamic susceptibility contrast MRI using Bookend and VASO steady-state CBV calibration: a comparison with pseudo-continuous ASL. *MAGMA Magn. Reson. Mater. Phys. Biol. Med.* 27, 487–499 (2014). doi:10.1007/s10334-014-0431-x.

67. Lemasson B. et al. MR vascular fingerprinting in stroke and brain tumors models. *Sci. Rep.* 6, 37071 (2016). doi:10.1038/srep37071.

68. Christen T. et al. MR vascular fingerprinting: A new approach to compute cerebral blood volume, mean vessel radius, and oxygenation maps in the human brain. *Neuroimage* 89, 262–270 (2014) doi:10.1016/j.neuroimage.2013.11.052.

69. Haaf P. et al. Cardiac T1 Mapping and Extracellular Volume, (ECV) in clinical practice: a comprehensive review. *J. Cardiovasc. Magn. Reson.* 18, 89 (2016). doi:10.1186/s12968-016-0308-4.

70. Wang S. et al. Arterial input functions, (AIFs) measured directly from arteries with low and standard doses of contrast agent, and AIFs derived from reference tissues. *Magn. Reson. Imaging* 34, 197–203 (2016). doi:10.1016/j.mri.2015.10.025.

71. Cron G. O. et al. Arterial input functions determined from MR signal magnitude and phase for quantitative dynamic contrast-enhanced MRI in the human pelvis. *Magn. Reson. Med.* 66, 498–504 (2011). doi:10.1002/mrm.22856.

72. Korporaal J. G. et al. Phase-based arterial input function measurements in the femoral arteries for quantification of dynamic contrast-enhanced, (DCE) MRI and comparison with DCE-CT. *Magn. Reson. Med.* 66, 1267–1274 (2011). doi:10.1002/mrm.22905.

73. Jajamovich G. H., Calcagno C., Dyvorne H. A., Rusinek H.,Taouli B. DCE-MRI of the liver: reconstruction of the arterial input function using a low dose pre-bolus contrast injection. *PLoS One* 9, e115667 (2014). doi:10.1371/journal.pone.0115667.

74. Lemasson B. et al. Monitoring blood-brain barrier status in a rat model of glioma receiving therapy: dual injection of low-molecular-weight and macromolecular MR contrast media. *Radiology* 257, 342–352 (2010). doi:10.1148/radiol.10092343.

75. Sorensen A. G. Science to practice: blood-brain barrier leakage—one size does not fit all. *Radiology* 257, 303–304 (2010). doi:10.1148/radiol.101691.

76. Marty B. et al. Dynamic study of blood-brain barrier closure after its disruption using ultrasound: a quantitative analysis. *J. Cereb. Blood Flow Metab.* 32, 1948–1958 (2012). doi:10.1038/jcbfm.2012.100.

77. Pernet-Gallay K. et al. Vascular permeability in the RG2 Glioma model can be mediated by macropinocytosis and be independent of the opening of the tight junction. *J. Cereb. Blood Flow Metab.* 37, 1264–1275 (2017). doi:10.1177/0271678X16654157.

78. Paulson E. S., Prah D. E., Schmainda K. M. Spiral perfusion imaging with consecutive echoes, (SPICE) for the simultaneous mapping of DSC- and DCE-MRI parameters in brain tumor patients: theory and initial feasibility. *Tomography* 2, 295–307 (2016). doi:10.18383/j.tom.2016.00217.

79. Beaumont M. et al. Characterization of tumor angiogenesis in rat brain using iron-based vessel size index MRI in combination with gadolinium-based dynamic contrast-enhanced MRI. *J. Cereb. Blood Flow Metab.* 29, 1714–1726 (2009).

80. Kim J. et al. Multiparametric characterization of response to anti-angiogenic therapy using USPIO contrast-enhanced MRI in combination with dynamic contrast-enhanced MRI. *J. Magn. Reson. Imaging* (2017). doi:10.1002/jmri.25898.

81. Detre J. A., Leigh J. S., Williams D. S., Koretsky A. P. Perfusion imaging. *Magn. Reson. Med.* 23, 37–45 (1992).

82. Alsop D. C., Detre J. A. Reduced transit-time sensitivity in noninvasive magnetic resonance imaging of human cerebral blood flow. *J. Cereb. Blood Flow Metab.* 16, 1236–1249 (1996). doi:10.1097/00004647-199611000-00019.

83. Buxton R. B. et al. A general kinetic model for quantitative perfusion imaging with arterial spin labeling. *Magn. Reson. Med.* 40, 383–396 (1998).

84. Barbier E. L., Lamalle L., Decorps M. Methodology of brain perfusion imaging. *J. Magn. Reson. Imaging* 13, 496–520 (2001).

85. Ferre J. C. et al. Arterial spin labeling, (ASL) perfusion: techniques and clinical use. *Diagn. Interv. Imaging* 94, 1211–1223 (2013). doi:10.1016/j.diii.2013.06.010.

86. Hernandez-Garcia L., Lahiri A., Schollenberger J. Recent progress in ASL. *Neuroimage* (2018). doi:10.1016/j.neuroimage.2017.12.095.

87. Edelman R. R. et al. Qualitative mapping of cerebral blood flow and functional localization with echo-planar MR imaging and signal targeting with alternating radio frequency. *Radiology* 192, 513–520 (1994). doi:10.1148/radiology.192.2.8029425.

88. Kwong K. K., Chesler D. A., Weisskoff R. M., Rosen B. R. Perfusion MR imaging. *Proc. SMR, 2nd Annual Meeting,* 1005 (1994).

89. Wong E. C., Buxton R. B., Frank L. R. Quantitative imaging of perfusion using a single subtraction, (QUIPSS and QUIPSS II). *Magn. Reson. Med.* 39, 702–708 (1998).

90. Williams D. S., Detre J. A., Leigh J. S., Koretsky A. P. Magnetic resonance imaging of perfusion using spin inversion of arterial water. *Proc. Natl. Acad. Sci. U. S. A.* 89, 212–216 (1992).

91. Dai W., Garcia D., de Bazelaire C., Alsop D. C. Continuous flow-driven inversion for arterial spin labeling using pulsed radio frequency and gradient fields. *Magn. Reson. Med.* 60, 1488–1497 (2008). doi:10.1002/mrm.21790.

92. Zhang W., Silva A. C., Williams D. S., Koretsky A. P. NMR measurement of perfusion using arterial spin labeling without saturation of macromolecular spins. *Magn. Reson. Med.* 33, 370–376 (1995).

93. Norris D. G., Schwarzbauer C. Velocity selective radiofrequency pulse trains. *J. Magn. Reson.* 137, 231–236 (1999). doi:10.1006/jmre.1998.1690.

94. Duhamel G., de Bazelaire C., Alsop D. C. Evaluation of systematic quantification errors in velocity-selective arterial spin labeling of the brain. *Magn. Reson. Med.* 50, 145–153 (2003). doi:10.1002/mrm.10510.

95. Wong E. C. et al. Velocity-selective arterial spin labeling. *Magn. Reson. Med.* 55, 1334–1341 (2006). doi:10.1002/mrm.20906.

96. Qin Q., van Zijl P. C. Velocity-selective-inversion prepared arterial spin labeling. *Magn. Reson. Med.* 76, 1136–1148 (2016). doi:10.1002/mrm.26010.

97. Ye F. Q., Frank J. A., Weinberger D. R., McLaughlin A. C. Noise reduction in 3D perfusion imaging by attenuating the static signal in arterial spin tagging, (ASSIST). *Magn. Reson. Med.* 44, 92–100 (2000).

98. Gunther M., Oshio K., Feinberg D. A. Single-shot 3D imaging techniques improve arterial spin labeling perfusion measurements. *Magn. Reson. Med.* 54, 491–498 (2005). doi:10.1002/mrm.20580.

99. Gunther M., Bock M., Schad L. R. Arterial spin labeling in combination with a look-locker sampling strategy: inflow turbo-sampling EPI-FAIR, (ITS-FAIR). *Magn. Reson. Med.* 46, 974–984 (2001).

100. Petersen E. T., Lim T., Golay X. Model-free arterial spin labeling quantification approach for perfusion MRI. *Magn. Reson. Med.* 55, 219–232 (2006). doi:10.1002/mrm.20784.

101. Yun T. J. et al. Transit time corrected arterial spin labeling technique aids to overcome delayed transit time effect. *Neuroradiology* 60, 255–265 (2018). doi:10.1007/s00234-017-1969-x.

102. Teeuwisse W. M., Schmid S., Ghariq E., Veer I. M.,van Osch M. J. Time-encoded pseudocontinuous arterial spin labeling: basic properties and timing strategies for human applications. *Magn. Reson. Med.* 72, 1712–1722 (2014). doi:10.1002/mrm.25083.

103. Jezzard P., Chappell M. A., Okell T. W. Arterial spin labeling for the measurement of cerebral perfusion and angiography. *J. Cereb. Blood Flow Metab.*, 271678X17743240 (2017). doi:10.1177/0271678X17743240.

104. Alsop D. C. et al. Recommended implementation of arterial spin-labeled perfusion MRI for clinical applications: A consensus of the ISMRM perfusion study group and the European consortium for ASL in dementia. *Magn. Reson. Med.* 73, 102–116 (2015). doi:10.1002/mrm.25197.

105. Mutsaerts H. J. et al. The spatial coefficient of variation in arterial spin labeling cerebral blood flow images. *J. Cereb. Blood Flow Metab.* 37, 3184–3192 (2017). doi:10.1177/0271678X16683690.

106. Herscovitch P., Raichle M. E. What is the correct value for the brain–blood partition coefficient for water? *J. Cereb. Blood Flow Metab.* 5, 65–69 (1985) doi:10.1038/jcbfm.1985.9.

107. Wong E. C., Buxton R. B., Frank L. R. A theoretical and experimental comparison of continuous and pulsed arterial spin labeling techniques for quantitative perfusion imaging. *Magn. Reson. Med.* 40, 348–355 (1998).

108. Hirschler L. et al. Interpulse phase corrections for unbalanced pseudo-continuous arterial spin labeling at high magnetic field. *Magn. Reson. Med.* 79, 1314–1324 (2018). doi:10.1002/mrm.26767.

109. Francis S. T., Bowtell R., Gowland P. A. Modeling and optimization of Look-Locker spin labeling for measuring perfusion and transit time changes in activation studies taking into account arterial blood volume. *Magn. Reson. Med.* 59, 316–325 (2008). doi:10.1002/mrm.21442.

110. MacIntosh B. J. et al. Assessment of arterial arrival times derived from multiple inversion time pulsed arterial spin labeling MRI. *Magn. Reson. Med.* 63, 641–647 (2010). doi:10.1002/mrm.22256.

111. Chappell M. A. et al. Separation of macrovascular signal in multi-inversion time arterial spin labelling MRI. *Magn. Reson. Med.* 63, 1357–1365 (2010). doi:10.1002/mrm.22320.

112. Parkes L. M. Quantification of cerebral perfusion using arterial spin labeling: two-compartment models. *J. Magn. Reson. Imaging* 22, 732–736 (2005). doi:10.1002/jmri.20456.

113. Mutsaerts H. J. et al. Multi-vendor reliability of arterial spin labeling perfusion MRI using a near-identical sequence: implications for multi-center studies. *Neuroimage* 113, 143–152 (2015). doi:10.1016/j.neuroimage.2015.03.043.

114. van Osch M. J. et al. Can arterial spin labeling detect white matter perfusion signal? *Magn. Reson. Med.* 62, 165–173 (2009). doi:10.1002/mrm.22002.

115. Cutajar M. et al. Comparison of ASL and DCE MRI for the non-invasive measurement of renal blood flow: quantification and reproducibility. *Eur. Radiol.* 24, 1300–1308 (2014). doi:10.1007/s00330-014-3130-0.

116. Do H. P. et al. Double-gated myocardial ASL perfusion imaging is robust to heart rate variation. *Magn. Reson. Med.* 77, 1975–1980 (2017). doi:10.1002/mrm.26282.

117. Peng Q., Zhang Y., Nateras O. S., van Osch M. J., Duong T. Q. MRI of blood flow of the human retina. *Magn. Reson. Med.* 65, 1768–1775 (2011). doi:10.1002/mrm.22763.

118. Miller G. W. et al. Advances in functional and structural imaging of the human lung using proton MRI. *NMR Biomed.* 27, 1542–1556 (2014). doi:10.1002/nbm.3156.

119. Lopez D. et al. Arterial spin labeling perfusion cardiovascular magnetic resonance of the calf in peripheral arterial disease: cuff occlusion hyperemia vs exercise. *J. Cardiovasc. Magn. Reson.* 17, 23 (2015). doi:10.1186/s12968-015-0128-y.

120. Debacker C. S. et al. Impact of tissue T1 on perfusion measurement with arterial spin labeling. *Magn. Reson. Med.* 77, 1656–1664 (2017). doi:10.1002/mrm.26255.

121. Hirschler L. et al. Transit time mapping in the mouse brain using time-encoded pCASL. *NMR Biomed.* 31 (2018). doi:10.1002/nbm.3855.

122. Romero C. A. et al. Noninvasive measurement of renal blood flow by magnetic resonance imaging in rats. *Am. J. Physiol. Renal. Physiol.* 314, F99-F106 (2018). doi:10.1152/ajprenal.00332.2017.

123. Larkin J. R. et al. Quantitative blood flow measurement in rat brain with multiphase arterial spin labelling magnetic resonance imaging. *J. Cereb. Blood Flow Metab.*, 271678X18756218 (2018). doi:10.1177/0271678X18756218.

124. Wong E. C. Vessel-encoded arterial spin-labeling using pseudocontinuous tagging. *Magn. Reson. Med.* 58, 1086–1091 (2007). doi:10.1002/mrm.21293.

125. Helle M. et al. Superselective pseudocontinuous arterial spin labeling. *Magn. Reson. Med.* 64, 777–786 (2010). doi:10.1002/mrm.22451.

126. Chappell M. A., Okell T. W., Jezzard P., Woolrich M. W. A general framework for the analysis of vessel encoded arterial spin labeling for vascular territory mapping. *Magn. Reson. Med.* 64, 1529–1539 (2010). doi:10.1002/mrm.22524.

127. Okell T. W. et al. Optimization of 4D vessel-selective arterial spin labeling angiography using balanced steady-state free precession and vessel-encoding. *NMR Biomed.* 29, 776–786 (2016). doi:10.1002/nbm.3515.

128. Liu P., Uh J., Lu H. Determination of spin compartment in arterial spin labeling MRI. *Magn. Reson. Med.* 65, 120–127 (2011). doi:10.1002/mrm.22601.

129. Gregori J., Schuff N., Kern R., Gunther M. T2-based arterial spin labeling measurements of blood to tissue water transfer in human brain. *J. Magn. Reson. Imaging* 37, 332–342 (2013). doi:10.1002/jmri.23822.

130. Lu H., Ge Y. Quantitative evaluation of oxygenation in venous vessels using T2-Relaxation-Under-Spin-Tagging MRI. *Magn. Reson. Med.* 60, 357–363 (2008) doi:10.1002/mrm.21627.

131. Bolar D. S., Rosen B. R., Sorensen A. G., Adalsteinsson E. Quantitative Imaging of eXtraction of oxygen and tissue consumption, (QUIXOTIC) using venular-targeted velocity-selective spin labeling. *Magn. Reson. Med.* 66, 1550–1562 (2011). doi:10.1002/mrm.22946.

132. Krainik A. et al. Functional imaging of cerebral perfusion. *Diagn. Interv. Imaging* 94, 1259–1278 (2013) doi:10.1016/j.diii.2013.08.004.

133. Mumford J. A., Hernandez-Garcia L., Lee G. R., Nichols T. E. Estimation efficiency and statistical power in arterial spin labeling fMRI. *Neuroimage* 33, 103–114 (2006). doi:10.1016/j.neuroimage.2006.05.040.

134. Steketee R. M. et al. Quantitative functional arterial spin labeling, (fASL) MRI–sensitivity and reproducibility of regional CBF changes using pseudo-continuous ASL product sequences. *PLoS One* 10, e0132929 (2015). doi:10.1371/journal.pone.0132929.

135. Li Z. et al. Effects of resting state condition on reliability, trait specificity, and network connectivity of brain function measured with arterial spin labeled perfusion MRI. *NeuroImage* 173, 165–175 (2018). doi:10.1016/j.neuroimage.2018.02.028.

136. Villien M. et al. Changes in cerebral blood flow and vasoreactivity to CO_2 measured by arterial spin labeling after 6 days at 4350 m. *Neuroimage* 72, 272–279 (2013). doi:10.1016/j.neuroimage.2013.01.066.

137. Rosen B. R., Belliveau J. W., Vevea J. M., Brady T. J. Perfusion imaging with NMR contrast agents. *Magn. Reson. Med.* 14, 249–265 (1990).

Section III

Clinical Applications of IVIM MRI

Part 1: Neurological Applications

Chapter 3

Clinical Applications of IVIM MRI to the Nervous System

C. Federau
Institute for Biomedical Engineering, ETH Zürich, Gloriastrasse 35, 8092 Zürich, Switzerland
Department of Radiology, University Hospital Basel, Petersgraben 4, 4031 Basel, Switzerland
federau@biomed.ee.ethz.ch

3.1 Introduction

Intravoxel incoherent motion (IVIM) refers to translational movements within a given voxel, which result in a distribution in position during measurement time [1] and can be measured using appropriate encoding gradients. The main application of this method was found to be the measurement of the restriction of thermal diffusion through the biological environment, using the concept of apparent diffusion coefficient. In particular, the observation that acute brain ischemia lesions [2] show a restriction in diffusion compared to normal parenchyma has been a tremendous breakthrough in the diagnosis and management of this disease.

Intravoxel Incoherent Motion (IVIM) MRI: Principles and Applications
Edited by Denis Le Bihan, Mami Iima, Christian Federau, and Eric E. Sigmund

ISBN 978-981-4800-19-8 (Hardcover), 978-0-429-42727-5 (eBook)
www.panstanford.com

Interesting information on cell density can also be extracted from the apparent diffusion coefficient (ADC), with important implications in cancer imaging, permitting the recognition of lesions with increased cellular density, such as lymphoma [3]. The ADC also permits the evaluation of the maturation of myelination processes and disease thereof in the white matter of newborns [4]. Diffusion is a three-dimensional process and varies in space according to direction because of the presence of anisotropic obstacles, which limit molecular movement, such as the axon of neurons. This led to the introduction of diffusion tensor imaging [5] and to the possibility of following noninvasively fiber tracks in the brain in vivo, assuming that the direction of fastest diffusion is followed.

There is an additional very interesting property of this method, which is the observation that incoherent motions are also produced by blood components flowing in the microvascular network [6]. This implies that perfusion information can be obtained from a few diffusion-weighted images, without contrast injection, using a biexponential signal equation model to separate perfusion effects from thermal effects, as follows:

$$\frac{S(b)}{S_0} = fe^{-bD^*} + (1-f)e^{-bD},$$

where D stands for the diffusion coefficient, D^* for the pseudodiffusion coefficient, b for the b value, and f for the perfusion fraction. This so-called IVIM signal equation model can be seen as a two-compartment extension of the ADC single-exponential signal decay model. In the brain, where this method was first applied, this model is valid for b values between 0 and 1000 s/mm^2. At b values above 1000 s/mm^2, additional effects due to motion restrictions of water molecules through biological barriers such as cell membranes and organelles are visible, resulting in non-Gaussian diffusive behavior [7].

In practice, multiple b value images are acquired, usually around 10 to 30, and the IVIM biexponential signal equation is fitted, typically by using a two-step method. First, a single-exponential equation is fitted for b values above the threshold of 200 s/mm^2, which is the threshold above which the perfusion effects on the IVIM signal is thought to be vanishing. In a second step, the full biexponential signal equation is fitted. Interestingly, several reports [8–10] suggest that using only a few b values, even as few as two nonzero b value images, might be sufficient to extract clinically significant perfusion information in many organs, suggesting that only a minimal amount of additional scan time to a standard diffusion-weighted acquisition is necessary to obtain additional perfusion information. In the brain, because the IVIM perfusion signal is only a small percentage of the total "diffusion signal" in a voxel, around 5%, data should be acquired at the optimal signal-to-noise ratio and with a maximal reduction of susceptibility and motion artifacts.

The perfusion fraction f relates to the microvascular blood volume, or, to be more exact, to the "incoherently flowing" blood volume. D^* holds information on blood speed and should be understood as the measured diffusion coefficient of the microvascular compartment, which also includes thermal motion of the blood constituents. Finally fD^*, which is the multiplication of the perfusion fraction and the pseudodiffusion coefficient, is thought to be related to blood flow [11] or, in other words, to the quantity of blood flowing through a unit tissue per unit time. The perfusion fraction maps are generally less noisy in the brain compared to the D^* and fD^* maps, and for this reason, most clinical studies have concentrated on this parameter.

The sources of incoherent motion in a biological tissue can be multiple, and the IVIM perfusion parameters should be interpreted with this knowledge in mind. For example, in the brain, partial volume between the cerebrospinal fluid compartment and brain cortex might lead to an intravoxel biexponential behavior because the apparent diffusion coefficient of the cerebrospinal fluid is larger than that of the brain. Cerebrospinal fluid pulsation itself can lead to incoherent motion, most prominently in the sulci in the sylvian cistern and at the level of the foramen of Monro (Fig. 3.1). The cerebrospinal fluid signal can be nulled using an inversion recovery pulse, such as in the widely used fluid attenuation inversion recovery (FLAIR) sequence, but due to the relative comparable T1 of blood to the cerebrospinal fluid, the signal of blood is also reduced significantly, to one-third of the total blood signal. By using a T2-prep inversion pulse compared to a conventional 180° inversion pulse, 50% more signal from blood can be recovered [12]. Such a T2-prep inversion pulse allows a significant increase in the contrast of high-grade tumors compared to the underlying normal brain parenchyma (Fig. 3.2). The pulsatility properties of the cerebrospinal fluid can also be directly investigated with IVIM [13].

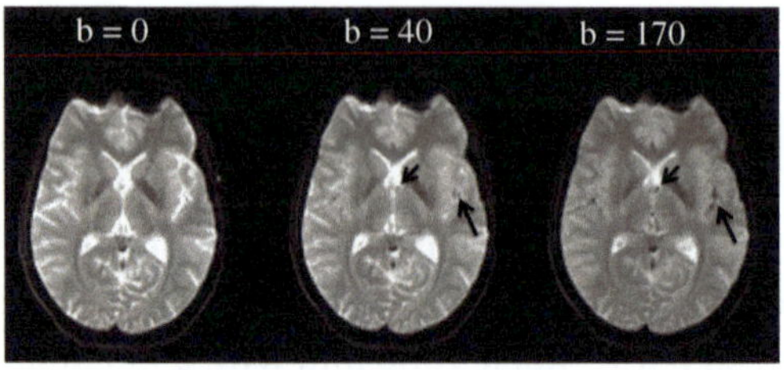

Figure 3.1 Cerebrospinal fluid pulsations can have a strong intravoxel incoherent effect. A *b* value of as small as 40 s/mm^2 is enough to dephase most of the protons at the level of the foramen of Monro (small arrow) as well as in the sulci of the sylvian cistern (long arrow).

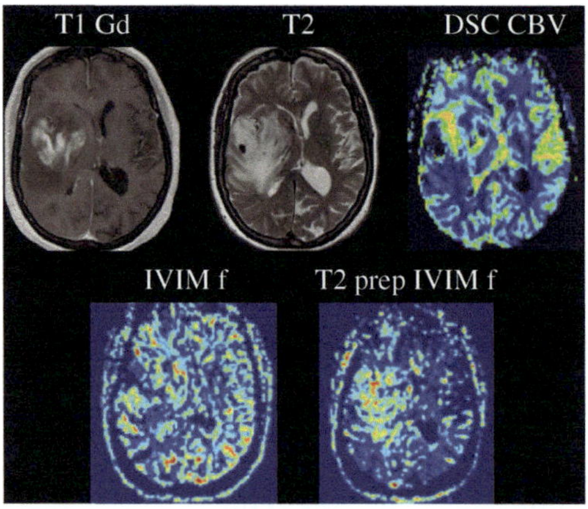

Figure 3.2 Nulling cerebrospinal fluid signal permits a significant increase in the contrast of high-grade tumors compared to the underlying normal brain parenchyma, as shown in the example of a glioblastoma centered in the right insular region. Using a T2-preparation inversion pulse permits the recovery of 50% more signal from the blood compared to using a conventional 180° inversion pulse.

The IVIM perfusion method is of interest, firstly because its methodology is essentially different than other perfusion methods, in the sense that it provides perfusion information that is specific to the local microvasculature, and the method might therefore be additional and complementary to other perfusion methods. Several recent reports have indeed been published suggesting that IVIM might provide additional perfusion information not available with other techniques about diseases such as vasospasm after subarachnoid hemorrhage (SAH) [14], cerebral small vessel disease [15], or anterior ischemic optic neuropathy [16] (see below for more details). Further, it permits the acquisition of perfusion maps without the need to inject a contrast agent, which is of particular interest given the recent discoveries of gadolinium deposition in various part of the brain after repeated intravenous (IV) gadolinium-based contrast injection [17].

3.2 Validations Studies of IVIM Perfusion Imaging in the Brain

Several important validation studies of the IVIM perfusion method have been performed and all of those studies showed positive results. First, in two independent experiments by Neil and Ackerman [18] and by Henkelman et al. [19], blood of rats was replaced with a ^{19}F-containing perfluorocarbon blood substitute, which does remain purely intravascular in the brain because it does not cross the blood–brain barrier, and a pseudodiffusion signal was measured in the brain with fluorine nuclear magnetic resonance (NMR). In addition, under hypercapnia, which can be experimentally induced by inhalation of a gas mix with an increased amount of carbon dioxide and with the well-known effect of dilatation of the brain vessels, an increase in IVIM perfusion parameters could be observed in both rats [20] and humans [21]. Interestingly, the IVIM perfusion parameters have also been found to be dependent on the cardiac cycle and to correlate with blood speed measured with phase contrast in a proximal brain artery [22]. Finally, an effect on the signal at low b values was visible in the primary visual cortex after a visual activation paradigm [23, 24], similar to functional imaging with blood-oxygen-level-dependent magnetic resonance imaging (BOLD MRI) and in accordance with the well-known local increase in blood flow under specific tasks (for more details on this topic, see Chapter 5, on fMRI IVIM).

A simple, linear relationship between the standard perfusion parameters and the IVIM perfusion parameters can be derived, assuming a random capillary network and a sufficiently long diffusion time [11] (for more details, see Chapter 1, "Introduction to IVIM MRI"). Using this relationship, several studies found a fair to good correlation between the perfusion fraction f and blood volume as measured with the clinically most used MRI perfusion method dynamic susceptibility contrast [25]. The results concerning the correlation of the other perfusion parameters, that is, between IVIM and dynamic contrast-enhanced perfusion parameters as well as arterial spin labeling are currently less conclusive, in part because of the sparse number of studies on a range of organs and pathologies and in part due to contradictory results of the published studies [25]. Certainly, additional work on the exact relationship between the IVIM perfusion parameters, the microvascular network structure, and the blood flow and blood speed is necessary. Indeed, many additional factors might be relevant, such as the viscosity of blood, turbulent and pulsating flow, flow restrictions through vessel wall components, and variability of the capillary network structure. Finally, a study comparing directly the IVIM perfusion method to an accepted quantitative gold standard perfusion method, such as positron emission tomography (PET) or single-photon emission computed tomography (SPECT), would be of great interest.

3.3 Clinical Application of IVIM Perfusion Imaging in the Brain

The potential clinical applications of IVIM in the brain include all perfusion-related diseases. In addition, because of its particular properties compared to other perfusion methods, IVIM might provide specific microvascular perfusion information not available otherwise, which could be of particular interest in diseases concerning the microvasculature.

3.3.1 Stroke

Perfusion imaging plays a major role in therapeutic decision making in the context of acute stroke. It is currently thought to be the best method to evaluate the tissue at risk to die if nothing is done to salvage this tissue, which is also called the penumbra. The infarct core, that is, the irreversibly damaged brain parenchyma, can also be assessed with perfusion imaging. Whether IVIM perfusion imaging can play a role in therapeutic decision making in stroke remains to be established, but the property of the IVIM perfusion method to be essentially local, in the sense that because both excitation and readout are done in the same plane, is particularly interesting in cases of slow blood flow. This might be particularly useful in cerebral stroke or severe carotid artery stenosis, in which local blood flow might be nevertheless conserved through appropriate collaterals. In three independent studies, a significant decrease in f was measured in the infarct core compared to the contralateral hemisphere in acute stroke [26–28] (Fig. 3.3). It is important to note that in regions where the perfusion compartment is vanishing, caution is advised when interpreting D^*, because D^* becomes the pseudodiffusion coefficient of an "empty compartment" and is therefore not properly defined [28]. In interesting preliminary results in hyperacute stroke imaged within 6 h after symptom onset, the IVIM microvascular perfusion was found to be retained in the penumbra (infarct core excluded) compared to the healthy contralateral side but was decreased in the infarct core, demonstrating that microvascular perfusion is retained through collateral flow in the not-yet-infarcted tissue at risk [29]. This suggests that IVIM perfusion imaging might be a marker of the quality of the collateral blood flow in the penumbra in hyperacute stroke patients.

3.3.2 Cerebral Death

The determination of irreversible total brain damage is obviously extremely important, with significant implications for discussion with families of patients under life support in the context of organ donation. The definitive diagnosis of brain death is based on clinical criteria, including coma, absence of brain-stem reflexes, and apnea [30], but additional noninvasive quantitative methods are of interest, especially in critically ill patients under anesthesia, in whom clinical assessment is difficult or not possible. In this context, tests demonstrating the absence of cerebral blood flow are commonly used, including conventional angiography, transcranial Doppler ultrasound, and perfusion methods using computed tomography (CT) or radionuclides. Cerebral perfusion in patients with brain death has also been shown to vanish with IVIM [31]. The local nature of the measurement (i.e., independent of the inflow parameters) is of particular interest in brain death evaluation because the absence of brain perfusion cannot be caused by delayed inflow effect, as could possibly occur in a method like arterial spin labeling. The absence of the need of contrast media injection is also of particular interest in those critically ill patients because they often present with reduced renal function.

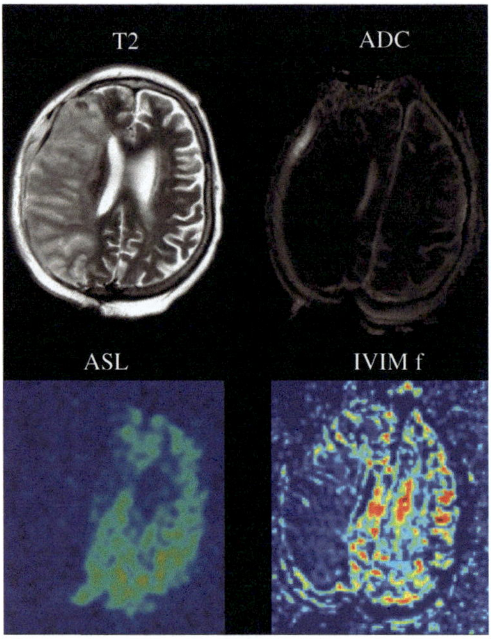

Figure 3.3 Acute stroke of the territory of the right middle cerebral artery, with a clear hyperintense signal on the T2-weighted image (T2), and a reduced apparent diffusion coefficient (ADC). The perfusion of the right middle cerebral artery territory is clearly vanishing, as demonstrated with both method arterial spin labeling cerebral blood flow (ASL) and IVIM perfusion fraction *f*.

3.3.3 Detection of Vasospasms Related Perfusion Anomalies

SAH secondary to the rupture of a cerebral aneurysm is a relatively common disease, with an incidence of around 10 per 100,000 people [32], with significant associated morbidity and mortality. An important, frequent, and feared complication is the development of delayed cerebral ischemia due to an arterial vasospasm, usually occurring 7 to 10 days after the subarachnoid bleeding and usually resolving spontaneously 2 weeks later [32]. Frequent neurologic clinical examinations, transcranial Doppler ultrasound, and CT with angiography and perfusion are the typical methods to detect early signs of delayed cerebral ischemia but with a relatively low specificity and sensitivity. Interestingly, some patients with severe large-artery vasospasms might never become symptomatic and never show signs of ischemia and other patients with only subtle large-artery vasospasms might develop large zones of infarction, suggesting that distal microcirculatory failure might play an important role in some patients [33]. In this context, in a recent initial report in 16 patients, Heit et al. [14] found an interesting significant decrease in IVIM perfusion fraction f and blood flow–related parameter fD^* in the brains of patients who developed delayed cerebral ischemia following cerebral aneurysm ruptures, suggesting that IVIM might be used as an early noninvasive marker of this disease. This is of particular importance because aggressive treatment in those patients has been shown to lead to improved functional outcomes [32].

3.3.4 Cerebral Small Vessel Disease

Cerebral small vessel disease is a widespread disease and an important contributor to cognitive impairment and dementia. It is thought to be due to chronic microstructural damage of the microvascular network, inducing reduced cerebral perfusion and resulting in microinfarctions, white matter hyperintensities, and lacunae. Interestingly, Zhang et al. [15] found that lower fD^* in the normal appearing white matter and cortical gray matter was associated with lower cognition function, suggesting that IVIM might be able to measure anomalies in this disease not visible with conventional MRI methods.

3.3.5 Neoangiogenesis in Brain Tumors

Abnormalities in the microvasculature are an important diagnostic marker of brain tumors, and it is well known that characteristic neoangiogenesis produced in high-grade brain tumors shows irregular, leaky vessels with a disordered network structure. The dependence of the IVIM method on the microvasculature makes it an interesting method to probe the regularity and order of the capillary network. Indeed, a fair to good correlation between perfusion fraction *f* and histological microvascular density was found in a rat brain glioma model [34] and in patients with meningiomas [35]. Further, a significant increase in the perfusion fraction *f* was observed in high-grade gliomas compared to low-grade gliomas (Fig. 3.4) in three independent studies [36–38]. It is important to understand that most low-grade gliomas will sooner or later evolve into high-grade gliomas, after a variable amount of time. Typical changes can then be observed on imaging, such as contrast uptake and increase in tumor size. Perfusion imaging has a particular role in this context because of the so-called angiogenic switch, which is the observation of an increase in perfusion in a low-grade glioma before any other changes can be observed on conventional imaging and which is highly suggestive of an evolution to a higher aggressive tumor. This angiogenic switch is observable with IVIM perfusion imaging, although to our knowledge only a single case has been published so far (see Fig. 5 in Ref. [39]). Further, while it is well known that the survival prognosis of patients with brain tumors decreases with histologic grading, two independent studies found that in the highest-grade group, an initial increased perfusion fraction might be an additional deleterious parameter for survival [40, 41] (although the p-value in both studies was slightly above statistical significance), suggesting that *f* might be of additional value to histology in this context. In addition, a significant decrease in perfusion fraction was observed in brain lymphoma compared to normal brain parenchyma [42], in good accordance with the well-known low vascularity of those tumors, suggesting that IVIM might be of value in the diagnosis of brain expending lesions (Fig. 3.5). Finally and importantly, in brain metastases treated with stereotactic radiotherapy IVIM has been shown to be of value in differentiating radiation necrosis from tumor progression [43].

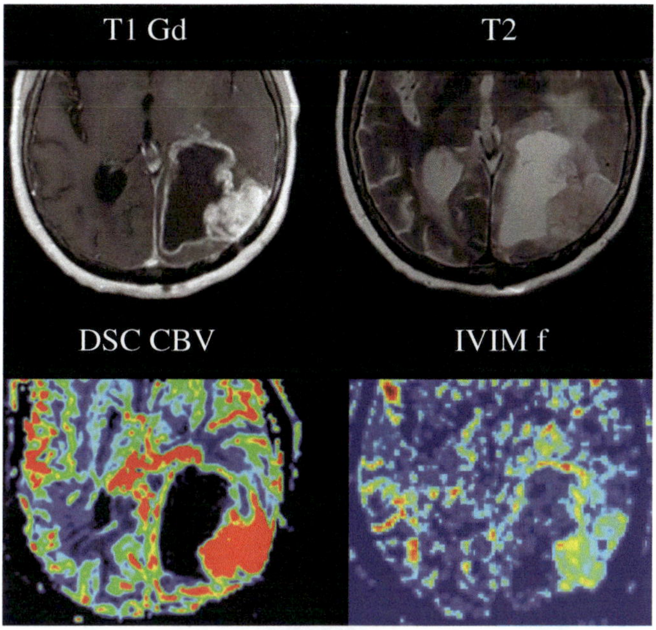

Figure 3.4 Gliomastoma (grade IV glial brain tumor) of the left parieto-occipital region, with a nodular, gadolinium-chelate uptaking region in the lateral portion of the tumor (T1 Gd), and a more cystic region in the medial part of the tumor (T2). The mass shows a marked hyperperfusion on both dynamic susceptibility contrast cerebral blood volume (DSC CBV) and on IVIM perfusion fraction *f*.

3.3.6 Detection of Perfusion Anomalies in the Papilla of the Optic Nerve

Anterior ischemic optic neuropathy refers to a specific infarction of the optic nerve at the level of the optic disc, resulting in sudden, painless vision loss. In clinical practice, conventional MRI provides little information on the microcirculation disorders underlying this disease, probably because of the small region involved in a distal perfusion region. This might not be a problem for IVIM perfusion imaging because of the local nature of the method. Indeed, in an impressive study, Lu et al. [16] found a significant reduction in the IVIM perfusion fraction in the optic disc affected by anterior ischemic optic neuropathy compared to the nonaffected contralateral side, as well as compared to normal control. They suggest that IVIM could be helpful for the diagnosis as well as for the assessment of the treatment efficacy or prognosis of this disease.

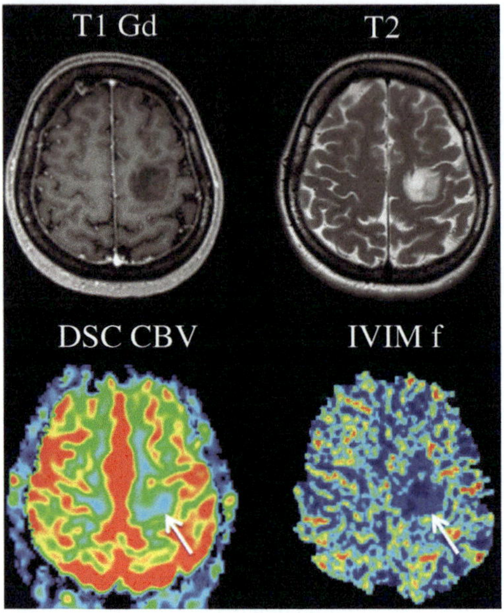

Figure 3.5 Pathologically proven large B cell lymphoma of the brain, with only little Gadolinium chelate contrast uptake (T1 Gd), and an intermediate T2-weighted signal (T2). Those tumors are made of densely packed B cells and are therefore typically hypoperfused, as seen in both dynamic susceptibility contrast cerebral blood volume (DSC CBV) and IVIM perfusion fraction *f* (white arrow).

References

1. Le Bihan D. et al. MR imaging of intravoxel incoherent motions: application to diffusion and perfusion in neurologic disorders. *Radiology* 161, 401–407 (1986).
2. Moseley M. E. et al. Early detection of regional cerebral ischemia in cats: Comparison of diffusion- and T2-weighted MRI and spectroscopy. *Magn. Reson. Med.* 14, 330–346 (1990).
3. Guo A. C., Cummings T. J., Dash R. C., Provenzale J. M. Lymphomas and high-grade astrocytomas: comparison of water diffusibility and histologic characteristics. *Radiology* 224, 177–183 (2002).

4. Song S.-K. et al. Dysmyelination revealed through MRI as increased radial (but unchanged axial) diffusion of water. *NeuroImage* 17, 1429–1436 (2002).
5. Basser P. J., Mattiello J., LeBihan D. MR diffusion tensor spectroscopy and imaging. *Biophys. J.* 66, 259–267 (1994).
6. Le Bihan D. et al. Separation of diffusion and perfusion in intravoxel incoherent motion MR imaging. *Radiology* 168, 497–505 (1988).
7. Jensen J. H., Helpern J. A. MRI quantification of non-Gaussian water diffusion by kurtosis analysis. *NMR Biomed.* 23, 698–710 (2010).
8. Sasaki M. et al. Simple and reliable determination of intravoxel incoherent motion parameters for the differential diagnosis of head and neck tumors. *PloS One* 9, e112866 (2014).
9. Conklin J. et al. A simplified model for intravoxel incoherent motion perfusion imaging of the brain. *AJNR Am. J. Neuroradiol.* 37, 2251–2257 (2016).
10. Pang Y. et al. Intravoxel incoherent motion MR imaging for prostate cancer: an evaluation of perfusion fraction and diffusion coefficient derived from different b-value combinations. *Magn. Reson. Med.* 69, 553–562 (2013).
11. Le Bihan D., Turner R. The capillary network: a link between IVIM and classical perfusion. *Magn. Reson. Med.* 27, 171–178 (1992).
12. Federau C., O'Brien K. Increased brain perfusion contrast with T_2-prepared intravoxel incoherent motion (T2prep IVIM) MRI. *NMR Biomed.* 28, 9–16 (2015).
13. Becker A. S. et al. Investigation of the pulsatility of cerebrospinal fluid using cardiac-gated intravoxel incoherent motion imaging. *NeuroImage* 169, 126–133 (2017).
14. Heit J. J. et al. Reduced intravoxel incoherent motion microvascular perfusion predicts delayed cerebral ischemia and vasospasm after aneurysm rupture. *Stroke* 49, 741–745 (2018).
15. Zhang C. E. et al. Intravoxel incoherent motion imaging in small vessel disease: microstructural integrity and microvascular perfusion related to cognition. *Stroke* 48, 658–663 (2017).
16. Lu P. et al. Assessment of nonarteritic anterior ischemic optic neuropathy with intravoxel incoherent motion diffusion-weighted imaging using readout-segmented echo-planar imaging, parallel imaging, and 2D navigator-based reacquisition. *J. Magn. Reson. Imaging JMRI* 46, 1760–1766 (2017).

17. Errante Y. et al. Progressive increase of T1 signal intensity of the dentate nucleus on unenhanced magnetic resonance images is associated with cumulative doses of intravenously administered gadodiamide in patients with normal renal function, suggesting dechelation. *Invest. Radiol.* 49, 685–690 (2014).
18. Neil J. J., Ackerman J. J. H. Detection of pseudodiffusion in rat brain following blood substitution with perfluorocarbon. *J. Magn. Reson.* 1969 97, 194–201 (1992).
19. Henkelman R. M., Neil J. J., Xiang Q. S. A quantitative interpretation of IVIM measurements of vascular perfusion in the rat brain. *Magn. Reson. Med.* 32, 464–469 (1994).
20. Neil J. J., Bosch C. S., Ackerman J. J. An evaluation of the sensitivity of the intravoxel incoherent motion (IVIM) method of blood flow measurement to changes in cerebral blood flow. *Magn. Reson. Med.* 32, 60–65 (1994).
21. Federau C. et al. Quantitative measurement of brain perfusion with intravoxel incoherent motion MR imaging. *Radiology* 265, 874–881 (2012).
22. Federau C. et al. Dependence of brain intravoxel incoherent motion perfusion parameters on the cardiac cycle. *PloS One* 8, e72856 (2013).
23. Song A. W., Woldorff M. G., Gangstead S., Mangun G. R., McCarthy G. Enhanced spatial localization of neuronal activation using simultaneous apparent-diffusion-coefficient and blood-oxygenation functional magnetic resonance imaging. *NeuroImage* 17, 742–750 (2002).
24. Federau C. et al. Functional mapping of the human visual cortex with intravoxel incoherent motion MRI. *PloS One* 10, e0117706 (2015).
25. Federau C. Intravoxel incoherent motion MRI as a means to measure in vivo perfusion: A review of the evidence. *NMR Biomed.* 30, (2017).
26. Suo S. et al. Stroke assessment with intravoxel incoherent motion diffusion-weighted MRI. *NMR Biomed.* 29, 320–328 (2016).
27. Yao Y. et al. Intravoxel incoherent motion diffusion-weighted imaging in stroke patients: initial clinical experience. *Clin. Radiol.* 71, 938.e11–e16 (2016).
28. Federau C. et al. Intravoxel incoherent motion perfusion imaging in acute stroke: initial clinical experience. *Neuroradiology* 56, 629–635 (2014).

29. Federau C. et al. Intravoxel incoherent motion (IVIM) perfusion imaging in hyperacute stroke: Initial results. *Proc Int Soc Magn Res Med 2018, Paris*

30. Wijdicks E. F. M. The diagnosis of brain death. *N. Engl. J. Med.* 344, 1215–1221 (2001).

31. Federau C., Nguyen A., Christensen S., Saba L., Wintermark M. Cerebral perfusion measurement in brain death with intravoxel incoherent motion imaging. *Neurovasc. Imaging* 2, 9 (2016).

32. Connolly E. S. et al. Guidelines for the management of aneurysmal subarachnoid hemorrhage: a guideline for healthcare professionals from the American Heart Association/American Stroke Association. *Stroke* 43, 1711–1737 (2012).

33. Vergouwen M. D. I. et al. Definition of delayed cerebral ischemia after aneurysmal subarachnoid hemorrhage as an outcome event in clinical trials and observational studies: proposal of a multidisciplinary research group. *Stroke* 41, 2391–2395 (2010).

34. Iima M. et al. Characterization of glioma microcirculation and tissue features using intravoxel incoherent motion magnetic resonance imaging in a rat brain model. *Invest. Radiol.* 49, 485–490 (2014).

35. Togao O. et al. Measurement of the perfusion fraction in brain tumors with intravoxel incoherent motion MR imaging: validation with histopathological vascular density in meningiomas. *Br. J. Radiol.* 20170912 (2018). doi:10.1259/bjr.20170912

36. Bisdas S. et al. Intravoxel incoherent motion diffusion-weighted MR imaging of gliomas: feasibility of the method and initial results. *Neuroradiology* 55, 1189–1196 (2013).

37. Federau C., Meuli R., O'Brien K., Maeder P., Hagmann P. Perfusion measurement in brain gliomas with intravoxel incoherent motion MRI. *AJNR Am. J. Neuroradiol.* 35, 256–262 (2014).

38. Togao O. et al. Differentiation of high-grade and low-grade diffuse gliomas by intravoxel incoherent motion MR imaging. *Neuro-Oncol.* 18, 132–141 (2016).

39. Federau C., O'Brien K., Meuli R., Hagmann P., Maeder P. Measuring brain perfusion with intravoxel incoherent motion (IVIM): initial clinical experience. *J. Magn. Reson. Imaging JMRI* 39, 624–632 (2014).

40. Puig J. et al. Intravoxel incoherent motion metrics as potential biomarkers for survival in glioblastoma. *PloS One* 11, e0158887 (2016).

41. Federau C. et al. IVIM perfusion fraction is prognostic for survival in brain glioma. *Clin. Neuroradiol.* 27, 485–492 (2017).

42. Suh C. H. et al. Atypical imaging features of primary central nervous system lymphoma that mimics glioblastoma: utility of intravoxel incoherent motion MR imaging. *Radiology* 272, 504–513 (2014).

43. Detsky J. S. et al. Differentiating radiation necrosis from tumor progression in brain metastases treated with stereotactic radiotherapy: utility of intravoxel incoherent motion perfusion MRI and correlation with histopathology. *J. Neurooncol.* 134, 433–441 (2017).

Chapter 4

IVIM MRI: A Window to the Pathophysiology Underlying Cerebral Small Vessel Disease

Jacobus F. A. Jansen, Sau May Wong, and Walter H. Backes
Department of Radiology, Maastricht University Medical Center, PO Box 5800, Maastricht, 6202 AZ, The Netherlands
jacobus.jansen@mumc.nl

To investigate the pathophysiology underlying cerebral small vessel disease (cSVD), novel advanced functional MRI techniques, such as intravoxel incoherent motion (IVIM), are very promising. Thus far, in vivo imaging of cSVD has been extensively performed with a focus on morphological abnormalities and blood perfusion. MRI has the advantage that it can reveal various types of small morphological abnormalities using various image contrasts together with information on blood perfusion and other physiological properties in one imaging session. IVIM, in particular, can provide physiological information in terms of quantitative measures on the microvascular and parenchymal integrity. This chapter reviews some (early) applications of IVIM in cSVD (and its related condition, stroke) and provides a methodological and clinical context.

Intravoxel Incoherent Motion (IVIM) MRI: Principles and Applications
Edited by Denis Le Bihan, Mami Iima, Christian Federau, and Eric E. Sigmund

ISBN 978-981-4800-19-8 (Hardcover), 978-0-429-42727-5 (eBook)
www.panstanford.com

4.1 Cerebral Small Vessel Disease

Cerebral small vessel disease (cSVD) is an umbrella term for pathologies with various etiologies that affect small arteries, arterioles, venules, and capillaries of the brain [1, 2]. This disease is strongly associated with ageing and cardiovascular risk factors. It contributes to up to 25% of all ischemic strokes and 45% of all dementias, causing cognitive, physical, and psychiatric disabilities [1]. Various pathologies underlie this disease, among which the most prevailing pathologies are cerebral amyloid angiopathy and arteriolosclerosis. A common form is arteriolosclerotic cSVD, which clinically manifests mostly as lacunar stroke or vascular cognitive impairment [1]. Employing conventional magnetic resonance imaging (MRI) methods to visualize structural abnormalities of the brain (i.e., T1w and T2w; e.g., fluid attenuated inversion recovery (FLAIR) imaging), morphological abnormalities of the brain can be visualized in cSVD [3] (Fig. 4.1). In the clinic, the motivation to perform imaging in the acute situation is often to evaluate early infarcts and to differentiate between irreversibly affected brain tissue and reversibly impaired tissue, whereas imaging in the chronic phase (i.e., cSVD) is more aimed at helping elucidate the mechanisms underlying cognitive decline, gait disturbances, and mobility difficulties. Commonly observed abnormalities include white matter hyperintensities (WMHs), visible perivascular spaces (PVSs), small subcortical infarcts, lacunae, microbleeds, and brain atrophy. The visualization and assessment of these morphological abnormalities have significantly improved the characterization of the disease over the last years [3]. Until recently, the typical application of MRI in cSVD was to evaluate morphological abnormalities, which typically constitute the end state of damage to the microvessels. However, with advancement in functional MRI techniques, subtle abnormalities beyond the scope of macrostructure become visible, as functional MRI techniques potentially allow for earlier detection of abnormalities. Noninvasive imaging plays an important role in the management of cSVD, as it can provide in vivo pathophysiological information, without your having to rely on histopathology. The pathophysiological sequence leading to these abnormalities remains largely unknown. A better understanding of the pathophysiological mechanisms is crucial for developing effective treatment for patients with cSVD and risk assessment for cerebrovascular events.

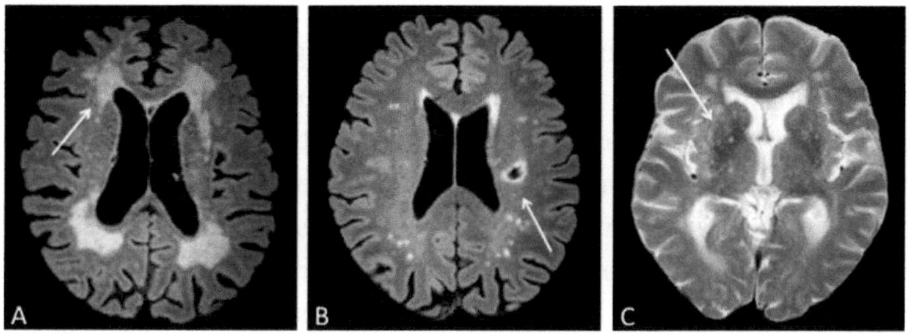

Figure 4.1 Morphological abnormalities in cSVD visible in an MRI, such as white matter hyperintensities (A), lacunae (B), and enlarged perivascular spaces (C), which are indicated by the white arrows.

4.2 Impairment of Cerebral Blood Flow

An important mechanism in the pathophysiology of cSVD is the impairment of cerebral blood flow (CBF). The autoregulation of CBF is carried out by mural cells (i.e., pericytes and vascular smooth muscle cells) [4]. Through interactions with other elements of the neurovascular unit (NVU), they regionally regulate CBF by means of vessel contraction and dilation. For example, interneurons and endothelial cells have been shown to release nitric oxide, which relaxes the vascular smooth muscle cells and leads to vessel dilation [5]. In addition, astrocytes have also shown to be involved in the contraction and relaxation of pericytes [6]. Several changes in cSVD can contribute to the impairment of CBF. For example, cSVD is associated with the loss of smooth muscle cells and also the degeneration of the vessel wall composition [1]. Furthermore, pericytes have been shown to be affected [7]. The resulting malfunction in CBF autoregulation can cause persisting hypoperfusion [8]. This results in the depletion of nutrients and ultimately deterioration of brain tissue. However, hypoperfusion in itself is not a unique feature of cSVD, as many other neuronal and (systemic) cardiovascular disorders can contribute to impairment of CBF. Therefore, characterization of cSVD should focus on the properties of the vasculature and its interrelationship with parenchyma and not solely on blood flow.

4.3 Intravoxel Incoherent Motion Imaging Metrics as a Marker of Pathophysiology

IVIM imaging is a diffusion-weighted imaging (DWI) technique that has the potential to quantitatively describe the microstructural tissue environment and has received great attention in recent years [9]. DWI measures the diffusion properties of water molecules in living tissue. From these properties, structural information can be derived of the tissue microstructure in which the water molecules move. DWI has already shown its credible contribution by identifying tissue that might be salvaged after ischemic stroke [10]. IVIM imaging is characterized by the inclusion of low diffusion-sensitizing b values (i.e., $<200\ \mathrm{s/mm^2}$), where the b value represents the amount of diffusion sensitization (i.e., a combination of applied field gradient strength and duration) during image acquisition [11, 12]. As the MRI measurement for the IVIM contrast is largely derived from attenuation measurements with relatively low b values, it is sensitive to water molecules that diffuse with no or relatively little hindrance. The IVIM signal was initially assumed to arise from water movements from two compartments: a microvascular compartment and a parenchymal one. In the microvascular compartment, water molecules flowing through a randomly orientated microvasculature give rise to the intravascular pseudodiffusivity D^*, which is relatively large compared to parenchymal diffusivity D and has diffusion restrictions of the cell and matrix structures. Furthermore, the perfusion volume fraction f represents the volume fraction that gives rise to the intravascular diffusivity. Finally, the composite measure $f{\cdot}D^*$ is sometimes used to represent blood flow. These quantitative measures can concurrently provide surrogate markers of both microvascular blood perfusion and parenchymal microstructure without the use of a (exogeneous) contrast agent. This technique seems ideal for studying the pathophysiology of cSVD, since both microvasculature and brain parenchyma are impaired in this disease. Therefore, IVIM imaging can be used to investigate affected microvascular blood perfusion and the extent to which the surrounding brain parenchyma is disintegrated.

4.4 Applications of IVIM in cSVD

In 17 patients with acute stroke, Federau et al. investigated the feasibility of IVIM perfusion imaging [13]. Patients presenting with symptoms of acute hemispheric stroke, which constitutes a rather critical form of cSVD as the blood flow to an area of the brain is cut off, were included. IVIM perfusion maps showed an area of decreased perfusion fraction f in the region of decreased diffusion coefficient D (indicative of cell swelling) and that both f and D were significantly lower compared with the contralateral side. As they observed a significantly reduced perfusion fraction (i.e., hypoperfusion) in the visible infarct, they concluded that IVIM perfusion imaging is feasible in acute stroke.

In a population of 15 patients with acute ischemic stroke, Hu et al. compared CBF metrics, obtained using arterial spin labeling, with IVIM metrics D and D^* [14]. They found that D^*, though not D, in the ischemic penumbras was significantly lower than those of the contralateral normal brain regions. Furthermore, a significant correlation was detected between D^* and ASL-derived CBF. It was concluded that D^* might be indicative of perfusion.

Yao et al. set out to investigate the feasibility of using IVIM to measure variations in diffusion and perfusion metrics in 38 stroke patients [15]. They reported positive correlations between f and CBF (as obtained through arterial spin labeling) as well as fD^* and CBF. Quantitative analysis showed a significant decrease in D, D^*, f, fD^*, and CBF of the lesions compared with the contralateral side. It was concluded that IVIM analysis allowed separation of the perfusion contribution from parenchymal diffusion and thus provided an evaluation of both variations in perfusion and diffusion metrics during stroke, which might further elucidate the mechanisms of ischemic stroke.

Van Bussel et al. investigated hippocampal microvascular and microstructural changes in relationship with verbal memory performance in a population with diabetes mellitus type 2 (T2DM), a known risk factor for cSVD [16]. For the microvasculature, the blood perfusion volume (f) was larger in participants with T2DM, f and blood flow (fD^*) increased with higher fasting blood glucose (FBG) levels, and microvascular pseudodiffusion (D^*) and fD^*, which are indicative of altered (vasodilated) microvasculature, were higher in participants with both relatively high FBG levels and low memory performance. For the parenchyma, the diffusion (*D*) was higher in T2DM, indicative of an injured microstructure, with reduced memory performance. It was concluded that the microvascular properties of the hippocampus were altered in participants with both T2DM and memory decrements and possibly hint at an underlying vascular mechanism, which complies with the notion that T2DM is a risk factor for cSVD, in addition to other cardiovascular morbidities.

Sun et al. used IVIM imaging in 32 subjects with visible WMHs to study the microvasculature and microstructure integrity and their association with cognitive performance [17]. They reported a decreased D^* (indicative of a decreased blood flow) and an increased *D* (indicative of parenchymal degeneration) and *f* (showing increased microvascular volume) in both periventricular and deep WMH. Poorer cognitive performance was related to a decrease in *f*. With the latter finding, it was proposed that an elevated *f* could serve as a protective (i.e., compensatory) mechanism against cognitive decline, though this bold statement was not backed up with solid evidence.

Wong et al. performed a study in which IVIM imaging at 3T was used to measure both microvascular perfusion and parenchymal diffusivity in 73 patients with cSVD and 39 controls [18] (Fig. 4.2). The authors used inversion recovery IVIM [19], which suppresses contamination of the CSF signal using inversion recovery preparation. Patients had a higher *D* (indicating microstructural tissue disintegration) and a larger *f* in normal appearing white matter (NAWM) compared to controls. Both *f* and *D* in NAWM and gray matter increased with disease severity, that is, the WMH load, suggesting that IVIM imaging might be able to provide a surrogate marker for the progression of cSVD. Zhang et al. studied the same group as Wong et al. but related IVIM measures *D* and fD^* with cognitive performance [20]. They found in the patients that a lower fD^* was associated with lower overall cognition, executive function, and processing speed. The relationship of higher *D* with lower cognitive scores disappeared after careful correction of covariates. It was concluded that perfusion in both cortical gray matter and NAWM may play a role in the pathophysiology of cognitive dysfunction in cSVD.

Furthermore, Wong et al. investigated the reproducibility and clinical feasibility of inversion recovery IVIM in cerebrovascular disease [21]. Good reproducibility of inversion recovery IVIM was found in normal appearing tissue and lesion areas in patients with cerebrovascular disease, which indicates that this technique provides the feasibility to monitor disease progression or treatment response in the clinic. Wong et al. provided values of repeatability coefficients in the NAWM of 0.15×10^{-2} and 0.10 mm^2/s for perfusion volume fraction and parenchymal diffusivity, which may serve as threshold values to identify significant changes during follow-up and therapeutic trials.

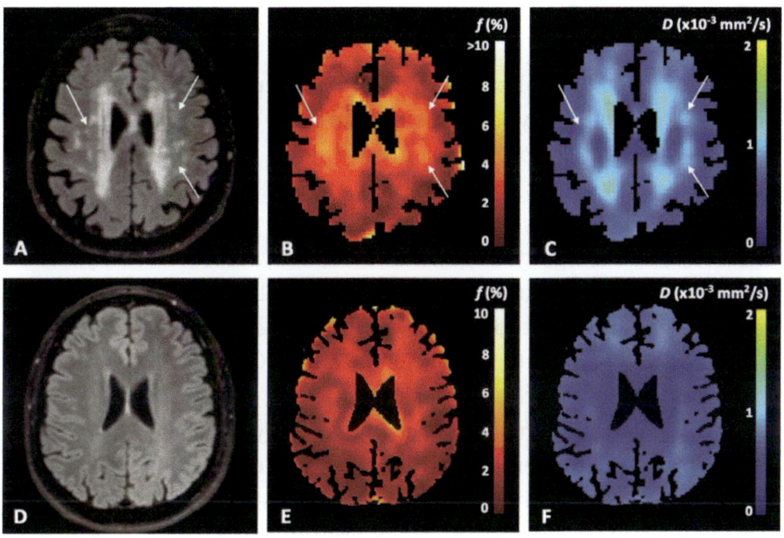

Figure 4.2 Example of a FLAIR image (A, D) and IVIM maps of the perfusion volume fraction *f* (B, E) and parenchymal diffusivity *D* (C, F) for a patient with cSVD and a control, respectively. The white arrows in the images in the upper row indicate tissue with high values of perfusion volume fraction *f* and parenchymal diffusivity *D*, which appears normal in the FLAIR image (A). Figure reprinted from Ref. [18] with permission from Elsevier, copyright 2017.

Wong et al. also applied a spectral diffusion IVIM analysis in 63 cSVD patients and 35 controls [22]. A topic of interest was regions with enlarged PVSs. It was motivated that conventional IVIM, which assumes a two-compartment model, is not appropriate in the context of PVS, as water diffusion in the perivascular fluid might strongly contribute to the MRI signal, in addition to parenchymal diffusion and microvascular perfusion-driven pseudodiffusion. Therefore, regularized non-negative least squares was used to deconvolve the IVIM signal in multiple diffusion components [23]. An additional, intermediate component to the assumed parenchymal and perfusion components was revealed. It was shown that the fraction of this component was related to the amount of scored enlarged PVS. As visual quantification of PVS is a time-consuming process, this spectral diffusion method was suggested to aid the development of automatic quantification.

4.5 Discussion

Interestingly, the application of IVIM in acute stroke is typically aimed at detecting hypoperfusion, through f, D^*, or fD^* [13–15], whereas the application in the chronic phase (i.e., cSVD) [17, 18, 20, 22] has revealed that these metrics are not necessarily indicative of the classical perfusion (i.e., CBF) but are more indicative of the microvascular integrity. Degeneration of the vessel wall composition and damage to the mural cells have been observed in cSVD using postmortem histopathological methods [24]. Both have been suggested to contribute to dysregulation of CBF, which can lead to the deterioration of the white matter [24]. The microvasculature was studied in cSVD using IVIM imaging, by measuring the more or less random movement of water molecules that flow into the microvascular network [17, 18]. In both studies, a higher IVIM perfusion volume fraction f was found for patients, which is surprising at first sight as CBF is typically decreased in cSVD [8], which was also found using IVIM in acute stroke [13]. Hence, a reduction of CBF (ischemia) may precede the formation of WMHs and suggests the presence of hypoperfusion in the NAWM. Moreover, evidence from a cSVD study employing dynamic contrast-enhanced (DCE) MRI reported that the blood plasma volume, a measure related to perfusion, was lower in cSVD [25]. Whereas results with DCE MRI are in line with hypoperfusion in cSVD, results of IVIM imaging point toward hyperperfusion. These results seem contraindicative.

Three possible explanations can be provided for these conflicting findings. First, cSVD is likely to originate at some stage from focal ischemia to which the surrounding microvasculature responds with vasodilation as a compensatory mechanism, which likely persists for longer duration and thus can be picked up using IVIM. Second, IVIM perfusion may not measure "classic" convective blood perfusion and is potentially susceptible to the topology of the microvascular network. The vascular part of IVIM is sensitive to the phase dispersion arising from water molecules in blood undergoing many directional changes when flowing into the random-orientated microvasculature. Many directional changes result in stronger signal attenuation and hence contribute to a larger perfusion volume component. Therefore, whereas at first sight a higher perfusion volume fraction seems to imply hyperperfusion, it may actually indicate altered vascular architecture. For instance, increased vessel tortuosity has been shown in cSVD with retinal imaging [26] and agrees with the notion of reduced CBF since blood flowing in tortuous vessels is less efficient and contributes to more directional changes of the water molecules than blood flowing in straight vessels. Third, the nature of the IVIM perfusion volume fraction might not be solely vascular. An additional diffusion component, indicative for interstitial fluid, was shown to contribute to the overestimation of the perfusion volume fraction in the entire brain [22] (as explained above).

In the literature, results on the relation between reduced CBF and WMH formation are not consistent; on one hand lower CBF has been shown to be associated with more WMHs [27] and on the other hand it was demonstrated that WMHs precede reduced CBF as a result of a decreased metabolic demand [28]. Although more detailed studies of the vascular IVIM measures are needed regarding IVIM's precise interpretation, IVIM might also hint at hypoperfusion through an altered microvascular network [18].

4.6 Parenchymal Damage

Conventional DWI indicates that the condition of the parenchyma observed in WMHs is impaired compared with that of the NAWM [29]. This impairment includes the loosening of white matter tracts, reduction in the number of oligodendrocytes, subtotal loss of myelin and axons, and the degeneration of the extracellular matrix. Hence, an increased amount of interstitial fluid can be found in WMHs, which contributes to a larger parenchymal diffusivity of water molecules measured with DWI than measured in the NAWM. In addition to detecting injury in the WMHs, DWI can be used to detect parenchymal abnormalities in the NAWM [29]. IVIM-derived parenchymal diffusivity should not be contaminated by the microvasculature [16] and appeared to be stronger in all tissue regions in cSVD than in age-matched controls [18]. This demonstrates that IVIM can detect parenchymal abnormalities of the normal appearing tissue in cSVD. Using techniques to investigate the diffusion spectrum of the IVIM signal (non-negative least squares, NNLS), it was demonstrated (as explained above) that in the WMHs, the parenchymal component could be separated from an intermediate diffusion component, which is indicative of interstitial fluid [22]. NNLS might enable isolation and quantification of the damaged part of the parenchyma (i.e., an aberrant amount of interstitial fluid), which might be more sensitive than parenchymal diffusivity. An intermediate diffusion component was also observed in the NAWM and cortex and hence may serve as an early biomarker for parenchymal degeneration or as a (nonspecific) disease marker for cSVD [22].

4.7 On the Validity of IVIM Models

By using relatively low *b* values (<200 s/mm^2) IVIM imaging is advocated to detect water diffusion in both parenchyma and microvasculature [11, 12]. In line with this, a two-compartment model is typically employed to model the IVIM signal. However, more than two compartments can exist, as was demonstrated in the case of pathologic tissue; in Ref. [22], the NNLS method was introduced to analyze the IVIM signal in structural abnormalities in cSVD and revealed the presence of an additional component. Assumption regarding the number and nature of the compartments a priori can influence the interpretation of the derived measures. For example, it was shown that when assuming two compartments the perfusion volume fraction was not solely vascular, which may have clouded its interpretation as a perfusion-related measure. In contrast, when the IVIM signal is not forced to fit a fixed number of compartments, as employed in Refs. [22, 23], a less restrictive interpretation of the IVIM signal is allowed. The number and nature of compartments can be interpreted on the basis of the distribution of diffusivity values observed in the diffusion spectrum. Previous studies [30, 31] have interpreted the multiexponential behavior of a diffusion signal to be a result of different biological processes (e.g., water transport and macromolecule binding) in tissue and is not solely indicative of biological (spatially separated) compartments [32]. In addition to compartments, biological processes should be considered when interpreting the IVIM signal, which is especially relevant in diseases such as cSVD.

4.8 Clinical Implications

Current therapies of lacunar stroke, one of the most common clinical manifestations of cSVD [33], include antiplatelet therapy, blood pressure reduction, and statin therapy [34]. Quantitative IVIM imaging measures were associated with WMHs and may act as potential surrogate markers for structural damage in cSVD [17, 18, 20]. Tissue injury, including lacunae and WMHs, is linked to cognitive decline and physical and psychiatric disabilities [3]. Since the imaging measures may be potential surrogate markers of structural damages in cSVD, these measures can be employed as a neurobiological readout of treatment for patients with cSVD in the short term. For example, vascular risk factors (e.g., smoking, blood pressure, and diabetes) are known to be correlated with WMH severity and the occurrence of lacunae [35]. It can be investigated whether an intervention to improve the vascular condition could lead to less tissue injury in the future. However, prior to conducting this intervention study, which will likely require a long follow-up time, the effect of this intervention on the imaging measures can be studied in the shorter term to gain an early insight into biological responses. For this purpose, longitudinal studies are required to explore the role of imaging measures as surrogate markers of cSVD in more detail. These studies could evaluate whether functional impairment (e.g., abnormal microvasculature and/or parenchyma as shown through IVIM) indeed precedes morphological abnormalities.

4.9 Conclusions

The pathophysiology of cSVD remains to be largely elucidated, and advanced functional MRI techniques are advocated to unravel the underlying mechanisms. Using IVIM imaging, it can be shown that multiple aspects are concurrently affected in cSVD, such as hypoperfusion, abnormal microvasculature, and parenchyma. These abnormalities were found (in NAWM) to be associated with WMH formation or cognitive performance, suggesting that functional impairment precedes structural damage. Hence the corresponding imaging measures could potentially function as an early biomarker of the disease. IVIM techniques can aid the pursuit of a better understanding and hopefully treatment of cSVD.

References

1. Pantoni L. Cerebral small vessel disease: from pathogenesis and clinical characteristics to therapeutic challenges. *Lancet Neurol.*, 2010, 9(7), 689–701.
2. Rosenberg G. A., et al. Consensus statement for diagnosis of subcortical small vessel disease. *J. Cereb. Blood Flow Metab.*, 2016, 36(1), 6–25.
3. Wardlaw J. M., et al. Neuroimaging standards for research into small vessel disease and its contribution to ageing and neurodegeneration. *Lancet Neurol.*, 2013, 12(8), 822–838.
4. Kisler K., et al. Cerebral blood flow regulation and neurovascular dysfunction in Alzheimer disease. *Nat. Rev. Neurosci.*, 2017, 18(7), 419–434.
5. Mishra A., et al. Astrocytes mediate neurovascular signaling to capillary pericytes but not to arterioles. *Nat. Neurosci.*, 2016, 19(12), 1619–1627.
6. Biesecker K. R., et al. Glial cell calcium signaling mediates capillary regulation of blood flow in the retina. *J. Neurosci.*, 2016, 36(36), 9435–9445.
7. Fernandez-Klett F., et al. Early loss of pericytes and perivascular stromal cell-induced scar formation after stroke. *J. Cereb. Blood Flow Metab.*, 2013, 33(3), 428–439.
8. Knottnerus I. L., et al. Endothelial dysfunction in lacunar stroke: a systematic review. *Cerebrovasc Dis.*, 2009, 27(5), 519–526.
9. Iima M., Le Bihan D. Clinical intravoxel incoherent motion and diffusion MR imaging: past, present, and future. *Radiology*, 2016, 278(1), 13–32.
10. Latchaw R. E., et al. Recommendations for imaging of acute ischemic stroke: a scientific statement from the American Heart Association. *Stroke*, 2009, 40(11), 3646–3678.

11. Le Bihan D., et al. Separation of diffusion and perfusion in intravoxel incoherent motion MR imaging. *Radiology*, 1988, 168(2), 497–505.

12. Le Bihan D., et al. MR imaging of intravoxel incoherent motions: application to diffusion and perfusion in neurologic disorders. *Radiology*, 1986, 161(2), 401–407.

13. Federau C., et al. Intravoxel incoherent motion perfusion imaging in acute stroke: initial clinical experience.*Neuroradiology*, 2014, 56(8), 629–635.

14. Hu L. B., Hong N., Zhu W. Z. Quantitative measurement of cerebral perfusion with intravoxel incoherent motion in acute ischemia stroke: initial clinical experience. *Chin. Med. J. (Engl)*, 2015, 128(19), 2565–2569.

15. Yao Y., et al. Intravoxel incoherent motion diffusion-weighted imaging in stroke patients: initial clinical experience. *Clin. Radiol.*, 2016, 71(9), 938, e11–e16.

16. van Bussel F. C., et al. On the interplay of microvasculature, parenchyma, and memory in type 2 diabetes. *Diabetes Care*, 2015, 38(5), 876–882.

17. Sun J., et al. The relationship between microvasculature in white matter hyperintensities and cognitive function. *Brain Imaging Behav.*, 2017, 11(2), 503–511.

18. Wong S. M., et al. Simultaneous investigation of microvasculature and parenchyma in cerebral small vessel disease using intravoxel incoherent motion imaging. *Neuroimage Clin.*, 2017, 14, 216–221.

19. Hales P. W., Clark C. A. Combined arterial spin labeling and diffusion-weighted imaging for noninvasive estimation of capillary volume fraction and permeability-surface product in the human brain. *J. Cereb. Blood Flow Metab.*, 2013, 33(1), 67–75.

20. Zhang C. E., et al. Intravoxel incoherent motion imaging in small vessel disease: Microstructural integrity and microvascular perfusion related to cognition. *Strokc*, 2017, 48(3), 658–663.

21. Wong S. M., et al. On the reproducibility of inversion recovery intravoxel incoherent motion imaging in cerebrovascular disease. *AJNR Am. J. Neuroradiol.*, 2018, 39(2), 226–231.

22. Wong S. M., et al. Spectral diffusion IVIM analysis of enlarged perivascular spaces in cerebral small vessel disease. in *Proc. Intl. Soc. Mag. Reson. Med.* , 2017, 25, 4721, Honolulu, HI, USA.

23. Keil V. C., et al. Intravoxel incoherent motion MRI in the brain: Impact of the fitting model on perfusion fraction and lesion differentiability. *J. Magn. Reson. Imaging*, 2017, 46(4), 1187–1199.

24. Pantoni L., Garcia J. H. Pathogenesis of leukoaraiosis: a review. *Stroke*, 1997, 28(3), 652–659.

25. Zhang C. E., et al. Blood-brain barrier leakage is more widespread in patients with cerebral small vessel disease. *Neurology*, 2017, 88(5), 426–432.

26. Hilal S., et al. Microvascular network alterations in retina of subjects with cerebral small vessel disease. *Neurosci. Lett.*, 2014, 577, 95–100.

27. ten Dam V. H., et al. Decline in total cerebral blood flow is linked with increase in periventricular but not deep white matter hyperintensities. *Radiology*, 2007, 243(1), 198–203.

28. van der Veen P. H., et al. Longitudinal relationship between cerebral small-vessel disease and cerebral blood flow: the second manifestations of arterial disease-magnetic resonance study. *Stroke*, 2015, 46(5), 1233–1238.

29. Chabriat H., et al. Clinical severity in CADASIL related to ultrastructural damage in white matter: in vivo study with diffusion tensor MRI. *Stroke* 1999 30(12) 2637–2643.

30. Finkenstaedt T., et al. The IVIM signal in the healthy cerebral gray matter: A play of spherical and non-spherical components. *Neuroimage*, 2017, 152, 340–347.

31. Rydhog A. S., et al. Separating blood and water: Perfusion and free water elimination from diffusion MRI in the human brain. *Neuroimage*, 2017, 156, 423–434.

32. Novikov D. S., Kiselev V. G. Effective medium theory of a diffusion-weighted signal. *NMR Biomed.*, 2010, 23(7), 682–697.

33. Wardlaw J. M., Smith C., Dichgans M. Mechanisms of sporadic cerebral small vessel disease: insights from neuroimaging. *Lancet Neurol.*, 2013, 12(5), 483–497.

34. Bath P. M., Wardlaw J. M. Pharmacological treatment and prevention of cerebral small vessel disease: a review of potential interventions. *Int. J. Stroke*, 2015, 10(4), 469–478.

35. Staals J., et al. Stroke subtype, vascular risk factors, and total MRI brain small-vessel disease burden. *Neurology*, 2014, 83(14), 1228–1234.

Chapter 5

IVIM fMRI: Brain Activation with a High Spatial Specificity and Resolution

Allen W. Song, Iain Bruce, Christopher Petty, and Nan-Kuei Chen

Brain Imaging and Analysis Center, Duke University, Durham, North Carolina, USA

allen.song@duke.edu

More than three decades ago, intravoxel incoherent motion (IVIM) contrast was proposed as a potential mechanism sensitive to blood flow changes during brain activation. While not as widely used as the blood-oxygenation-level-dependent (BOLD) contrast, which arises from venous networks, IVIM may offer improved spatial localization to smaller vasculature (e.g., arterioles and capillaries) more closely tied to the sites of neural activity. However, inherent high spatial specificity can only be realized and demonstrated if the IVIM images can be acquired at high spatial resolutions. To date most prior work on IVIM fMRI relied on diffusion-weighted single-shot EPI techniques, which are constrained to low spatial resolutions. Recent advances in multishot diffusion MRI, such as

Intravoxel Incoherent Motion (IVIM) MRI: Principles and Applications

Edited by Denis Le Bihan, Mami Iima, Christian Federau, and Eric E. Sigmund

ISBN 978-981-4800-19-8 (Hardcover), 978-0-429-42727-5 (eBook)

www.panstanford.com

that using multiplexed sensitivity encoding (MUSE), have built a solid technical foundation to enable IVIM fMRI at much higher spatial resolutions. This new advancement can be incorporated with previous theoretical framework and acquisition strategies on IVIM to investigate functional motor activations at both high spatial resolutions and high spatial specificity in the finger homunculus. New results along this front are also illustrated in this chapter. It is hoped that such progress will allow IVIM-based functional brain activation in the cortical gray matter to be investigated in the finest-grained detail, further complementing the current fMRI practice based on the BOLD contrast.

5.1 Introduction

The contrast mechanism based on the IVIM [1] has seen extensive growth over the past three decades, reaching far beyond the original realm of diffusion magnetic resonance imagery (MRI). Within the realm of functional MRI (fMRI) [2–7], IVIM contrast has provided unique contributions thanks to its high sensitivity to moving proton pools, for example, blood flow changes, upon brain activation.

Over the past 20 some years, BOLD contrast [4] has been extensively used in fMRI. However, its spatial specificity can be influenced mostly by large veins [8] where the oxygenation level changes are the greatest, which are often spatially distant from the sites of neural activity. Using invasive optical imaging intraoperatively in humans in vivo, Hochman and Haglund [9] have shown that blood-oxygenation-level changes primarily occur in large veins, while blood volume changes are more focal in small vessels and spatially colocalized with neuronal activities (Fig. 5.1).

Within the fMRI community, parallel development in cerebral blood flow (CBF) and cerebral blood volume (CBV) contrasts has been developed and applied over the past two decades. Specifically, by employing an arterial spin labeling (ASL) scheme [10–12], perfusion-weighted images can be made sensitive to the CBF changes from upstream arterial networks to the capillaries. Because of the exchange mechanism in the capillaries and the diminishing sensitivity in large veins due to T1 recovery, optimized perfusion contrast is believed to have a better spatial localization ability [12, 13] compared to BOLD imaging methods. This finding was also confirmed in animal models, which demonstrated the existence of the orientation columns in the visual cortex of cats [14]. However, perfusion imaging does have limitations, most notably the necessity for the wait time for the labeled upstream blood to arrive at the imaging plane, the often-undetermined mean transit time, and the inevitable T1 recovery, all of which lead to a low temporal resolution and limited spatial coverage. Researchers have also developed CBV contrast to image brain activation [15, 16], which are believed to be originated from small-vessel networks (e.g., arterioles). While these techniques have been shown to provide improved spatial colocalization with neuronal activities, they may be limited by temporal throughput (due to the use of inversion pulse) or require contrast agents.

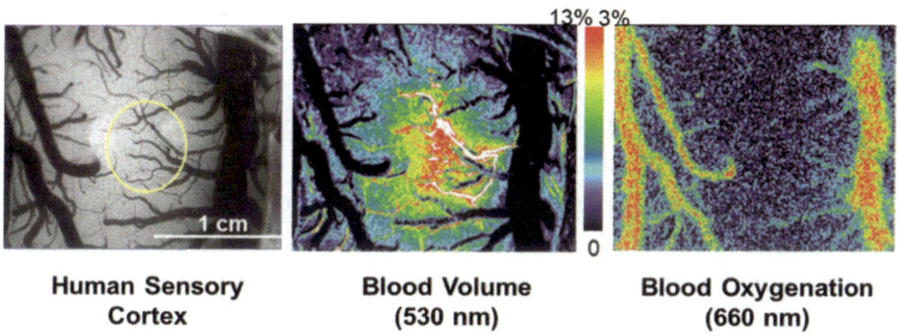

Figure 5.1 Derived from optical imaging in the human sensory cortex during sensory stimulation, contrast in blood volume is spatially colocalized to upstream small vessels and neuronal activities, while blood-oxygenation-level changes are predominantly located in the venous network.

Similar to CBF and CBV contrasts, the IVIM mechanism can be made sensitive to functional changes in the vasculature. The apparent diffusion coefficients (ADCs) derived at low b values include perfusion-driven IVIM effects. This differs from the ADC derived at very high b values [17, 18] where direct neuronal activation related to potential cell swelling was probed. At low b values, a simple signal classification based on the static ADC can be used to differentiate highly mobile proton pools (e.g., those in large vessels and cerebrospinal fluid [CSF]) from those that are less mobile (e.g., those in brain tissue and small vessels), as illustrated in Fig. 5.2. Thus, if the ADC increases upon brain activation due to higher blood flow and volume, it is possible to apply dynamic ADC imaging to capture this increase.

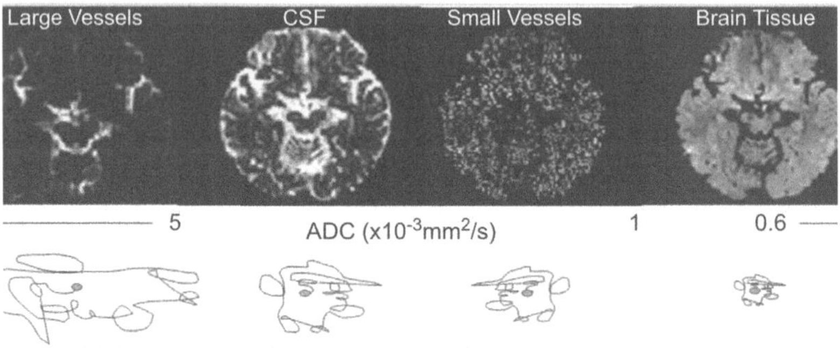

Figure 5.2 A simple signal classification based on static ADC values generally clustered in large vessels, CSF, small vessels, and brain tissues.

A number of groups, including ours, reported that dynamic ADC imaging at low *b* values can be used for image changes in blood flow upon brain activation [19–22]. Such dynamic use of the moderate diffusion weighting strategies is sensitive to the IVIM and differs from early studies that simply employed static weighting strategies to eliminate proton pools of large mobility [23, 24]. In addition, it is not sensitive to the extravascular component of large vessels as the parenchyma tissue near large vessels does not change mobility over time. Furthermore, it is possible that, by setting an appropriate *b* factor range for IVIM weighting, ADC contrast can be made uniquely sensitive to the capillary networks where the increased flow within the lumen and exchange with the interstitial space give rise to significant ADC changes. Compared to the traditional BOLD methods, dynamic ADC contrast is advantageous in that (i) it does not require an ultrahigh field, as it is detecting the blood mobility changes, (ii) it has a higher contrast-to-noise ratio (CNR) and lower power consumption compared to the spin-echo BOLD method, which is believed to be another alternative for capillary localization, and (iii) it has the potential to be sensitive to small-vessel networks if the appropriate *b* factor range is used. Dynamic ADC contrast is also advantageous compared to another popular fMRI method using CBF contrast in that (i) it does not require the long transit and exchange time between tagging and image acquisition and thus could afford much higher temporal throughput and (ii) it intrinsically has a much larger spatial coverage.

As shown in previous reports (e.g., Ref. [22]), appropriate ranges of low *b* values can generate IVIM contrast highly sensitive to brain activation. Specifically, moderate diffusion weighting (i.e., with *b* factors ranging from 0 to $\sim$200 s/mm^2) has been shown to be primarily sensitive to the IVIM changes in the vasculature. Furthermore, IVIM activations can be classified on the basis of their ADC values to infer the origins of their large or small vessels (Fig. 5.3).

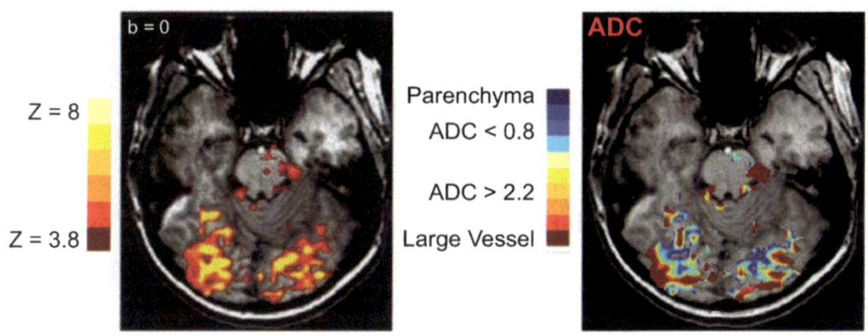

Figure 5.3 Concurrent BOLD and ADC activation maps, with ADC values classified in various ranges, from small to large vessels.

Further evidence of the IVIM origin of ADC contrast has been obtained through temporal analysis of ADC activation. Studies [21, 25] have shown that peak ADC activation temporally precedes peak BOLD activation by approximately 2 s (shown in Fig. 5.4), with both overlapping and spatially distinct activated regions, suggesting that it mainly originates from capillaries and upstream arterial networks, as opposed to BOLD contrast, which originates from capillaries and downstream venous networks. By selecting an appropriate baseline *b* factor (e.g., 20 s/mm^2), the signal contributions from large arteries with a high blood velocity can be eliminated. By acquiring two or more *b* factors across an appropriate range, the ADC contrast can then be tuned to increase the sensitivity toward small-vessel networks (i.e., arterioles and capillaries). These networks are more closely tied to the sites of neural activity and can thus achieve improved functional localization [25, 26].

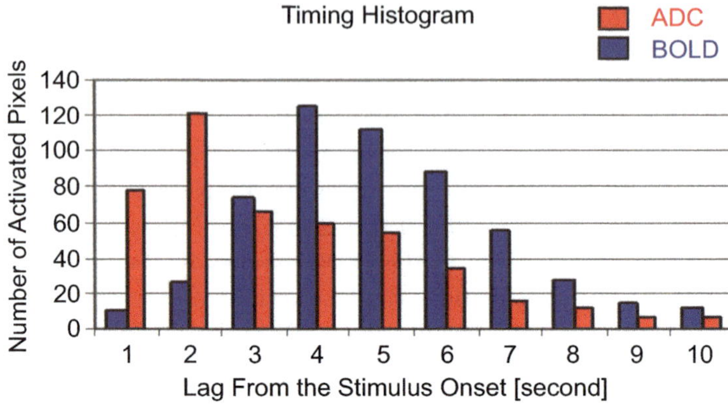

Figure 5.4 Temporal histogram of ADC and BOLD activation across all pixels. The peak ADC activation precedes peak BOLD activation by approximately 2 s, confirming its upstream origin toward the arterial side.

To this end, it was concluded that the IVIM contrast mechanism can complement the existing BOLD contrast in fMRI studies, thereby improving the colocalization with the underlying neuronal activities and enabling the investigation of small-vessel networks.

5.2 IVIM fMRI Needs a High Spatial Resolution

While the IVIM contrast mechanism has the advantage of improved spatial localization in small-vessel networks, earlier applications relied on the traditional single-shot diffusion-weighted echo-planar imaging (EPI) technique to acquire the time-course images while preventing severe motion-induced artifacts. Due to transverse relaxation, the data readout window in EPI acquisitions is limited in duration, making it difficult to achieve the high spatial resolution needed to realize the full benefit in spatial specificity for IVIM fMRI using single-shot EPI. Parallel imaging at a high acceleration factor can potentially reach a very high spatial resolution, but at the cost of a reduced SNR. Ideally, if multiple excitations (shots) can be used, it would remove the constraints on the spatial resolution and SNR. However, due to a heightened motion sensitivity inherent in diffusion weighted acquisitions, shot-to-shot phase variations would result in motion-induced artifacts that render the final images unusable.

Over the last decade, remarkable progress has been made in achieving high-resolution diffusion MRI using multiple excitations, such as multishot EPI. Techniques using a segmented readout window or navigator echoes [27, 28] have been highly effective in reducing the phase variation between shots, but with the potential cost of increased imaging time. A new class of multishot diffusion MRI, termed multiplexed sensitivity encoding (MUSE) [29], takes advantage of the now-common large phased-array coils to generate inherent phase maps to account for intershot motion artifacts in an efficient manner. A simple example using a two-shot diffusion-weighted EPI acquisition, shown in Fig. 5.5, graphically illustrates the effectiveness of phase correction using the MUSE technique. Specifically, the advent of receive coil arrays allows researchers to construct images with partially sampled data through sensitivity encoding (SENSE) [30]. As a result, the k-space data in each individual excitation from a multishot acquisition is identical to a SENSE-accelerated scan; thus, it can be reconstructed into a complete image using SENSE in a straightforward manner, shown in the left column of Fig. 5.5 for each segment of the two-shot EPI acquisition. Subsequently, the maps of phase discrepancy can be determined on the basis of these two individually reconstructed images (blue box, middle column). This map of phase discrepancy can then be fed back into the original data to improve the conditioning of the matrix inversion to generate the final high-quality image (green box, right column). This final image offers a drastic improvement in image quality as compared to the original image without corrections (red box, middle column).

The use of MUSE diffusion MRI acquisition offers a number of advantages for fMRI. For example, it does not rely on real-time rejection of acquisitions with severe phase errors such as that used in RESOLVE (REadout Segmentation Of Long Variable Echo trains), which can be challenging in fMRI applications; nor does it require additionally acquired navigator echoes, which would reduce temporal resolution. Finally, since MUSE employs regular EPI trajectories, it can take advantage of recent advances in EPI acquisition, such as reverse-polarity gradient distortion correction.

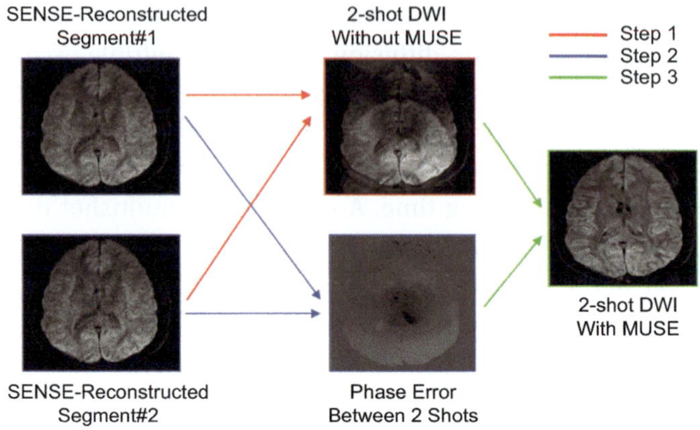

Figure 5.5 Illustration of MUSE reconstruction using a two-shot diffusion-weighted EPI as an example.

5.3 IVIM fMRI during Motor Activation at a High Spatial Resolution

Building onto the advances in high-resolution diffusion MRI, it is now straightforward to integrate IVIM with MUSE to generate high-resolution diffusion-weighted MR images and investigate IVIM fMRI at its intended high spatial resolution.

To demonstrate the initial promise, we designed our activation paradigm using alternating thumb- and finger-tapping tasks to illustrate the well-known and separate spatial representation of thumb and index finger in the motor homunculus. Healthy adult volunteers, who provided written informed consent as approved by our Institutional Review Board, were studied on a General Electric MR750 3 T whole-body MRI scanner (GE Healthcare, Waukesha, WI) equipped with a 50 mT/m maximum amplitude and 200 T/m/s slew rate gradient system. Images were acquired using an eight-channel head coil. Six axial slices covering the primary motor cortex were acquired using a spin-echo two-shot MUSE EPI sequence: repetition time (TR) = 1 s, TE = 39.1 ms, field of view 19.2 cm, matrix size 192 × 192, and slice thickness 4 mm. High-resolution T1-weighted images were also acquired using a 3D fast SPGR (SPoiled Gradient Recalled) sequence with an isotropic resolution of 1 × 1 × 1 mm^3

for anatomical reference. Automatic whole-volume high-order shimming was used to minimize the global B_0 inhomogeneity.

Dynamic IVIM-ADC imaging was achieved by applying diffusion-weighting gradients with three *b* factors, 20, 120, and 220 s/mm^2, along with a dynamic BOLD experimental run with the *b* factor set at 0. A dynamic IVIM-ADC time course was generated by fitting a monoexponential decay to the three image volume time series acquired at each *b* factor. Note here that an initial *b* factor of 20 s/mm^2 was chosen to remove the signal contributions from large vessels with high blood velocities (i.e., the vast majority of signals from vessels with a velocity >2.3 cm/s) and thus sensitize the ADC contrast to small vessels [25].

The activation paradigm was a block design consisting of one 12 s resting period at the beginning, followed by three cycles of task periods (24 s thumb tapping, 12 s resting, 24 s index finder tapping, 12 s resting). Subjects were instructed through visual cues delivered through an MR-compatible back projection system (Resonance Technology, Inc., Northridge, CA). After 4 s of dummy scans to allow magnetizations to reach an equilibrium, a total of 114 volumes (at 2 s per volume) were acquired for each *b* factor.

The resultant time course was then motion-corrected using MCFLIRT [31], linearly detrended, and temporally aligned, before an exponential fitting algorithm was performed to derive the dynamic ADC time course. Statistical activation maps were generated for both BOLD and ADC time-course images using fMRI Expert Analysis Tool (FEAT) in FMRIP's Software Library (FSL, www.fmrib.ox.ac.uk/fsl) in which a multiplicative mean intensity normalization was performed at each point in the time course and high-pass temporal filtering was conducted in the time course of each voxel using a Gaussian-weighted least-squares strait line fit, with sigma = 36 s. To investigate the spatial characteristics in the finger homunculus, a cluster-*z*-statistics criterion was applied to narrow the BOLD activation in the finger/thumb area of the motor cortex. This focal ROI (region of interest) was derived using a $z \geq 3.0$ threshold and then used to further investigate the spatial characteristics of the ADC activation on the basis of the IVIM contrast in the same region.

Representative results for the same subject in the finger homunculus are shown in Fig. 5.6. BOLD activation maps for the index finger (in red) and thumb (in blue) are shown separately in the

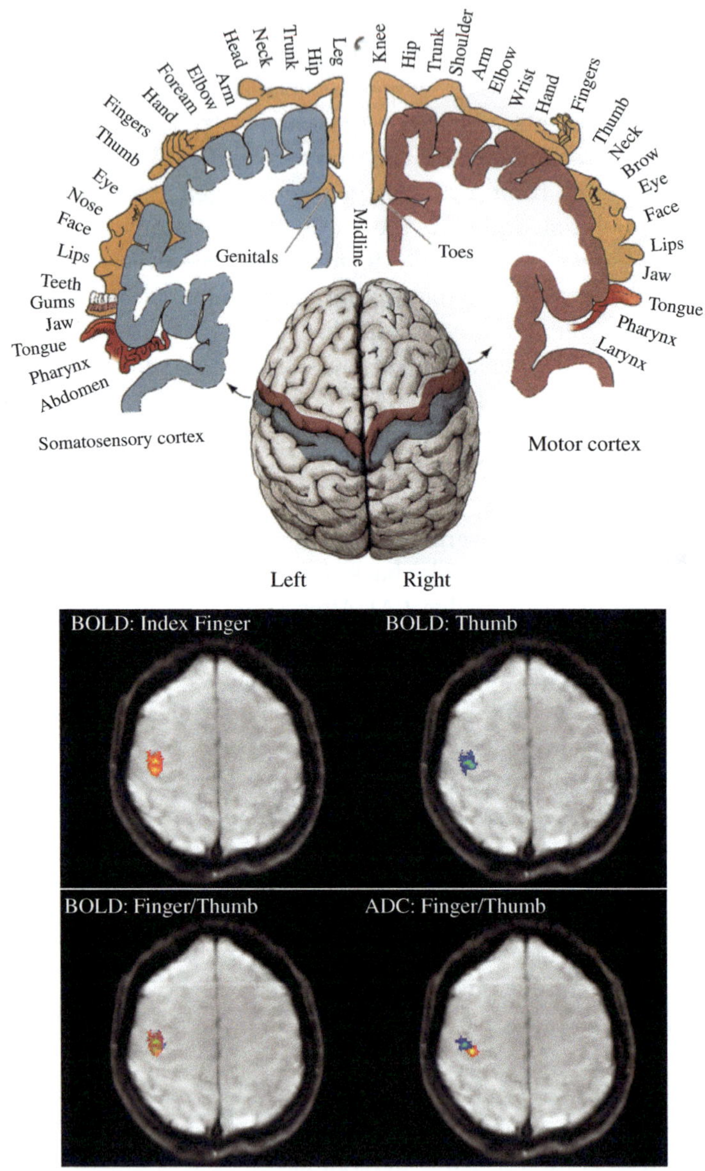

Figure 5.6 Cortical representation of sensory and motor functions (left); BOLD and IVIM ADC activation maps during thumb- and index-finger-tapping tasks: BOLD activations shared significant spatial overlap between the two digits, while ADC activations (devoid of large-vessel effects) show better spatial discrimination between the two, with the index finger exhibiting more medial activation.

top row of Fig. 5.6. A combination of the close proximity between the finger and thumb regions of the motor cortex and the contributions from both large and small vessels to the BOLD contrast results in a significant overlap between the two areas of activation, even at the high statistical threshold used (shown with $z \geq 2.0$), as illustrated in the combined finger/thumb BOLD activation map (lower left). In comparison, the absence of a large-vessel effect in the ADC time course results in an IVIM activation map (lower right) with a distinct spatial separation of thumb activation (in blue) on the lateral side and index finger activation (in red) on the medial side, as predicted by the homunculus organization for thumb and index fingers.

In addition to illustrating the fine-grained spatial organizations (e.g., finger and thumb representations in the motor homunculus shown here), high-resolution IVIM can also be used to investigate the depth dependence and layeral architecture of the cortical activation, as previously reported in the human visual cortex, confirming the predominant IVIM sensitivity to midcortical layers (shown in Fig. 5.7; also see Ref. [32]). A parallel study in the animal model using CBV contrast also reported similar findings [15]. It is anticipated that MUSE-based IVIM fMRI can be further developed to achieve even higher temporal and spatial resolutions (well into the submillimeter range), thus allowing whole-brain analysis of layeral cortical activation, with the potential to further identify the true neuronal origins (e.g., pyramidal cells in the cortical gray matter).

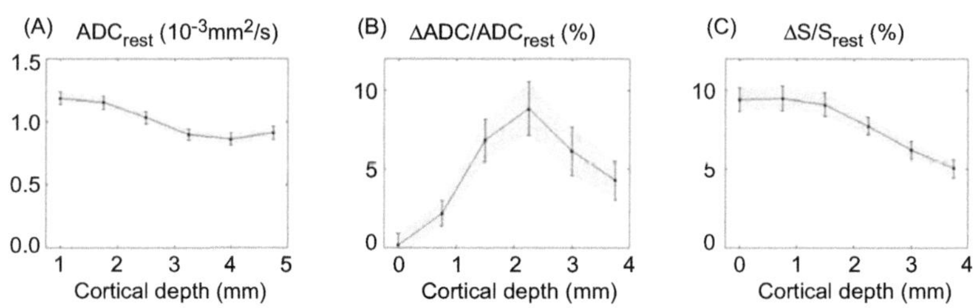

Figure 5.7 Cortical depth dependence of the baseline ADC (A), functional ADC change (B), and BOLD signal change (C) averaged across all ROIs, indicating the peak activation in the midcortical layers for ADC IVIM contrast.

5.4 Discussions and Conclusions

In this chapter, we have made a systematic yet succinct introduction to our prior work using IVIM as a complementary contrast to the traditional BOLD mechanism, with the goal to improve spatial specificity. To further realize the full benefit of this improvement, recent advances in high-resolution diffusion MRI using the MUSE technique were also incorporated to illustrate the separate finger representations in the motor homunculus. We have demonstrated in a comprehensive manner the improved spatial colocalization from the known characteristics of spatial organization, temporal behavior, and cortical layeral distribution of brain activations when taken together.

As the BOLD contrast mechanism is about to approach its 30-year anniversary, alternative contrast mechanisms have not been nearly as dominant due to their respective limitations. Even with the demonstrated promise in IVIM fMRI, there are still a number of bottlenecks that limit its practice use. For example, dynamic ADC imaging has typically been performed by using repeated excitations with different *b* factors, reducing the temporal resolution and throughput, and potentially introducing inaccuracies in the ADC derivation resulting from signal changes due to subject motion, physiological noise, and/or system instabilities occurring between successive excitations. To address these limitations, a single-shot ADC imaging technique [33], in which a gradient echo and two diffusion-weighted spin echoes are acquired within a single excitation to generate an ADC map, has shown improved efficiency and accuracy. This technique can be further improved by integrating recent advances in parallel imaging and MUSE to reach a much-improved functional localization both temporally and spatially.

To further improve acquisition speed and efficiency, recent progress using multiband (MB) or simultaneous multislice (SMS) imaging [34–37] can be incorporated with IVIM acquisition. With these improved acquisition approaches that are more efficient and sensitive, optimized *b* factors could be further determined to reduce the number of *b* factors required to localize the small-vessel network, thereby further improving the temporal resolution with the same high spatial specificity.

In conclusion, IVIM fMRI has shown strong promise where selectively mapping brain activation in the small-vessel networks with potentially high temporal throughput and without the use of an external contrast agent is concerned, making it especially suitable for wide human applications in vivo. Coupled with the recent advances in image acquisition hardware and software with greatly improved spatial and temporal resolutions, IVIM fMRI may reach a critical threshold for routine use in brain studies that will provide the finest-grained delineation of the cortical functional organization.

References

1. Le Bihan D., Breton E., Lallemand D., Grenier P., Cabanis E., Laval-Jeantet M. MR imaging of intravoxel incoherent motions: application to diffusion and perfusion in neurologic disorders, *Radiology* 161, 401–407, 1986.
2. Kwong K. K., Belliveau J. W., Chesler D. A., Goldberg I. E., Weisskoff R. M., Poncelet B. P., et al. Dynamic magnetic resonance imaging of human brain activity during primary sensory stimulation. *Proc. Natl. Acad. Sci. U. S. A.* 89, 5675–5679, 1992.
3. Bandettini P. A., Wong E. C., Hinks R. S., Tikofsky R. S., Hyde J. S. Time course EPI of human brain function during task activation. *Magn. Reson. Med.* 25, 390–397, 1992.
4. Ogawa S., Tank D. W., Menon, R., Ellerman J. M., Kim S.-G., Merkle H., Ugurbil K. Intrinsic signal changes accompanying sensory stimulation: functional brain mapping with magnetic resonance imaging. *Proc. Natl. Acad. Sci. U. S. A.* 89, 5951–5955, 1992.
5. Ogawa S., Menon R. S., Tank D. W., Kim S.-G., Merkle H., Ellerman J. M., et al. Functional brain mapping by blood oxygenation level-dependent contrast magnetic resonance imaging. *Biophys. J.* 64, 803–812, 1993.
6. Menon R., Ogawa S., Tank D. W., Ugurbil K. 4 Tesla gradient recalled echo charateristics of photic stimulation-induced signal changes in the human primary visual cortex. *Magn. Reson. Med.* 30, 380–386, 1993.
7. Turner R., Jezzard P., Wen H., Kwong K. K., LeBihan D., Zeffiro T., et al. Functional mapping of the human visual cortex at 4 and 1.5 Tesla using deoxygenated contrast EPI. *Magn. Reson. Med.* 29, 277–279, 1993.
8. Lai S. A., Hopkins L., Haacke E. M., Li D., Wasserman B. A., Buckley P., Friedman L., et al. Identification of vascular structures as a major source of signal contrast in high resolution 2D and 3D functional

activation imaging of the motor cortex at 1.5 T: preliminary results. *Magn. Reson. Med.* 30, 387–392, 1993.

9. Haglund M. M., Hochman D. W. Optical imaging of epileptiform activitity in human neocortex. *Epilepsia* 45 (Suppl 4), 43–47, 2004.
10. Kim S. G. Quantification of relative cerebral blood flow changes by flow-sensitive alternating inversion recovery (FAIR) technique: application to functional mapping. *Magn. Reson. Med.* 34, 293–301, 1995.
11. Alsop D. C., Detre J. A. Reduced transit time sensitivity in noninvasive magnetic resonance imaging of human cerebral blood flow. *J. Cereb. Blood Flow Metab.* 16, 1236–1249, 1996.
12. Detre J. A., Wang J. Technical aspects and utility of fMRI using BOLD and ASL. *Clin. Neurophysiol.* 113(5), 621–634, 2002.
13. Luh W. M., Wong E. C., Bandettini P. A., Ward B. D., Hyde J. S. Comparison of simultaneously measured perfusion and BOLD signal increases during brain activation with T1-based tissue identification. *Magn. Reson. Med.* 44(1), 137–143, 2000.
14. Duong T. Q., Kim D. S., Ugurbil K., Kim S. G. Localized cerebral blood flow response at submillimeter columnar resolution. *Proc. Natl. Acad. Sci. U. S. A.* 98(19), 10904–10909, 2001.
15. Zhao F., Wang P., Hendrich K., Ugurbil K., Kim S. G. Cortical layer-dependent BOLD and CBV responses measured by spin-echo and gradient-echo fMRI: insights into hemodynamic regulation. *NeuroImage* 30(4), 1149–1160, 2006.
16. Lu H., Hua J., van Zijl P. C. M. Noninvasive functional imaging of cerebral blood volume with vascular-space-occupancy (VASO) MRI. *NMR Biomed.* 26, 932–948, 2013.
17. Darquie A., Poline J.-B., Poupon C., Saint-Jalmes H., Le Bihan D. Transient decrease in water diffusion observed in human occipital cortex during visual stimulation. *Proc. Natl. Acad. Sci. U. S. A.* 98, 9391–9395, 2001.
18. Le Bihan D., Urayama S., Aso T., Hanakawa T., Fukuyama H. Direct and fast detection of neuronal activation in the human brain with diffusion MRI. *Proc. Natl. Acad. Sci. U. S. A.* 103(21), 8263–8268, 2006.
19. Song, A. W., Popp, C. A., fMRI using ADC-dependent contrast. *Proc. ISMRM* 6, 1438, 1998.
20. Darquie A., Clark C. A., Van de Moortele P. F., Le Bihan D. Comparison of BOLD and IVIM event-related fMRI. *Proc. ISMRM* 7, 447, 1999.
21. Gangstead S. L., Song A. W. On the timing characteristics of the apparent diffusion coefficient contrast in fMRI. *Magn. Reson. Med.* 48, 385–388, 2002.

22. Song A. W., Woldorff M. G., Gangstead S. L., Mangun G. R., McCarthy G. Enhanced spatial localization of neuronal activation using simultaneous apparent-diffusion-coefficient and blood-oxygenation functional MRI. *NeuroImage* 17, 742–750, 2002.
23. Boxerman J. L., Bandettini P. A., Kwong K. K., Baker J. R., Davis T. L., Rosen B. R., et al. The intravascular contribution to fMRI signal change: monte carlo modeling and diffusion weighted studies *in vivo*. *Magn. Reson. Med.* 34, 4–10, 1995.
24. Song A. W., Wong E. C., Tan S. G., Hyde J. S. Diffusion weighted fMRI at 1.5 T. *Magn. Reson. Med.* 35, 155–158, 1996.
25. Song A. W., Gangstead S. L. The spatial and temporal characteristics of the apparent-diffusion-coefficient-dependent fMRI signal changes during visual stimulation. *J. Neural. Eng.* 1, 32–38, 2004.
26. Song A. W., Harshbarger T., Li T., Kim K. H., Ugurbil K., Mori S., et al. Functional activation using apparent diffusion coefficient-dependent contrast allows better spatial localization to the neuronal activity: evidence using diffusion tensor imaging and fiber tracking. *Neuroimage* 20, 955–961, 2003.
27. Atkinson D., Counsell S., Hajnal J. V., Batchelor P. G., Hill D. L. G., Larkman D. J. Nonlinear phase correction of navigated multi-coil diffusion images. *Magn. Reson. Med.* 56(5), 1135–1139, 2006.
28. Porter D.A., Heidemann R. M. High resolution diffusion-weighted imaging using readout-segmented echo-planar imaging, parallel imaging and a two-dimensional navigator-based reacquisition. *Magn. Reson. Med.* 62(2), 468–475, 2009.
29. Chen N. K., Guidon A., Chang H. C., Song A. W. A robust multi-shot scan strategy for high-resolution diffusion weighted MRI enabled by multiplexed sensitivity-encoding (MUSE). *NeuroImage* 72, 41–47, 2013.
30. Pruessmann K. P., Weiger M., Scheidegger M. B., Boesiger P. SENSE: sensitivity encoding for fast MRI. *Magn. Reson. Med.* 42, 952–962, 1999.
31. Jenkinson, M., Bannister, P., Brady, M., Smith, S., Improved optimization for the robust and accurate linear registration and motion correction of brain images, *NeuroImage* 17(2), 825–841, 2002
32. Truong T. K., Guidon A., Song A. W. Cortical depth dependence and implications on the neuronal specificity of the functional apparent diffusion coefficient contrast. *NeuroImage* 47(1), 65–68, 2009.

33. Song A. W., Guo, H., Truong T.-K. Single-shot ADC imaging for fMRI. *Magn. Reson. Med.* 57, 417–422, 2007.

34. Larkman D. J., Hajnal J. V., Herlihy A. H., Coutts G. A., Young I. R., et al., Use of multicoil arrays for separation of signal from multiple slices simultaneously excited. *J. Magn. Reson. Imaging* 13, 313–317, 2001.

35. Breuer F. A., Blaimer M., Heidemann R. M., Mueller M. F., Griswold M. A., et al., Controlled aliasing in parallel imaging results in higher acceleration (CAIPIRINHA) for multi-slice imaging. *Magn. Reson. Med.* 53, 684–691, 2005.

36. Moeller S., Yacoub E., Olman C. A., Auerbach E., Strupp J., et al. Multiband multislice GE-EPI at 7 Tesla, with 16-fold acceleration using partial parallel imaging with application to high spatial and temporal whole-brain fMRI. *Magn. Reson. Med.* 63, 1144–1153, 2010.

37. Setsompop K., Cohen-Adad J., Gagoski B. A., Raij T., Yendiki A., et al. Improving diffusion MRI using simultaneous multi-slice echo planar imaging. *NeuroImage* 63, 569–580, 2012.

Section III

Clinical Applications of IVIM MRI

Part 2: Body IVIM MRI

Chapter 6

IVIM in the Body: A General Overview

Matthew R. Orton,[a] Neil P. Jerome,[b] Mihaela Rata,[a] and Dow-Mu Koh[c]

[a]*Cancer Research UK Cancer Imaging Centre, Division of Radiotherapy & Imaging, The Institute of Cancer Research, London, SM2 5NG, UK*

[b]*Department of Circulation and Medical Imaging, Norwegian University of Science and Technology (NTNU), Trondheim, Norway Clinic of Radiology and Nuclear Medicine, St. Olavs Hospital, Trondheim, Norway*

[c]*Department of Radiology, Royal Marsden Hospital, Sutton, Surrey, UK*

dowmukoh@icr.ac.uk

6.1 Introduction

Diffusion-weighted imaging (DWI) performed using multiple *b* values is attractive as a technique to derive functional information from tissues on the basis of the principles of intravoxel incoherent motion (IVIM). Although the technique has been applied for some time in the brain, it is only in the past decade or so that has seen its wider investigation and application in the body. In this chapter, we review the technical considerations for performing IVIM DWI in the body, discuss measurement repeatability for IVIM-derived parameters, and survey the potential clinical applications of the technique.

Intravoxel Incoherent Motion (IVIM) MRI: Principles and Applications
Edited by Denis Le Bihan, Mami Iima, Christian Federau, and Eric E. Sigmund

ISBN 978-981-4800-19-8 (Hardcover), 978-0-429-42727-5 (eBook)
www.panstanford.com

6.2 Technical Considerations

6.2.1 Selection of *b* Values

Modern scanners have had the capability of delivering practical IVIM acquisitions for around 20 years [1], but despite this, the consensus on the choice of *b* values for different organs, pathologies, and applications is still being refined. The persistent difficulty of reliably estimating the pseudodiffusion coefficient seems to underlie this lack of consensus and is due to an incomplete understanding of the IVIM process in biological tissues.

Some researchers argue that since estimates of the pseudodiffusion coefficient are not sufficiently accurate for routine use, the acquisition should not even attempt to measure it and in so doing the selection of *b* values is greatly simplified [2–5]. To obtain estimates of the pseudodiffusion volume fraction and tissue diffusion coefficient (and the amplitude scaling), a minimum of just three *b* values is required, and these would normally include (i) $b = 0\ \text{s/mm}^2$, (ii) an intermediate *b* value that is just large enough to ensure the signal attenuation of the pseudodiffusion compartment is complete (e.g., $b \approx 200\text{–}400\ \text{s/mm}^2$ [6]), and (iii) a *b* value large enough to capture the tissue attenuation while being above the rectified noise floor (e.g., $b > 500\ \text{s/mm}^2$). When estimates of the pseudodiffusion coefficient are also required, at least one more *b* value is required, and this will typically be less than $100\ \text{s/mm}^2$, depending on the tissue of interest. Having selected three or four *b* values, the number of averages can then be chosen to make a direct trade-off between acquisition time and parameter accuracy, although it may be advantageous to use a larger number of averages at higher *b* values where the signal-to-noise ratio (SNR) is lower. This minimal approach is of utility where the range of IVIM parameters for the tissues or pathologies of interest has already been established, for example, to differentiate between two (or more) diagnoses using IVIM, which may be further confirmed by validation studies using other techniques.

Using a minimal number of *b* values is less applicable in exploratory studies where the IVIM parameter ranges are not known a priori and also where the presence or magnitude of any confounding factors is unknown. With a minimal number of *b* values, the estimation accuracy will deteriorate rapidly as the IVIM parameters move away from the region for which the *b* values are optimal. As the number of *b* values increases, the range of IVIM parameter values over which acceptable estimation accuracy will be obtained is increased, which is clearly desirable in exploratory studies. Six or more *b* values that depend on the organ of interest are typically appropriate [7–10], with some studies employing up to 32 *b* values [11]. The work of Lemke et al. [12] used Monte Carlo simulations of three prototype tissues to propose an ordered list of 16 *b* values that can be truncated to give close-to-optimal *b*-value protocols. The truncation point determines the trade-off between acquisition time and parameter estimation accuracy, and the authors recommend that 10 or more *b* values be used in practice. In another study looking at the choice of low *b* values for measuring IVIM in liver, it was concluded that at least two *b* values below 50 s/mm^2 are required for a reliable estimation of the pseudodiffusion coefficient [13].

Another advantage of using more than the minimum number of *b* values is that voxel-wise information about noise levels is preserved in the image data, and this can be further improved by retaining any repeat measurements as separate images rather than returning averaged images. This is particularly important for techniques that require or benefit from the parameter uncertainty in each voxel to be measurable, such as hierarchical Bayesian modeling [14] and Markov random field modeling [15]. In both these cases the overall parameter inference is governed by a loss function that is the weighted sum of a data consistency term and a regularization term, where the two weights relate to the measurement noise standard deviation and some statistical property of the regularization (determined by the choice of regularization). Obtaining a sufficiently large number of *b* values and/or retaining repeat measurements as separate images implies that the measurement noise (and therefore the data consistency weight) can be inferred from the data, which is required for the hierarchical Bayesian modeling approach to work. In this case, the regularization weight will be the covariance of the IVIM parameters across the ROI, and this can also be inferred from the data. Inferring the data consistency weight from the data is not essential for the Markov random field modeling, but if it is possible, the regularization weight is then the expected difference in the IVIM parameter values between neighboring voxels, and this property is useful in selecting an appropriate regularization weight.

The ability to flexibly specify *b* values on most magnetic resonance imaging (MRI) platforms has improved over the years, which is an important step toward wider clinical use of such techniques. Specifying low *b* values was historically a significant limitation on many platforms, where the lowest *b* value available was often insufficiently low to probe the IVIM effect and the *b* value selection was quantized to a very limited number of *b* values below 100 s/mm^2. It should be borne in mind that the presence of imaging gradients implies that the effective *b* value is never actually zero and for the very low *b* values that are used in more recent studies it may be necessary to correct for this effect in the future [16].

Most diffusion-weighted MR sequences employ trapezoidal diffusion-sensitizing gradient lobes placed on either side of a 180° refocusing pulse. Although their net effect is summarized via the Stejskal–Tanner equation as the *b* value, there is increasing evidence that the duration and spacing of the gradient lobes have a separate effect on the attenuation observed in IVIM systems [17]. While many studies do not aim to examine the effect of the diffusion timing, in order to meaningfully interpret differences between published studies it is nevertheless crucial that the gradient timing parameters be also disclosed in published works [18].

More advanced diffusion gradient profiles are also feasible, and their application to IVIM measurement is dealt with in more detail in other chapters in this book. Bipolar gradients can be used instead of the more standard monopolar gradients, and these have reduced eddy current artifacts, but at the expense of SNR due to the need for longer echo times. In organs such as the liver that have short T_2 values, the benefits have been shown to outweigh the SNR loss for measuring diffuse liver disease with IVIM [19]. Further studies on liver and pancreas comparing IVIM parameters obtained with monopolar, bipolar, and flow-compensated acquisitions have shed light on the nature of the IVIM phenomenon in these organs, including the velocity and length scales that can be probed with these measurements [17].

6.2.2 Motion Control

MRI outside the brain is challenging due to motion arising from breathing, cardiac activity, and peristalsis, and these confounders have a range of effects that are particular to DWI. In the context of IVIM imaging, these effects can be especially deleterious because the perfusion-related signal can be hard to detect—it may be small in amplitude or be present for a small range of low *b* values or both.

In the context of IVIM (but also for the apparent diffusion coefficient [ADC] measurement), images with multiple contrasts must be acquired, which leads to the possibility of image misregistration. This is particularly problematic for IVIM measurements where a large number of *b* values are required and acquisition duration extends to several minutes. Another important issue is that bulk tissue motion during the application of paired diffusion gradient lobes causes unrecoverable dephasing of the signal. This leads to a signal loss that is difficult to distinguish from attenuation arising from the tissue microstructure and is more pronounced with larger diffusion probing gradients. Although the IVIM effect is inferred from low-*b*-value images that are less sensitive to this effect, the necessity of also acquiring images with high *b* values implies any bias will be propagated into the IVIM parameter estimates when signal dropouts occur at high *b* values. Since it is not feasible to correct images affected in this way, one must either detect and remove such images prior to IVIM model fitting, as is done with DTI [20, 21], or incorporate the signal dropout process into the noise model, as was achieved by Murphy et al. [22] using a beta log-normal error model.

Most MR platforms are now available with DWI sequences that use triggered acquisition techniques to initiate repetitive image capture segments, with the aim of acquiring data when the relevant anatomy of the subject is static and in the same position. In principle such techniques will minimize not only image misregistration but also signal dropouts due to bulk motion. However, the use of triggering means that not all of the scanning time is used in collecting data and, in the context of IVIM, the proportionate increase in scan times can be prohibitive. In addition, the scan time is not known a priori and can vary widely between subjects, which would be particularly problematic in a clinical context. Free-breathing acquisitions have the advantage that the scan time is fully utilized but further post processing may be necessary to handle motion and signal dropouts. These competing issues mean that the choice between free-breathing and respiratory triggered techniques is not straightforward and the context of any proposed study (exploratory/clinical, volunteers/patients, etc.) introduces extra factors that must be considered when making such a choice.

There is a useful body of recent literature comparing the performance of free-breathing and respiratory-triggered IVIM acquisitions [19, 23, 24] and also exploring the use of cardiac triggering to limit the localized effect of cardiac motion on the left lobe of the liver [25]. While these publications do not collectively reach a clear consensus, they are a useful resource for designing new studies. Developments in simultaneous slice (SS) acquisition techniques that give speedup factors of around 3 show great promise for IVIM measurement [26]. A recent comparison of free-breathing and respiratory triggered methods with SS for ADC measurement found no advantage with the use of triggering [26, 27], although a similar comparison has yet to be performed for IVIM measurements. It is also worth noting that existing studies comparing motion control techniques have used either subjective image quality assessments or quantitative metrics (including reproducibility) based on summary statistics such as the mean or median on which to base their comparisons. However, there is increasing interest in the potential of higher-order univariate statistics (standard deviation, skewness, kurtosis, etc.) and spatial statistics (measures of image texture) for radiomic analysis of images [28–30]. Such analyses will have more stringent requirements for IVIM measurement techniques in relation to motion control, compared to analysis using the mean or median, and so evaluations of motion control techniques may need to be repeated where radiomic analyses are proposed.

Whether a free-breathing or triggered acquisition is used, in practice there will always be some degree of motion between individual image frames and this can only be properly accounted for with image registration techniques. Having said that, when multiple averages are acquired a much simpler technique that nevertheless has good performance is to combine the images at a given b value using the median (or trimmed mean) over the repeated measurements instead of the mean [31]. While this method does not explicitly account for motion or signal dropouts, it is nevertheless robust to both effects and can be used with free-breathing or respiratory triggered acquisitions.

Directly accounting for subject motion with image registration is challenging for IVIM measurements for a number of reasons. DWI uses 2D acquisitions, where the in-plane voxel dimensions are typically smaller than the slice thickness. Handling through-plane motion is therefore problematic; for this reason many studies in the abdomen have used coronal imaging so that the dominant motion direction due to breathing (superior-inferior) is in the imaging plane. This is particularly beneficial with free-breathing techniques because the amount of motion is sufficiently large for substantial improvements to be obtained with simple 2D image registration. When regional analysis is to be used it may be sufficient to apply local affine transformations, but nonrigid transformations may be necessary where whole organ or global analysis is used. Since real subject motion is a 3D process one may expect that nonrigid 3D registration techniques would show the most promise, but this makes the assumption that the IVIM measurement yields coherent 3D data volumes. Figure 6.1 shows an example of a number of image volumes acquired coronally under free breathing. Figure 6.1a is a case where the subject motion happened to be very small while all 16 slices were acquired, whereas Figs. 6.1b and 6.1c (at two different *b* values) show examples where there is significant motion during the acquisition. These images reveal the interleaved scheme used by many DWI sequences, where odd-indexed slices followed by even-indexed slices are measured sequentially in order to minimize crosstalk between adjacent slices due to imperfect slice profiles. These figures clearly demonstrate why simple 3D registration of DW images is highly challenging under free breathing, and even when noninterleaved slice acquisition schemes are used, the same effect is still present but may not be as apparent as in the figure. Registration techniques for interleaved acquisition schemes have been developed [32] but have yet to be applied to IVIM measurements.

The difference in image contrast between the lowest and highest *b* values, and in addition the low SNR for high *b* values, is another challenge when registering IVIM data. Techniques involving the sequential acquisition of high- and low-*b*-value images have been proposed [33], where deformations are determined from the low-*b*-value (high SNR) images, which are then applied to the adjacent high-

b-value images on the assumption that there is negligible motion between the adjacent frames. Combining IVIM signal modeling with image registration is also feasible, [34] and this relies on using the IVIM model itself to generate target images for the registration so that they should automatically have the appropriate contrast for the given *b* value.

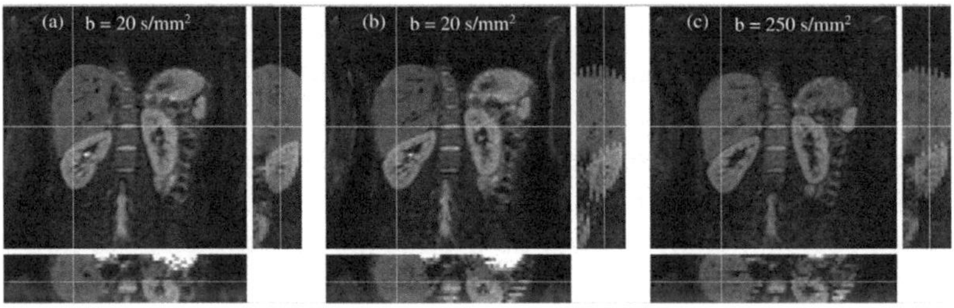

Figure 6.1 An example showing a number of image volumes acquired coronally under free breathing. Panel (a) is a case where the subject motion happened to be very small while all 16 slices were acquired, whereas panels (b) and (c) (at two different *b* values) show examples where there is significant motion during the acquisition.

6.2.3 Measurement Repeatability

The utility of quantitative biomarkers in clinical decision making, such as those derived from DWI, is tied not only to their sensitivity and specificity to underlying physiology and microstructure but also to the stability of the measurement itself. The ability to meaningfully measure or detect changes in the pseudodiffusion and tissue diffusion components of the IVIM signal therefore relies not only on the properties of the system being observed but also on the performance of the MR scanner hardware and acquisition strategies being used. Significant advancements in technology since the first description of the IVIM experiment have facilitated the clinical use of the IVIM acquisition extracranially, demonstrating the phenomenon clearly for healthy and diseased abdominal organs [35, 36] as well as neoplasms [37, 38].

DWI is a challenging MR modality; it is notable, though not unique, among MR techniques in that contrast is introduced by actively destroying signal, specifically through diffusion-sensitizing gradients. When quantitative diffusion measurements are required, one must therefore be mindful of the available SNR and how it may influence signal modeling. Well-documented challenges of DWI are the dependence of minimum echo times on the maximum *b* value, distortion in echo-planar imaging (EPI) readouts from susceptibility boundaries, and artifacts arising from both cardiac and respiratory motion for extracranial targets.

These challenges, notwithstanding the IVIM model (and corresponding acquisition strategy) have received wide attention and application in literature. Articles that employ a repeatability assessment for IVIM are scarcer, however, and it is necessary for the radiologist to balance the promise of the IVIM acquisition with the additional confounding factors that accompany it. In particular, the mathematical fitting of a biexponential model is not trivial, and the specific choices of *b* values and fitting algorithm that are fertile areas for discussion and disagreement [8, 13, 39–43] are less critical for the single-exponential ADC model. Such technical considerations and their implications have been discussed in the previous section. Here we consider experimental methods for estimating the errors that affect real-world IVIM measurements, in particular, the use of repeatability studies, as recommended by the quantitative imaging biomarkers alliance [44].

There are alternative ways of quantifying repeatability, and without a standardized approach it is not always possible to directly compare across studies. Many studies report the repeat-measures coefficient of variation (CoV, expressed as a percentage), which quantifies the error expected in the parameter value estimate [45]. Another commonly reported measure is the limit of agreement (LoA), described by Bland and Altman, derived from the variance of the difference of repeated measures, such that 95% of observed discrepancies between measures are expected to be within those limits from the average value [46]. In both cases, smaller numbers represent improved repeatability, which implies greater stability and thus usability.

Table 6.1 summarizes some recent studies (2008–2018) that have assessed repeatability of IVIM measurements by performing the same DWI measurement twice on the same object, with a delay between 1 h and 7 days [8, 25, 37, 38, 47–56]. While it is more common to perform repeatability studies on volunteers, a number of articles report repeatability for pathological as well as normal tissue from patients, which provides a more clinically relevant assessment. Many of these studies also report the repeatability of the ADC derived from the same data, giving a comparison to a simpler, well-established biomarker that is known to be robust [57].

Across the studies analyzed, comparison of the within-study repeatability measures shows that the IVIM tissue diffusion coefficient D commonly has a higher CoV than the corresponding ADC, although it is likely that this arises from the reduced data used in the calculation, and in general D shows good repeatability, with the CoV of D above 20% in only a few studies (Fig. 6.2a). In contrast, the CoVs observed for the pseudodiffusion parameters f and D^* are consistently higher, with the former commonly reaching higher than 20% and the latter having a substantially larger range (Fig. 6.2b). The same observation is reflected in the LoA data where, while it is conceivable that these measures could differentiate pathologic conditions or be changed under intervention to this degree, such a degree of variation intrinsic to a measurement is at least an indication of the need for cautious interpretation. It is notable that the studies reporting the lowest variation in repeated measurement are intracranial, where the pseudodiffusion component contributes less to the overall signal than in the body (Fig. 6.3).

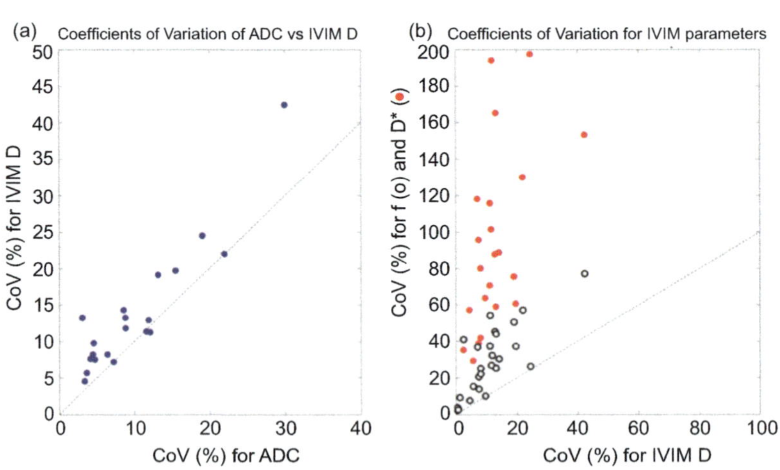

Figure 6.2 Comparisons from studies reporting coefficients of variation (CoVs) for ADC and IVIM parameters showing that (a) ADC and IVIM D are similar in showing acceptable CoV whereas (b) the pseudodiffusion parameters f and D^* show a substantially higher CoV.

Table 6.1 Results from literature discussing extracranial IVIM repeatability, including studies reporting coefficients of variation (CoVs) and Bland–Altman 95% limits of agreement (LoA)

Name	Year	Organ	Delay	n	Field (T)	b-values	Tissue	CoV (± LoA, %) ADC	D	f	D*
Wong et al	2017	Brain	48 hrs	16	3	15	NAWM		0.5	2.3	
							cortex		0.7	2.9	
							DGM		0.5	3.7	
							WMH		0.7	2.5	
							VL		1.3	9.2	
Pan et al	2017	Kidney	24 - 48 hrs	25	3	9	tumour	13.2 (-42.1, 51.1)	19.1 (-61.2, 44.5)	50.5 (-87.5, 127.3)	75.5 (-210.4, 134.8)
						16	tumour	8.8 (-33.1, 30.0)	11.8 (-46.7, 48.8)	26.8 (-72.7, 78.7)	101.4 (-198.3, 151.6)
				23		9	cortex	8.6 (-24.4, 22.5)	14.3 (-41.7, 40.9)	30.4 (-81.7, 94.2)	88.7 (-158.1, 131.9)
						16	cortex	6.4 (-18.1, 18.1)	8.2 (-19.7, 25.3)	25.1 (-78.4, 64.1)	80.0 (-162.3, 166.8)
						9	medulla	11.6 (-32.3, 30.4)	11.3 (-32.6, 29.1)	54.2 (-130.2, 140.9)	115.7 (-266.6, 239.9)
						16	medulla	7.3 (-20.3, 21.1)	7.2 (-23.3, 18.1)	36.8 (-94.9, 79.4)	117.9 (-203.0, 271.6)
Jiang et al	2017	Lung	1 hr	50	3	10	tumour	12.1 (-26.9, 31.6)	11.2 (-27.5, 34.5)	37.4 (-129.9, 122.4)	70.6 (-158.6, 174.5)
Lecler et al	2017	Orbit	17 min	22	3	15	tumour	22.0 (-69.0, 70.0)	22.0 (-33.0, 31.0)	57.0 (-159.0, 147.0)	130.0 (-10.0, 11.0)
Sun et al	2017	Rectal	20-30 mins	26	3	8	tumour	19.1 (-16.7, 21.5)	24.5 (-19.2, 29.8)	26.3 (-147.9, 104.7)	197.4 (-176.7, 218.1)
		Prostate		16			healthy	11.9 (-12.0, 11.8)	12.9 (-12.0, 13.7)	45.3 (-49.0, 41.4)	87.7 (-92.4, 83.0)
Kang et al	2017	Head/Neck	14 mins	9	1.5	4	healthy	4.8 (-23.6, 21.7)	7.5 (-33.4, 34.3)	20.5 (-73.6, 75.9)	38.7 (-127.3, 154.9)
			14 mins			4*	healthy	3.7 (-17.2, 15.1)	5.7 (-280.0, 23.5)	15.3 (-58.0, 63.6)	29.2 (-105.2, 104.4)
			14 mins			17	healthy	4.5 (-19.9, 30.0)	8.2 (-38.1, 42.4)	22.1 (-89.5, 77.1)	41.8 (-138.4, 153.2)
			10 mins	5		4*	tumour	3.7 (-2.8, 10.2)	5.7 (-3.2, 12.2)	15.3 (-25.3, 22.3)	29.2 (-76.2, 102.3)
			10 mins			17	tumour	4.5 (-65.1, 109.1)	8.2 (-64.3, 113.1)	22.1 (-216.6, 177.4)	41.8 (-243.1, 207.1)
Dyvorne et al	2014	Liver	7 days	53	1.5	16	mixed		12.0	32.3	193.3
Lee et al	2015	Liver	5 mins	12	1.5	9	healthy	4.2 (-2.7, 5.6)	7.6 (-3.5, 11.7)	13.8 (-9.5, 18.2)	95.6 (-56.3, 134.9)
						9*	healthy	3.4 (-1.8, 5.1)	4.5 (-3.0, 6.1)	7.6 (-5.8, 9.4)	57.1 (-40.0, 74.1)
						9*	healthy	4.6 (-1.2, 7.9)	9.7 (-4.5, 14.9)	10.1 (-4.9, 15.2)	63.7 (-27.9, 99.6)
Song et al	2014	Breast	5 mins	11	3	9	tumour§	(-12.2, 11.5)	(-11.5, 10.7)	(-34.9, 30.3)	(-15.9, 10.1)
Kakite et al	2015	Liver	5 days	11	3	16	healthy	8.8 (-28.7, 15.7)	13.2 (-32.8, 28.4)	25.3 (-74.6, 56.4)	59.0 (-151.2, 132.7)
				15			tumour	15.6 (-38.2, 17.4)	19.7 (-57.4, 36.3)	37.3 (-66.2, 101.0)	60.6 (-161.6, 135.3)
Andreou et al	2013	Liver	1 hr	14	1.5	8	healthy	(-4.3, 6.8)	(-5.1, 8.1)	(-24.3, 25.1)	(-31.2, 59.1)
							tumour	(-14.7, 13.8)	(-20.8, 25.3)	(-75.3, 241.0)	(-89.0, 2120.0)
Jerome et al	2016	Tumour	1 day	15	1.5	6	tumour		2.5 (-1.8, 4.0)	41.0 (-29.4, 68.6)	35.1 (-25.4, 57.9)
Miyazaki et al	2015	Tumour	1 day	15	1.5	6	tumour	3.7 (-7.1, 7.6)			
Winfield et al	2015	Ovarian	3 days	31	1.5	10	tumour	3.1	13.2	44.0	165.1

* indicates the DWI included a differential triggering strategy within the study
§ indicates a preclinical study

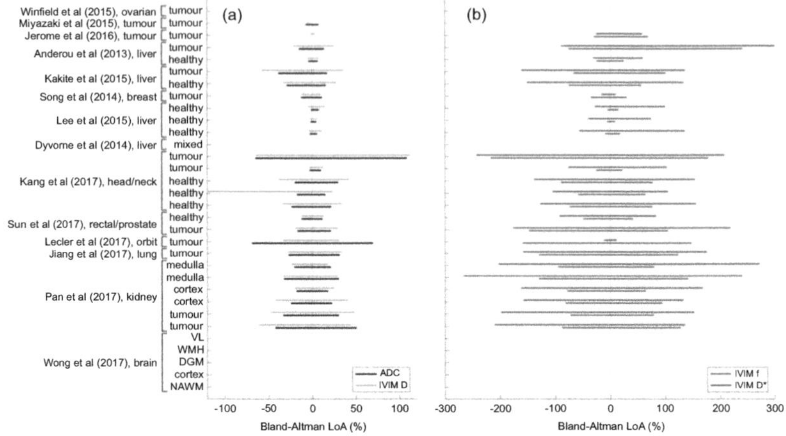

Figure 6.3 Results from studies that report Bland–Altman limits of agreement (LoA, 95%) for (a) diffusion parameters ADC and IVIM *D* and (b) pseudodiffusion parameters *f* and *D** provided by IVIM repeatability studies. Note the extended axes in plot (b). Studies reporting only the CoV are shown as blank entries.

Sources of variation in derived IVIM parameters, aside from noise associated with the scanner hardware (e.g., electrical noise and field inhomogeneity), and the scan procedure (e.g., coil and patient positioning), arise from the diffusion sequence itself. It should be remembered that, exactly like the ADC, IVIM parameters are *empirical* and that the assumptions of the model are not necessarily or consistently valid, for example, the incoherence of capillary direction, the lack of influence from larger vessels that may contribute a pulsatile or coherent flow component, and a lack of spin exchange between the two compartments. Lemke et al. demonstrated that a difference in the T_2 between the two compartments considered in the IVIM model leads to a bias in the estimation of *f* related to the choice of echo time (TE) [58]. A useful extension of the model to include the estimation of T_2 values by Jerome et al. mitigates this effect at the expense of some additional acquisitions [59]. This work also demonstrates that the bias in *f* in healthy liver can be over 100%. Further, it has been shown that the diffusion time (i.e., the spacing of the diffusion-weighting gradients) also influences estimates of the pseudodiffusion fraction *f* [60].

Reproducibility, by contrast, is more difficult to infer from these studies, since using different MR hardware may necessarily incorporate differences in protocol. In this sense, the simplicity of the ADC model, both in practical application as well as sensitivity, will remain a challenge for the widespread acceptance of IVIM [61]. While the development of a robust IVIM phantom [62] may assist in the practicalities of conducting reproducibility measurements, the standardization of the IVIM acquisition, including but not limited to repetition time, echo time, diffusion b values, and diffusion times, remains a significant target and a critical step in maximizing the utility of IVIM-derived parameters.

6.3 Overview of the Clinical Applications of IVIM in the Body

The notion of IVIM is highly attractive as a clinical tool for disease evaluation in the body. As IVIM measurements can provide potential information that reflects capillary perfusion, tubular flow, and glandular secretion, these measurements have been applied to detect disease, characterize lesions, evaluate organ function, and assess treatment response of diseases.

One of the perceived advantages of IVIM measurement is that the technique does not require the administration of an exogenous contrast medium to obtain information that reflects tissue perfusion. This is attractive given the recent concerns of gadolinium contrast deposition in the brain. Hence, the avoidance of or reduction in contrast use, particularly in the pediatric population or where repeated contrast dosing is anticipated, would be welcomed. The potential disadvantage of IVIM measurement is the longer MR examination time (required to acquire images of a sufficiently high SNR, images of multiple b values, or the use of techniques to overcome respiratory and/or cardiac motion where appropriate) compared with a DWI examination to derive the ADC using two or three b values. Furthermore, as previously discussed, the perfusion-sensitive measurements of perfusion fraction and pseudodiffusion coefficient are less robust with poorer measurement repeatability and reproducibility compared to the true diffusion coefficient or the ADC [63].

In the following section, we present some current clinical and research applications of body IVIM measurements for disease assessment. However, for an in-depth discussion of specific areas, the reader should refer to the individual chapters.

6.3.1 Disease Detection

The use of high-*b*-value DWI and ADC maps has improved the detection of cellular disease across the body [64]. However, in some studies, the use of IVIM DWI has also improved the detection of prostate [65, 66] and pancreatic [67, 68] cancers (Fig. 6.4) in patients. In nasopharyngeal cancers, one study showed that IVIM parameters are useful for discriminating disease but not conventional ADC measurements [69]. The technique has also been applied to detect diffuse disease, such as liver cirrhosis [70–73], but the IVIM parameters appear to lack the sensitivity for early disease detection [74].

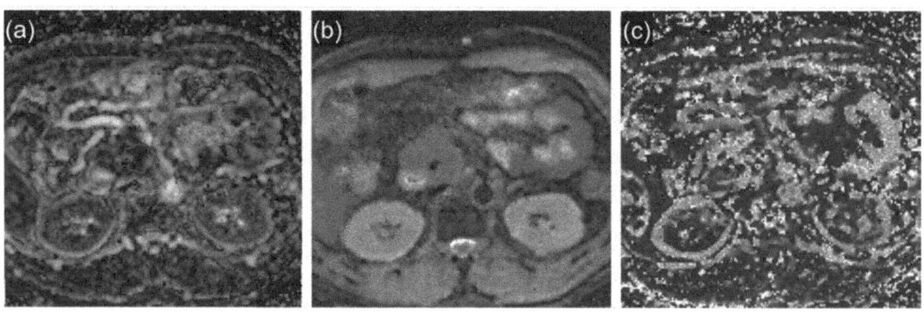

Figure 6.4 Detection of pancreatic cancer. IVIM DWI–derived maps of *f* (a), *D* (b), and D^* (c) in a middle-aged man with pancreatic head adenocarcinoma. Note that the tumor shows a lower perfusion fraction compared with the normal pancreas. MRI was performed using nine *b* values (0 to 1500 s/mm^2) on a 1.5 T imaging scanner.

In the post-therapy setting, while IVIM has been helpful in discriminating between disease recurrence and pseudoprogression in patients with brain metastases treated with stereotactic radiotherapy [74, 75], the use of IVIM has not been widely investigated for disease recurrence elsewhere within the body.

6.3.2 Lesion Characterization

Quantitative ADC values have been used for lesion characterization across the body. Likewise, IVIM measurements have been applied to specific areas to improve tissue and lesion characterization. In the pancreas, differences have been found between the perfusion fraction and the pseudodiffusion coefficient of pancreatic carcinoma and pancreatic neuroendocrine tumors [2, 76, 77] and also between pancreatic carcinoma and pancreatitis [78, 79]. However, in the liver, the role of IVIM parameters for lesion characterization appears less clear. Some studies showed limited values of IVIM parameters for characterizing focal liver lesions [61, 80–82], while other studies showed differences between the perfusion fraction and pseudodiffusion coefficient values of hypervascular and hypovascular liver lesions [83].

In the breast, studies have shown that IVIM parameters can distinguish between benign and malignant breast lesions, with higher perfusion fractions [84–87] and/or pseudodiffusion coefficients [88] observed in malignant lesions. Differences were also observed between breast cancers of different histologies [89, 90]. A few studies have shown correlations between IVIM measurements with quantitative dynamic contrast–enhanced magnetic resonance imaging (DCE MRI)-derived parameters [86, 91].

Others studies have evaluated the specific applications of IVIM for disease characterization, such as differentiating uterine fibroid from focal adenomyosis [92], distinguishing benign and malignant lymph nodes [93–97], and distinguishing between different salivary gland tumors.

6.3.3 Evaluation of Organ Function

The use of IVIM measurement to evaluate kidney function has been assessed in native and transplanted kidneys because the fast component of water diffusion arising from vascular perfusion and tubular flow can be quantified and characterized by the technique. IVIM parameters have been shown to be reduced in renal impairment resulting from early disease [97], chronic parenchymal disease [97–99], and renal obstruction [100, 101]. IVIM has also been used to evaluate the function of renal transplants [102, 103], with a reduction in the perfusion-sensitive parameters seen in transplant rejection.

6.3.4 Evaluation of Treatment Response

There is considerable interest in the application of IVIM parameters for the evaluation of treatment response. Several studies have been conducted in patients with metastatic breast cancer to evaluate the response to conventional chemotherapy and radioembolization treatment [104]. In this regard, both mean and histogram parameters have been used to determine changes in IVIM parameters for treatment, as well as to provide predictive and/or prognostic information associated with these measurements [30, 104–106].

Other studies have been conducted in patients with rectal cancer [107, 108], gastrointestinal stromal tumors [109], hepatocellular carcinoma [110], liver metastases, cervical cancer [111], head and neck cancers [112], and bone marrow infiltration [112, 113]. Several studies have also assessed the use of IVIM measurement to evaluate the effectiveness of antiangiogenic [112–115] and antivascular [116] therapies. Overall, these studies do not show consistent results, particularly with regard to predictive and prognostic biomarkers, where different parameters or combinations of parameters have been found to be associated with improved treatment outcomes. Clearly, these need to be further validated with future studies.

6.3.5 Clinical Challenges and Future Work

One of the greatest challenges to the wider use of IVIM measurements in the clinical setting is its ability to inform on individual patient management or treatment outcomes. Most of the current published studies have demonstrated differences between IVIM-derived parameters in study cohorts that are too small for the current measurement acquisition and data analysis technique to confidently detect because of the relatively large associated measurement repeatability and reproducibility. For these reasons, IVIM measurements can appear successful in single-center studies but are unable to cross the translation gap into the multicenter setting to be widely applied. Likewise, although there are reports of potential predictive and prognostic biomarkers arising from IVIM measurements, well-conducted validation cohort studies have not been undertaken to show that biomarker values obtained from one study cohort can be directly applied to another unrelated cohort with a resultant similar predictive, prognostic, or diagnostic performance.

There is a clear need to better understand and minimize measurement uncertainties so that IVIM-derived parameters can be measured with confidence, precision, and accuracy. In this regard, clinicians utilizing and investigating the technique need to work closely with their physicists to design imaging sequences that are appropriate for the scope of the examinations, balancing the number of *b* values/signal averages within an acceptable MR examination time. Where possible, the uncertainty of the signal measurements should be characterized so that IVIM quantification is not derived or reported from areas with very high levels of measurement uncertainty.

As we move increasingly into an era of artificial intelligence (AI) and machine learning, it may be appropriate to investigate the emerging roles of these approaches in both data acquisition and data analysis to help improve our measurement confidence and help cross the multicenter translational gap. Currently, there is also a significant interest in characterizing intralesional and interlesional disease heterogeneity, which may reflect differences in the biology of various diseases and their treatment behavior. It is likely that we can also apply AI and machine learning to characterize disease behavior in IVIM measurements on a regional basis so that such biologically meaningful information can be harnessed for the treatment planning and management decisions of patients.

References

1. Yamada I., Aung W., Himeno Y., Nakagawa T., Shibuya H. Diffusion coefficients in abdominal organs and hepatic lesions: evaluation with intravoxel incoherent motion echo-planar MR imaging. *Radiology*, 1999, 210(3), 617–623.
2. Concia M., Sprinkart A. M., Penner A.-H., Brossart P., Gieseke J., Schild H. H., et al. Diffusion-weighted magnetic resonance imaging of the pancreas: diagnostic benefit from an intravoxel incoherent motion model-based 3 b-value analysis. *Invest. Radiol.*, 2014, 49(2), 93–100.
3. Penner A.-H., Sprinkart A. M., Kukuk G. M., Gütgemann I., Gieseke J., Schild H. H., et al. Intravoxel incoherent motion model-based liver

lesion characterisation from three b-value diffusion-weighted MRI. *Eur. Radiol.*, 2013, 23(10), 2773–2783.

4. Meeus E. M., Novak J., Dehghani H., Peet A. C. Rapid measurement of intravoxel incoherent motion (IVIM) derived perfusion fraction for clinical magnetic resonance imaging. *MAGMA*, 2018, 31(2), 269–283.
5. Gurney-Champion O. J., Froeling M., Klaassen R., Runge J. H., Bel A., van Laarhoven H. W. M., et al. Minimizing the acquisition time for intravoxel incoherent motion magnetic resonance imaging acquisitions in the liver and pancreas. *Invest. Radiol.*, 2016, 51(4), 211–220.
6. Iima M., Le Bihan D. Clinical intravoxel incoherent motion and diffusion MR imaging: past, present, and future. *Radiology*, 2016, 278(1), 13–32.
7. Cho G. Y., Moy L., Zhang J. L., Baete S., Lattanzi R., Moccaldi M., et al. Comparison of fitting methods and b-value sampling strategies for intravoxel incoherent motion in breast cancer. *Magn. Reson. Med.*, 2015, 74(4), 1077–1085.
8. Dyvorne H., Jajamovich G., Kakite S., Kuehn B., Taouli B. Intravoxel incoherent motion diffusion imaging of the liver: optimal b-value subsampling and impact on parameter precision and reproducibility. *Eur. J. Radiol.*, 2014, 83(12), 2109–2113.
9. Wu Q., Wang Y., Shi L., Dong L., Liu M., Dou S., et al. Intravoxel incoherent motion diffusion-weighted magnetic resonance imaging of cervical cancer with different b-values. *J. Comput. Assist. Tomogr.*, 2017, 41(4), 592–598.
10. Pang Y., Turkbey B., Bernardo M., Kruecker J., Kadoury S., Merino M. J., et al. Intravoxel incoherent motion MR imaging for prostate cancer: an evaluation of perfusion fraction and diffusion coefficient derived from different b-value combinations. *Magn. Reson. Med.*, 2013, 69(2), 553–562.
11. Orton M. R., Jerome N. P., Kaza E., Collins D. J., Koh D.-M., Kuehn B., Leach M. O. Use of a multi-exponential attenuation model for sequential registration of diffusion weighted imaging in the abdomen and pelvis. In: *Proceedings of the ISMRM.*, 2015, p. 6341.
12. Lemke A., Stieltjes B., Schad L. R., Laun F. B. Toward an optimal distribution of *b* values for intravoxel incoherent motion imaging. *Magn. Reson. Imaging*, 2011, 29(6), 766–776.
13. Cohen A. D., Schieke M. C., Hohenwalter M. D., Schmainda K. M. The effect of low *b*-values on the intravoxel incoherent motion derived pseudodiffusion parameter in liver. *Magn. Reson. Med.*, 2015, 73(1), 306–311.

14. Orton M. R., Collins D. J., Koh D.-M., Leach M. O. Improved intravoxel incoherent motion analysis of diffusion weighted imaging by data driven Bayesian modeling. *Magn. Reson. Med.*, 2014, 71(1), 411–420.

15. Freiman M., Perez-Rossello J. M., Callahan M. J., Voss S. D., Ecklund K., Mulkern R. V., et al. Reliable estimation of incoherent motion parametric maps from diffusion-weighted MRI using fusion bootstrap moves. *Med. Image Anal.*, 2013, 17(3), 325–336.

16. Güllmar D., Haueisen J., Reichenbach J. R. Analysis of *b*-value calculations in diffusion weighted and diffusion tensor imaging. *Concepts Magn. Reson. Part A Bridg. Educ. Res.*, 2005, 25A(1), 53–66.

17. Wetscherek A., Stieltjes B., Laun F. B. Flow-compensated intravoxel incoherent motion diffusion imaging. *Magn. Reson. Med.*, 2015, 74(2), 410–419.

18. Padhani A. R., Liu G., Koh D. M., Chenevert T. L., Thoeny H. C., Takahara T., et al. Diffusion-weighted magnetic resonance imaging as a cancer biomarker: consensus and recommendations. *Neoplasia*, 2009, 11(2), 102–125.

19. Dyvorne H. A., Galea N., Nevers T., Fiel M. I., Carpenter D., Wong E., et al. Diffusion-weighted imaging of the liver with multiple *b* values: effect of diffusion gradient polarity and breathing acquisition on image quality and intravoxel incoherent motion parameters—a pilot study. *Radiology.*, 2013, 266(3), 920–929.

20. Li Y., Shea S. M., Lorenz C. H., Jiang H., Chou M.-C., Mori S. Image corruption detection in diffusion tensor imaging for post-processing and real-time monitoring. *PLoS One*, 2013, 8(10), e49764.

21. Zhou Z., Liu W., Cui J., Wang X., Arias D., Wen Y., et al. Automated artifact detection and removal for improved tensor estimation in motion-corrupted DTI data sets using the combination of local binary patterns and 2D partial least squares. *Magn. Reson. Imaging*, 2011, 29(2), 230–242.

22. Murphy P., Wolfson T., Gamst A., Sirlin C., Bydder M. Error model for reduction of cardiac and respiratory motion effects in quantitative liver DW-MRI. *Magn. Reson. Med.*, 2013, 70(5), 1460–1469.

23. Jerome N. P., Orton M. R., d'Arcy J. A., Collins D. J., Koh D.-M., Leach M. O. Comparison of free-breathing with navigator-controlled acquisition regimes in abdominal diffusion-weighted magnetic resonance images: Effect on ADC and IVIM statistics. *J. Magn. Reson. Imaging*, 2014, 39(1), 235–240.

24. Shan Y., Zeng M.-S., Liu K., Miao X.-Y., Lin J., Fu C. X., et al. Comparison of free-breathing with navigator-triggered technique in diffusion

weighted imaging for evaluation of small hepatocellular carcinoma: effect on image quality and intravoxel incoherent motion parameters. *J. Comput. Assist. Tomogr.*, 2015, 39(5), 709–715.

25. Lee Y., Lee S. S., Kim N., Kim E., Kim Y. J., Yun S.-C., et al. Intravoxel incoherent motion diffusion-weighted MR imaging of the liver: effect of triggering methods on regional variability and measurement repeatability of quantitative parameters. *Radiology.*, 2015, 274(2), 405–415.

26. Boss A., Barth B., Filli L., Kenkel D., Wurnig M. C., Piccirelli M., et al. Simultaneous multi-slice echo planar diffusion weighted imaging of the liver and the pancreas: Optimization of signal-to-noise ratio and acquisition time and application to intravoxel incoherent motion analysis. *Eur. J. Radiol.*, 2016, 85(11), 1948–1955.

27. Taron J., Martirosian P., Erb M., Kuestner T., Schwenzer N. F., Schmidt H., et al. Simultaneous multislice diffusion-weighted MRI of the liver: Analysis of different breathing schemes in comparison to standard sequences. *J. Magn. Reson. Imaging*, 2016, 44(4), 865–879.

28. Zhang X., Yan L.-F., Hu Y.-C., Li G., Yang Y., Han Y., et al. Optimizing a machine learning based glioma grading system using multi-parametric MRI histogram and texture features. *Oncotarget*, 2017, 8(29), 47816–47830.

29. Aerts H. J. W. L., Velazquez E. R., Leijenaar R. T. H., Parmar C., Grossmann P., Carvalho S., et al. Decoding tumour phenotype by noninvasive imaging using a quantitative radiomics approach. *Nat. Commun.*, 2014, 5, 4006.

30. Cho G. Y., Gennaro L., Sutton E. J., Zabor E. C., Zhang Z., Giri D., et al. Intravoxel incoherent motion (IVIM) histogram biomarkers for prediction of neoadjuvant treatment response in breast cancer patients. *Eur. J. Radiol Open*, 2017, 4, 101–107.

31. Jerome N. P., Orton M. R., d'Arcy J. A., Feiweier T., Tunariu N., Koh D.-M., et al. Use of the temporal median and trimmed mean mitigates effects of respiratory motion in multiple-acquisition abdominal diffusion imaging. *Phys. Med. Biol.*, 2015, 60(2), N9–N20.

32. Guyader J.-M., Bernardin L., Douglas N. H. M., Poot D. H. J., Niessen W. J., Klein S. Influence of image registration on apparent diffusion coefficient images computed from free-breathing diffusion MR images of the abdomen. *J. Magn. Reson. Imaging*, 2015, 42(2), 315–330.

33. Mazaheri Y., Do R. K. G., Shukla-Dave A., Deasy J. O., Lu Y., Akin O. Motion correction of multi-b-value diffusion-weighted imaging in the liver. *Acad Radiol.*, 2012, 19(12), 1573–1580.

34. Kurugol S., Freiman M., Afacan O., Domachevsky L., Perez-Rossello J. M., Callahan M. J., et al. Motion-robust parameter estimation in abdominal diffusion-weighted MRI by simultaneous image registration and model estimation. *Med. Image Anal.*, 2017, 39, 124–132.

35. Koh D.-M., Collins D. J., Orton M. R. Intravoxel incoherent motion in body diffusion-weighted MRI: reality and challenges. *AJR Am. J. Roentgenol.*, 2011, 196(6), 1351–1361.

36. Sigmund E. E., Vivier P.-H., Sui D., Lamparello N. A., Tantillo K., Mikheev A., et al. Intravoxel incoherent motion and diffusion-tensor imaging in renal tissue under hydration and furosemide flow challenges. *Radiology*, 2011, 196(6), 1351–1361.

37. Jerome N. P., Miyazaki K., Collins D. J., Orton M. R., d'Arcy J. A., Wallace T., et al. Repeatability of derived parameters from histograms following non-Gaussian diffusion modelling of diffusion-weighted imaging in a paediatric oncological cohort. *Eur. Radiol.*, 2017, 27(1), 345–353.

38. Winfield J. M., deSouza N. M., Priest A. N., Wakefield J. C., Hodgkin C., Freeman S., et al. Modelling DW-MRI data from primary and metastatic ovarian tumours. *Eur. Radiol.*, 2015, 25(7), 2033–2040.

39. Meeus E. M., Novak J., Withey S. B., Zarinabad N., Dehghani H., Peet A. C. Evaluation of intravoxel incoherent motion fitting methods in low-perfused tissue. *J. Magn. Reson. Imaging*, 2017, 45(5), 1325–1334.

40. ter Voert E. E. G. W., Delso G., Porto M., Huellner M., Veit-Haibach P. Intravoxel incoherent motion protocol evaluation and data quality in normal and malignant liver tissue and comparison to the literature. *Invest. Radiol.*, 2017, 45(5), 1325–1334.

41. Wurnig M. C., Donati O. F., Ulbrich E., Filli L., Kenkel D., Thoeny H. C., et al. Systematic analysis of the intravoxel incoherent motion threshold separating perfusion and diffusion effects: Proposal of a standardized algorithm. *Magn. Reson. Med.*, 2015, 74(5), 1414–1422.

42. While P. T. A comparative simulation study of bayesian fitting approaches to intravoxel incoherent motion modeling in diffusion-weighted MRI. *Magn. Reson. Med.* , 2017, 78(6), 2373–2387.

43. Fusco R., Sansone M., Petrillo A. A comparison of fitting algorithms for diffusion-weighted MRI data analysis using an intravoxel incoherent motion model. *MAGMA*., 2017, 30(2), 113–120.

44. Kessler L. G., Barnhart H. X., Buckler A. J., Choudhury K. R., Kondratovich M. V., Toledano A., et al. The emerging science of quantitative imaging biomarkers terminology and definitions for scientific studies and regulatory submissions. *Stat. Methods Med. Res.*, 2015, 24(1), 9–26.

45. Jerome N. P., Papoutsaki M.-V., Orton M. R., Parkes H. G., Winfield J. M., Boss M. A., et al. Development of a temperature-controlled phantom for magnetic resonance quality assurance of diffusion, dynamic, and relaxometry measurements. *Med. Phys.*, 2016, 43(6), 2998–3007.

46. Martin Bland J., Altman D. Statistical methods for assessing agreement between two methods of clinical measurement. *Lancet*, 1986, 327(8476), 307–310.

47. Wong S. M., Backes W. H., Zhang C. E., Staals J., van Oostenbrugge R. J., Jeukens CRLPN, et al. On the reproducibility of inversion recovery intravoxel incoherent motion imaging in cerebrovascular disease. *AJNR Am. J. Neuroradiol.*, 2018, 39(2), 226–231.

48. Pan J., Zhang H., Man F., Shen Y., Wang Y., Zhong Y., et al. Measurement and scan reproducibility of parameters of intravoxel incoherent motion in renal tumor and normal renal parenchyma: a preliminary research at 3.0 T MR. *Abdom Radiol.* (NY), 2017, http://dx.doi.org/10.1007/s00261-017-1361-7

49. Jiang J., Yin J., Cui L., Gu X., Cai R., Gong S., et al. Lung cancer: Short-term reproducibility of intravoxel incoherent motion parameters and apparent diffusion coefficient at 3T. *J. Magn. Reson. Imaging*, 2018, 47(4) 1003–1012.

50. Lecler A., Savatovsky J., Balvay D., Zmuda M., Sadik J.-C., Galatoire O., et al. Repeatability of apparent diffusion coefficient and intravoxel incoherent motion parameters at 3.0 Tesla in orbital lesions. *Eur. Radiol.*, 2017, 27(12), 5094–5103.

51. Sun H., Xu Y., Xu Q., Shi K., Wang W. Rectal cancer: Short-term reproducibility of intravoxel incoherent motion parameters in 3.0T magnetic resonance imaging. *Medicine*, 2017, 96(19), e6866.

52. Kang K. M., Choi S. H., Kim D. E., Yun T. J., Kim J.-H., Sohn C.-H., et al. Application of cardiac gating to improve the reproducibility of intravoxel incoherent motion measurements in the head and neck. *Magn. Reson. Med. Sci.*, 2017, 16(3), 190–202.

53. Song Y. S., Park C. M., Lee S. M., Park S. J., Cho H. R., Choi S. H., et al. Reproducibility of histogram and texture parameters derived from intravoxel incoherent motion diffusion-weighted MRI of FN13762 rat breast Carcinomas. *Anticancer Res.*, 2014, 34(5), 2135–2144.

54. Kakite S., Dyvorne H., Besa C., Cooper N., Facciuto M., Donnerhack C., et al. Hepatocellular carcinoma: short-term reproducibility of apparent diffusion coefficient and intravoxel incoherent motion parameters at 3.0T. *J. Magn. Reson. Imaging*, 2015, 41(1), 149–156.

55. Andreou A., Koh D. M., Collins D. J., Blackledge M., Wallace T., Leach M. O., et al. Measurement reproducibility of perfusion fraction and pseudodiffusion coefficient derived by intravoxel incoherent motion diffusion-weighted MR imaging in normal liver and metastases. *Eur. Radiol.*, 2013, 23(2), 428–434.

56. Miyazaki K., Jerome N. P., Collins D. J., Orton M. R., d'Arcy J. A., Wallace T., et al. Demonstration of the reproducibility of free-breathing diffusion-weighted MRI and dynamic contrast enhanced MRI in children with solid tumours: a pilot study. *Eur. Radiol.*, 2015, 25(9), 2641–2650.

57. Winfield J. M., Tunariu N., Rata M., Miyazaki K., Jerome N. P., Germuska M., et al. Extracranial soft-tissue tumors: repeatability of apparent diffusion coefficient estimates from diffusion-weighted MR imaging. *Radiology*, 2017, 284(1), 88–99.

58. Lemke A., Laun F. B., Simon D., Stieltjes B., Schad L. R. An in vivo verification of the intravoxel incoherent motion effect in diffusion-weighted imaging of the abdomen. *Magn. Reson. Med.*, 2010, 64(6), 1580–1585.

59. Jerome N. P., d'Arcy J. A., Feiweier T., Koh D.-M., Leach M. O., Collins D. J., et al. Extended T2-IVIM model for correction of TE dependence of pseudo-diffusion volume fraction in clinical diffusion-weighted magnetic resonance imaging. *Phys. Med. Biol.*, 2016, 61(24), N667–N680.

60. Thian Y., Orton M. R., Collins D. J., d'Arcy J. A., Leach M. O., Feiweier T., et al. Effect of diffusion time on intravoxel incoherent motion parameters in abdominal organs. In: *Proc 22nd Scientific Meeting, Int Society for Magnetic Resonance in Medicine.*, 2014, vol 22, p. 4457.

61. Klauss M., Mayer P., Maier-Hein K., Laun F. B., Mehrabi A., Kauczor H.-U., et al. IVIM-diffusion-MRI for the differentiation of solid benign and malign hypervascular liver lesions—Evaluation with two different MR scanners. *Eur. J. Radiol.*, 2016, 85(7), 1289–1294.

62. Cho G. Y., Kim S., Jensen J. H., Storey P., Sodickson D. K., Sigmund E. E. A versatile flow phantom for intravoxel incoherent motion MRI. *Magn. Reson. Med.* 2011, 67(6), 1710–1720.

63. Barbieri S., Donati O. F., Froehlich J. M., Thoeny H. C. Comparison of intravoxel incoherent motion parameters across MR imagers and field strengths: evaluation in upper abdominal organs. *Radiology*, 2016, 279(3) 784–794.

64. Koh D.-M., Collins D. J. Diffusion-weighted MRI in the body: applications and challenges in oncology. *Am. J. Roentgenol.*, 2007, 188(6), 1622–1635.

65. Valerio M., Zini C., Fierro D., Giura F., Colarieti A., Giuliani A., et al. 3T multiparametric MRI of the prostate: Does intravoxel incoherent motion diffusion imaging have a role in the detection and stratification of prostate cancer in the peripheral zone? *Eur. J. Radiol.*, 2016, 85(4), 790–794.

66. Pesapane F., Patella F., Fumarola E. M., Panella S., Ierardi A. M., Pompili G. G., et al. Intravoxel incoherent motion (IVIM) diffusion weighted imaging (DWI) in the periferic prostate cancer detection and stratification. *Med. Oncol.*, 2017, 34(3), 35.

67. Re T. J., Lemke A., Klauss M., Laun F. B., Simon D., Grünberg K., et al. Enhancing pancreatic adenocarcinoma delineation in diffusion derived intravoxel incoherent motion f-maps through automatic vessel and duct segmentation. *Magn. Reson. Med.*, 2011, 66(5), 1327–1332.

68. Lemke A., Laun F. B., Klauss M., Re T. J., Simon D., Delorme S., et al. Differentiation of pancreas carcinoma from healthy pancreatic tissue using multiple b-values: comparison of apparent diffusion coefficient and intravoxel incoherent motion derived parameters. *Invest. Radiol.*, 2009, 44(12), 769–775.

69. Zhang S.-X., Jia Q.-J., Zhang Z.-P., Liang C.-H., Chen W.-B., Qiu Q.-H., et al. Intravoxel incoherent motion MRI: emerging applications for nasopharyngeal carcinoma at the primary site. *Eur. Radiol.*, 2014, 24(8), 1998–2004.

70. Sandrasegaran K., Territo P., Elkady R. M., Lin Y., Gasparis P., Borthakur G., et al. Does intravoxel incoherent motion reliably stage hepatic fibrosis, steatosis, and inflammation? *Abdom. Radiol. (NY)*, 2018, 43(3), 600–606.

71. Wu C.-H., Ho M.-C., Jeng Y.-M., Liang P.-C., Hu R.-H., Lai H.-S., et al. Assessing hepatic fibrosis: comparing the intravoxel incoherent motion in MRI with acoustic radiation force impulse imaging in US. *Eur. Radiol.*, 2015, 25(12), 3552–3559.

72. Yoon J. H., Lee J. M., Baek J. H., Shin C.-I., Kiefer B., Han J. K., et al. Evaluation of hepatic fibrosis using intravoxel incoherent motion in diffusion-weighted liver MRI. *J. Comput. Assist. Tomogr.*, 2014, 38(1), 110–116.

73. Zhang B., Liang L., Dong Y., Lian Z., Chen W., Liang C., et al. Intravoxel incoherent motion mr imaging for staging of hepatic fibrosis. *PLoS One*, 2016, 11(1), e0147789.

74. Li Y. T., Cercueil J.-P., Yuan J., Chen W., Loffroy R., Wáng Y. X. J. Liver intravoxel incoherent motion (IVIM) magnetic resonance imaging: a comprehensive review of published data on normal values and

applications for fibrosis and tumor evaluation. *Quant. Imaging Med. Surg.*, 2017, 7(1), 59–78.

75. Detsky J. S., Keith J., Conklin J., Symons S., Myrehaug S., Sahgal A., et al. Differentiating radiation necrosis from tumor progression in brain metastases treated with stereotactic radiotherapy: utility of intravoxel incoherent motion perfusion MRI and correlation with histopathology. *J. Neurooncol.*, 2017, 134(2), 433–441.
76. Kang K. M., Lee J. M., Yoon J. H., Kiefer B., Han J. K., Choi B. I. Intravoxel incoherent motion diffusion-weighted MR imaging for characterization of focal pancreatic lesions. *Radiology*, 2014, 270(2), 444–453.
77. Klau M., Mayer P., Bergmann F., Maier-Hein K., Hase J., Hackert T., et al. Correlation of histological vessel characteristics and diffusion-weighted imaging intravoxel incoherent motion-derived parameters in pancreatic ductal adenocarcinomas and pancreatic neuroendocrine tumors. *Invest. Radiol.*, 2014, 270(2), 444–453.
78. Klauss M., Lemke A., Grünberg K., Simon D., Re T. J., Wente M. N., et al. Intravoxel incoherent motion MRI for the differentiation between mass forming chronic pancreatitis and pancreatic carcinoma. *Invest. Radiol.*, 2011, 46(1), 57–63.
79. Klauß M., Maier-Hein K., Tjaden C., Hackert T., Grenacher L., Stieltjes B. IVIM DW-MRI of autoimmune pancreatitis: therapy monitoring and differentiation from pancreatic cancer. *Eur. Radiol.*, 2016, 26(7), 2099–2106.
80. Doblas S., Wagner M., Leitao H. S., Daire J.-L., Sinkus R., Vilgrain V., et al. Determination of malignancy and characterization of hepatic tumor type with diffusion-weighted magnetic resonance imaging: comparison of apparent diffusion coefficient and intravoxel incoherent motion-derived measurements. *Invest. Radiol.*, 2013, 48(10), 722–728.
81. Watanabe H., Kanematsu M., Goshima S., Kajita K., Kawada H., Noda Y., et al. Characterizing focal hepatic lesions by free-breathing intravoxel incoherent motion MRI at 3.0 T. *Acta Radiol.*, 2014, 55(10), 1166–1173.
82. Zhu L., Cheng Q., Luo W., Bao L., Guo G. A comparative study of apparent diffusion coefficient and intravoxel incoherent motion-derived parameters for the characterization of common solid hepatic tumors. *Acta Radiol.*, 2014, 55(10), 1166–1173.
83. Yoon J. H., Lee J. M., Yu M. H., Kiefer B., Han J. K., Choi B. I. Evaluation of hepatic focal lesions using diffusion-weighted MR imaging: comparison of apparent diffusion coefficient and intravoxel incoherent motion-derived parameters. *J. Magn. Reson. Imaging*, 2014, 39(2), 276–285.

84. Bokacheva L., Kaplan J. B., Giri D. D., Patil S., Gnanasigamani M., Gregory Nyman C., et al. Intravoxel incoherent motion diffusion-weighted MRI at 3.0 T differentiates malignant breast lesions from benign lesions and breast parenchyma. *J. Magn. Reson. Imaging*, 2013, 40(4), 813–823.

85. Liu C., Liang C., Liu Z., Zhang S., Huang B. Intravoxel incoherent motion (IVIM) in evaluation of breast lesions: comparison with conventional DWI. *Eur. J. Radiol.*, 2013, 82(12), e782–e789.

86. Liu C., Wang K., Chan Q., Liu Z., Zhang J., He H., et al. Intravoxel incoherent motion MR imaging for breast lesions: comparison and correlation with pharmacokinetic evaluation from dynamic contrast-enhanced MR imaging. *Eur. Radiol.*, 2016, 26(11), 3888–3898.

87. Suo S., Lin N., Wang H., Zhang L., Wang R., Zhang S., et al. Intravoxel incoherent motion diffusion-weighted MR imaging of breast cancer at 3.0 tesla: Comparison of different curve-fitting methods. *J. Magn. Reson. Imaging*, 2014, 42(2), 362–370.

88. Ma D., Lu F., Zou X., Zhang H., Li Y., Zhang L., et al. Intravoxel incoherent motion diffusion-weighted imaging as an adjunct to dynamic contrast-enhanced MRI to improve accuracy of the differential diagnosis of benign and malignant breast lesions. *Magn. Reson. Imaging*, 2017, 36, 175–179.

89. Kawashima H., Miyati T., Ohno N., Ohno M., Inokuchi M., Ikeda H., et al. Differentiation between Luminal-A and Luminal-B breast cancer using intravoxel incoherent motion and dynamic contrast-enhanced magnetic resonance imaging. *Acad. Radiol.*, 2017, 24(12), 1575–1581.

90. Iima M., Kataoka M., Kanao S., Onishi N., Kawai M., Ohashi A., et al. Intravoxel incoherent motion and quantitative non-gaussian diffusion MR imaging: evaluation of the diagnostic and prognostic value of several markers of malignant and benign breast lesions. *Radiology*, 2018, 287(2), 432–441.

91. Sigmund E. E., Cho G. Y., Kim S., Finn M., Moccaldi M., Jensen J. H., et al. Intravoxel incoherent motion imaging of tumor microenvironment in locally advanced breast cancer. *Magn. Reson. Med.*, 2011, 65(5), 1437–1447.

92. Tian T., Zhang G.-F., Zhang H., Liu H. Intravoxel incoherent motion diffusion-weighted imaging in differentiating uterine fibroid from focal adenomyosis: initial results. *Springerplus*, 2016, 5(1), http://dx.doi.org/10.1186/s40064-015-1635-x

93. Qi L.-P., Yan W.-P., Chen K.-N., Zhong Z., Li X.-T., Cai K., et al. Discrimination of malignant versus benign mediastinal lymph nodes using diffusion MRI with an IVIM model. *Eur. Radiol.*, 2018, 28(3), 1301–1309.

94. Rong D., Mao Y., Hu W., Xu S., Wang J., He H., et al. Intravoxel incoherent motion magnetic resonance imaging for differentiating metastatic and non-metastatic lymph nodes in pancreatic ductal adenocarcinoma. *Eur. Radiol.*, 2018, http://dx.doi.org/10.1007/s00330-017-5259-0
95. Ye X., Chen S., Tian Y., You B., Zhang W., Zhao Y., et al. A preliminary exploration of the intravoxel incoherent motion applied in the preoperative evaluation of mediastinal lymph node metastasis of lung cancer. *J. Thorac. Dis.*, 2017, 9(4), 1073–1080.
96. Yu X.-P., Wen L., Hou J., Bi F., Hu P., Wang H., et al. Discrimination between metastatic and nonmetastatic mesorectal lymph nodes in rectal cancer using intravoxel incoherent motion diffusion-weighted magnetic resonance imaging. *Acad. Radiol.*, 2016, 23(4), 479–485.
97. Deng Y., Yang B., Peng Y., Liu Z., Luo J., Du G. Use of intravoxel incoherent motion diffusion-weighted imaging to detect early changes in diabetic kidneys. *Abdom. Radiol.* (NY), 2018, http://dx.doi.org/10.1007/s00261-018-1521-4
98. Mao W., Zhou J., Zeng M., Ding Y., Qu L., Chen C., et al. Chronic kidney disease: Pathological and functional evaluation with intravoxel incoherent motion diffusion-weighted imaging. *J. Magn. Reson. Imaging*, 2018, 47(5), 1251–1259.
99. Mao W., Zhou J., Zeng M., Ding Y., Qu L., Chen C., et al. Intravoxel incoherent motion diffusion-weighted imaging for the assessment of renal fibrosis of chronic kidney disease: A preliminary study. *Magn. Reson. Imaging*, 2018, 47, 118–124.
100. Hennedige T., Koh T. S., Hartono S., Yan Y. Y., Song I. C., Zheng L., et al. Intravoxel incoherent imaging of renal fibrosis induced in a murine model of unilateral ureteral obstruction. *Magn. Reson. Imaging*, 2015, 33(10), 1324–1328.
101. Pons M., Leporq B., Ali L., Alison M., Albuquerque M., Peuchmaur M., et al. Renal parenchyma impairment characterization in partial unilateral ureteral obstruction in mice with intravoxel incoherent motion-MRI. *NMR Biomed.*, 2018, 31(2), http://dx.doi.org/10.1002/nbm.3858
102. Rheinheimer S., Schneider F., Stieltjes B., Morath C., Zeier M., Kauczor H. U., et al. IVIM-DWI of transplanted kidneys: reduced diffusion and perfusion dependent on cold ischemia time. *Eur. J. Radiol.*, 2012, 81(9), e951–e956.
103. Schneider M. J., Dietrich O., Ingrisch M., Helck A., Winter K. S., Reiser M. F., et al. Intravoxel incoherent motion magnetic resonance imaging in partially nephrectomized kidneys. *Invest. Radiol.*, 2016, 51(5), 323–330.

104. Kim Y., Kim S. H., Lee H. W., Song B. J., Kang B. J., Lee A., et al. Intravoxel incoherent motion diffusion-weighted MRI for predicting response to neoadjuvant chemotherapy in breast cancer. *Magn. Reson. Imaging*, 2018, 48, 27–33.

105. Pieper C. C., Sprinkart A. M., Meyer C., König R., Schild H. H., Kukuk G. M., et al. Evaluation of a simplified intravoxel incoherent motion (IVIM) analysis of diffusion-weighted imaging for prediction of tumor size changes and imaging response in breast cancer liver metastases undergoing radioembolization. *Medicine*, 2016, 95(14), e3275.

106. Pieper C. C., Willinek W. A., Meyer C., Ahmadzadehfar H., Kukuk G. M., Sprinkart A. M., et al. Intravoxel incoherent motion diffusion-weighted MR imaging for prediction of early arterial blood flow stasis in radioembolization of breast cancer liver metastases. *J. Vasc. Interv. Radiol.*, 2016, 27(9), 1320–1328.

107. Lu W., Jing H., Ju-Mei Z., Shao-Lin N., Fang C., Xiao-Ping Y., et al. Intravoxel incoherent motion diffusion-weighted imaging for discriminating the pathological response to neoadjuvant chemoradiotherapy in locally advanced rectal cancer. *Sci. Rep.*, 2017, 7(1), 8496.

108. Petrillo A., Fusco R., Granata V., Setola S. V., Sansone M., Rega D., et al. MR imaging perfusion and diffusion analysis to assess preoperative Short Course Radiotherapy response in locally advanced rectal cancer: Standardized Index of Shape by DCE-MRI and intravoxel incoherent motion-derived parameters by DW-MRI. *Med. Oncol.*, 2017, 34(12), 198.

109. Pan F., Den J., Zhang C., Wang H., Cheng J., Wu W., et al. The therapeutic response of gastrointestinal stromal tumors to imatinib treatment assessed by intravoxel incoherent motion diffusion-weighted magnetic resonance imaging with histopathological correlation. *PLoS One*, 2016, 11(12), e0167720.

110. Shirota N., Saito K., Sugimoto K., Takara K., Moriyasu F., Tokuuye K. Intravoxel incoherent motion MRI as a biomarker of sorafenib treatment for advanced hepatocellular carcinoma: a pilot study. *Cancer Imaging*, 2016, 16, 1.

111. Wang Y.-C., Hu D.-Y., Hu X.-M., Shen Y.-Q., Meng X.-Y., Tang H., et al. Assessing the early response of advanced cervical cancer to neoadjuvant chemotherapy using intravoxel incoherent motion diffusion-weighted magnetic resonance imaging: a pilot study. *Chin. Med. J.*, 2016, 129(6), 665–671.

112. Noij D. P., Martens R. M., Marcus J. T., de Bree R., Leemans C. R., Castelijns

J. A., et al. Intravoxel incoherent motion magnetic resonance imaging in head and neck cancer: A systematic review of the diagnostic and prognostic value. *Oral Oncol.*, 2017, 68, 81–91.

113. Niu J., Li W., Wang H., Wu W., Gong T., Huang N., et al. Intravoxel incoherent motion diffusion-weighted imaging of bone marrow in patients with acute myeloid leukemia: a pilot study of prognostic value. *J. Magn. Reson. Imaging*, 2017, 46(2), 476–482.

114. Cui Y., Zhang C., Li X., Liu H., Yin B., Xu T., et al. Intravoxel incoherent motion diffusion-weighted magnetic resonance imaging for monitoring the early response to ZD6474 from nasopharyngeal carcinoma in nude mouse. *Sci. Rep.*, 2015, 5(1). http://dx.doi.org/10.1038/srep16389

115. Granata V., Fusco R., Catalano O., Filice S., Amato D. M., Nasti G., et al. Early assessment of colorectal cancer patients with liver metastases treated with antiangiogenic drugs: the role of intravoxel incoherent motion in diffusion-weighted imaging. *PLoS One*, 2015, 10(11), e0142876.

116. Shi C., Liu D., Xiao Z., Zhang D., Liu G., Liu G., et al. Monitoring tumor response to antivascular therapy using non-contrast intravoxel incoherent motion diffusion-weighted MRI. *Cancer Res.*, 2017, 77(13), 3491–3501.

Chapter 7

Head and Neck IVIM MRI

Takashi Nakamura and Misa Sumi
Department of Radiology and Cancer Biology,
Nagasaki University Graduate School of Biomedical Sciences,
1-7-1 Sakamoto, Nagasaki 852-8588, Japan
taku@nagasaki-u.ac.jp

7.1 Authentic and Geographic Estimations of Perfusion and Diffusion Properties for Head and Neck IVIM MRI

IVIM imaging can be characterized by three parameters: pure diffusion coefficient (D), microvascular volume fraction (f), and perfusion-related incoherent microcirculation (D^*) [1, 2]. In general, the perfusion/diffusion parameters can be determined by using the least-squares method from a multiexponential signal decay curve obtained with multiple b values, usually ≥8, including a b value of 0 s/mm^2 and spanning from low (<200 s/mm^2) to high (200–1000 s/mm^2) values. As many numbers of b values less than 200 s/mm^2 as possible should be used for precisely characterizing

Intravoxel Incoherent Motion (IVIM) MRI: Principles and Applications
Edited by Denis Le Bihan, Mami Iima, Christian Federau, and Eric E. Sigmund

ISBN 978-981-4800-19-8 (Hardcover), 978-0-429-42727-5 (eBook)
www.panstanford.com

the decay curve, which is predominantly influenced by tissue perfusion. However, increases in the number of b values used will extend the scan time and increase the chances of patient motion.

In brief, D can be obtained by the least-squares method using signals in logarithm at high b values (e.g., $\ln S_{200}$, $\ln S_{300}$, $\ln S_{400}$, and $\ln S_{800}$, as in Fig. 7.1a,b). To estimate f, an initial f value is calculated as $(S_0 - S_{\text{inter}})/S_0$, where S_0 is the signal intensity at $b = 0$ s/mm^2 and S_{inter} is the interception of the logarithmic regression line obtained by using b values of 200, 300, 400, and 800 s/mm^2 with the y axis.

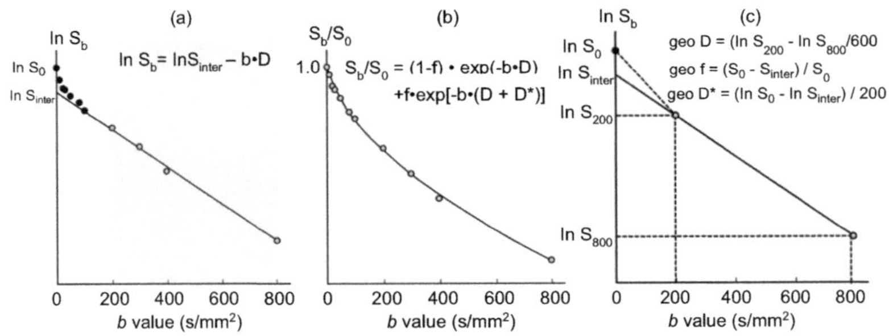

Figure 7.1 IVIM parameter determination by the least-squares or geometric methods. (a, b) The least-squares method. The left panel (a) shows a representative signal decay curve obtained by using 11 b values (0, 10, 20, 30, 50, 80, 100, 200, 300, 400, and 800 s/mm^2). First, D (fit D) can be obtained by the least-squares method using $\ln S_{200}$, $\ln S_{300}$, $\ln S_{400}$, and $\ln S_{800}$, and the initial f value is calculated as $(S_0 - S_{\text{inter}})/S_0$, where S_{inter} is the interception of the logarithmic regression line obtained by using b values of 200, 300, 400, and 800 s/mm^2 with the y axis. The middle panel (b) shows the relationship between S_b/S_0 and varying b values. When fit D and initial f and D^* values are given, f (fit f) and D^* (fit D^*) values can be obtained by the least-squares method on the basis of the equation $S_b/S_0 = (1-f)\cdot\exp(-bD) + f\cdot[-b(D+D^*)]$. (c) The geometric method. The graph shows geometric determination of IVIM parameters using 3 (0, 200, and 800 s/mm^2) of the 11 b values. D is calculated by the equation geo $D = (\ln S_{200} - \ln S_{800})/600$. f is estimated by the equation geo $f = (S_0 - S_{\text{inter}})/S_0$, and geo D^* is estimated by the equation geo $D^* = (\ln S_0 - \ln S_{\text{inter}})/200$.

The initial D^* value of 0.01 was successfully used for assessing the IVIM of salivary gland tumors [3]. When the D, initial f, and initial D^* values are given, f (fit f) and D^* (fit D^*) values can be obtained using a nonlinear regression algorithm based on the following equation:

$$S_b/S_0 = (1-f)\cdot\exp(-bD) + f\cdot[-b(D+D^*)]. \tag{7.1}$$

Fit *f* and fit D^* values can be obtained after substituting the initial *f* and D^* values into the Levenberg–Marquardt algorithm [4].

IVIM analysis using the least-squares method is cumbersome and time consuming and thus may not be suitable for routine clinical use. Accordingly, several techniques have been developed to simplify the procedures for estimating the diffusion and perfusion properties [5–8]. These simplified techniques may have some shortcomings in precisely determining IVIM parameters compared to the analysis using the least-squares method. However, a comparative study has recently demonstrated that the geometric estimation of IVIM parameters using a limited number of *b* values is a simple and reliable technique for diagnosing a wide spectrum of head and neck tumors [9]. In the simplified geometric method (geo), the number of *b* values used can be limited to as few as three (e.g., $b = 0$, 200, and 800 s/mm^2, as shown in Fig. 7.1c). By using logarithmic plots, *D* can be estimated as a decline between $b = 200$ s/mm^2 and $b = 800$ s/mm^2:

$$\text{geo } D = (\ln S_{200} - \ln S_{800})/600\,. \tag{7.2}$$

When an estimated *D* value is given, we can then estimate the tissue perfusion fraction by geometrically determining *f* as follows:

$$\text{geo } f = (S_0 - S_{\text{inter}})/S_0\,, \tag{7.3}$$

where S_0 is the signal intensity at $b = 0$ s/mm^2 and S_{inter} is the interception of the logarithmic regression line obtained by using *b* values of 200 and 800 s/mm^2 with the *y*-axis. The perfusion property geo D^* can also be geometrically estimated as follows:

$$\text{geo} D^* = (\ln S_0 - \ln S_{\text{inter}})/200\,. \tag{7.4}$$

In the least-squares method, we can use fit D^* for estimating the perfusion properties of a tissue. However, the perfusion parameter geo D^* is heavily weighted toward the extravascular space. Therefore, geo D^* is basically different from fit D^* [9]. However, as mentioned in the later section of this chapter, geo *D* and geo *f* are very close to the corresponding parameters fit *D* and fit *f*, respectively, in terms of the value levels as well as diagnostic efficacy for different types of head and neck tumors.

7.2 Head and Neck Squamous Cell Carcinomas

7.2.1 Perfusion and Diffusion Characteristics of Head and Neck Squamous Cell Carcinomas

Squamous cell carcinomas are the most common malignancy of the head and neck, occurring in the oral cavity, nasopharynx, oropharynx, hypopharynx, larynx, and paranasal sinuses. Several researchers have attempted to evaluate the usefulness of IVIM models in characterizing perfusion and diffusion properties of head and neck squamous cell carcinomas. Among them, Sumi and Nakamura [8, 10] effectively characterized head and neck squamous cell carcinomas in comparison with the other types of head and neck tumors using geometrically determined microvascular volume fraction (geo *f*) and pure diffusion coefficient (geo *D*) based on the IVIM model obtained with *b* values of 0, 500, and 1000 s/mm^2. These studies have shown that the geo *f* and geo *D* values are significantly different among the malignant as well as benign tumors (lymphomas, squamous cell carcinomas, and benign and malignant salivary gland tumors) (Fig. 7.2). Distinctive histological structures of particular types of head and neck tumors may successfully explain the differences in geo *f* and geo *D* values among the different types of head and neck tumors; for instance, lymphomas exclusively contain dense proliferations of lymphoid cells with scarce amounts of stromal tissues between the tumor cells, both restraining the water diffusivity within the tumors. However, squamous cell carcinomas have varying amounts of stromal tissues depending on the tumor grade, ranging from poor or undifferentiated to well-differentiated histology. Large stromal tissue areas within squamous cell carcinoma may increase the tumor perfusion. Aberrant perfusion with dysfunctional capillaries within the solid tumor would produce hypoxic microenvironments and resultant areas of necrosis, developing into areas with varying degrees of higher diffusivity depending on the necrotic contents (liquefaction or coagulation necrosis) [11]. Keratin deposits in the stromal tissues in squamous cell carcinomas could also influence the water diffusivity.

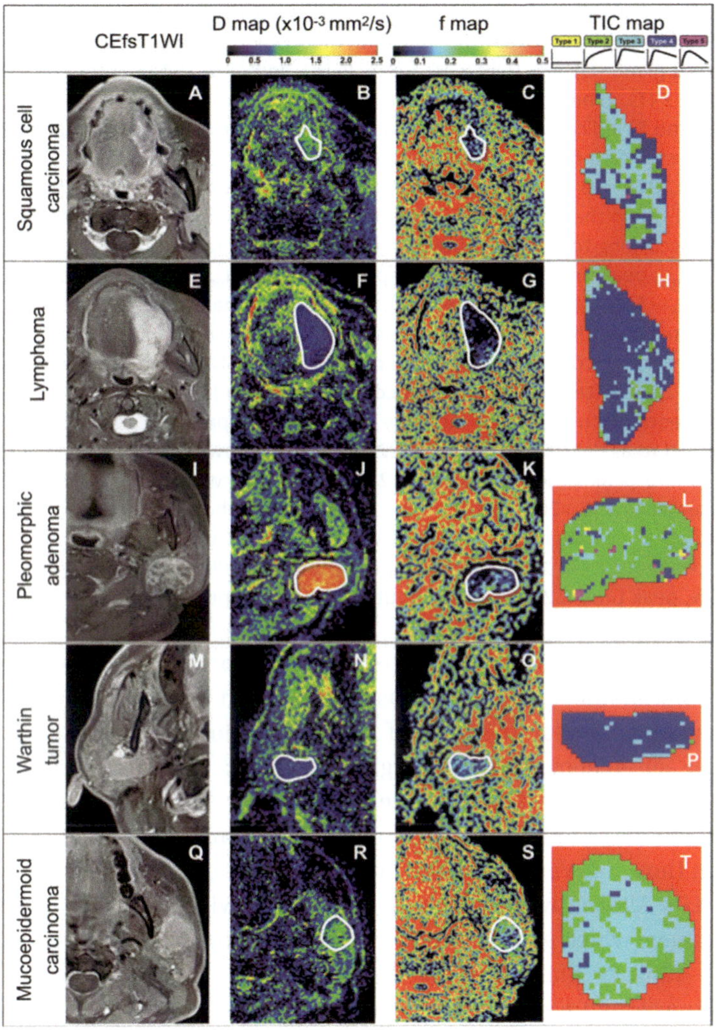

Figure 7.2 Representative contrast-enhanced fat-suppressed T1-weighted MR images (CEfsT1WI) and geo D, geo f, and TIC maps of squamous cell carcinoma, lymphoma, pleomorphic adenoma, Warthin tumor, and mucoepidermoid carcinoma. (**A–D**)A 56-year-old man with SCC in the tongue (**A**). $D = 0.85 \times 10^{-3}$ mm^2/s (**B**), geo $f = 0.097$ (**C**), and overall TIC profile = Type 3 (**D**). (**E–H**) An 80-year-old woman with non-Hodgkin lymphoma (large B-cell lymphoma) in the tongue (**E**). $D = 0.46 \times 10^{-3}$ mm^2/s (**F**), geo $f = 0.031$ (**G**), and overall TIC profile = Type 4(**H**). (**I–L**) A 66-year-old woman with a pleomorphic adenoma in the left parotid gland (**I**). $D = 2.25 \times 10^{-3}$ mm^2/s (**J**), geo $f = 0.083$ (**K**), and TIC profile = Type 2 (**L**). (**M–P**) A 69-year-old man with a Warthin tumor in the right

(*continued on next page*)

parotid gland (**M**). $D = 0.56 \times 10^{-3}$ mm^2/s (**N**), geo $f = 0.124$ (**O**), and TIC profile = Type 4 (**P**). (**Q–T**) A 53-year-old man with mucoepidermoid carcinoma in the left parotid gland (**Q**). $D = 0.89 \times 10^{-3}$ mm^2/s (**R**), geo $f = 0.154$ (**S**), and TIC profile = Type 3 (**T**). White demarcations on *D* (**B**, **F**, **J**, **N**, and **R**) and geo *f* maps (**C**, **G**, **K**, **O**, and **S**) indicate tumor areas. Tumor areas are cropped on TIC maps (**D**, **H**, **L**, **P**, and **T**).Geo *D* and *f* values were calculated using *b* values of 500 and 1000 s/mm^2. TICs in each pixel of the tumor area can be categorized into five types (Type 1–5) on the basis of the increment ratio, the peak time, and the washout ratio according to the following formulas: Increment ratio (%) = $(SI_{peak} - SI_{pre}) \times 100/SI_{pre}$, peak time (*s*) = time corresponding to the SI_{peak}, and washout ratio (%) = $(SI_{peak} - SI_{3min}) \times 100/(SI_{peak} - SI_{pre})$. SI_{peak} is the signal intensity at peak, SI_{pre} is the signal intensity of pre-enhancement, SI_{3min} is the signal intensity 180 s after the start of the contrast medium injection, T_{pre} is the time at pre-enhancement, $T_{3min}$is 180 s after the start of the contrast medium injection, and T_{peak} is the time required to reach the intensity peak. The TIC patterns are, for example, referred to as flat (increment ratio ≤20%; Type 1), slow uptake (increment ratio >20% and peak time ≥120 s; Type 2), rapid uptake with a low washout ratio (increment ratio >20%, peak time <120 s, and washout ratio <30%; Type 3), rapid uptake with a high washout ratio (increment ratio >20%, peak time <120s, and washout ratio ≥30%/<70%; Type 4), and miscellaneous (increment ratio >20%, peak time<120 s, and washout ratio ≥70%; Type 5).

The *D* values of squamous cell carcinomas are significantly larger than those of lymphomas, smaller than those of pleomorphic adenomas, similar to those of Warthin tumors, and smaller than those of malignant salivary gland tumors; and the *f* values of squamous cell carcinomas are significantly larger than those of lymphomas, similar to those of pleomorphic adenomas, and smaller than those of Warthin tumors and malignant salivary gland tumors [8, 10]. Alternatively, schwannomas have a wide spectrum of *f* and *D* values, which greatly overlap those of squamous cell carcinomas and salivary gland tumors. Schwannomas are characteristically composed of mixtures of cellular Antoni type A areas with Verocay bodies and hypocellular Antoni type B areas. The Antoni type B areas often contain small ectatic vessels. This histological diversity in schwannomas is well correlated with the wide spectrum of the IVIM parameters [8].

The large overlaps in the *f* and *D* values of head and neck tumors may diminish the value of these parameters in differentiating between tumors with different histological types. This is partly because the other IVIM perfusion parameter *D** is less precise and less informative in diagnosing different tumor types with different perfusion characteristics. However, additional perfusion information, for example, perfusion kinetic parameters obtained by time intensity curve (TIC) analysis from dynamic contrast–enhanced (DCE) MRI, could improve the ability of the IVIM parameters to differentiate between some types of head and neck tumors. This concept is based on the fact that some TIC kinetic parameters are useful for differentiating between some types of head and neck tumors and the parameters are well correlated with the IVIM perfusion parameters [12–16]. The strategy for the combined use of TIC and IVIM parameters may differ between different sets of tumor types; however, a successful approach has been reported as follows: First, tumors can be classified into those with Type 2, Type 3, Type 4, or Type 5 profiles (see legends for Fig. 7.2). Then, the tumors in each category with a distinctive TIC profile can be further classified into particular tumor types according to the f and D value levels based on the cluster analysis [10]. This stepwise approach using TIC profiles and IVIM parameters with varying thresholds can effectively differentiate between benign and malignant tumors with 97% accuracy and diagnose different tumor types with 89% accuracy in that study.

7.2.2 Metastatic vs. Nonmetastatic Lymph Nodes in the Neck

Lymph node metastasis is a critical prognostic factor in patients with head and neck squamous cell carcinoma. The presence of one or more metastatic nodes in the neck greatly affects the locoregional control, the treatment strategy, and even patient survival [17]. MRI has been evaluated as a diagnostic tool for neck diseases in patients with head and neck squamous cell carcinoma [11, 18, 19]. However, the application of IVIM imaging to the diagnosis of metastatic nodes in the neck has been very limited, mainly because metastatic nodes are often small in size (<10 mm), with potentially poor precision in measuring IVIM parameters using multiple b values, and partly because the whole neck is often outside the scope of IVIM MRI for primary tumors so as to avoid unfavorably extended scan times.

Information about extranodal spread (ENS) has been recently included in staging patients with head and neck cancer [20, 21].

Actually, ENS is a dominant risk factor for survival in patients with head and neck squamous cell carcinoma [22]. Although the usefulness of IVIM imaging in detecting ENS has not been evaluated, pathognomonic changes in perfusion and diffusion parameters can be assumed in ENS-positive metastatic nodes, where the TIC profiles largely shift from dominant Type 3 rapid uptake with a low washout ratio or Type 4 rapid uptake with a high washout ratio pattern into dominant Type 2 slow uptake patterns [23] (Fig. 7.3).

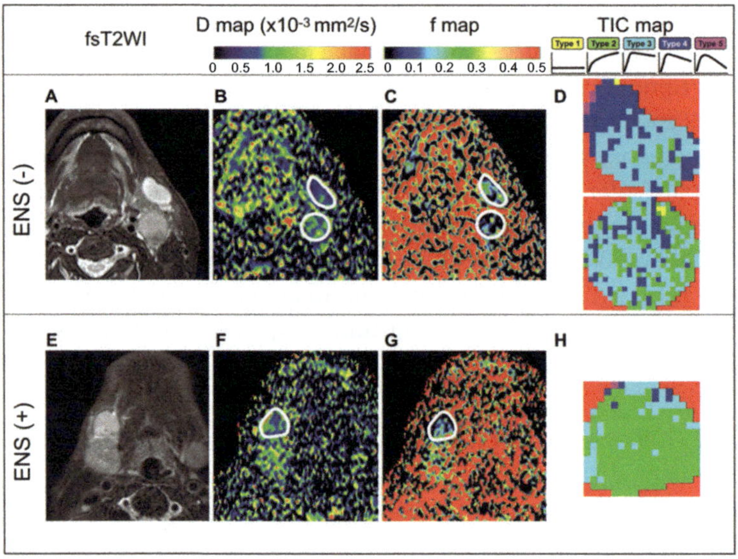

Figure 7.3 Representative fat-suppressed T2-weighted MR images (fsT2WI) and geo *D*, geo *f*, and TIC maps of metastatic nodes with or without extranodal spread (ENS). (**A–D**) A 55-year-old man with SCC in the oropharynx and ENS-negative, ENS (–), metastatic nodes in the neck levels IB and IIA (**A**), $D = 0.60 \times 10^{-3}$ mm^2/s (IB) and 0.64×10^{-3} mm^2/s (IIA) (**B**), geo $f = 0.207$ (IB) and 0.131 (IIA) (**C**), and overall TIC profile = Type 3 (IB) and Type 3 (IIA) (**D**). Geo *D* and *f* values were calculated using *b* values of 500 and 1000 s/mm^2. (**E–H**) A 74-year-old man with SCC in the floor of the mouth and ENS-positive, ENS (+), metastatic node in the neck level IB (**E**). $D = 0.74 \times 10^{-3}$ mm^2/s (**F**), geo $f = 0.115$ (**G**), and overall TIC profile = Type 2 (**H**). White demarcations on geo *D* (**C**, **G**) and geo *f* maps (**D**, **H**) indicate areas of metastatic nodes with (**G**) or without (**C**) ENS. Note that nodal areas with a Type 2 TIC profile are predominant in an ENS (+) node (**H**); however, nodal areas with Type 3 or 4 TIC profiles are predominant in ENS (–) nodes (**D**). Geo *D* and *f* values were calculated using *b* values of 500 and 1000 s/mm^2.

7.2.3 Prediction of Treatment Response in Head and Neck Cancer

One of the major issues in the clinical application of IVIM MRI in patients with head and neck carcinoma is the potential of the MR technique for predicting treatment responses. Several researchers have attempted to evaluate the usefulness of IVIM parameters in predicting responses of the primary tumors or metastatic nodes to chemoradiotherapy/nonadjuvant chemotherapy [24–29]. The general consensus among these studies is that the baseline and interval changes of some IVIM parameters may be useful for predicting treatment responses of the primary tumors and metastatic lymph nodes in the necks of patients with head and neck cancer. For example, the baseline D values of nasopharyngeal carcinomas (NPCs) in responders to nonadjuvant chemotherapy are significantly lower than those of the cancer in nonresponders, with the best cutoff threshold of $D = 0.911 \times 10^{-3}$ mm^2/s; and the interval changes in D, f, and D^* values of responders during treatment periods are significantly greater than those of nonresponders [24]. Another study using a cohort of patients with human papillomavirus (HPV)-positive or HPV-negative head and neck cancers of the oropharynx and unknown in origin showed that interval changes in D values during chemoradiotherapy are significantly higher for a complete response (CR) group than those for a non-CR group [25]. A tumor that is epithelial in origin with a low baseline D value is supposedly composed of densely packed small cancer cells with poorly differentiated characteristics, which is considered to be more sensitive to chemoradiotherapy compared with a tumor with a higher D value. Increases in f and D^* values during radiochemotherapy may be caused by improved vascular network within the solid tumors, which will lead to improved vascular microenvironments and accelerated immune responses of the host. On the other hand, greater increases in D values during the treatment indicate higher rates of cell death in tumors of responders.

Similar findings with IVIM parameters have been reported for the prediction of treatment responses in metastatic nodes of patients with head and neck cancer. In patients with locally advanced head and neck carcinomas who had undergone chemoradiotherapy without surgical intervention, high baseline f values and higher interval changes in f and $f \times D^*$ values in the lymph nodes can be predictors of successful locoregional control in the neck [27, 29]. Locoregional failure of primary laryngeal and hypopharyngeal cancers can also be predicted by IVIM estimation of tumor diffusion and perfusion properties. In this case, D values and f values in recurrent tumors are significantly lower than those of post-therapeutic changes, supporting the idea that estimating D and f values can effectively differentiate between these malignant and inflammatory lesions [30]. These results are consistent with the notion that tumor capillaries are leaky and insufficient, while inflammatory lesions are characterized by dilated capillaries and vascular hyperpermeability. Therefore, the tumor microenvironment is associated with decreases in fast-moving blood pools, and the inflammatory lesions contain more pools of fast-moving blood and increased water content in the interstitial tissues. Both D and f values are significantly different between malignant and inflammatory lesions. However, the f value may be the best for differentiating between malignant and inflammatory lesions, considering its higher sensitivity (94% vs. 78%) and accuracy (80% vs. 74%) [30].

7.3 Lymphomas

7.3.1 Perfusion and Diffusion Characteristics of Nodal/Extranodal Lymphomas

Lymphomas can be classified into several subtypes on the basis of the morphology, immunophenotype, molecular and genetic characteristics, and clinical presentation and course [31]. Classification at the initial stage of patient management is mandatory because not all lymphomas share the same clinical course and the treatment depends on specific histologic features.

Lymphomas have common MRI features, including characteristically homogeneous signals on T1- and fat-suppressed T2-weighted MR images and low D values [8, 10] (Fig. 7.2). These

MRI features reflect the histological features of lymphomas largely comprising dense and exclusive proliferation of several types of lymphoid cells. However, some (~20%) lymphoma nodes (nodal lymphomas) contain nonenhanced areas in contrast-enhanced MR images [11] (Fig. 7.4). *D* values of lymphoma nodes without focal defects, which were determined as signal declines between *b* values of 500 and 1000 s/mm^2, were significantly smaller than those of metastatic nodes without focal defects (0.45 ± 0.10 vs. 0.96 ± 0.31 × 10^{-3} mm^2/s, respectively). Although *D* value levels of focal defects in lymphoma nodes were also significantly smaller than those of focal defects in metastatic nodes, the values for lymphomas as well as metastatic nodes were widely distributed and greatly overlapped with each other (1.09 ± 0.41 for lymphomas vs. 1.42 ± 0.53 × 10^{-3} mm^2/s for metastatic nodes) (Fig. 7.4). The broad range of *D* values in metastatic nodes may be attributable to the different viscosity of coagulation and liquefaction necrosis in the metastatic nodes, with the former type having lower *D* values compared to the latter. On the other hand, necrotic tissues in lymphoma nodes may represent necrotizing granulomas mimicking tuberculosis with a high viscosity of caseous materials [32]. As a result, the *D* values of lymphoma nodes with focal defects were at levels similar to those of metastatic nodes with focal defects (1.09 ± 0.41 vs. 1.42 ± 0.53 × 10^{-3} mm^2/s, respectively). Accordingly, the *D* value cutoff threshold of 0.6 × 10^{-3} mm^2/s for the entire node was the best for discriminating between lymphoma from metastatic nodes without focal defects; and the *D* value cutoff threshold of 1.45 × 10^{-3} mm^2/s for focal defects was the best for differentiating between lymphomas and metastatic nodes with focal defects [11]. The presence or absence of focal defects and the nature of the defects in lymphoma nodes may be an important prognostic indicator in patients with non-Hodgkin lymphoma [33].

Perfusion levels of lymphomas as assessed by *f* values are the smallest among different types of head and neck tumors [8]. These results may be explained by the differences in the relative areas of stromal tissues among the head and neck tumors, with lymphomas exclusively comprising condensed proliferating lymphoma cells and scarce amounts of stromal tissues between tumor cells [34].

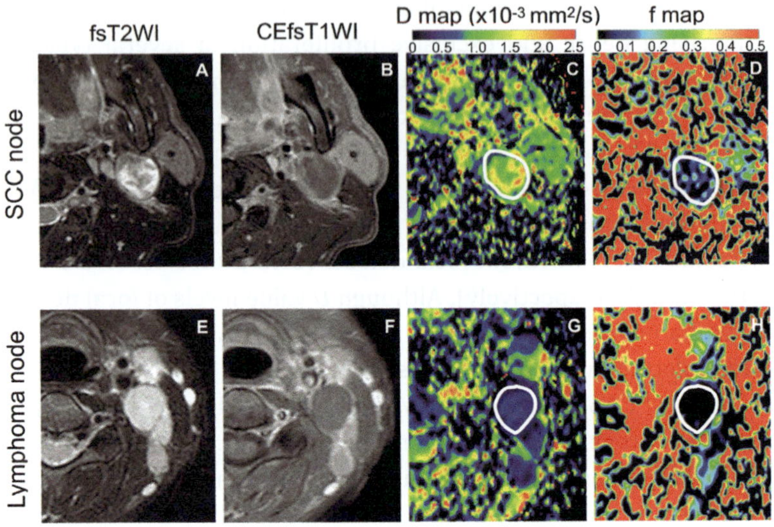

Figure 7.4 Representative fat-suppressed T2-weighted (fsT2WI) and contrast-enhanced fat-suppressed T1-weighted (CEfsT1WI) MR images and geo *D* and geo *f* maps of metastatic (SCC node) and lymphoma nodes with focal defects. (**A–D**) A 52-year-old man with SCC in the tongue. A metastatic node in the neck level IIA (**A**) contains a large nonenhanced area (**B**) with $D = 1.32 \times 10^{-3}$ mm^2/s (**C**) and geo $f = 0.092$ (**D**). (**E–H**) A 50-year-old woman with adult T-cell leukemia lymphoma. A lymphoma node in the neck level IIA (**E**) contains a large nonenhanced area (**F**), with $D = 0.47 \times 10^{-3}$ mm^2/s (**G**) and geo $f = 0$ (**H**). White demarcations on geo *D* (**C, G**) and geo *f* maps (**D, H**) indicate areas of focal defect (nonenhanced areas) within the nodes. Note that some perfusion activity remains in the focal defect of the metastatic node (**D**) but apparent perfusion signals are not detected in that of lymphoma node (**H**). Geo *D* and *f* values were calculated using *b* values of 500 and 1000 s/mm^2.

7.3.2 Differential Diagnosis from Nasopharyngeal Cancer

IVIM imaging is useful in differentiating between primary central nervous system lymphomas (PCNSLs) and glioblastomas that have some common conventional MRI findings [35–37]. The maximum values of microvascular volume fraction (f_{max}) of glioblastomas, which were determined from multiple regions of interest (ROIs) placed within the tumor areas of brain diffusion-weighted (DW) MR images, were significantly greater than those of PCNSLs. However, the results were controversial among the studies for minimum values of pure diffusion (D_{min}).

Glioblastomas are to PCNSLs what NPCs are to extracranial head and neck lymphomas (ECHNLs). These head and neck tumors have indistinguishable MRI features on T1- and fat-suppressed T2-weighted MR images and have similar levels of apparent diffusion coefficient (ADC) values [38]. NPCs encompass differentiated or undifferentiated nonkeratinized carcinomas, keratinizing squamous cell carcinomas, and basaloid squamous cell carcinomas. Of these NPC subtypes, the majority (75%–99%) are nonkeratinized carcinomas, which are histologically characterized by sheets of densely proliferating carcinoma cells separated by an attenuated infiltrate of lymphocytes and plasma cells [39]. Therefore, with respect to tissue cellularity, NPCs may have histological characteristics very akin to those of lymphomas.

A separate study has shown that NPCs have significantly higher f and D^* values than lymphomas [40]. These results are consistent with the notion that lymphomas are composed of low-perfusion tissues compared with NPCs. In contrast to the aforementioned study [36], this study reported that the D values of lymphomas are significantly smaller than those of NPCs (0.53 ± 0.11 vs. $0.73 \pm 0.19 \times 10^{-3}$ mm^2/s). The discrepancy in the levels of NPC and lymphoma D values between these two studies may be explained by the differences in distributions of histological types of NPC and/or lymphoma cells. For instance, differences in the proportions of tumor areas having undifferentiated or differentiated features could affect the D values of the tumors since nonkeratinizing carcinoma cells with undifferentiated phenotypes are larger in size and their nuclear-to-cytoplasmic ratios are greater compared with the carcinoma cells with differentiated phenotypes [39]. The amounts of lymphocyte infiltration into the tumor areas may also influence the tumor D values.

7.4 Salivary Gland Tumors

7.4.1 Diffusion and Perfusion Characteristics of Salivary Gland Tumors

Most salivary gland tumors are of epithelial origin and composed of mixed areas of various cell types, including acinar, ductal, myoepithelial, and lymphoid cells, with varying degrees of differentiation, as well as cysts, necrosis, and myxomatous tissues. Therefore, there can be a broad range of morphological diversity between different salivary gland tumor types and sometimes within an individual salivary gland tumor type [39]. The histological diversity of salivary gland tumors makes the preoperative differential diagnosis of malignant from benign salivary gland tumors and of different subtypes of tumors very challenging.

Basically, conventional T1- and T2-weighted MRI features of the salivary glands are nonspecific. An alternative approach to differentiating between benign and malignant salivary gland tumors and desirably between different types of salivary gland tumors is to understand the distinctive perfusion and diffusion properties of salivary gland tumors. In this regard, some types of tumor tissues with specific diffusion and/or perfusion properties are predominant components of particular tumor types, and thus assessing these tumor properties may be useful for preoperative differential diagnosis of salivary gland tumors. Actually, extensive studies have demonstrated that DW and DCE MRI can provide a clue for discriminating malignant from benign salivary gland tumors and for differentiating between some subtypes of benign or malignant salivary gland tumors [12, 15, 41–43]. Accordingly, the tissue characterization of salivary gland tumors using high-resolution DW MRI and subsequent *D* value mapping analysis allows the effective discrimination of malignant from benign tumors [41]. However, due to an overlap within benign and malignant tumor groups and even between these groups, the precise diagnosis may be difficult on the basis of *D* values solely [42].

A related but more effective strategy for improving the diagnostic performance of benign and malignant salivary gland tumors may be the combined use of DW and DCE MRI techniques for predicting both diffusion and perfusion properties of salivary gland tumors. A stepwise approach using diffusion and perfusion MRI parameters accurately discriminated 18 malignant from 52 benign salivary gland tumors [44]. Similar attempts using the multiparametric MRI technique have also effectively differentiated between different types of sinonasal tumors and tumor-like lesions or between benign and malignant thyroid nodules [13, 45].

7.4.2 IVIM MRI–Based Differentiation of Benign and Malignant Salivary Gland Tumors

The diffusion and perfusion characteristics are physiologically and biologically different phenomena, with the former largely depending on the cell density and the latter being an important marker of many physiologic and pathologic processes. In addition, these tissue properties may be distinctive in some types of salivary gland tumors. Therefore, concomitant estimations of these two distinctive phenomena in tumor tissues may be helpful for the preoperative diagnosis of salivary gland tumors. However, performing both DW and DCE MRI at a single examination would be very time consuming. Moreover, the use of gadolinium-based contrast agents may be contraindicated in some patients with acute and/or chronic kidney insufficiency with low estimated glomerular filtration rate (eGFR) values [46]. In this regard, IVIM MRI allows concomitant estimations of the physiologically and biologically different phenomena of tissue diffusion and perfusion by a single examination of DW MRI using multiple *b* values.

One of the very early studies using IVIM MRI for diagnosing salivary gland tumors showed that the *f* values of Warthin tumors were significantly larger than those of pleomorphic adenomas (0.16 ± 0.04 vs. 0.07 ± 0.03), the *D* values of malignant salivary gland tumors ($0.96 \pm 0.22 \times 10^{-3}$ mm^2/s) were significantly smaller than those of pleomorphic adenomas ($1.38 \pm 0.30 \times 10^{-3}$ mm^2/s) and were significantly larger than those of Warthin tumors ($0.61 \pm 0.11 \times 10^{-3}$ mm^2/s), and the *D** values of malignant tumors were significantly smaller than those of Warthin tumors ($21.99 \pm 19.01 \times 10^{-3}$ mm^2/s vs. $42.64 \pm 20.17 \times 10^{-3}$ mm^2/s) [3]. Accordingly, a stepwise approach using different combinations of *D* and *D** values provided the best diagnostic accuracy (100%) for differentiating among the three tumor types [3] (Fig. 7.5). Among the three types of salivary gland tumors, Warthin tumors have abundant lymphoid components, thereby more severely restricting the water diffusion than the pleomorphic adenomas and malignant salivary gland tumors, which contain large areas of cystic and fibromyxoid connective tissue components (pleomorphic adenomas), or proliferating cancer cells in the varying areas of stromal tissues (malignant salivary gland tumors). D^* is considered proportional to the mean capillary segment length and average blood velocity [1]. Previous studies using contrast-enhanced MRI showed that Warthin tumors are characterized by rapid-enhancement kinetics and pleomorphic adenomas by delayed-enhancement kinetics [12, 44]. On the other hand, some malignant salivary gland tumors (adenoid cystic carcinomas and carcinoma ex pleomorphic adenomas) exhibit delayed kinetics, while the other types exhibit rapid enhancement. Therefore, the low D^* cutoff threshold for pleomorphic adenomas ($D^* < 12 \times 10^{-3}$ mm^2/s) may reflect relatively low vascularity, with small blood flow and blood volume values, and the high D^* cutoff threshold for Warthin tumors ($D^* > 23 \times 10^{-3}$ mm^2/s) may reflect relatively high vascularity, with large blood flow and blood volume values of these tumors. The wide range of D^* values in malignant salivary gland tumors ($D^* = 12 - 23 \times 10^{-3}$ mm^2/s) are consistent with varying tumor vascularity among the malignant tumor subtypes [12, 15, 41–43].

The f value did not contribute to the best differentiation hierarchy of the stepwise processes in the aforementioned IVIM study [3]. The best f value cutoff threshold ($f \leq 0.10$) can distinguish between pleomorphic adenomas (0.07 ± 0.03) and Warthin tumors (0.16 ± 0.04) with 83% sensitivity, 100% specificity, and 90% accuracy. However, the f value alone was not able to effectively differentiate between benign and malignant salivary gland tumors. Similar results with the f value were obtained in differentiating between different types of head and neck tumors, where the varying f value cutoff thresholds were useful only in combinations with the different perfusion parameters that were determined by DCE MRI [10]. The f value can be defined as the fractional volume of capillary blood flow in each voxel [47]. Therefore, the f value may be proportional to the amount of normal angiogenesis with intact vascular permeability in the tissues. Equation 7.1 can be transformed as follows:

$$S_b = S_0 \cdot (1-f) \cdot \exp(-bD) + S_0 \cdot f \cdot \exp[-b(D + D^*)], \quad (7.5)$$

where $S_0 \cdot (1-f)$ indicates the signal intensity of a tumor excluding the blood capillaries at $b = 0$ (S_{ti}) and $S_0 \cdot f$ indicates the signal intensity of the blood capillaries in the tumor (S_{ca}), that is:

$$S_{ti} = S_0 \cdot (1-f) \quad (7.6)$$

and

$$S_{ca} = S_0 \cdot f \quad (7.7)$$

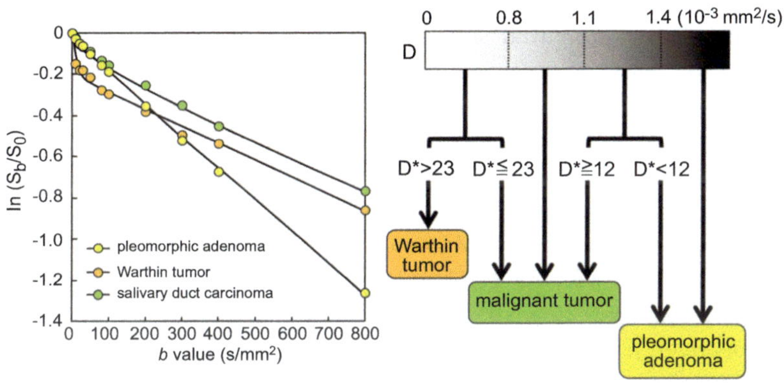

Figure 7.5 Differentiation of salivary gland tumors based on IVIM imaging. (**A**) IVIM diffusion decay curves obtained from a 62-year-old female patient with a pleomorphic adenoma (*D*, *f*, and *D** values = 1.50×10^{-3} mm²/s, 0.065, and 9.623 $\times 10^{-3}$ mm²/s, respectively); a 56-year-old male patient with a Warthin tumor (*D*, *f*, and *D** values = 0.78×10^{-3} mm²/s, 0.194, and 78.20×10^{-3} mm²/s, respectively); and a 55-year-old male patient with salivary duct carcinoma (*D*, *f*, and *D** values = 0.84×10^{-3} mm²/s, 0.093, and 15.59×10^{-3} mm²/s, respectively). (**B**) A schematic drawing shows an IVIM parameter–based strategy for differentiating between pleomorphic adenomas, Warthin tumors, and malignant tumors of the salivary glands. The combined use of *D* ($\times 10^{-3}$ mm²/s) and *D** ($\times 10^{-3}$ mm²/s) cutoff points achieves effective (100% accuracy) differentiation of the tumors in the present cohort. Geo *D* and *f* values were calculated using *b* values of 400 and 800 s/mm².

Accordingly, we can obtain the following formula:

$$f = S_{ca}/(S_{ca} + S_{ti}). \quad (7.8)$$

Therefore, the f value is defined as the signal intensity ratio of blood capillaries and tumor tissues. In the f value estimation, all relaxation effects are ignored. This assumption is acceptable as long as the relaxation times of tissues and blood capillaries are similar. However, T2 contributions from tumor tissues and blood capillaries are often greatly different [48]. It is well known that the T2 of tumor tissue tends to increase. Prolonged T2 of tumor tissue will lead to underestimation of the f value, which is further worsened by a longer echo time and an increased difference in T2 between the capillary blood and the tumor tissue. Therefore, one should carefully interpret the meaning of calculated f values. The IVIM parameters of salivary gland tumors can also be determined using geometrical analysis of the multiexponential signal decay curves instead of using the authentic least-squares method. Recently, IVIM values determined by geometric analysis or the authentic least-squares method have been compared for their diagnostic abilities for differentiating between different types of salivary gland tumors [9]. As expected, geo D^* values were greatly different from those determined by the least-squares method in pleomorphic adenomas ($0.35 \pm 0.19 \times 10^{-3}$ mm^2/s vs. $15.16 \pm 17.15 \times 10^{-3}$ mm^2/s, respectively), Warthin tumors ($0.70 \pm 0.20 \times 10^{-3}$ mm^2/s vs. $36.23 \pm 28.61 \times 10^{-3}$ mm^2/s, respectively), and malignant salivary gland tumors ($0.47 \pm 0.22 \times 10^{-3}$ mm^2/s vs. $18.38 \pm 17.84 \times 10^{-3}$ mm^2/s, respectively). However, f and D values were very similar between the two techniques for all the salivary gland tumor types: geo D and fit D values were $1.41 \pm 0.28 \times 10^{-3}$ mm^2/s and $1.40 \pm 0.28 \times 10^{-3}$ mm^2/s, respectively, for pleomorphic adenomas; $0.80 \pm 0.27 \times 10^{-3}$ mm^2/s and $0.79 \pm 0.27 \times 10^{-3}$ mm^2/s, respectively, for Warthin tumors; and $0.93 \pm 0.20 \times 10^{-3}$ mm^2/s and $0.94 \pm 0.22 \times 10^{-3}$ mm^2/s, respectively, for malignant salivary gland tumors. Geo f and fit f values were $0.07 \pm 0.04 \times 10^{-3}$ mm^2/s and $0.09 \pm 0.04 \times 10^{-3}$ mm^2/s, respectively, for pleomorphic adenomas; $0.13 \pm 0.04 \times 10^{-3}$ mm^2/s and $0.13 \pm 0.03 \times 10^{-3}$ mm^2/s, respectively, for Warthin tumors; and $0.09 \pm 0.04 \times 10^{-3}$ mm^2/s and $0.08 \pm 0.03 \times 10^{-3}$ mm^2/s, respectively, for malignant salivary gland tumors. Similar results were obtained for other types of head and neck tumors (lymphomas and squamous cell carcinomas). Accordingly, stepwise approaches using combinations of geo D and geo D^* values, geo D and geo f values, or fit D and fit D^* values differentiated between pleomorphic adenomas, Warthin tumors, and malignant salivary gland tumors with the same efficacy (91% accuracy). However, a stepwise differentiation using fit D and fit f values was less effective (83% accuracy). Considering cumbersome procedures and lower precisions (higher inter- and intraobserver errors) for determining the IVIM parameters with the least-squares method [9], the simple geometric analysis for IVIM parameters could be an alternative to the least-squares method in the clinic.

7.5 Masticator Muscles

7.5.1 Perfusion and Diffusion Kinetics of the Masticator Muscles during Clenching

The masseter, medial and lateral pterygoid, and temporal muscles are the primary masticator muscles. The masseter, medial pterygoid, and temporal muscles are involved in elevating the mandible, while the lateral pterygoid muscles participate in protruding (superior head) and depressing (inferior head) the mandible. The medial and lateral pterygoid and masseter muscles also participate in the lateral movement of the mandible. The mylohyoid, geniohyoid, and digastric muscles also participate in opening the mouth. Effective mastication can be achieved by the coordinate action of these muscles. In clenching, for example, the masseter, temporal, and medial pterygoid muscles are all involved in the process, but the lateral pterygoid muscles are not.

Application of IVIM imaging to the masticator muscles has been very limited. In a recent study, DW MRI was performed with healthy subjects at rest, and then the second MRI examination was performed after clenching a disposable bite block that was placed on the molars of the right side of the mandible (clenching side) [49]. After clenching, the f and D^* values of the masseter muscles on the clenching sides increased significantly from the resting states ($f = 0.17 \pm 0.10$ vs. 0.29 ± 0.11; $D^* = 21.3 \pm 18.5 \times 10^{-3}$ mm^2/s vs. $42.1 \pm 33.3 \times 10^{-3}$ mm^2/s). The f values of the medial pterygoid muscles also increased significantly on the clenching sides (0.20 ± 0.09 vs. 0.30 ± 0.09), but not the D^* values. On the balancing (opposite) sides, the f values of the masseter muscles (0.19 ± 0.12 vs. 0.30 ± 0.12)

and medial pterygoid muscles (0.20 ± 0.09 vs. 0.29 ± 0.11) increased significantly during clenching, implying that they work cooperatively with the muscles on the clenching side. In contrast, the IVIM values of the lateral pterygoid muscles, which do not participate in clenching, did not change on the clenching or balancing sides. Interestingly, the D values of the three masticator muscles (the masseters and the medial and lateral pterygoids) did not change during clenching. These results are consistent with the notion that the masticator muscles work via isometric contraction without changes in muscle length during clenching [49, 50]. In contrast, the extremity muscles work by means of isotonic contraction, thereby decreasing the sarcomere length and increasing the diameters of the fibers and microfibrils. These morphologic changes will increase the D values [51, 52].

The physiologic relevance of changes in f and D^* values during clenching has not been fully understood. Perfusion allows the delivery of oxygen and metabolic substrates that are needed for the muscles to maintain functional integrity. Further, a strong muscle contraction can induce a transient hypoxic state owing to mechanical compression [53]. Therefore, adequate adaptation of muscle perfusion to the local demands may be an important physiological process. In addition, the assessment of muscle perfusion is essential for understanding the disease states of muscle dysfunction, including temporomandibular joint dysfunction [54].

References

1. Le Bihan D., Breton E., Lallemand D., Aubin M. L., Vignaud, J., Laval-Jeantet M. (1988). Separation of diffusion and perfusion in intravoxel incoherent motion MR imaging. *Radiology,* 168, 497–505.
2. Luciani A., Vignaud A., Cavet M., Nhieu J. T., Mallat A., Ruel. L., et al. (2008). Liver cirrhosis: intravoxel incoherent motion MR imaging—pilot study. *Radiology*, 249, 891–899.
3. Sumi M., Van Cauteren M., Sumi T., Obara M., Ichikawa Y., Nakamura T. (2012). Salivary gland tumors: use of intravoxel incoherent motion MR imaging for assessment of diffusion and perfusion for the differentiation of benign from malignant tumors. *Radiology*, 263, 770–777.

4. Zhou X. J., Gao Q., Abdullah O., Magin R. L. (2010). Studies of anomalous diffusion in the human brain using fractional order calculus. *Magn. Reson. Med.*, 63, 562–569.
5. Moteki T., Horikoshi H. (2006). Evaluation of hepatic lesions and hepatic parenchyma using diffusion-weighted echo-planar MR with three values of gradient b-factor. *J. Magn. Reson. Imaging*, 24, 637–645.
6. Lewin M., Fartoux L., Vignaud A., Arrivé L., Menu Y., Rosmorduc O. (2011). The diffusion-weighted imaging perfusion fraction f is a potential marker of sorafenib treatment in advanced hepatocellular carcinoma: a pilot study. *Eur. Radiol.*, 21, 281–290.
7. Mazaheri Y., Vargas H. A., Akin O., Goldman D. A., Hricak H. (2012). Reducing the influence of b-value selection on diffusion-weighted imaging of the prostate: evaluation of a revised monoexponential model within a clinical setting. *J. Magn. Reson. Imaging*, 35, 660–668.
8. Sumi M., Nakamura T. (2013). Head and neck tumors: assessment of perfusion-related parameters and diffusion coefficients based on the intravoxel incoherent motion model. *AJNR Am. J. Neuroradiol.*, 34, 410–416.
9. Sasaki M., Sumi M., Eida S., Katayama I., Hotokezaka Y., Nakamura T. (2014). Simple and reliable determination of intravoxel incoherent motion parameters for the differential diagnosis of head and neck tumors. *PLoS One*, 9(11), e112866.
10. Sumi M., Nakamura T. (2014). Head and neck tumours: combined MRI assessment based on IVIM and TIC analyses for the differentiation of tumors of different histological types. *Eur. Radiol.*, 24, 223–231.
11. Sumi M., Nakamura T. (2009). Diagnostic importance of focal defects in the apparent diffusion coefficient-based differentiation between lymphoma and squamous cell carcinoma nodes in the neck. *Eur. Radiol.*, 19, 975–981.
12. Eida S., Ohki M., Sumi M., Yamada T., Nakamura T. (2008). MR factor analysis: improved technology for the assessment of 2D dynamic structures of benign and malignant salivary gland tumors. *J. Magn. Reson. Imaging*, 27, 1256–1262.
13. Sasaki M., Sumi M., Eida S., Ichikawa Y., Sumi T., Yamada T., et al. (2011). Multiparametric MR imaging of sinonasal diseases: time-signal intensity curve- and apparent diffusion coefficient-based differentiation between benign and malignant lesions. *AJNR Am. J. Neuroradiol.*, 32, 2154–2159.

14. Eida S., Sumi M., Nakamura T. (2010). Multiparametric magnetic resonance imaging for the differentiation between benign and malignant salivary gland tumors. *J. Magn. Reson. Imaging,* 31, 673–679.
15. Yabuuchi H., Fukuya T., Tajima T., Hachitanda Y., Tomita K., Koga M. (2003). Salivary gland tumors: diagnostic value of gadolinium-enhanced dynamic MR imaging with histopathologic correlation. *Radiology,* 226, 345–354.
16. Zhou N., Chu C., Dou X., Li M., Liu S., Zhu L., et al. (2016). Early evaluation of irradiated parotid glands with intravoxel incoherent motion MR imaging: correlation with dynamic contrast-enhanced MR imaging. *BMC Cancer,* 16, 865.
17. Amit M., Yen T. C., Liao C. T., Binenbaum Y., Chaturvedi P., Agarwal J. P., et al. (2013). Clinical nodal stage is a significant predictor of outcome in patients with oral cavity squamous cell carcinoma and pathologically negative neck metastases: results of the international consortium for outcome research. *Ann. Surg. Oncol.,* 20, 3575–3581.
18. Sumi M., Kimura Y., Sumi T., Nakamura T. (2007). Diagnostic performance of MRI relative to CT for metastatic nodes of head and neck squamous cell carcinomas. *J. Magn. Reson. Imaging,* 26, 1626–1633.
19. Nakamura T., Sumi M. (2007). Nodal imaging in the neck: recent advances in US, CT and MR imaging of metastatic nodes. *Eur. Radiol.,* 17, 1235–1241.
20. Amin M. B., Edge S.B, Greene F. L., Byrd D. R., Brookland R. K., Washington M. K., et al. eds. (2017) *AJCC Cancer Staging Manual* 8th Ed. (Springer, New York).
21. Brierley J. D., Gospodarowicz M. K., Witterkind C., O'Sullivan B., Mason M., Asamura H., et al. eds. (2017) *TNM Classification of Malignant Tumours* (Willey Blackwell, UK).
22. Sumi M., Eida S., Nakamura T. (2017). Extranodal spread of primary and secondary metastatic nodes: The dominant risk factor of survival in patients with head and neck squamous cell carcinoma. *PLoS One,* 12(8), e0183611.
23. Sumi M., Nakamura T. (2011). Extranodal spread in the neck: MRI detection on the basis of pixel-based time-signal intensity curve analysis. *J. Magn. Reson. Imaging,* 33, 830–838.
24. Xiao Y., Pan J., Chen Y., Chen Y., He Z., Zheng X. (2015). Intravoxel incoherent motion-magnetic resonance imaging as an early predictor of treatment response to neoadjuvant chemotherapy in locoregionally

advanced nasopharyngeal carcinoma, *Medicine (Baltimore)*, 94(24), e973.

25. Paudyal R., Oh J.H., Riaz N., Venigalla P., Li J., Hatzoglou V. et al. (2017). Intravoxel incoherent motion diffusion-weighted MRI during chemoradiation therapy to characterize and monitor treatment response in human papillomavirus head and neck squamous cell carcinoma. *J. Magn. Reson. Imaging*, 45, 1013–1023.
26. Fujima N., Yoshida D., Sakashita T., Homma A., Tsukahara A., Shimizu Y., et al. (2017). Prediction of the treatment outcome using intravoxel incoherent motion and diffusional kurtosis imaging in nasal or sinonasal squamous cell carcinoma patients. *Eur. Radiol.*, 27, 956–965.
27. Hauser T., Essig M., Jensen A., Laun F. B., Münter M., Maier-Hein K. H., et al. (2014). Prediction of treatment response in head and neck carcinomas using IVIM-DWI: Evaluation of lymph node metastasis. *Eur. J. Radiol.*, 83, 783–787.
28. Lu L., Li Y., Li W. (2016). The role of intravoxel incoherent motion MRI in predicting early treatment response to chemoradiation for metastatic lymph nodes in nasopharyngeal carcinoma. *Adv. Ther.*, 33, 1158–1168.
29. Marzi S., Piludu F., Sanguineti G., Marucci L., Farneti A., Terrenato I., et al. (2017).The prediction of the treatment response of cervical nodes using intravoxel incoherent motion diffusion-weighted imaging. *Eur. J. Radiol.*, 92, 93–102.
30. Tshering Vogel D. W., Zbaeren P., Geretschlaeger A., Vermathen P., De Keyzer F., Thoeny, H.C. (2013). Diffusion-weighted MR imaging including bi-exponential fitting for the detection of recurrent or residual tumour after (chemo)radiotherapy for laryngeal and hypopharyngeal cancers. *Eur. Radiol.*, 23, 562–569.
31. Campo E., Swerdlow S. H., Harris N. L., Pileri S., Stein H., Jaffe E.S. (2011). The 2008 WHO classification of lymphoid neoplasms and beyond: evolving concepts and practical applications. *Blood*, 117, 5019–5032.
32. Hall P.A., Kingston J., Stansfeld A.G. (1988). Extensive necrosis in malignant lymphoma with granulomatous reaction mimicking tuberculosis. *Histopathology*, 13, 339–346.
33. Saito A., Takashima S., Takayama F., Kawakami S., Momose M., Matsushita T. (2001). Spontaneous extensive necrosis in non-Hodgkin lymphoma: prevalence and clinical significance. *J. Comput. Assist. Tomogr.* 25 482–486.

34. Swerdlow S. H., Campo E., Haris N. L., Jaffe E. S., Pileri S. A., Stein H., et al. eds. (2008) *WHO Classification of Tumours of Haematopoietic and Lymphoid Tissues* 4th Ed. (IARC Press, Lyon).

35. Suh C. H., Kim H. S., Lee S. S., Kim N., Yoon H. M., Choi C. G., et al. (2014). Atypical imaging features of primary central nervous system lymphoma that mimics glioblastoma: utility of intravoxel incoherent motion MR imaging. *Radiology* , 272, 504–513.

36. Shim W. H., Kim H. S., Choi C. G., Kim S.J. (2015). Comparison of apparent diffusion coefficient and intravoxel incoherent motion for differentiating among glioblastoma, metastasis, and lymphoma focusing on diffusion-related parameter. *PLoS One*, 10(7), e0134761.

37. Yamashita K., Hiwatashi A., Togao O., Kikuchi K., Kitamura Y., Mizoguchi M., et al. (2016). Diagnostic utility of intravoxel incoherent motion MR imaging in differentiating primary central nervous system lymphoma from glioblastoma multiforme. *J. Magn. Reson. Imaging*, 44, 1256–1261.

38. Ichikawa Y., Sumi, M, Sasaki M., Sumi T., Nakamura T. (2012). Efficacy of diffusion-weighted imaging for the differentiation between lymphomas and carcinomas of the nasopharynx and oropharynx: correlations of apparent diffusion coefficients and histologic features. *AJNR Am. J. Neuroradiol.*, 33, 761–766.

39. Barnes L., Eveson J. E., Reichart P., Sidransky D. eds. (2005) *Pathology and Genetics of Head and Neck Tumours* (IARC Press, Lyon).

40. Yu X. P., Hou J., Li F. P., Wang H., Hu P. S., Bi F., et al. (2016). Intravoxel incoherent motion diffusion-weighted magnetic resonance imaging for differentiation between nasopharyngeal carcinoma and lymphoma at the primary site. *J. Comput. Assist. Tomogr.*, 40, 413–418.

41. Eida S., Sumi M., Sakihama N., Takahashi H., Nakamura T. (2007). Apparent diffusion coefficient mapping of salivary gland tumors: prediction of the benignancy and malignancy. *AJNR Am J Neuroradiol.*, 28, 116–121.

42. Habermann C. R., Arndt C., Graessner J., Diestel L., Petersen K. U., Reitmeier F., et al. (2009). Diffusion-weighted echo-planar MR imaging of primary parotid gland tumors: is a prediction of different histologic subtypes possible? *AJNR Am. J. Neuroradiol.*, 30, 591–596.

43. Katayama I., Eida S., Fujita S., Hotokezaka Y., Sumi M., Nakamura T. (2017). Perfusion MR imaging detection of carcinoma arising from preexisting salivary gland pleomorphic adenoma by computer-assisted analysis of time-signal intensity maps. *PLoS One*, 12(5), e0178002

44. Eida S., Sumi M., Nakamura T. (2010). Multiparametric magnetic resonance imaging for the differentiation between benign and malignant salivary gland tumors. *J. Magn. Reson. Imaging*, 31, 673–679.

45. Sasaki M., Sumi M., Kaneko K., Ishimaru K., Takahashi H., Nakamura T. (2013). Multiparametric MR imaging for differentiating between benign and malignant thyroid nodules: initial experience in 23 patients. *J. Magn. Reson. Imaging*, 38, 64–71.

46. Tsai L. L., Grant A. K., Mortele K. J., Kung J. W., Smith M.P. (2015). A practical guide to MR imaging safety: What radiologists need to know. *Radiographics*, 35, 1722–1737.

47. Le Bihan D., Turner R. (1992). The capillary network: a link between IVIM and classical perfusion. *Magn. Reson. Med.*, 27, 171–178.

48. Clark C. A., Le Bihan D. (2000). Water diffusion compartmentation and anisotropy at high b values in the human brain. *Magn. Reson. Med.*, 44, 852–859.

49. Sasaki M., Sumi M., Van Cauteren M., Obara M., Nakamura T. (2013). Intravoxel incoherent motion imaging of masticatory muscles: pilot study for the assessment of perfusion and diffusion during clenching. *AJR Am. J. Roentgenol.*, 201, 1101–1107.

50. Karampinos D. C., King K. F., Sutton B. P., Georgiadis J. G. (2010). Intravoxel partially coherent motion technique: characterization of the anisotropy of skeletal muscle microvasculature. *J. Magn. Reson. Imaging*, 31, 942–953.

51. Deux J. F., Malzy P., Paragios N., Bassez G., Luciani A., Zerbib P., et al. (2008). Assessment of calf muscle contraction by diffusion tensor imaging. *Eur. Radiol.*, 18, 2303–2310.

52. Schraml C., Schwenzer N. F., Martirosian P., Claussen C. D., Schick F. (2011). Temporal course of perfusion in human masseter muscle during isometric contraction assessed by arterial spin labeling at 3T. *MAGMA*, 24, 201–209.

53. Filli L., Boss A., Wurnig M. C., Kenkel D., Andreisek G., Guggenberger R. (2015). Dynamic intravoxel incoherent motion imaging of skeletal muscle at rest and after exercise. *NMR Biomed.*, 28, 240–246.

54. Nguyen A., Ledoux J. B., Omoumi P., Becce F., Forget J., Federau C. (2017). Selective microvascular muscle perfusion imaging in the shoulder with intravoxel incoherent motion (IVIM). *Magn. Reson. Imaging*, 35, 91–97.

Chapter 8

IVIM MRI of the Breast

Mami Iima [a,b] **and Masako Kataoka** [a]
[a]*Department of Diagnostic Imaging and Nuclear Medicine, Graduate School of Medicine, Kyoto University, Kyoto 606-8507, Japan*
[b]*The Hakubi Center for Advanced Research, Kyoto University 54 Shogoin-kawaharacho, Sakyo-ku, Kyoto 606-8501, Japan*
mamiiima@kuhp.kyoto-u.ac.jp

Breast cancer is one of the most common neoplasms among women worldwide [1]. Tumor angiogenesis plays a crucial role in local tumor growth and distant metastasis and is considered an important prognostic factor in breast cancer [2, 3]. The intravoxel incoherent motion (IVIM) model can investigate both tissue diffusivity and tissue microcapillary perfusion without the need for contrast agents, which are currently essential in breast magnetic resonance imaging (MRI) in clinical practice. This approach was explored in human brain and bone by Le Bihan et al. in the 1980s [4] and now is experiencing a dramatic revival in neuroimaging and oncology.

The IVIM model was first investigated in breast cancer patients by Sigmund et al. in 2011 [5]. They found some nonsignificant

Intravoxel Incoherent Motion (IVIM) MRI: Principles and Applications
Edited by Denis Le Bihan, Mami Iima, Christian Federau, and Eric E. Sigmund

ISBN 978-981-4800-19-8 (Hardcover), 978-0-429-42727-5 (eBook)
www.panstanford.com

variations in perfusion fraction, fp (which is equivalent to flowing blood volume fraction, f_{IVIM}), between invasive ductal carcinoma and other histologic subtypes (10.5 ± 5.0% vs. 6.9 ± 2.9%, $p = 0.06$). Since then, numerous studies with larger cohorts have been initiated by these authors and others to investigate the perfusion and diffusion characteristics of different breast lesions.

Recent developments in MRI hardware have enabled the acquisition of higher *b* values (larger than 600 s/mm^2) compared with those in the 1980s. At the same time, the original analysis of the IVIM signal component has been updated to account for non-Gaussian DWI and noise floor effects observed at high *b* values (especially with values larger than 1000 s/mm^2). Accordingly, the combination of IVIM and non-Gaussian DWI has recently been explored [6, 7]. In addition to IVIM parameters, non-Gaussian diffusion can be investigated using appropriate models, such as the kurtosis model, which provides estimates of ADC_0; the theoretical "free diffusion" ADC (apparent diffusion coefficient), which would be obtained at a *b* value of 0 s/mm^2; and *K*, the kurtosis parameter that quantifies the non-Gaussian diffusion effect.

8.1 Using IVIM to Distinguish Malignant from Benign Lesions and Normal Breast Tissue

Some studies have revealed that the fp in malignant lesions is significantly higher than that in benign lesions and normal breast tissue [7–9]; however, there is a large overlap with benign lesions. Examples of typical malignant and benign breast lesions are shown in Figs. 8.1 and 8.2. A combination of high flowing blood volume fraction (f_{IVIM})/high kurtosis (*K*)/low ADC_0 is often observed at the periphery of tumors, while the necrotic central part exhibits an opposite pattern, in good agreement with contrast-enhanced (CE) images in Fig. 8.1.

Fibroadenomas display a low f_{IVIM}/high ADC_0/low *K* combination, with weak and slow/persistent kinetics in the lesion on dynamic contrast-enhanced magnetic resonance imaging (DCE MRI, Fig. 8.2).

Nine studies of IVIM in breast tumor patients, totaling 714 women, are summarized in a review on breast diffusion-weighted imaging (DWI) [10]. According to this review, malignant lesions had significantly lower tissue diffusivity (Dt) values than benign lesions in all five studies that compared malignant to benign lesions, yielding a mean sensitivity of 86 ± 13%, specificity of 81 ± 19%, and accuracy of 84 ± 12%. Malignant lesions had significantly higher fp values in 4 of 5 studies, with a mean sensitivity of 82 ± 8%, specificity of 81 ± 20%, and accuracy of 84 ± 2% compared with benign lesions. An updated review comprises 15 studies [5, 7–9, 11–21] on IVIM metrics or analysis in human breast cancer lesions, with a total of 1089 patients. Among these studies, 8 showed significantly lower Dt in malignant lesions (for 7 reporting studies, sensitivity 87±10% and specificity 79±17%) and 7 showed significantly higher fp in malignant lesions (for 6 reporting studies, average sensitivity 81±7% and specificity 75±13%). In all studies reporting diagnostic performance [8, 9, 11, 12, 21], IVIM outperformed ADC. The approach of combining parameters to improve diagnostic accuracy has been also explored [11, 22–24].

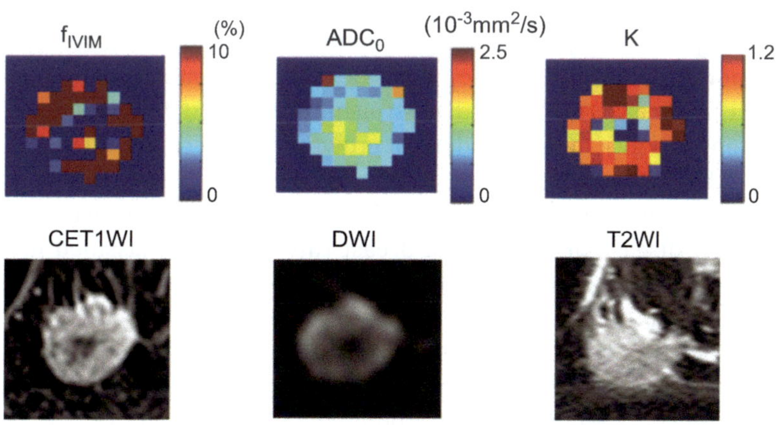

Figure 8.1 f_{IVIM}, ADC_0 (theoretical ADC at *b* value of 0 s/mm^2), and *K* (kurtosis) maps and the conventional MR images of an invasive ductal carcinoma in a 44-year-old woman. (Upper row) f_{IVIM}, ADC_0, and *K* maps. (Lower row), contrast-enhanced (CE) T1-weighted images (T1WI), DWI, and T2-weighted images (T2WI).

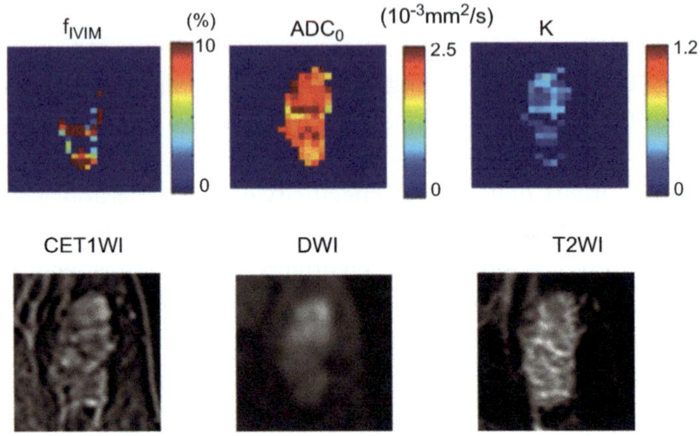

Figure 8.2 f_{IVIM}, K, and ADC_0 maps and conventional MR images of a fibroadenoma in a 63-year-old woman. (Upper row) f_{IVIM}, K, and ADC_0 maps. (Lower row) CE T1WI, DWI, and T2WI.

8.2 IVIM for Identification of Prognostic Factors/Subtypes in Breast Cancers

Improvements in breast cancer treatment highlight the increasing importance of prognostic factors [25]. Immunohistochemistry (IHC) biomarkers, such as the estrogen receptor (ER), progesterone receptor (PgR), human epidermal growth factor receptor 2 (HER2), and the proliferation marker Ki-67, together with clinicopathologic features, are conventionally used to classify breast cancer and predict disease outcome [26]. Breast cancer can be classified into several subtypes on the basis of these molecular markers, that is, Luminal A, Luminal B and HER2 negative, Luminal B and HER2 positive, HER2 enriched, and triple negative. Stratification of breast cancer by clinically relevant subtypes is required for treatment planning [27]. More and more studies have investigated this [11, 13, 14, 19, 23, 24, 28]. Interestingly, some researchers have estimated the histogram metrics of IVIM. The findings from each of the above-mentioned studies are summarized in Table 8.1. Some groups found that IVIM and diffusion parameters and their histogram metrics differed depending on ER or PgR expression. Cho et al. reported that fp and pseudodiffusivity (Dp) were significantly correlated with hormonal factor expression (ER or PgR) [11]. They also found that the histogram IVIM parameters might show less vendor system variability and higher combined performance compared to mean IVIM values alone, when comparing data acquired at different MR vendor systems [29]. Suo and colleagues found that the fast component of diffusion (Df) was significantly correlated with Ki-67 expression, while ADC, the slow component of diffusion (Ds), the fraction of fast diffusion (*f*), the distributed diffusion coefficient (DDC), and the mean diffusivity (MD) were significantly correlated with ER expression [19].

Some IVIM parameters were found to be significantly linked to different tumor subtypes. Iima et al. have found that synthetic ADC ($sADC_{200-1500}$) (calculated using b = 200 and 1500 s/mm^2) was significantly different among tumor subtypes (p = 0.006) [30]. Kim et al. and Kawashima et al. found that both Dt and ADC values in luminal B cancers were significantly lower in luminal A cancers and other tumor subtypes [13, 28].

8.3 The Multiparametric Approach: IVIM in Combination with Dynamic Contrast–Enhanced MRI, DWI, or Positron-Emission Tomography/MRI

DCE MRI has been established as a valuable tool in breast cancer diagnosis, with excellent sensitivity and variable specificity [31, 32]. Multiparametric MRI, including IVIM, has been developed to overcome the limitations in the specificity of DCE MRI [33, 34].

The correlation between IVIM and DCE MRI parameters has been investigated. Liu and colleagues found that combined microvascular volume fraction (*f*) values had a moderate correlation with the blood volume fraction (V_p) (r = 0.692) and a poor correlation with the volume transfer constant (K^{trans}) (r = 0.456) in 36 malignant and 23 benign breast lesions [15]. Jiang and colleagues found that areas under the curve (AUCs) of *f* plus pseudodiffusion coefficient (D^*) (0.834) were not significantly different from the AUCs of DCE-derived parameters (0.876–0.904) [35] in 31 malignant and

Table 8.1 Correlation of IVIM and DWI parameters with molecular prognostic factors in breast cancers. All studies were conducted using 3T MRI scanners

Author [Reference]	*b* values	Cases (n)	Hormonal receptor	Subtype
Cho 2016 [11]	0, 30, 70, 100, 150, 200, 300, 400, 500, 800	50	ADCmax, Dmax, DtSD, Dp kurtosis, Dp skewness for ER ADCmin, Dtmin, DtSD, Dp max, Dp skewness, fp kurtosis, fp skewness for PgR	Dp average, Dp skewness, Dp kurtosis significantly differentiated ER+HER2− from ER+HER2+
Kim 2016 [13]	0, 30, 70, 100, 150, 200, 300, 400, 500, 800	275	Dt significantly lower in high-Ki-67 than low Ki-67 tumors	Dt and ADC significantly lower in luminal B
Iima 2017 [23]	5, 10, 20, 30, 50, 70, 100, 200, 400, 600, 800, 1000, 1500, 2000, 2500	76 (training) 76 (validation)	$sADC_{200\text{-}1500}$ for PgR	$sADC_{200\text{-}1500}$ significantly different among subtypes
Vidić 2017 [24]	0, 10, 20, 30, 40, 50, 70, 90, 120, 150, 200, 400, 700	28	N/A	Combined model distinguished ER+HER2− from vER+HER2+ with high accuracy (0.90)
Lee 2017 [14]	0, 25, 50, 75, 100, 150, 200, 300, 500, 800	72	Dslow 50th, 75th, and 90th significantly lower in ER+ compared to ER− Dslow 75th percentile a significant differentiator of Ki-67 grouping	Dslow 75th percentile a significant differentiator of tumor subtype
Suo 2017 [19]	0, 10, 30, 50, 100, 150, 200, 500, 800, 1000, 1500, 2000, 2500	57	ADC, Ds, f, DDC, and MD for ER; Df and α significantly correlated with Ki-67 expression compared with luminal A	N/A
Kawashima 2017 [28]	0, 20, 40, 80, 120, 200, 400, 600, 800	134	N/A	D and ADC were significantly lower in luminal B

35 benign breast lesions. However, a correlation between IVIM parameters and microvascular density obtained from CD31 stain was not observed in a chemically induced rat model of mammary carcinoma [36]. Conversely, numerous studies found a correlation between microvessel density and IVIM parameters in other organs; a correlation was observed between microvessel density and IVIM perfusion measures Dp and fp in mouse colorectal cancer [37] and gastric cancer [38] models and between microvessel density and fp in a rat brain glioma model [6] and a mouse model of hepatocellular carcinoma (HCC) [39], pancreatic ductal adenocarcinomas and pancreatic neuroendocrine tumors [40], and meningiomas [41]. D^* and fD^* values had correlation with the mean vessel diameter (MVD) in patients with rectal cancer [42]. Dp was significantly correlated with MVD in abdominal organs of mice ($r = 0.90$, $p = 0.037$) [43].

Wang and colleagues investigated several indicators, including the initial enhancement ratio (IER), the time-signal intensity curve (TIC), ADC, the diffusion coefficient (D), D^*, and f in 23 benign and 31 malignant breast tumors [44]. They found that D derived from IVIM had the highest AUC in distinguishing malignant from benign breast tumors. Both D and TIC were identified as independent predictors of malignancy, with the combination of D and TIC providing an AUC of up to 0.990. Ma et al. assessed the diagnostic performance of DCE MRI and combined DCE MRI and IVIM DWI for 47 benign and 81 malignant breast tumors [16]. DCE MRI provided 90.1% sensitivity, 70.2% specificity, and 82.8% accuracy. The combination of DCE MRI and IVIM DWI provided 88.8% sensitivity, 85.1% specificity, and 87.5% accuracy. The authors concluded that IVIM DWI may be helpful as an adjunct to DCE MRI to improve specificity and accuracy. Dijkstra et al. reported that the combined diagnostic approach of DCE MRI and IVIM improved specificity significantly when compared with DCE MRI alone (from 30.4% to 56.5%; $p = 0.016$) as a problem solver for distinguishing BI-RADS 3 and 4 lesions in 139 breast lesions (including 7 BI-RADS 3 and 19 BI-RADS 4 lesions) [45].

The clinical usefulness of using IVIM in 18-fluorodeoxyglucose positron-emission tomography/MRI (FDG-PET/MRI) has also been investigated. Ostenson and colleagues found that the correlation coefficient of the standardized uptake value (SUV) and Dt was a significant indicator for distinguishing between treated and nontreated patients. The correlation of SUV and fp was negative for all cohorts, suggesting the possibility that lesions with stronger limited diffusion and greater negative correlation coefficients of SUV with fp might indicate more aggressive tumor growth [17].

The merit of IVIM in combination with other techniques, such as DCE MRI or FDG-PET/MRI, includes the potential to improve the diagnostic accuracy or predict the treatment response of breast cancers without any gadolinium contrast agents. The multiparametric approach can be applied using only DWI-related parameters. Recent studies have shown improved diagnostic performance for differentiation between malignant and benign breast tumors using an IVIM and DWI multiparametric method with a support vector machine [24, 46]. Combined IVIM parameters provided significantly better specificity than ADC alone (43.5%–52.5% vs. 13.0%–21.7%, $p \leq 0.0034$), using a semiautomated method in 139 breast lesions [12].

It has been shown that a multiparametric approach combining only IVIM and non-Gaussian DWI is almost as accurate as the current diagnostic performance for the differentiation of malignant and benign breast tumors using BI-RADS for MRI [30]. Our study comprised 199 patients with breast tumors. Multiparametric threshold scores or probabilities using Bayesian analysis were established to maximize the diagnostic ability of flowing blood volume fraction (f_{IVIM}), ADC_0, and K parameters. Sensitivity and specificity with two independent radiologists interpreting ranges between 89.5%–96.1% and 66.7%–88.3%, respectively, for the multiparametric DWI approach, which is comparable to those for BI-RADS (100% sensitivity and 79.2% specificity). These diffusion MRI-derived approaches have the potential to be an appealing alternative to DCE MRI in patients in whom contrast agents are contraindicated, such as pregnant patients or patients with renal dysfunction. This is also an important feature to consider given the accumulating evidence of gadolinium deposition in the brain [47].

8.4 IVIM for Prediction of the Treatment Response

The performance of IVIM in the prediction of the treatment response (mainly neoadjuvant chemotherapy [NAC]) in breast cancer has been recently explored. Cho and colleagues found that the pretreatment average, skewness, and K of Dp were significant differentiators of responders from nonresponders in 32 lesions [48]. Kim and colleagues assessed 46 patients with stage II or III breast cancer and found that pretreatment IVIM histogram parameters, including the mean, 25th percentile, 50th percentile, and 75th percentile of D obtained from the histogram of the whole tumor (D_{mean}, D_{25}, D_{50}, and D_{75}, respectively), were significantly higher in good responders than in poorer responders [49]. Che et al. showed that the f value before NAC of patients with a pathologic complete response (pCR) was significantly larger than that of non-pCR patients and the change in f after two cycles of NAC was also significantly larger than that in the non-pCR group in 28 patients with locally advanced breast cancer [50]. These IVIM values and histogram metrics might serve as prognostic biomarkers for the selection of neoadjuvant treatment.

IVIM has also been investigated for the evaluation of radiotherapy response in bone metastases from breast cancer [51] or prediction of the outcome [52], early arterial blood flow stasis, or tumor size change and RECIST response [53] in radioembolization of liver metastases from breast cancer.

8.5 IVIM in Lactation

Evaluation of the lactating breast by DCE MRI is challenging due to marked background parenchymal enhancement. IVIM might be a promising alternative method in this context, yet baseline data are currently limited. Breast appearance in lactation depends upon milk content (i.e., pre- or post-breastfeeding). Nissan et al. have reported a significant change in diffusion tensor imaging (DTI) parameters (larger MD and lower fractional anisotropy [FA]) in lactating compared with postweaning women [54]. However, no evidence exists on the optimal timing to scan lactating breasts (i.e., pre- or post-breastfeeding) so far. We have investigated the effect of breastfeeding on IVIM and non-Gaussian diffusion (NGD) parameters in lactating women (Fig. 8.3). A significant increase in f_{IVIM} values after breastfeeding (1.97 vs. 2.97%, $p < 0.01$) was found [55], consistent with increased milk flow in ducts, as milk production is stimulated by breastfeeding [56]. Significant decreases in ADC_0

and sADC values, as well as increases in *K* values, in post- compared with pre-breastfeeding were found in the study.

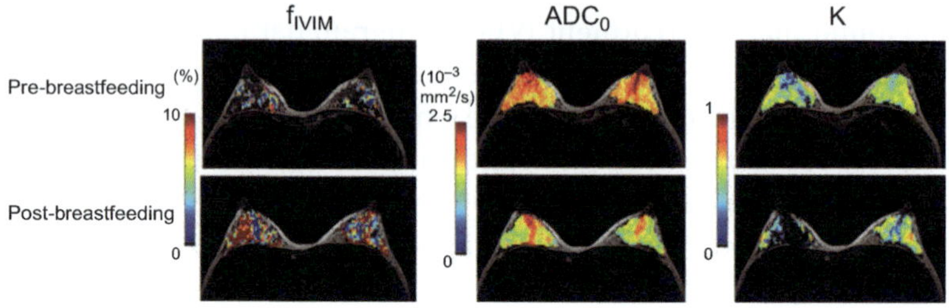

Figure 8.3 Increase in post-breastfeeding f_{IVIM} and decrease in post-breastfeeding ADC_0 values can be observed compared with pre-breastfeeding values.

8.6 Optimal Fitting Method and Choice of *b* Values

Conventional IVIM assumes the biexponential model, which can be numerically challenging without special care in fitting. Several approaches have been explored to overcome this challenge, and IVIM parameters were compared using different curve-fitting methods [57, 58]. Cho and colleagues have compared "free" (conventional biexponential) and "segmented" (two-step) fitting both for conventional (0, 30, 70, 100, 150, 200, 300, 400, 500, and 800 s/mm^2) and optimized (0 and 3 repetitions of 20, 300, and 800 s/mm^2) *b* value datasets. They found that segmented fitting with optimized *b* values provided higher precision and accuracy in 14 patients with breast cancer. Relative bias in fp and Dt was reduced significantly with segmented compared with free-fitting approaches. Notably, their simulations and patient experiments indicate that fp values estimated with free fitting (20.39%–21.41%) were more than twice as high as those estimated with segmented fitting (6.00%–7.89%), with a signal-to-noise ratio (SNR) = 10 in breast cancer (see more detailed results along different SNR values in Table 1 by Cho et al., Ref. [57]).

Similar results was found by Suo and colleagues [58]. They used seven *b* values (0, 50, 100, 150, 200, 500, and 800 s/mm^2) and reported that the precision of D^* and f determination was maximized with Method 2 (first estimation of D and then estimation of f and D^*) and Method 3 (first estimation of D and f and then estimation of D^*). They also found that the f value with (conventional) direct fitting with a biexponential model (Method 1; 16.33 ± 5.21%) was significantly larger than with segmented fitting (Method 2; 7.61 ± 2.33%; Method 3; 6.10 ± 3.19%). Moreover, f estimated using Method 2 showed moderate correlation with the relative enhancement ratio (RER) and the initial area under the curve (iAUC) from DCE MRI. Investigating 29 breast tumors, Yuan et al. have reported that the biexponential model does not necessarily better represent the DWI signal decay compared with the monoexponential model [20]; however, they used b values up to 1000 s/mm^2, and the analysis might have been partially confounded by non-Gaussian effects observed at high b values. It is important to be aware that non-Gaussian DWI (kurtosis) and noise floor effects are observed at high b values and b needs to be kept low enough to keep the signal free from these effects (Fig. 8.4) [59]. b values reached up to approximately 200 s/mm^2 when the initial IVIM model was developed by Le Bihan et al. [4]; thus NGD effects when using medium or high b values were not considered at that time. The IVIM effect can be overestimated when using higher b values, as shown in Fig. 8.4, and those high IVIM (f, fp, f_{IVIM}) values likely reflect residual tissue diffusion non-Gaussianity. The artifactual IVIM effect will increase with increasing b values. More importantly, malignant tissues have more curvature in the signal decay, so the artifactual IVIM effect will be greater for malignant lesions than benign lesions or normal tissue where curvature is less expected (the estimation of both IVIM and non-Gaussian DWI with noise correction is described in Ref. [71]).

A recent simulation study of the breast and liver by While indicated that Bayesian modeling approaches performed better than the least-squares approach with lower relative error and deviation [60]. Still, coefficients of variation in IVIM parameters (f, fp, and f_{IVIM}) tend to be higher compared with diffusion parameters (Dt, D, and ADC$_0$) [57, 58, 61, 62] and further investigation is needed to calculate D^* appropriately [18]. These studies clearly indicate that special care (e.g., the segmented two-step method) needs to be taken in IVIM analysis in clinical settings, where an insufficient SNR is often expected. The conventional biexponential model is susceptible to image noise and might be reliable only when a sufficient SNR is present on DWI.

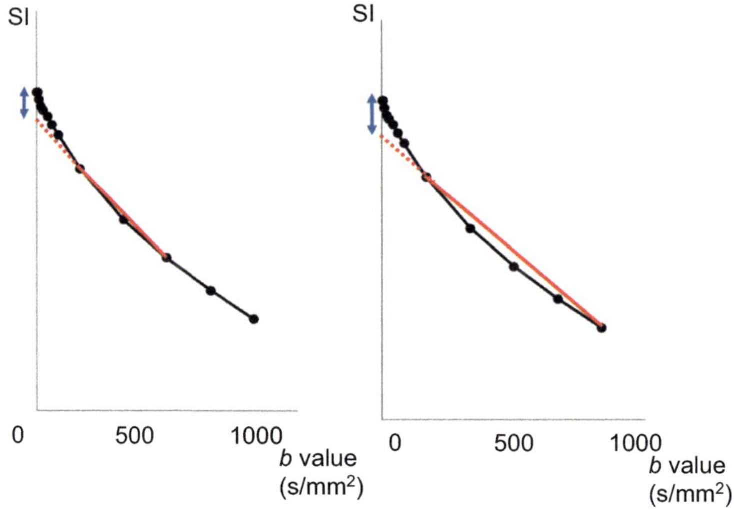

Figure 8.4 Pitfalls in the estimation of IVIM parameters illustrated by example data. An example of signal attenuation in typical malignant breast tissue. IVIM estimation includes *b* values up to 600 s/mm^2 (left) and 1000 s/mm^2 (right). The red line indicates apparent diffusion coefficient between *b* values of 200 and 600 s/mm^2 (left), and between *b* values of 200 and 1000 s/mm^2 (right). The IVIM effect is exaggerated (the blue arrow in the figure on the right compared to that in the figure on the left) if one includes larger *b* values (>800–1000 s/mm^2), because of the lower degree of signal attenuation at high *b* values due to the non-Gaussian DWI and noise floor effects. SI: signal intensity

The choice of optimal *b* values for accurate IVIM estimation is also important, as this could significantly affect the calculated IVIM and DWI parameter values. Sigmund et al., Iima et al., and many other scholars have used 200 s/mm^2 as a threshold in previous IVIM studies. Chen et al. recently reported the optimal *b* value to separate perfusion and diffusion effects to be 300 s/mm^2 through the investigation of 28 patients with breast cancer [63]. More work with a larger cohort is necessary before optimal *b* values can be confirmed.

8.6.1 Exhaustive (or Dictionary-Based) Approach without Fitting

To overcome the pitfalls mentioned above with the usual data fitting algorithms, a new approach has been proposed, called the "exhaustive approach" [7]. This method can also be seen as a dictionary-based approach. The raw signal profile is compared with that of a database of simulated signals using an exhaustive set of all parameter combinations (i.e., f, D^*, D, and the signal at $b = 0$ s/mm^2) instead of fitting. A distance is calculated between the measured signal attenuation profile and each simulated signal of the database. The parameter combination resulting in the shortest distance is deemed to represent the searched parameter estimates. The database can be built using this exhaustive set of parameter combinations. The exhaustive method might work better than fitting as fitting might stop at the local minima, while the exhaustive search approach will find the real minimum among all minima and give a better estimation of the parameters. A drawback is that the processing takes a long time, especially if a large database is used to ensure accuracy of estimation. Implementation of the algorithm on graphic cards may be helpful.

8.6.2 Simplified Approach without Fitting

Some other simplified approaches have recently been explored without the need for fitting [64, 65]. Teruel and colleagues have introduced relative enhanced diffusivity (RED) [65], the relative increase of ADC values at low *b* values (i.e., 200 s/mm^2) with respect to ADC values at high *b* values (i.e., 700 s/mm^2), which is defined as follows:

$$\mathrm{RED}(\%) = 100\frac{\mathrm{ADC}_{\mathrm{perf}}}{\mathrm{ADC}_{200,700}} = 100\left[\frac{\mathrm{ADC}_{0,200}}{\mathrm{ADC}_{200,700}} - 1\right] \tag{8.1}$$

RED is directly calculated from the signal intensity with three *b* values, with resulting reductions in both scanning time and processing time. They found a correlation of RED with the iAUC calculated from DCE MRI (Spearman rank correlation of 0.61). RED also had an accuracy of 90% (88% sensitivity and 92% specificity) for distinguishing 34 malignant from 27 benign breast tumors. RED parameters are weighted both on diffusion and perfusion; however, higher RED values were found in malignant compared with benign breast tumors and a similar trend was also found in previous IVIM studies [10]. A recent simulation study indicated linear proportionality between RED and IVIM parameter f and inverse proportionality between RED and D. Use of a b value of 100 s/mm^2 has also been suggested in analysis of RED of the breast [66]. There have been several papers published on the utility of RED for the diagnosis of breast lesions, and these results look promising; however, further investigation with a larger cohort is needed. A potential drawback is that in the presence on NGD, ADC_{0-200} is higher than $ADC_{200-700}$ (please see Chapter 1), resulting in positive RED values that are not related to IVIM and perfusion effects. Indeed, ADC values obtained from just three b values at low (e.g., ADC_{0-200}) and higher b values (e.g., $ADC_{200-700}$) can be combined into an NGD index to reflect the degree of NGD [67].

8.7 Conclusions

The seeds of IVIM, planted in the 1980s, have germinated and bloomed in the 2010s regarding breast imaging. They range from distinguishing between malignant and benign breast tumors and identifying histologic subtypes to the prediction of treatment response. IVIM might also characterize the physiological changes in lactating breasts.

The multiparametric approach using IVIM and DWI could be completely noninvasive in patients in whom contrast agents are contraindicated. The potential of IVIM for the diagnosis of breast lesions is huge; however, there are some issues that need to be kept in mind for IVIM estimation to be optimally utilized. The biexponential IVIM model developed in the 1980s assumed only moderate b values (i.e., 200 s/mm^2). Thus, if one uses a classical IVIM model using a high b value (i.e., 1000 s/mm^2), and if special care is not taken with fitting (including the two-step segmented approach) an artifactual (higher) IVIM effect will appear and be exaggerated in malignant lesions. IVIM is susceptible to noise, and sufficient SNR is crucial. IVIM parameters (especially D^*) tend to be more variable than ADC. There is still room for refinement of the IVIM model to reduce the variability of IVIM parameters in lesions.

IVIM is a still-evolving field, however, and the previously published results suggest that IVIM has great potential in playing an important clinical role as a functional MRI parameter in breast cancer assessment, prognostication, and treatment planning.

Acknowledgment

We acknowledge Dr. Eric E. Sigmund and Dr. Denis Le Bihan for their valuable and inspiring advice on this chapter. We acknowledge all the patients and volunteers who participated in the breast IVIM studies.

References

1. Torre L. A., Islami F., Siegel R. L., Ward E. M., Jemal A. Global cancer in women: burden and trends. *Cancer Epidemiol. Biomark. Prev.*, 2017, 26(4), doi: 10.1158/1055-9965.
2. Folkman J. Tumor angiogenesis: therapeutic implications. *N. Engl. J. Med.*, 1971, 285(21), 1182–1186.
3. Toi M., Inada K., Suzuki H., Tominaga T. Tumor angiogenesis in breast cancer: its importance as a prognostic indicator and the association with vascular endothelial growth factor expression. *Breast Cancer Res. Treat.*, 1995, 36(2), 193–204.
4. Le Bihan D., Breton E., Lallemand D., Aubin M. L., Vignaud J., Laval-Jeantet M. Separation of diffusion and perfusion in intravoxel incoherent motion MR imaging. *Radiology*, 1988, 168(2), 497–505.
5. Sigmund E., Cho G., Kim S., Finn M., Moccaldi M., Jensen J., et al. Intravoxel incoherent motion imaging of tumor microenvironment in locally advanced breast cancer. *Magn. Reson. Med.*, 2011, 65(5), 1437–1447.
6. Iima M., Reynaud O., Tsurugizawa T., Ciobanu L., Li J-R, Geffroy F., et al. Characterization of glioma microcirculation and tissue features using intravoxel incoherent motion magnetic resonance imaging in a rat brain model. *Invest. Radiol.*, 2014, 49(7), 485–490.
7. Iima M., Yano K., Kataoka M., Umehana M., Murata K., Kanao S., et al. Quantitative non-gaussian diffusion and intravoxel incoherent motion magnetic resonance imaging: differentiation of malignant and benign breast lesions. *Invest. Radiol.*, 2015, 50(4), 205–211.

8. Bokacheva L., Kaplan J. B., Giri D. D., Patil S., Gnanasigamani M., Nyman C. G., et al. Intravoxel incoherent motion diffusion-weighted MRI at 3.0 T differentiates malignant breast lesions from benign lesions and breast parenchyma. *J. Magn. Reson. Imaging*, 2014, 40(4), 813–823.
9. Liu C., Liang C., Liu Z., Zhang S., Huang B. Intravoxel incoherent motion (IVIM) in evaluation of breast lesions: comparison with conventional DWI, *Eur J. Radiol.*, 2013, 82(12), e782–e789.
10. Partridge S. C., Nissan N., Rahbar H., Kitsch A. E., Sigmund E. E. Diffusion-weighted breast MRI: Clinical applications and emerging techniques. *J. Magn. Reson. Imaging*, 2017, 45(2), 337–355.
11. Cho G. Y., Moy L., Kim S. G., Baete S. H., Moccaldi M., Babb J. S., et al. Evaluation of breast cancer using intravoxel incoherent motion (IVIM) histogram analysis: comparison with malignant status, histological subtype, and molecular prognostic factors. *Eur Radiol.*, 2016, 26(8), 2547–2558.
12. Dijkstra H., Dorrius M. D., Wielema M., Jaspers K., Pijnappel R. M., Oudkerk M., et al. Semi-automated quantitative intravoxel incoherent motion analysis and its implementation in breast diffusion-weighted imaging. *J. Magn. Reson. Imaging*, 2016, 43(5), 1122–1131.
13. Kim Y., Ko K., Kim D., Min C., Kim S. G., Joo J., et al. Intravoxel incoherent motion diffusion-weighted MR imaging of breast cancer: association with histopathological features and subtypes. *Br. J. Radiol.*, 2016, 89(1063), 20160140.
14. Lee Y. J., Kim S. H., Kang B. J., Kang Y. J., Yoo H., Yoo J., et al. Intravoxel incoherent motion (IVIM)-derived parameters in diffusion-weighted MRI: Associations with prognostic factors in invasive ductal carcinoma. *J. Magn. Reson. Imaging*, 2017, 45(5), 1394–1406.
15. Liu C., Wang K., Chan Q., Liu Z., Zhang J., He H., et al. Intravoxel incoherent motion MR imaging for breast lesions: comparison and correlation with pharmacokinetic evaluation from dynamic contrast-enhanced MR imaging. *Eur Radiol.*, 2016, 26(11), 3888–3898.
16. Ma D., Lu F., Zou X., Zhang H., Li Y., Zhang L., et al. Intravoxel incoherent motion diffusion-weighted imaging as an adjunct to dynamic contrast-enhanced MRI to improve accuracy of the differential diagnosis of benign and malignant breast lesions. *Magn. Reson. Imaging*, 2017, 36, 175–179.
17. Ostenson J., Pujara A. C., Mikheev A., Moy L., Kim S. G., Melsaether A. N., et al. Voxelwise analysis of simultaneously acquired and spatially correlated (18) F-fluorodeoxyglucose (FDG)-PET and intravoxel incoherent motion metrics in breast cancer. *Magn. Reson. Med.*, 2017, 78(3) 1147–1156.

18. Panek R., Borri M., Orton M., O'Flynn E., Morgan V., Giles S. L., et al. Evaluation of diffusion models in breast cancer. *Med. Phys.,* 2015, 42(8), 4833–4839.

19. Suo S., Cheng F., Cao M., Kang J., Wang M., Hua J., et al. Multiparametric diffusion-weighted imaging in breast lesions: association with pathologic diagnosis and prognostic factors. *J. Magn. Reson. Imaging,* 2017, 46(3), 740–750.

20. Yuan J., Wong O. L., Lo G. G., Chan H. H., Wong T. T., Cheung P. S. Statistical assessment of bi-exponential diffusion weighted imaging signal characteristics induced by intravoxel incoherent motion in malignant breast tumors. *Quant. Imaging Med. Surg.,* 2016, 6(4), 418–429.

21. Lin N., Chen J., Hua J., Zhao J., Zhao J., Lu J. Intravoxel incoherent motion MR imaging in breast cancer: quantitative analysis for characterizing lesions. *Int. J. Clin. Exp. Med.,* 2017, 10(1), 1705–1714.

22. Bokacheva L., Kaplan J. B., Giri D. D., Patil S., Gnanasigamani M., Nyman C. G., et al. Intravoxel incoherent motion diffusion-weighted MRI at 3.0 T differentiates malignant breast lesions from benign lesions and breast parenchyma. *J. Magn. Reson. Imaging,* 2014, 40(4), 813–823.

23. Iima M., Kataoka M., Kanao S., Onishi N., Kawai M., Ohashi A., et al. Intravoxel incoherent motion and quantitative non-gaussian diffusion MR imaging: evaluation of the diagnostic and prognostic value of several markers of malignant and benign breast lesions. *Radiology,* 2018, 287(2), 432–441

24. Vidić I, Egnell L., Jerome N. P., Teruel J. R., Sjøbakk T. E., Østlie A., et al. Support vector machine for breast cancer classification using diffusion-weighted MRI histogram features: Preliminary study. *J. Magn. Reson. Imaging,* 2018, 47(5), 1205–1216

25. Rakha E. A., Reis-Filho J. S., Baehner F., Dabbs D. J., Decker T., Eusebi V., et al. Breast cancer prognostic classification in the molecular era: the role of histological grade. *Breast Cancer Res.,* 2010, 12(4), 207.

26. Blows F. M., Driver K. E., Schmidt M. K., Broeks A., Van Leeuwen F. E., Wesseling J., et al. Subtyping of breast cancer by immunohistochemistry to investigate a relationship between subtype and short and long term survival: a collaborative analysis of data for 10,159 cases from 12 studies. *PLOS Med.,* 2010, 7(5), e1000279.

27. Goldhirsch A., Wood W. C., Coates A. S., Gelber R. D., Thürlimann B., Senn H-J, et al. Strategies for subtypes—dealing with the diversity of breast cancer: highlights of the St Gallen International Expert Consensus on the Primary Therapy of Early Breast Cancer 2011. *Ann. Oncol.,* 2011, 22(8), 1736–1647.

28. Kawashima H., Miyati T., Ohno N., Ohno M., Inokuchi M., Ikeda H., et al. Differentiation between luminal-A and luminal-B breast cancer using intravoxel incoherent motion and dynamic contrast-enhanced magnetic resonance imaging. *Acad. Radiol.*, 2017, 24(12), 1575–1581.

29. Cho G. Y., Sutton E. J., Moy L., Gennaro L., Mikheev A., Rusinek, H., et al. (eds.) Multicenter study of intravoxel incoherent motion (IVIM) metrics in breast cancer with software comparison. *International Society for Magnetic Resonance in Medicine* 2017, Honolulu, HI, USA.

30. Iima M., Kataoka M., Kanao S., Onishi N., Kawai M., Ohashi A., et al. Intravoxel incoherent motion and quantitative non-Gaussian diffusion MR imaging: evaluation of the diagnostic and prognostic value of several markers of malignant and benign breast lesions. *Radiology,* 2018, 287(2), 432–441.

31. Leithner D., Wengert G. J., Helbich T. H., Thakur S., Ochoa-Albiztegui R. E., Morris E. A., et al. Clinical role of breast MRI now and going forward. *Clin. Radiol.*, 2018, 73(8), 700-714.

32. Morrow M., Waters J., Morris E. MRI for breast cancer screening, diagnosis, and treatment. The *Lancet,* 2011, 378(9805), 1804–1811.

33. Pinker K., Helbich T. H., Morris E. A. The potential of multiparametric MRI of the breast. *Br. J. Radiol.*, 2016, 90(1069), 20160715.

34. Marino M. A., Helbich T., Baltzer P., Pinker-Domenig K. Multiparametric MRI of the breast: A review. *J. Magn. Reson. Imaging*, 2018, 47(2), 301–315.

35. Jiang L., Lu X., Hua B., Gao J., Zheng D., Zhou Y. Intravoxel incoherent motion diffusion-weighted imaging versus dynamic contrast-enhanced magnetic resonance imaging: comparison of the diagnostic performance of perfusion-related parameters in breast. *J. Comput. Assist. Tomogr.*, 2018, 42(1), 6–11.

36. Jerome N. P., Boult J. K., Orton M. R., d'Arcy J. A., Nerurkar A., Leach M. O., et al. Characterisation of fibrosis in chemically-induced rat mammary carcinomas using multi-modal endogenous contrast MRI on a 1.5 T clinical platform. *Eur Radiol.*, 2018, 28(4), 1642–1653.

37. Lee H. J., Rha S. Y., Chung Y. E., Shim H. S., Kim Y. J., Hur J., et al. Tumor perfusion-related parameter of diffusion-weighted magnetic resonance imaging: Correlation with histological microvessel density. *Magn. Reson. Med.*, 2014, 71(4), 1554–1558.

38. Song X. L., Kang H. K., Jeong G. W., Ahn K. Y., Jeong Y. Y., Kang Y. J., et al. Intravoxel incoherent motion diffusion-weighted imaging for

monitoring chemotherapeutic efficacy in gastric cancer. *World J. Gastroenterol.*, 2016, 22(24), 5520–5531.

39. Lee Y., Lee S. S., Cheong H., Lee C. K., Kim N., Son W. C., et al. Intravoxel incoherent motion MRI for monitoring the therapeutic response of hepatocellular carcinoma to sorafenib treatment in mouse xenograft tumor models. *Acta Radiol.*, 2017, 58(9), 1045–1053.

40. Klau M., Mayer P., Bergmann F., Maier-Hein K., Hase J., Hackert T., et al. Correlation of histological vessel characteristics and diffusion-weighted imaging intravoxel incoherent motion-derived parameters in pancreatic ductal adenocarcinomas and pancreatic neuroendocrine tumors. *Invest. Radiol.*, 2015, 50(11), 792–797.

41. Togao O., Hiwatashi A., Yamashita K., Kikuchi K., Momosaka D., Yoshimoto K., et al. Measurement of the perfusion fraction in brain tumors with intravoxel incoherent motion MR imaging: validation with histopathological vascular density in meningiomas. *Br. J. Radiol.*, 2018, 91(1085), 20170912.

42. Surov A., Meyer H. J., Hohn A. K., Behrmann C., Wienke A., Spielmann R. P., et al. Correlations between intravoxel incoherent motion (IVIM) parameters and histological findings in rectal cancer: preliminary results. *Oncotarget*, 2017, 8(13), 21974–21983.

43. Eberhardt C., Wurnig M. C., Wirsching A., Rossi C., Rottmar M., Ozbay P. S., et al. Intravoxel incoherent motion analysis of abdominal organs: computation of reference parameters in a large cohort of C57Bl/6 mice and correlation to microvessel density. *MAGMA (New York, NY)*, 2016, 29(5), 751–763.

44. Wang Q., Guo Y., Zhang J., Wang Z., Huang M., Zhang Y. Contribution of IVIM to conventional dynamic contrast-enhanced and diffusion-weighted MRI in differentiating benign from malignant breast masses. *Breast Care* (Basel, Switzerland), 2016, 11(4), 254–258.

45. Dijkstra H., Dorrius M. D., Wielema M., Pijnappel R. M., Oudkerk M., Sijens P. E. Quantitative DWI implemented after DCE-MRI yields increased specificity for BI-RADS 3 and 4 breast lesions. *J. Magn. Reson. Imaging*, 2016, 44(6), 1642–1649.

46. Chen F., Chen P., Hamid Muhammed H., Zhang J. Intravoxel incoherent motion diffusion for identification of breast malignant and benign tumors using chemometrics. *BioMed Res. Int.*, 2017, 2017, 3845409.

47. Pullicino R., Radon M., Biswas S., Bhojak M., Das K. A Review of the current evidence on gadolinium deposition in the brain. *Clin. Neuroradiol.*, 2018, 28(2), 159–169.

48. Cho G. Y., Gennaro L., Sutton E. J., Zabor E. C., Zhang Z., Giri D., et al. Intravoxel incoherent motion (IVIM) histogram biomarkers for prediction of neoadjuvant treatment response in breast cancer patients. *Eur. J. Radiol. Open*, 2017, 4, 101–107.
49. Kim Y., Kim S. H., Lee H. W., Song B. J., Kang B. J., Lee A., et al. Intravoxel incoherent motion diffusion-weighted MRI for predicting response to neoadjuvant chemotherapy in breast cancer. *Magn. Reson. Imaging*, 2018, 48, 27–33.
50. Che S., Zhao X., Ou Y., Li J., Wang M., Wu B., et al. Role of the intravoxel incoherent motion diffusion weighted imaging in the pre-treatment prediction and early response monitoring to neoadjuvant chemotherapy in locally advanced breast cancer. *Medicine*, 2016, 95(4), e2420.
51. Gaeta M., Benedetto C., Minutoli F., D'Angelo T., Amato E., Mazziotti S., et al. Use of diffusion-weighted, intravoxel incoherent motion, and dynamic contrast-enhanced MR imaging in the assessment of response to radiotherapy of lytic bone metastases from breast cancer. *Acad. Radiol.*, 2014, 21(10), 1286–1293.
52. Pieper C. C., Meyer C., Sprinkart A. M., Block W., Ahmadzadehfar H., Schild H. H., et al. The value of intravoxel incoherent motion model-based diffusion-weighted imaging for outcome prediction in resin-based radioembolization of breast cancer liver metastases. *OncoTargets Ther.*, 2016, 9, 4089–4098.
53. Pieper C. C., Sprinkart A. M., Meyer C., König R., Schild H. H., Kukuk G. M., et al. Evaluation of a simplified intravoxel incoherent motion (IVIM) analysis of diffusion-weighted imaging for prediction of tumor size changes and imaging response in breast cancer liver metastases undergoing radioembolization: a retrospective single center analysis. *Medicine*, 2016, 95(14), e3275.
54. Nissan N., Furman-Haran E., Shapiro-Feinberg M., Grobgeld D., Degani H. Monitoring in-vivo the mammary gland microstructure during morphogenesis from lactation to post-weaning using diffusion tensor MRI. *J. Mammary Gland Biol. Neoplasia*, 2017, 22(3), 193–202.
55. Iima M., Kataoka M., Sakaguchi R., Kanao S., Onishi N., Kawai M., et al. Intravoxel incoherent motion (IVIM) and non-Gaussian diffusion MRI of the lactating breast. *Eur J. Radiol. Open*, 2018, 5, 24–30.
56. Geddes D. T. Inside the lactating breast: the latest anatomy research. *J. Midwifery Women's Health*, 2007, 52(6), 556–563.
57. Cho G. Y., Moy L., Zhang J. L., Baete S., Lattanzi R., Moccaldi M., et al. Comparison of fitting methods and b-value sampling strategies for

intravoxel incoherent motion in breast cancer. *Magn. Reson. Med.*, 2015, 74(4), 1077–1085.

58. Suo S., Lin N., Wang H., Zhang L., Wang R., Zhang S., et al. Intravoxel incoherent motion diffusion-weighted MR imaging of breast cancer at 3.0 Tesla: Comparison of different curve-fitting methods. *J. Magn. Reson. Imaging*, 2015, 42(2), 362-370.

59. Iima M., Le Bihan D. Clinical intravoxel incoherent motion and diffusion MR imaging: past, present, and future. *Radiology*, 2016, 278(1), 13–32.

60. While P. T. A comparative simulation study of bayesian fitting approaches to intravoxel incoherent motion modeling in diffusion-weighted MRI. *Magn. Reson. Med.*, 2017, 78(6), 2373–2387.

61. Iima M., Kataoka M., Kanao S., Kawai M., Onishi N., Koyasu S., et al. Variability of non-Gaussian diffusion MRI and intravoxel incoherent motion (IVIM) measurements in the breast. *PLoS One*, 2018, 13(3), e0193444.

62. Song Y. S., Park C. M., Lee S. M., Park S. J., Cho H. R., Choi S. H., et al. Reproducibility of histogram and texture parameters derived from intravoxel incoherent motion diffusion-weighted MRI of FN13762 rat breast Carcinomas. *Anticancer Res.*, 2014, 34(5), 2135–2144.

63. Chen W., Zhang J., Long D., Wang Z., Zhu J. M. Optimization of intra-voxel incoherent motion measurement in diffusion-weighted imaging of breast cancer. *J. Appl. Clin. Med. Phys.*, 2017, 18(3), 191–199.

64. Thoeny H. C., De Keyzer F., Vandecaveye V., Chen F., Sun X., Bosmans H., et al. Effect of vascular targeting agent in rat tumor model: dynamic contrast-enhanced versus diffusion-weighted MR imaging. *Radiology*, 2005, 237(2), 492–499.

65. Teruel J. R., Goa P. E., Sjøbakk T. E., Østlie A., Fjøsne H. E., Bathen T. F. A simplified approach to measure the effect of the microvasculature in diffusion-weighted MR imaging applied to breast tumors: preliminary results. *Radiology*, 2016, 281(2), 373–381.

66. While P. T., Teruel J. R., Vidić I, Bathen T. F., Goa P. E. Relative enhanced diffusivity: noise sensitivity, protocol optimization, and the relation to intravoxel incoherent motion. *Magnetic Resonance Materials in Physics, Biology and Medicine*, 2018, 31(3), 425–438.

67. Le Bihan D., Ichikawa S., Motosugi U. Diffusion and intravoxel incoherent motion MR imaging–based virtual elastography: a hypothesis-generating study in the liver. *Radiology*, 2017, 285(2), 609–619.

Chapter 9

Cardiac IVIM MRI

Zhiyong Li[a] and Anna Mou[b]
[a]*Department of Radiology, First Affiliated Hospital of Dalian Medical University, No. 222 Zhongshan Road, Dalian 116011, China*
[b]*Department of Radiology, Sichuan Provincial People's Hospital, No. 32 Yihuan Road, Chengdu 610031, China*
zjy_lzy@126.com

Intravoxel incoherent motion (IVIM) proposed by Le Bihan et al. in 1986 has been developing for several decades. It has been widely used to assess pathological characteristics of multiple organs, such as the brain, abdominal organs, and breasts, including animal experiments and clinical research. However, only a few studies have investigated cardiac IVIM.

9.1 Implementation of Cardiac IVIM

The development of echo-planar imaging (EPI) made cardiac IVIM possible by greatly reducing the scan time. Formerly, Pop et al. [1] used a custom fast spin echo (FSE) sequence to scan the total heart, which took approximately 10 h for only one b value (500 s/mm^2).

Intravoxel Incoherent Motion (IVIM) MRI: Principles and Applications
Edited by Denis Le Bihan, Mami Iima, Christian Federau, and Eric E. Sigmund

ISBN 978-981-4800-19-8 (Hardcover), 978-0-429-42727-5 (eBook)
www.panstanford.com

Using an EPI sequence, currently one needs just 10 s to complete one slice of a cardiac IVIM scan with nine *b* values [2, 3]. Nowadays, a spin-echo echo-planar imaging (SE-EPI) sequence is usually used in cardiac IVIM.

Diffusion-weighted imaging (DWI) is very sensitive to motion, including respiratory, cardiac, and gastrointestinal peristaltic movements, which can induce signal loss at a low signal intensity and reduce the signal-to-noise ratio (SNR). Bulk motion is the most challenging motion type for cardiac IVIM. Therefore, strategies are being developed to minimize physiological motion during the acquisition.

The first study of microcirculation in canine heart using IVIM was performed by Callot et al. in 2003 [4]. To remove the influence of cardiac motion, they used a correction long-axis stimulated echo acquisition mode (STEAM) sequence. Encoding and rewinding gradients of the STEAM sequence were placed at exactly the same point of the cardiac cycle, to measure water movement between the same end-diastolic points of two consecutive heartbeats when the position and shape of the heart were the same. STEAM could shorten the acquisition time, enhance spatial resolution and temporal resolution, and improve image quality.

Implementing motion-compensated (MOCO) diffusion-encoding gradient waveforms can mitigate sensitivity to bulk motion. Gamper et al. [5] used flow-compensated diffusion gradients in combination with a reduced field of view to increase the SNR without using the STEAM technique. Aliotta et al. [6] recently demonstrated that the convex optimized diffusion encoding (CODE) DWI can reduce the echo time (TE) and enhance the SNR of the DWI map as well as compensate for bulk motion; they did this by comparing CODE DWI with the conventional MOCO diffusion spin-echo encoding by nulling first- and/or second-order gradient moments (M1, M1 + M2) to mitigate bulk motion [6].

Rapacchi et al. [10] proposed a method to minimize motion-induced signal loss by principal component analysis filtering and temporal maximum intensity projection (PCATMIP) techniques. The PCATMIP algorithm was used with a set of 10 repetitions (acquired with time shifts of 10 ms) for each *b* value to capture the moment when motion-induced signal loss was minimized. Studies demonstrated that the PCATMIP postprocessing was beneficial for signal recovery, increasing the SNR. This method was also shown to be robust enough to be independent of the RR irregularity and might therefore be the solution of choice for patients with arrhythmic cardiac cycles [2, 8–10]. In addition, the IVIM parameters had a good reproducibility with PCATMIP both in-between free breathing and in breath-hold acquisitions [8].

There is a certain degree of water exchange between the intra- and extravascular compartments. Lemke et al. [7] proposed a refinement of the DWI signal model that accounts for the T1 and T2 relaxation of blood and tissue as well as the TE and repetition time (TR) sequence parameters:

$$SI = S_0 \left[\frac{(1-f)\times(1-e^{-TR/\mathrm{T1}_{\mathrm{tissue}}})\times e^{-TE/\mathrm{T2}_{\mathrm{tissue}}}\times e^{-bD} + f\times(1-e^{-TR/\mathrm{T1}_{\mathrm{blood}}})\times e^{-TE/\mathrm{T2}_{\mathrm{blood}}}\times e^{-b(D+D^*)}}{(1-f)\times(1-e^{-TR/\mathrm{T1}_{\mathrm{tissue}}})\times e^{-TE/\mathrm{T2}_{\mathrm{tissue}}} + f\times(1-e^{-TR/\mathrm{T1}_{\mathrm{tissue}}})\times e^{-TE/\mathrm{T2}_{\mathrm{blood}}}} \right]$$

Here $\mathrm{T1}_{\mathrm{tissue/blood}}$ and $\mathrm{T2}_{\mathrm{tissue/blood}}$ are the longitudinal and transverse relaxation parameters of the tissue and blood, respectively. This model was used in studies by Moulin et al. and Delattre et al. [2, 8].

All cardiac IVIM imaging studies were performed on the left ventricular short axis. Cardiac triggering is necessary in cardiac IVIM, and a stable RR cycle and a normal heart rate play an important part in the acquisition, as a higher heart rate reduces the quality of IVIM imaging [3]. Cardiac IVIM acquisitions are usually performed at end-expiration breath-hold because it gives a reproducible slice position. The best time window to acquire the images is during the most quiescent cardiac phase in end diastole, corresponding to minimal motion in the cardiac cycle.

9.2 Choice of *b* Values

To extract perfusion and diffusion information in tissue, at least four *b* values should be used to characterize the IVIM biexponential signal attenuation, although a larger number of *b* values would provide more data to analyze the physiologic characteristic of tissues using more sophisticated methods. A larger number of *b* values requires a longer scan time, which might become unacceptable for patients and might not be clinically feasible. We suggest acquiring six to eight *b* values [11]. In the study by Delattre et al. [2], they found that 9 *b* values instead of 13 would be sufficient for the analysis of IVIM parameters and this would reduce the scan time while providing the same results.

Higher *b* values are more stable and reproducible, but the reproducibility of low *b* values is poor [12]. This suggests that the combination of fewer high *b* values (two to three) and more low *b* values (four or more) could be optimal for measuring the challenging effects of perfusion. Lower *b* values (<200 s/mm^2) are more sensitive to microcirculation in the capillary network [12]. Higher *b* values are more reflective of tissue diffusion. However, there is no consensus on the optimal choice and magnitude of *b* values, which might depend on the individualized tissue and the clinical needs. The myocardial signal does attenuate with an increasing *b* value, which results from extending the duration and interval time of the gradient pulse.

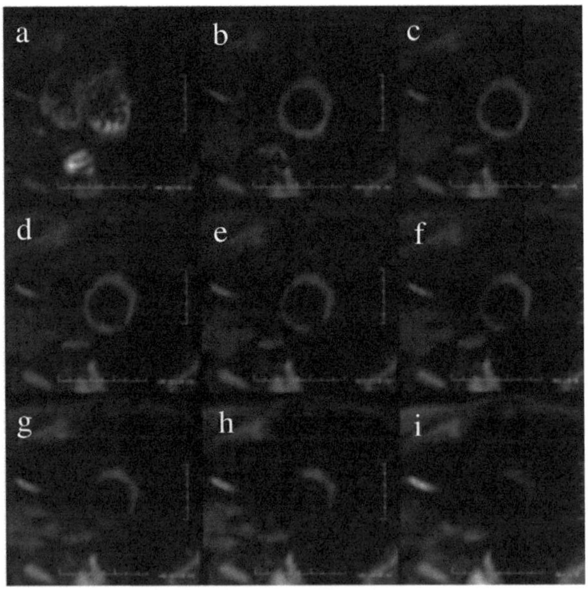

Figure 9.1 Example of IVIM raw images of the base-ventricular short-axis slices in a healthy volunteer: (a–i) *b* values = 0, 20, 50, 80, 100, 120, 200, 300, and 500 s/mm^2, respectively. The signal of the left ventricle attenuated with *b* value increment and got lost for *b* values above 300 s/mm^2.

In cardiac IVIM, typically nine values were used, with a higher concentration of lower *b* values, for example, 0, 15, 30, 50 ,75, 100,

200, 300, and 400 s/mm^2 in the study by Delattre et al. [2] and 0, 20, 50, 80, 100, 120, 200, 200, and 500 s/mm^2 by Mou et al. (Fig. 9.2) [3]. Importantly, in the latter study, they described that the signal intensity in the in vivo myocardium was too low to be observed for b > 300 s/mm^2 (Fig. 9.1) [3]. The b values should be chosen for the entire acquisition to be performed in a reasonable amount of time with adequate breath-hold duration.

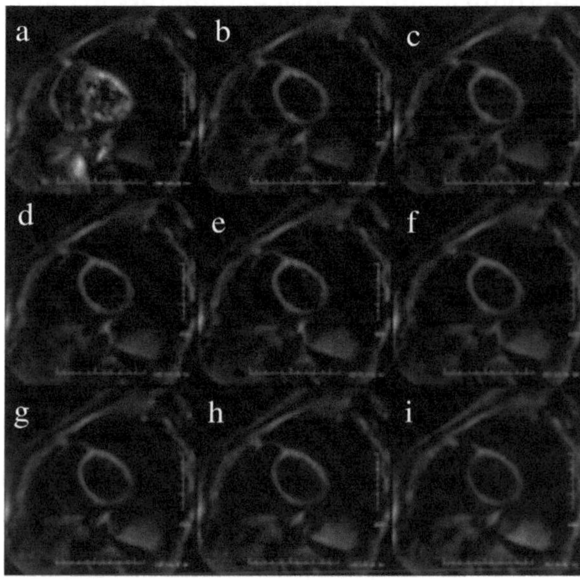

Figure 9.2 Example of IVIM raw images of the central base-ventricular short-axis slices in a healthy volunteer: (a–i) b values = 0, 20, 50, 80, 100, 120, 200, 300, and 500 s/mm^2, respectively.

9.3 Assessment of IVIM Quality and Quantitative Analysis

There are currently no clear criteria to assess the quality of IVIM images. IVIM parameters (D, D*, and f) are usually measured on commercial magnetic resonance imaging (MRI) systems and calculated automatically. Regions of interest are usually chosen close to the midwall area, avoiding the papillary muscles, intracardiac blood flow, and the edge pixels to minimize the impact of partial volume effects when measuring [2–4, 8].

A few published articles have mentioned the quality of cardiac DWI images [3, 13], assessing signal attenuation of myocardium, the SNR, the contrast-on-noise ratio (CNR), geometric distortion artifacts, ventricular wall delineation, and blood suppression.

9.3.1 Reproducibility of IVIM Parameters in Cardiac IVIM

Moulin et al. performed cardiac IVIM with a free-breathing acquisition protocol using nine *b* values from 0 to 400 s/mm^2 [8] in 10 healthy human hearts. The perfusion fraction *f* and the water diffusion coefficient *D* had high reproducibility, precision, and accuracy, but though the pseudodiffusion coefficient *D** had a good accuracy, it was found to be less reproducible. On the other hand, all IVIM parameters, *f*, *D*, and *D**, were found to be well reproducible and consistent in 22 patients and 15 heart-damaged patients [3].

9.3.2 Normal Values of CMR IVIM Parameters

Callot et al. [4] observed three-directional anisotropy (circumferential, radial, and longitudinal) of IVIM parameters in diffusion and flow movements parallel (*z*, in the long direction) and perpendicular (*x* and *y*, in the short-axis plane) to the myofiber orientation. At rest, the *D* and *f* values were the highest in the circumferential encoding and *f* was the lowest in the longitudinal direction: $f_{circ} > f_{rad} > f_{long}$ (0.111 ± 0.022 vs. 0.083 ± 0.026 vs. 0.053 ± 0.017) and $D_{circ} > D_{long} > D_{rad}$ (1.64 ± 0.18 vs. 1.17 ± 0.18 vs. 0.99 ± 0.14, mm^2/s). *D** had no statistically significant directional anisotropy (13.35 ± 4.93 vs. 11.16 ± 5.48 vs. 14.09 ± 2.18, mm^2/s). This phenomenon is consistent with the capillary morphology and high-order branches in the myocardium. The capillaries are oriented along the myofibers (circumferential), and the small vessels are mainly spread in the short-axis plane (radial/longitudinal). Compared with *f*, *D** is less dependent on the gradient direction.

Mou et al. studied 22 healthy volunteers and found no significant difference in the IVIM parameters acquired on the left ventricle short axis at the level of the apex, the midventricle, and the base [3].

Few published articles have investigated normal cardiac IVIM, and large cohort data are missing. We listed the published normal IVIM parameters, which are all from a small sample (no more than 30) (Table 8.1). It is worth noting that the study by Callot et al. was performed on dog hearts using a STEAM sequence with 14 *b* values up to 600 s/mm^2 [4]. The result of the study by Mou et al. was higher than the results of others. The discrepancy may be related to the acquisition techniques, different multi-*b* values, diffusion gradients, diffusion strengths, fitting methods, and sample variability.

Table 9.1 Summary of cardiac IVIM parameters in normal animals or humans

	Callot et al. [4]	Delattre et al. [2]	Moulin et al. [8]	Mou et al. [3]
D (10^{-3} mm^2/s)	1.26 ± 0.10	2.43 ± 0.98	1.41 ± 0.09	3.33 ± 0.85
D^* (10^{-3} mm^2/s)	12.87 ± 2.56	76.3	43.6 ± 9.25	132.43 ± 20.23
f	0.082 ± 0.013	0.150 ± 0.046	0.122 ± 0.013	0.31 ± 0.07

9.4 Clinical Application of CMR IVIM

IVIM, as an endogenous contrast technique to distinguish between water diffusion and perfusion, can reflect microcirculation and detect directional anisotropy in the capillary morphology in the myocardium without a contrast agent by measuring the vascular volume fraction and the microflow velocity.

In the study by Callot et al. [4], the values of D were unchanged in all three directions after adenosine infusion. The value of D decreased in the postmortem measurement, which might be due to postmortem physiological changes that lead to a change in water mobility. D^* increased in all three directions (19.3% circumferential, 13.8% radial, and 11.7% longitudinal), and f also increased (23.2% circumferential, 25.9% radial, and 27.1% longitudinal) after adenosine infusion. Finally, the product fD^* increased by 44% after adenosine administration. f and D^* values could therefore reflect cardiac vascular volume, microflow velocity, and directional anisotropy. Another potential application of IVIM may be monitoring of blood vessel growth during angiogenesis in the heart, using anisotropy as an indicator of capillary organization.

In the study by Mou et al. [3], cardiac magnetic resonance (CMR) IVIM was performed successfully on 22 healthy volunteers and 15 patients, including 7 hypertrophic cardiomyopathy (HCM) and 8 patients with combined diabetes and hypertension. The D^* values of the HCM group and the diabetes and/or hypertension group were significantly lower than that of the healthy group (83.12 ± 22.33 vs. 103.02 ± 21.10 vs. 132.43 ± 20.23, $P < 0.05$, 10^{-3} mm^2/s). CMR IVIM could therefore monitor the hypoperfusion injury in the myocardium and could be used in clinic.

In conclusion, with improvements in MRI techniques, IVIM has been shown to be useful in estimating microcirculation in the myocardium. It can provide quantitative values of vascular volume and blood velocity in a noninvasive way without contrast media. Bulk motion remains the major challenge in cardiac IVIM imaging, and further work should address this issue.

References

1. Pop M., Ghugre N. R., Ramanan V., Morikawa L., Stanisz G., Dick A. J., Wright G. A. (2013). Quantification of fibrosis in infarcted swine hearts by ex vivo late gadolinium-enhancement and diffusion-weighted MRI methods. *J. Phys. Med. Biol.*, 58(15), 5009–5028.
2. Delattre B. M., Viallon M., Wei H., Zhu Y. M., Feiweier T., Pai V. M., Wen H., Croisille P. (2012). In vivo cardiac diffusion-weighted magnetic resonance imaging: quantification of normal perfusion and diffusion coefficients with intravoxel incoherent motion imaging. *J. Invest. Radiol.*, 47(11), 662–670.
3. Mou A., Zhang C., Li M., Jin F., Song Q., Liu A., Li Z. (2017). Evaluation of myocardial microcirculation using intravoxel incoherent motion imaging. *J. Magn. Reson. Imaging*, 46(6), 1818–1828.
4. Callot V., Bennett E., Decking U. K., Balaban R. S., Wen H. (2003). In vivo study of microcirculation in canine myocardium using the IVIM method. *J. Magn. Reson. Med.*, 50(3), 531–540.
5. Gamper U., Boesiger P., Kozerke S. (2007). Diffusion imaging of the in vivo heart using spin echoes-consideration on bulk motion sensitivity. *J. Magn. Reson. Med.*, 57(2), 331–337.

6. Aliotta E., Wu H. H., Ennis D. B. (2017). Convex optimized diffusion encoding (CODE) gradient waveforms for minimum echo time and bulk motion-compensated diffusion-weighted MR. *J. Magn. Reson. Med.*, 77(2), 717–729.

7. Lemke A., Laun F. B., Simon D., Stieltjes B., Schad L. R. (2010). An in vivo verification of the intravoxel incoherent motion effect in diffusion-weighted imaging of the abdomen. *J. Magn. Reson. Med.*, 64(6), 1580–1585.

8. Moulin K., Croisille P., Feiweier T., Delattre B. M., Wei H., Robert B., et al. (2016). In vivo free-breathing DTI and IVIM of the whole human heart using a real-time slice-followed SE-EPI navigator–based sequence: A reproducibility study in healthy volunteers. *J. Magn. Reson. Med.*, 76(1), 70–82.

9. Pai V. M., Rapacchi S., Kellman P., Croisille P., Wen H. (2011). PCATMIP: enhancing signal intensity in diffusion-weighted magnetic resonance imaging. *J. Magn. Reson. Med.*, 65(6), 1611–1619.

10. Rapacchi S., Wen H., Viallon M., Grenier D., Kellman P., Croisille P., Pai V. M. (2011). Low *b*-value diffusion-weighted cardiac magnetic resonance imaging initial results in humans using an optimal time window imaging approach. *J. Invest. Radiol.*, 46(12), 751–758.

11. Koh D. M., Collins D. J., Orton M. R. (2011). Intravoxel incoherent motion in body diffusion-weighted MRI: reality and challenges. *AJR Am. J. Roentgenol.*, 196(6), 1351–1361.

12. Koh D. M., Blackledge M., Collins D. J., Padhani A. R., Wallace T., Wilton B., et al. (2009). Reproducibility and changes in the apparent diffusion coefficients of solid tumours treated with combretastatin A4 phosphate and bevacizumab in a two centre phase I clinical trial. *J. Eur. Radiol.*, 19(11), 2728–2738.

13. Potet J., Rahmouni A., Mayer J., Vignaud A., Lim P., Luciani A., et al. (2013). Detection of myocardial edema with low-b-value diffusion-weighted echo-planar imaging sequence in patients with acute myocarditis. *J. Radiol.*, 269(2), 362–369.

Chapter 10

Liver Fibrosis

Shintaro Ichikawa and Utaroh Motosugi
Department of Radiology, University of Yamanashi,
1110 Shimokato, Chuo-shi, Yamanashi, 409-3898, Japan
si99006@yahoo.co.jp

10.1 Introduction

The stage of liver fibrosis is a strong determinant of the risk of hepatocellular carcinoma and its prognosis, so staging of hepatic fibrosis is important in the management of patients with chronic liver disease [1, 2]. End-stage liver fibrosis (cirrhosis) causes liver failure and is typically irreversible, whereas liver fibrosis in the early to intermediate stages can be treatable [3]. Therefore, early detection and staging of liver fibrosis are crucial for planning and monitoring the response to therapy. Liver biopsy followed by histopathologic assessment is commonly performed to stage liver fibrosis. However, biopsy may have severe complications, including hemorrhage and infection. Biopsy also has inherent drawbacks, including sampling error because of the small specimen sample, interobserver disagreement, and low patient acceptance [4–6]. Despite these limitations, biopsy is still considered the golden

Intravoxel Incoherent Motion (IVIM) MRI: Principles and Applications
Edited by Denis Le Bihan, Mami Iima, Christian Federau, and Eric E. Sigmund

ISBN 978-981-4800-19-8 (Hardcover), 978-0-429-42727-5 (eBook)
www.panstanford.com

standard for staging liver fibrosis. Therefore, noninvasive methods have been developed for assessing hepatic fibrosis, including serum markers and imaging-based methods.

10.2 Pathologic Features of Liver Fibrosis

When the liver parenchyma is damaged, regardless of the cause, which includes viral hepatitis, alcoholic or nonalcoholic steatohepatitis, or an autoimmune-related disorder, fibroblasts proliferate and produce collagen around the sinusoids. The collagen inhibits the molecular exchange between the sinusoids and hepatocytes. Abnormal communication between the hepatic arteries and veins or the portal vein is part of the pathologic state, and changes in diffusivity of molecules can be observed with diffusion-weighted imaging (DWI) or intravoxel incoherent motion (IVIM) imaging. Histopathologic assessment of liver fibrosis is usually performed using hematoxylin-eosin and Masson trichrome staining to determine the fibrosis stage (F score) using the METAVIR (meta-analysis of histological data in viral hepatitis) scoring system, that is, F0, no fibrosis; F1, portal fibrosis without bridging fibrosis; F2, portal fibrosis with bridging fibrosis; F3, portal and bridging fibrosis with deformity of hepatic lobules; and F4, cirrhosis [7, 8]. F2 and F3 are often called significant fibrosis and severe fibrosis, respectively.

10.3 ADC Value for Staging Liver Fibrosis

In general, the apparent diffusion coefficient (ADC) value (a monoexponential model-based diffusivity estimation) decreases with progression of liver fibrosis. Several studies have compared the ADC values of normal livers with those of cirrhotic livers. All five reports [9–13] listed in Table 10.1 show reduced ADC values in the cirrhotic liver. It is important to note that the ADC values of normal and cirrhotic livers vary according to the *b* values used in the study. The ADC value is mainly determined by two types of molecular movement, that is, molecular diffusion in solid tissue and microcirculation in vessels (perfusion) [14]. The liver is a highly vascularized organ, so perfusion-related effects are not negligible when assessing diffusivity by DWI. One of the above-mentioned reports concluded that DWI with a *b* value of 700 s/mm^2 had a higher ability than DWI with a *b* value of 1000 s/mm^2 to differentiate cirrhotic livers from normal livers (with Az values of 0.901 and 0.832, respectively) [13].

Table 10.1 Comparison of ADC values between normal and cirrhotic liver

			ADC value (10^{-3} mm^2/s)	
Authors	**Journal, year**	***b* value (s/mm^2)**	**Normal liver**	**Cirrhotic liver**
Koinuma, et al.	*JMRI*, 2005 (8)	0 / 128	3.45	1.98
Lewin, et al.	*Hepatology*, 2007 (9)	0–800	1.4	1.1
Sandrasegaran, et al.	*AJR*, 2009 (10)	50 / 400	1.26	0.99
Do, et al.	*AJR*, 2010 (11)	0–500	1.79	1.55
Taouli, et al.	*AJR*, 2007 (12)	0 / 500	1.60	1.22
		0 / 700	1.42	1.14
		0 / 1000	1.19	1.01

10.4 IVIM for Staging Liver Fibrosis

IVIM DWI is a biexponential model-based method that is used for simultaneous estimation of both perfusion-related (fast) and molecular diffusion–related (slow) diffusivity and analyzes the signal decay of multi-*b*-value diffusion-weighted images [14, 15]. The histopathologic structures of the liver are altered by fibrosis, so diffusivity measured by DWI or IVIM is strongly affected by the degree of fibrosis. Accumulation of collagen deposits increases the resistance of the portal system to blood flow, which in turn decreases the velocity of portal blood flow and increases the pressure in the portal system. IVIM is thought to be more suitable than DWI (monoexponential) in terms of precise estimation of the events occurring in a liver with fibrosis and uses the following three parameters: true diffusion, denoted by D; pseudodiffusion (perfusion), denoted by D^*; and the perfusion fraction, denoted by f [16].

10.4.1 Diagnostic Performance of IVIM for Liver Fibrosis

According to a recent systematic review and meta-analysis of studies that included DWI and IVIM [17], pooled sensitivity values with corresponding 95% confidence intervals (CIs) for liver fibrosis ≥F1, ≥F2, ≥F3, and F4 were 0.78 (95% CI 0.75–0.82), 0.81 (95% CI 0.78–0.84), 0.71 (95% CI 0.67–0.75), and 0.80 (95% CI 0.75–0.85), respectively. Pooled specificity values for liver fibrosis ≥F1, ≥F2, ≥F3, and F4 were 0.78 (95% CI 0.73–0.82), 0.80 (95% CI 0.76–0.83), 0.84 (95% CI 0.81–0.86), and 0.77 (95% CI 0.74–0.81), respectively. The area under the receiver-operating characteristic curve (Az) values that distinguished liver fibrosis ≥F1 from F0, ≥F2 from <F2, ≥F3 from <F3, and F4 from <F4 were 0.8554, 0.8770, 0.8836, and 0.8596, respectively. These results indicate that IVIM has good but not excellent diagnostic accuracy for staging of liver fibrosis (with Az values in the range of 0.8–0.9) when compared with magnetic resonance imaging (MRI) or ultrasound-based elastography (Table 10.2) [17–19].

Another meta-analysis [20] that included six papers focusing on IVIM only [21–26] showed that the weighted mean difference (WMD) values for D^* and D measurements were statistically significant in terms of distinguishing fibrosis stage (F0 vs. F1–4, WMD=2.46 [95% CI 0.83–4.09, $P = 0.006$] for D^* and 1.62 [95% CI 0.06–3.18, $P = 0.027$] for f; F0–1 vs. F2–3, 13.10 [95% CI 9.53–16.67, $P< 0.001$] for D^* and 5.63 [95% CI 2.74–8.52, $P< 0.001$] for f; F1–2 vs. F3–4, 14.34 [95% CI 10.26–18.42, $P< 0.001$] for D* and 3.30 [95% CI 2.10–4.50, $P< 0.001$] for f). However, the WMD values were not significant for the D and ADC measurements, except for the ADC of F1–2 versus F3–4 (WMD = 0.07 [95% CI 0.02–0.12, P=0.002]). This meta-analysis suggested that perfusion-related diffusivity (D^*) has a larger impact on reduced diffusivity than on true molecular diffusivity (D) in liver fibrosis. Considering the significant hemodynamic changes accompanying fibrosis of the liver, it seems reasonable that changes in D^* are substantial in cirrhosis (Figs.10.1–10.3).

Table 10.2 Diagnostic results of different liver fibrosis stages compared to magnetic resonance– or ultrasound-based elastography

	Sensitivity	Specificity	Positive likelihood ratio	Negative likelihood ratio	AUC
IVIM (17)					
≥ F1	0.78 (0.75–0.82)	0.78 (0.73–0.82)	3.24 (2.43–4.32)	0.29 (0.22–0.37)	0.86
≥ F2	0.81 (0.78–0.84)	0.80 (0.76–0.83)	3.72 (2.75–5.02)	0.25 (0.19–0.33)	0.88
≥ F3	0.71 (0.67–0.75)	0.84 (0.81–0.86)	4.44 (3.35–5.88)	0.28 (0.18–0.42)	0.88
= F4	0.80 (0.75–0.85)	0.77 (0.74–0.81)	3.30 (2.66–4.09)	0.31 (0.23–0.41)	0.86
MRE (18)					
≥ F1	0.83 (0.81–0.85)	0.91 (0.88–0.94)	10.27 (4.79–22.06)	0.19 (0.13–0.28)	0.93
≥ F2	0.92 (0.89–0.94)	0.92 (0.90–0.95)	9.44 (5.99–14.87)	0.12 (0.08–0.17)	0.95
≥ F3	0.88 (0.86–0.90)	0.92 (0.90–0.93)	10.28 (7.60–13.90)	0.15 (0.12–0.19)	0.94
= F4	0.88 (0.85–0.91)	0.91 (0.90–0.93)	9.45 (7.09–12.59)	0.15 (0.11–0.19)	0.92
SWE (19)					
≥ F1	0.76 (0.71–0.81)	0.92 (0.80–0.97)	9.28 (3.57–24.08)	0.26 (0.20–0.32)	0.85
≥ F2	0.84 (0.81–0.86)	0.83 (0.77–0.88)	4.92 (3.65–6.61)	0.20 (0.17–0.23)	0.87
≥ F3	0.89 (0.86–0.92)	0.86 (0.82–0.90)	6.40 (4.76–8.62)	0.13 (0.10–0.17)	0.93
= F4	0.89 (0.84–0.92)	0.88 (0.84–0.92)	7.68 (5.30–11.13)	0.13 (0.09–0.18)	0.94

AUC, area under ROC curve; MRE, magnetic resonance elastography; SWE, shear wave elastography

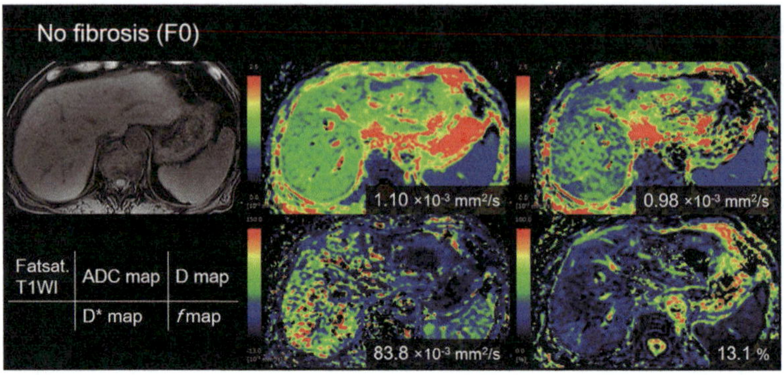

Figure 10.1 An 80-year-old man with no chronic liver disease (F0).

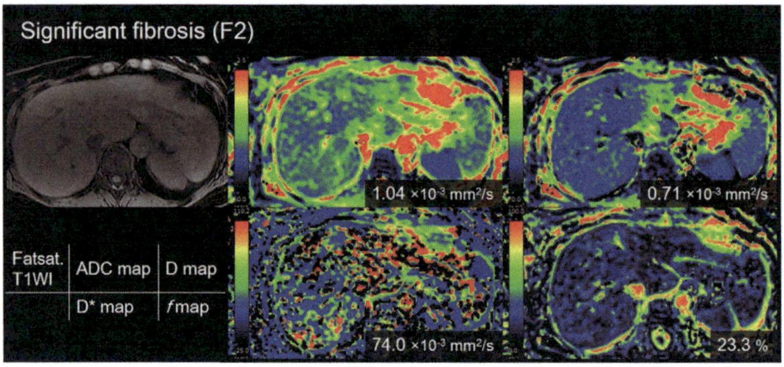

Figure 10.2 A 58-year-old-woman with chronic hepatitis type C (F2).

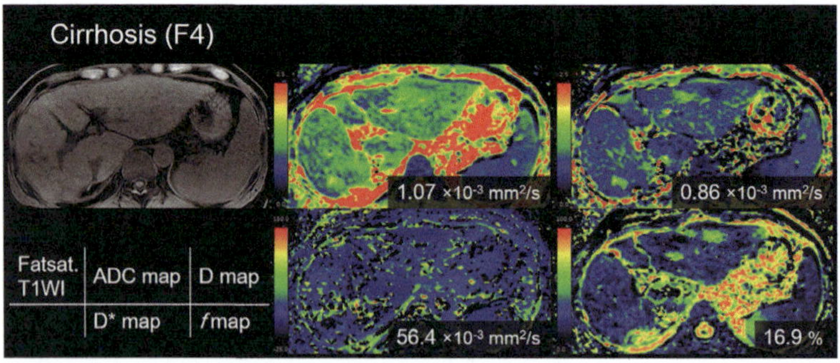

Figure 10.3 A 77-year-old-man with cirrhosis type C (F4). The *D** value of the liver decreased as the stage of the liver fibrosis progressed (from the red to the green area dominant in F0 and the blue area dominant in F4). There is no significant trend between the stage of fibrosis and other parameters (apparent diffusion coefficient, *D*, and *f* value).

Liver cirrhosis results in architectural changes in the liver parenchyma that have a direct effect on the microcirculation and macrocirculation in the liver. Portal perfusion decreases, while perfusion of the liver is partially compensated for by an increased hepatic arterial blood supply [27]. These changes in the hepatic circulation can be depicted in contrast-enhanced perfusion computed tomography (CT)/MRI as decreased portal flow and increased arterial flow in the liver [28]. There is a significant correlation between these perfusion CT/MRI-related parameters and the severity of chronic liver disease [28–30]. Reduced D^* in cirrhotic livers may represent these alterations in the hepatic circulation or perfusion [31]. In cirrhosis, the proportion of the volume of collagen fibers relative to that of hepatic sinuses could increase, which can reduce the f value. Although we have only collateral evidence, D^* and f measured by IVIM may be a biomarker for alteration of liver perfusion in the cirrhotic liver.

10.4.2 Factors Influencing IVIM Values

Magnetic field strength

Theoretically, DWI performed using a 3-T MR unit has the advantage of an improved signal-to-noise ratio in comparison with a 1.5-T MR unit [32]. However, a 3-T MR unit also has disadvantages, such as an increased number of magnetic susceptibility artifacts and eddy currents related to image distortion [33]. Cui et al. reported lower D and D^* values and a higher f value at 3 T when compared with values at 1.5 T and that the D and ADC values were reproducible between 1.5 T and 3 T MRI [34]. Barbieri et al. also reported a higher f value at 3 T than at 1.5 T [35]. At least, we should recognize the difference in measurement results attributable to field strength.

Number of *b* values

IVIM parameters depend on the choice of b values. Including more b values and applying an optimized b-value distribution reduce errors in IVIM parameter estimates [36]. A useful b-value distribution should have more b values in the range of 0–50 s/mm^2 and fewer in the midrange of 450–800 s/mm^2 and up to 1000 s/mm^2 [36]. The D^* value is more related to low b values. Li et al. constructed a graph of diffusion-weighted signals with respect to applied b values based on the values published for normal liver parenchyma. The curves are virtually parallel in the region of 100–800 s/mm^2, being almost exclusively influenced by the D value; however, they differ in the region of 0–100 s/mm^2, which is the most sensitive region for differentiation of the curves and the most difficult to fit reliably, especially in tissue with a high perfusion factor [37]. Lemke et al. reported that at least 10 optimally distributed b values should be measured for an IVIM experiment of high quality [36], whereas ter Voert et al. recommended 11 b values as an absolute minimum and preferably 16 [38]. At our hospital, we use 11 b values: 0, 10, 20, 30, 40, 50, 80, 100, 200, 500, and 1000 s/mm^2. The acquisition time for IVIM is 2–3 min., which is clinically acceptable. However, there is no consensus at this time regarding the choice of b values for liver IVIM.

Image postprocessing methods for IVIM parameters

Various methods have been used to calculate the IVIM parameters, including nonlinear least-squares fitting, combined linear and nonlinear least-squares fitting, and the Bayesian method. Presently, no conclusion can be drawn with regard to which of these methods is the best. However, it is clear that these parameters cannot be compared using values obtained by different postprocessing methods [37]. It should be recognized that IVIM parameters may vary depending on the fitting methods used. Different methods produce different results even though the same data are used. The D^* value, in particular, has been reported to show very wide variation because of the different postprocessing methods used [39].

Rapid motion caused by beating of the heart and respiration

Cardiac and respiratory movements are both bulk motions that are not supposed to cause intravoxel phase dispersion. However, they do cause motion artifact in images acquired in echo-planar acquisition. Furthermore, if these movements are rapid enough to be captured during motion encoding of the DWI acquisition, intravoxel phase dispersion occurs more often on images with a high b value than in those with a low b value (or $b = 0$). The effect of cardiac motion is more pronounced in the left lobe (resulting in a higher ADC [D^* and D] value in this lobe) than in the right lobe of the liver [40, 41]. Therefore, measurement (placement of the region of interest) in the right lobe is recommended for motion-robust measurement of diffusivity.

10.4.3 Drawbacks of IVIM for Staging Liver Fibrosis

As described above, IVIM is a useful noninvasive tool for staging hepatic fibrosis. However, there are some issues to be resolved.

Confounders

Inflammation may influence both ADC measurements and the IVIM parameters of diffusion and perfusion. The presence of concomitant fat and iron deposits in the liver parenchyma might also affect water diffusion. The *D* value can be influenced by fat and iron in the liver, which commonly coexist with liver fibrosis [42]. However, there have been no reports on staging the inflammatory activity of the liver by IVIM. Sandrasegaran et al. reported that IVIM parameters were not strongly predictive of hepatic fat content or inflammatory activity [43]. Moreover, Franca et al. reported that IVIM measurements were not accurate enough to stage necroinflammatory activity in diffuse liver disease [42].

Reproducibility

The poor reproducibility of the D^* value has been demonstrated in previous studies [42–46] and may reflect unstable signal acquisition or fitting uncertainty, as demonstrated in one published study [47]. This is the biggest issue associated with IVIM of the liver. Further technical refinement will be needed before IVIM can be used widely as a biomarker of liver fibrosis in the clinical setting.

10.5 Conclusion

DWI is an entirely noninvasive technique that can be performed routinely in a clinical MR protocol for the liver. IVIM MRI is worth studying further as a tool for staging liver fibrosis.

References

1. Nakagawa H., Maeda S., Yoshida H., et al. Serum IL-6 levels and the risk for hepatocarcinogenesis in chronic hepatitis C patients: an analysis based on gender differences. *Int. J. Cancer*, 2009, 125(10), 2264–2269.
2. Tsukuma H., Hiyama T., Tanaka S., et al. Risk factors for hepatocellular carcinoma among patients with chronic liver disease. *N. Engl. J. Med.*, 1993, 328(25), 1797–1801.

3. Marcellin P., Gane E., Buti M., et al. Regression of cirrhosis during treatment with tenofovir disoproxil fumarate for chronic hepatitis B: a 5-year open-label follow-up study. *Lancet*, 2013, 381(9865), 468–475.
4. Standish R. A., Cholongitas E., Dhillon A., Burroughs A. K., Dhillon A. P. An appraisal of the histopathological assessment of liver fibrosis. *Gut*, 2006, 55(4), 569–578.
5. Bravo A. A., Sheth S. G., Chopra S. Liver biopsy. *N. Engl. J. Med.*, 2001, 344(7), 495–500.
6. Regev A., Berho M., Jeffers L. J., et al. Sampling error and intraobserver variation in liver biopsy in patients with chronic HCV infection. *Am. J. Gastroenterol.*, 2002, 97(10), 2614–2618.
7. Intraobserver and interobserver variations in liver biopsy interpretation in patients with chronic hepatitis C. The French METAVIR Cooperative Study Group. *Hepatology*, 1994, 20(1Pt 1), 15–20.
8. Bedossa P., Poynard T. An algorithm for the grading of activity in chronic hepatitis C. The METAVIR Cooperative Study Group. *Hepatology*, 1996, 24(2): 289–293.
9. Koinuma M., Ohashi I., Hanafusa K., Shibuya H. Apparent diffusion coefficient measurements with diffusion-weighted magnetic resonance imaging for evaluation of hepatic fibrosis. *J. Magn. Reson. Imaging*, 2005, 22(1), 80–85.
10. Lewin M., Poujol-Robert A., Boelle P. Y., et al. Diffusion-weighted magnetic resonance imaging for the assessment of fibrosis in chronic hepatitis C. *Hepatology*, 2007, 46(3), 658–665.
11. Sandrasegaran K., Akisik F. M., Lin C., et al. Value of diffusion-weighted MRI for assessing liver fibrosis and cirrhosis. *AJR Am. J. Roentgenol.*, 2009, 193(6), 1556–1560.
12. Do R. K., Chandarana H., Felker E., et al. Diagnosis of liver fibrosis and cirrhosis with diffusion-weighted imaging: value of normalized apparent diffusion coefficient using the spleen as reference organ. *AJR Am. J. Roentgenol.*, 2010, 195(3), 671–676.
13. Taouli B., Tolia A. J., Losada M., et al. Diffusion-weighted MRI for quantification of liver fibrosis: preliminary experience. *AJR Am. J. Roentgenol.*, 2007, 189(4), 799–806.
14. Le Bihan D., Breton E., Lallemand D., Grenier P., Cabanis E., Laval-Jeantet M. MR imaging of intravoxel incoherent motions: application to diffusion and perfusion in neurologic disorders. *Radiology*, 1986, 161(2), 401–407.

15. Le Bihan D. Intravoxel incoherent motion perfusion MR imaging: a wake-up call. *Radiology*, 2008, 249(3), 748–752.

16. Le Bihan D., Breton E., Lallemand D., Aubin M. L., Vignaud J., Laval-Jeantet M. Separation of diffusion and perfusion in intravoxel incoherent motion MR imaging. *Radiology*, 1988, 168(2), 497–505.

17. Jiang H., Chen J., Gao R., Huang Z., Wu M., Song B. Liver fibrosis staging with diffusion-weighted imaging: a systematic review and meta-analysis. *Abdom. Radiol. (NY)*, 2017, 42(2), 490–501.

18. Kim Y. S., Jang Y. N., Song J. S. Comparison of gradient-recalled echo and spin-echo echo-planar imaging MR elastography in staging liver fibrosis: a meta-analysis. *Eur. Radiol.*, 2018, 28(4), 1709–1718.

19. Jiang T., Tian G., Zhao Q., et al. Diagnostic accuracy of 2D-shear wave elastography for liver fibrosis severity: a meta-analysis. *PLoS One*, 2016, 11(6), e0157219.

20. Zhang B., Liang L., Dong Y., et al. Intravoxel incoherent motion MR imaging for staging of hepatic fibrosis. *PLoS One*, 2016, 11(1), e0147789.

21. Chung S. R., Lee S. S., Kim N., et al. Intravoxel incoherent motion MRI for liver fibrosis assessment: a pilot study. *Acta Radiol.*, 2015, 56(12), 1428–1436.

22. Ichikawa S., Motosugi U., Morisaka H., et al. MRI-based staging of hepatic fibrosis: Comparison of intravoxel incoherent motion diffusion-weighted imaging with magnetic resonance elastography. *J. Magn. Reson. Imaging*, 2015, 42(1), 204–210.

23. Yoon J. H., Lee J. M., Baek J. H., et al. Evaluation of hepatic fibrosis using intravoxel incoherent motion in diffusion-weighted liver MRI. *J. Comput. Assist. Tomogr.*, 2014, 38(1), 110–116.

24. Leporq B., Saint-Jalmes H., Rabrait C., et al. Optimization of intra-voxel incoherent motion imaging at 3.0 Tesla for fast liver examination. *J. Magn. Reson. Imaging.*, 2015, 41(5), 1209–1217.

25. Lu P. X., Huang H., Yuan J., et al. Decreases in molecular diffusion, perfusion fraction and perfusion-related diffusion in fibrotic livers: a prospective clinical intravoxel incoherent motion MR imaging study. *PLoS One*, 2014, 9(12), e113846.

26. Wu C. H., Ho M. C., Jeng Y. M., et al. Assessing hepatic fibrosis: comparing the intravoxel incoherent motion in MRI with acoustic radiation force impulse imaging in US. *Eur. Radiol.*, 2015, 25(12), 3552–3559.

27. Moreno A. H., Rousselot L. M., Panke W. F., Burke M. L. The rate of hepatic blood flow in normal subjects and in patients with portal hypertension. *Surg. Gynecol. Obstet.*, 1960, 111, 443–450.

28. Van Beers B. E., Leconte I., Materne R., Smith A. M., Jamart J., Horsmans Y. Hepatic perfusion parameters in chronic liver disease: dynamic CT measurements correlated with disease severity. *AJR Am. J. Roentgenol.*, 2001, 176(3), 667–673.

29. Ronot M., Asselah T., Paradis V., et al. Liver fibrosis in chronic hepatitis C virus infection: differentiating minimal from intermediate fibrosis with perfusion CT. *Radiology*, 2010, 256(1), 135–142.

30. Hashimoto K., Murakami T., Dono K., et al. Assessment of the severity of liver disease and fibrotic change: the usefulness of hepatic CT perfusion imaging. *Oncol. Rep.*, 16(4), 677–683.

31. Le Bihan D., Turner R. The capillary network: a link between IVIM and classical perfusion. *Magn. Reson. Med.*, 1992, 27(1), 171–178.

32. Riffel P., Rao R. K., Haneder S., Meyer M., Schoenberg S. O., Michaely H. J. Impact of field strength and RF excitation on abdominal diffusion-weighted magnetic resonance imaging. *World J. Radiol.*, 2013, 5(9), 334–344.

33. Springer F., Martirosian P., Boss A., Claussen C. D., Schick F. Current problems and future opportunities of abdominal magnetic resonance imaging at higher field strengths. *Top Magn. Reson. Imaging*, 2010, 21(3), 141–148.

34. Cui Y., Dyvorne H., Besa C., Cooper N., Taouli B. IVIM Diffusion-weighted imaging of the liver at 3.0T: Comparison with 1.5T. *Eur. J. Radiol. Open*, 2015, 2, 123–128.

35. Barbieri S., Donati O. F., Froehlich J. M., Thoeny H. C. Comparison of intravoxel incoherent motion parameters across MR imagers and field strengths: evaluation in upper abdominal organs. *Radiology*, 2016, 279(3), 784–794.

36. Lemke A., Stieltjes B., Schad L. R., Laun F. B. Toward an optimal distribution of *b* values for intravoxel incoherent motion imaging. *Magn. Reson. Imaging*, 2011, 29(6), 766–776.

37. Li Y. T., Cercueil J. P., Yuan J., Chen W., Loffroy R., Wang Y. X. Liver intravoxel incoherent motion (IVIM) magnetic resonance imaging: a comprehensive review of published data on normal values and applications for fibrosis and tumor evaluation. *Quant Imaging Med Surg.*, 2017, 7(1), 59–78.

38. ter Voert E. E., Delso G., Porto M., Huellner M., Veit-Haibach P. Intravoxel incoherent motion protocol evaluation and data quality in normal and malignant liver tissue and comparison to the literature. *Invest. Radiol.*, 2016, 51(2), 90–99.

39. Ichikawa S., Motosugi U., Hernando D., et al. Histological grading of hepatocellular carcinomas with intravoxel incoherent motion diffusion-weighted imaging: inconsistent results depending on the fitting method. *Magn. Reson. Med. Sci.* 2017 Aug 16. doi: 10.2463/mrms.mp.2017-0047. [Epub ahead of print]

40. Nasu K., Kuroki Y., Fujii H., Minami M. Hepatic pseudo-anisotropy: a specific artifact in hepatic diffusion-weighted images obtained with respiratory triggering. *MAGMA*, 2007, 20(4), 205–211.

41. Kwee T. C., Takahara T., Niwa T., et al. Influence of cardiac motion on diffusion-weighted magnetic resonance imaging of the liver. *MAGMA*, 2009, 22(5), 319–325.

42. Franca M., Marti-Bonmati L., Alberich-Bayarri A., et al. Evaluation of fibrosis and inflammation in diffuse liver diseases using intravoxel incoherent motion diffusion-weighted MR imaging. *Abdom. Radiol. (NY)*, 2017, 42(2), 468–477.

43. Sandrasegaran K., Territo P., Elkady R. M., et al. Does intravoxel incoherent motion reliably stage hepatic fibrosis, steatosis, and inflammation? *Abdom. Radiol. (NY)*, 2018, 43(3), 600–606.

44. Andreou A., Koh D. M., Collins D. J., et al. Measurement reproducibility of perfusion fraction and pseudodiffusion coefficient derived by intravoxel incoherent motion diffusion-weighted MR imaging in normal liver and metastases. *Eur. Radiol.*, 2013, 23(2), 428–434.

45. Kakite S., Dyvorne H., Besa C., et al. Hepatocellular carcinoma: short-term reproducibility of apparent diffusion coefficient and intravoxel incoherent motion parameters at 3.0 T. *J. Magn. Reson. Imaging*, 2015, 41(1), 149–156.

46. Lee Y., Lee S. S., Kim N., et al. Intravoxel incoherent motion diffusion-weighted MR imaging of the liver: effect of triggering methods on regional variability and measurement repeatability of quantitative parameters. *Radiology*, 2015, 274(2), 405–415.

47. Dyvorne H. A., Galea N., Nevers T., et al. Diffusion-weighted imaging of the liver with multiple *b* values: effect of diffusion gradient polarity and breathing acquisition on image quality and intravoxel incoherent motion parameters—a pilot study. *Radiology*, 2013, 266(3), 920–929.

Chapter 11

Assessment of Liver Tumors with IVIM Diffusion-Weighted Imaging

Stefanie J. Hectors, Sara Lewis, and Bachir Taouli
Translational and Molecular Imaging Institute,
Icahn School of Medicine at Mount Sinai, New York, USA
Department of Radiology, Icahn School of Medicine at
Mount Sinai, New York, USA
bachir.taouli@mountsinai.org

Intravoxel incoherent motion diffusion-weighted imaging (IVIM DWI) is a noninvasive imaging method that probes the mobility of microscopic water molecules in biologic tissues and incorporates the contributions of microvascular perfusion and true cellular diffusion restriction. This method is well suited for investigation of focal liver lesions (FLL). Important technical considerations for IVIM include the selection of *b* values, acquisition technique, field strength, fitting algorithm, and postprocessing methods. Recent studies have explored the use of IVIM DWI for a variety of applications, including characterization of liver lesions, prediction of tumor grade, and

Intravoxel Incoherent Motion (IVIM) MRI: Principles and Applications
Edited by Denis Le Bihan, Mami Iima, Christian Federau, and Eric E. Sigmund

ISBN 978-981-4800-19-8 (Hardcover), 978-0-429-42727-5 (eBook)
www.panstanford.com

evaluation of the post-treatment response. This chapter will discuss in detail the promising early results of IVIM assessment of FLL.

11.1 Introduction

Given the increasing utilization of magnetic resonance imaging (MRI) and recent technological advances in hardware and software, FLL are being detected with increasing frequency in the clinical setting. Accurate detection and characterization is essential for diagnosis and appropriate management; and the superior soft-tissue contrast resolution of MRI is well suited for this purpose. There is increasing interest in the development and validation of advanced MRI methods to provide both anatomic and functional information. DWI has shown its value for a variety of clinical indications and is now widely adopted in most clinical abdominal protocols. IVIM has been recently implemented predominantly in the research setting, given the ability of this method to noninvasively and simultaneously probe several physiologic processes affecting tissues. An additional benefit of the use of DWI methods is the lack of intravenous gadolinium–based contrast administration, which is of increasing concern in the era of nephrogenic systemic fibrosis (NSF) [1] and given recent reports of gadolinium deposition in the central nervous system [2]. In this chapter, we will explore the use of the IVIM DWI technique in FLL, with an emphasis on technique, clinical applications, limitations, and future directions.

11.2 Background on Focal Liver Lesions

FLL are generally either benign or malignant, with rare premalignant lesions (hepatocellular adenomas [HCAs] and high-grade dysplastic nodules in cirrhosis). The most commonly encountered benign liver lesions are hemangiomas (reported prevalence 0.1%–20.0%), cysts (reported prevalence 0.06%–17.8%), focal nodular hyperplasia (FNH) (reported prevalence 0.8%–3.2%), and HCA (reported prevalence 0.4%–1.5%) [3]. The most frequently encountered malignant lesions are primary liver cancers, such as hepatocellular carcinoma (HCC) (reported incidence of 4.8 per 100,000/year), intrahepatic cholangiocarcinoma (ICC) (reported incidence of 1.6 per 100,000/year), and combined "bi-phenotypic" hepatocellular-cholangiocarcinoma (cHCC-ICC) [4]. The age-adjusted incidence of cHCC-ICC is not well known, as these lesions were only recently recognized by the World Health Organization (WHO) as a distinct subtype of ICC. However, they represent approximately 0.4%–14.5% of all primary liver cancers [5, 6]. Secondary (metastatic) cancers from a variety of primary cancer sites occur approximately 18 times more frequently than primary liver cancers [7]. It is essential to avoid unnecessary biopsy in patients with benign lesions, given the invasive nature and risk of complications associated with tissue sampling [8, 9]; and it is necessary to accurately diagnose malignant lesions for disease staging and directing patient management.

HCC is the sixth-most-common form of cancer and the third leading cause of cancer-related death [10]. HCC is the most common primary liver cancer and is closely linked to the presence of chronic liver disease, fibrosis, and cirrhosis, with an annual incidence ranging from 0.25% to 7.6%, depending on the etiology of the underlying liver disease and other risk factors [11]. HCC has high morbidity and mortality, with a five-year survival of <10% when detected after symptoms develop [12]. Accurate diagnosis is especially important as HCC is typically an imaging diagnosis, and tissue confirmation is only performed in a limited number of cases that demonstrate an atypical imaging appearance [13]. Depending on the tumor stage and the severity of the background liver disease, patients with HCC are generally treated with resection, liver transplantation, locoregional therapy (LRT), or systemic therapy using novel molecular-targeted agents [14]. Although arising less commonly, ICC and cHCC-ICC share common risk factors with HCC but will differ in both treatment strategy and prognosis [6, 15]. Currently, ICC and cHCC-ICC are considered relative contraindications to liver transplant and are also more sensitive to systemic chemotherapy, whereas systemic chemotherapy has not been shown to be effective for HCC [6, 16]. Therefore, it is essential that benign and malignant liver lesions are accurately detected and characterized, in order to inform management decisions.

11.3 Current Evidence on the Use of DWI and ADC for Liver Tumor Detection and Characterization

Multiphasic contrast-enhanced MRI (CEMRI) is currently the clinical standard for the assessment of FLL [17]. However, there is increasing interest in the validation of noninvasive and noncontrast methods, including DWI, for the evaluation of liver lesions. There is evidence of the potential added value of DWI for the detection and characterization of FLL. Low-*b*-value ($b<100$) DWI produces "black blood" images due to a suppressed vascular flow, leading to improved conspicuity of lesions, particularly for lesions adjacent to blood vessels [17].

11.3.1 DWI for Liver Lesion Detection

The diagnostic performance of DWI in liver lesion detection has been quite extensively compared with that of conventional sequences, such as T2-weighted imaging (T2WI) and CEMRI. Several studies have shown that DWI outperforms T2WI in terms of detection of FLL, including liver metastases, with accuracy values of 84.4%–92% reported for DWI versus 47%–70.1% reported for T2WI [18–20]. The detection rate of HCC in particular has also shown to be significantly higher using DWI compared to T2WI (80.5% vs. 53.9%) [19]. With respect to comparison with CEMRI, a recent meta-analysis by Vilgrain et al., which included 39 published articles with a total of 1989 patients, reported sensitivity values of 87.1%, 90.6%, and 95.5% for the detection of hepatic metastases using DWI, gadoxetic acid–enhanced MRI, and the combination of both methods, respectively. While DWI performed significantly worse than gadoxetic acid–enhanced MRI for lesion detection ($P = 0.0001$), it was shown that the combination of DWI with gadoxetic acid–enhanced MRI led to significantly better lesion detection compared to gadoxetic acid–enhanced MRI alone ($P < 0.0001$) [21]. For HCC, reported results on comparison between CEMRI and DWI have been mixed. Piana et al. showed improved sensitivity for HCC detection using DWI compared to CEMRI in 91 patients with 109 HCC lesions (72.5%–81.7% vs. 59.6%) [22], while Park et al. showed that DWI was outperformed by CEMRI (75.8% vs. 87.9%) for HCC detection in 52 patients with 72 HCC lesions (using explant correlation) [23]. Another study reported that combined DWI and CEMRI yielded improved sensitivity (95.2%) for the detection of small HCC lesions (<2 cm) in a cohort of 130 patients [24]. It is likely that the presence of background liver fibrosis and cirrhosis, which commonly coexist with HCC, contributes to lower tumor detection rates [25]. Reports of DWI for the detection of ICC are limited. A study by Park et al. showed that target appearance on DWI (a hyperintense rim with a central hypointense area) was the only significant predictor of ICC versus HCC among other features based on gadoxetic acid-enhanced MRI and DWI [26]. This study indicates the potential value of DWI for the detection of ICC, although this needs to be validated in a separate study.

11.3.2 DWI for Lesion Characterization

The apparent diffusion coefficient (ADC) measured with DWI has been extensively investigated as a parameter to differentiate between types of FLL. Several studies have assessed the diagnostic performance of ADC for differentiation between benign and malignant liver lesions. Using ADC cutoff values of 1.5–1.6 × 10^{-3} mm^2/s, sensitivity values of 63.5%–87% and specificity values of 77.3%–90% have been reported for the diagnosis of malignant liver lesions [19, 27–29]. In a large DWI study involving 542 FLL in 382 patients, it was found that cysts could be easily distinguished from other lesions but that there was significant overlap between ADC values of benign and malignant liver lesions [28]. Recent studies for HCC, ICC, and metastatic disease have also demonstrated the value of ADC measurement in predicting tumor grade, with an inverse relationship of ADC with increasing tumor grade [30–32].

In summary, DWI is increasingly being employed for the detection and characterization of liver lesions. While results have been promising, DWI cannot be used as a standalone technique for liver cancer imaging because of the overall lower detection rate of hepatic lesions compared to CEMRI and the substantial overlap between ADC values of benign and malignant lesions. More advanced DWI methods, including IVIM DWI, may potentially improve the sensitivity of DWI to liver lesion malignancy.

11.4 IVIM DWI for the Assessment of Liver Lesions: Technical Considerations

Because IVIM incorporates the contributions of microvascular perfusion and true cellular diffusion restriction, it has attracted much attention for the assessment of liver lesions. However, IVIM DWI for the detection and characterization of liver lesions is challenging, given the generally long acquisition times and respiratory motion. IVIM parameter quantification may be affected by several factors, including *b* values, acquisition scheme, field strength, and processing methods. Several technical considerations need to be taken into account to improve the accuracy of IVIM DWI for the imaging of liver lesions and are discussed in detail below.

11.4.1 Acquisition

Selection of *b* values

IVIM DWI employs a biexponential fitting model to extract three different variables from multi-*b*-value DWI data: pseudodiffusion coefficient D^* (or D_{fast}), (true) diffusion coefficient D (or D_t), and perfusion fraction (f or PF). A detailed description of the IVIM DWI technique can be found in Chapter 1, "Introduction to IVIM MRI." Due to the fitting of a larger number of variables compared to monoexponential fitting, the IVIM model is overall less stable than the monoexponential diffusion model that is used to extract ADC. While in theory four *b* values would be sufficient to fit the three IVIM parameters, the use of more *b* values improves parameter estimation. Dyvorne et al. showed that the use of an optimal set of four *b* values (0, 15, 150, and 800 s/mm^2) led to estimation errors that were below the test-retest repeatability of IVIM parameters in the liver [33]. Ter Voert et al. found that the use of 16 *b* values ranging from 0 to 1000 s/mm^2 yielded accurate results of IVIM for the characterization of liver lesions [34]. However, in light of restricted acquisition time in clinical applications, using at least 11 *b* values may be sufficient since the largest gain in error reduction was seen when moving from 4 to 11 *b* values [34].

Signal-to-noise ratio

DWI images with a sufficiently high signal-to-noise ratio (SNR) need to be obtained in order to allow for reliable fitting of IVIM DWI parameters. Using Monte Carlo simulations it was found that the accuracy of IVIM parameter estimation depends strongly and nonlinearly on the SNR and that an SNR value of at least 8 is required for IVIM DWI of tissues with high IVIM perfusion, such as the liver [35]. For low-perfused tissues, an SNR of at least 40 has been recommended [36]. Low perfusion may occur in tumor tissues, particularly when (treatment induced) necrosis is present. Therefore, an SNR of at least 40 would be advisable for reliable IVIM DWI of liver lesions.

Acquisition scheme

Published studies on IVIM for the evaluation of FLL have used a mix of respiratory-triggered (RT) [34, 37–50], free-breathing (FB) [51–57], and breath-hold [58–60] DWI techniques for IVIM acquisition. However, reports on the effect of the breathing scheme on IVIM DWI parameters in hepatic lesions are scarce. In a study of 30 patients with 37 small HCC lesions (range 0.5–2.0 cm), it was found that, while image quality with RT IVIM DWI was superior to FB IVIM DWI ($P = 0.02$), IVIM DWI parameters in HCC lesions were not significantly different between the acquisitions ($P > 0.24$) [61]. These results indicate that RT IVIM DWI is not advantageous for the quantification of IVIM DWI parameters in HCC except for a better image quality. Since FB acquisition schemes generally allow for faster IVIM acquisitions, FB IVIM DWI may be the best option in time-constrained clinical applications of IVIM DWI of liver lesions.

Field strength

While it has been reported that IVIM DWI parameters vary significantly between MR scanners in abdominal organs, including liver [62], the effect of field strength as a single variable on IVIM DWI parameter estimation in the liver has been scarcely studied. In a study of 19 subjects, it was found that all liver IVIM parameters were significantly different between 1.5T and 3.0T, except for the ADC ($P = 0.748$) [63]. While the use of 3.0T for IVIM DWI would appear advantageous due to an improved SNR compared to 1.5T, 3.0T IVIM

DWI images may be affected by increased magnetic susceptibility artifacts and eddy current–related distortions [64]. No studies have assessed differences in image quality and IVIM DWI parameters when using field strength of different values for hepatic lesions. Therefore, further investigation is warranted to determine which field strength is most suitable for IVIM DWI of hepatic lesions.

11.4.2 Postprocessing

Fitting algorithms

Since the accuracy of IVIM parameter estimation is strongly dependent on factors such as image quality and SNR, IVIM analysis requires a robust fitting method. Least-squares optimization is the mostly used fitting algorithm for IVIM modeling. However, it has been shown that Bayesian methods yield more stable and accurate IVIM parameters than least-squares methods [65, 66]. Unlike the least-squares method, which minimizes error residuals, the Bayesian methods determine the uncertainty of each parameter in the model and use a priori distributions of the IVIM parameters to determine joint posterior probability over all parameters. Superior fitting quality, as measured by variability and uncertainty estimates, of Bayesian versus least-squares methods has been demonstrated in the liver tissue of 20 patients with colorectal liver metastases [65]. While both fitting methods have not yet been compared in liver tumor tissue, it is expected that Bayesian modeling of IVIM data in liver tumors provides more stable and accurate parameter estimation. Nevertheless, only a few studies that used IVIM modeling of liver tumors have employed Bayesian modeling for the analysis of the IVIM data [40, 53]. Widespread implementation of Bayesian fitting algorithms for IVIM fitting may therefore be of value to improve parameter accuracy and stability.

Region of interest vs. parametric mapping

While most studies employed parametric mapping for IVIM analysis of liver lesions, several studies have used analysis of mean signal intensities in regions of interest (ROIs) within the lesion [39, 40, 50, 52, 53, 55, 58]. ROI-based analysis may be favorable in SNR-limited

IVIM DWI acquisitions as it increases the SNR for IVIM parameter fitting [52]. However, care must be taken using this approach for the analysis of heterogeneous or cystic/necrotic tumors, for which the averaged ROI signal will contain diffusion signals from different tissue types with distinct diffusion properties. The observed biexponential diffusion behavior in such cases may arise from the presence of tissue components with distinct diffusion coefficients rather than from pure diffusion and pseudodiffusion effects, leading to incorrect IVIM parameter estimates.

A summary of recommendations based on technical considerations for acquisition and postprocessing of IVIM DWI of liver lesions can be found in Table 11.1.

Table 11.1 Recommendations for acquisition and postprocessing of IVIM DWI data of liver lesions

Variable	Recommendation
Acquisition	
- *b* values	At least 11 *b* values
- SNR	At least 40
- Acquisition scheme	Free breathing
- Field strength	Either 1.5T or 3T
Postprocessing	
- Fitting algorithm	Bayesian
- ROI-based vs. parametric mapping	Parametric mapping

11.4.3 Quality Control

Reproducibility and repeatability of IVIM parameters

Several studies have assessed IVIM parameter measurement repeatability and reproducibility. Grouped results for reported coefficient of variations (CVs) for test-retest repeatability of IVIM parameters for FLL have shown that D^* and PF demonstrate poor measurement repeatability whereas the ADC and D generally show acceptable repeatability: ADC (8.3%–27.36%), D (8.7%–27.99%), D^* (11.9%–73.84%), and PF (13.7%–43.41%) [40, 42, 53, 67]. Interestingly, Kakite et al. showed that IVIM parameter repeatability was generally better for HCCs located in the right lobe compared to those in the left lobe [53]. With respect to parameter reproducibility, a recent study has assessed the reproducibility of IVIM parameters in HCC and FNH by two different 1.5T scanners [58]. While no significant difference in the measurement values of PF and D was observed, D^* for HCC and ADC for FNH were significantly different between the two MRIs (both $P = 0.02$) [58]. Results from these studies indicate that D^* suffers from the weakest repeatability and reproducibility, which could be secondary to a combination of physiologic and hemodynamic variability and technical limitations inherent to IVIM.

11.5 Applications of IVIM for the Assessment of FLL

11.5.1 Characterization of Benign and Malignant Liver Lesions

Early studies have shown mixed results regarding the performance of IVIM parameters for making the distinction between solid benign versus malignant liver lesions (Figs. 11.1–11.3). Malignant lesions are in theory well suited for investigation using IVIM, given the more complicated tissue microstructure, increased tumor cellularity, decreased extracellular space, accumulation of macromolecules, and altered intratumoral vascularity/perfusion. Grouped results of average IVIM parameter values for benign and malignant lesions from prior studies are summarized in Table 11.2. Several studies have shown that D (reflecting true diffusion restriction) is significantly lower in malignant lesions compared to benign lesions [42, 43, 50, 51, 55]. Results for the perfusion parameters PF and D^* have been mixed for the same studies. Furthermore, the added value of IVIM parameters compared to standard monoexponential ADC has also been mixed, with superior performance of ADC over IVIM parameters shown in some studies [51, 55]. Overall, the area under the curve (AUC) to accurately discriminate malignant from benign lesions ranges from 0.75 to 0.971 for D and from 0.75 to 0.983 for ADC [42, 43, 50, 51, 55, 57, 58].

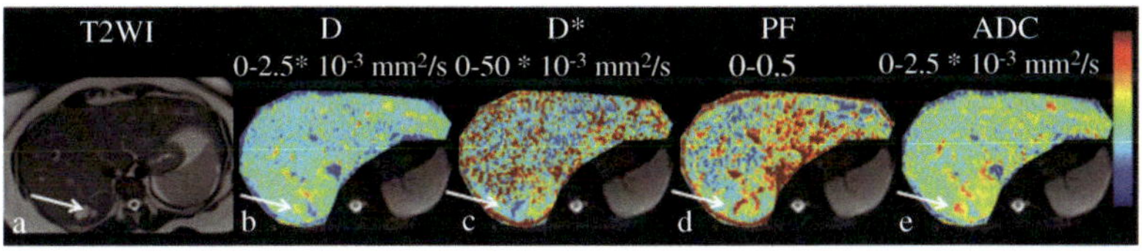

Figure 11.1 A 52-year-old female with NASH fibrosis (stage 3), steatosis, and a benign liver lesion. A 2.7 cm segment 7 hemangioma was identified at MRI with T2 and IVIM DWI performed with *b* values of 0–800 (arrows). *D*/*D**/PF/ADC values for the lesion were 1.4/17.6/0.27/1.7. ADC, *D*, and *D** values were expressed as 10^{-3} mm^2/s, and the PF is expressed as a fraction.

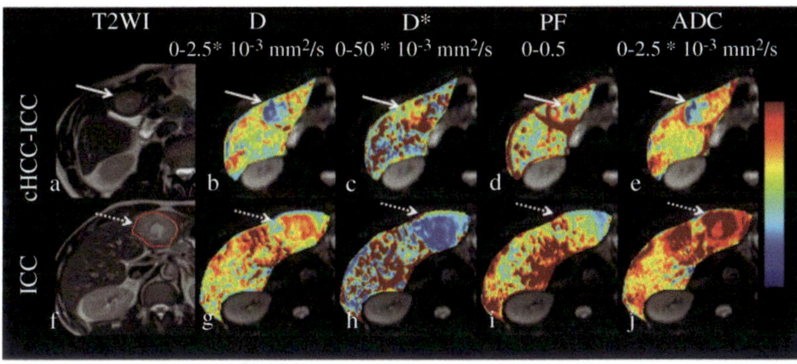

Figure 11.2 Primary liver cancers assessed with IVIM DWI. A 51-year-old male with synchronous segment 2 ICC (arrow) and segment 4 combined HCC-ICC (cHCC-ICC) (dashed arrow) that were incidentally detected at follow-up PET imaging for the history of laryngeal carcinoma. AFP was found to be elevated to 828.2 ng/mL. The patient underwent subsequent MRI, including T2 and IVIM DWI, showing the liver lesions (cHCC-ICC, top row of images, a–e; ICC, bottom row of images, f–j). IVIM DWI parameters (*D*/*D**/PF/ADC) for the cHCC-ICC and ICC were 0.8/40.3/0.30/1.1 and 1.7/11.5/0.29/2.4, respectively. The higher *D* and ADC values in the segment 2 ICC are explained by the presence of a large central necrosis within the lesion (red circle). ADC, *D*, and *D** values were expressed as 10^{-3} mm^2/s, and the PF is expressed as a fraction.

Furthermore, a potential role for IVIM to provide added value for lesion characterization lies in the assessment of hypervascular liver lesions, appearances of which can overlap on conventional imaging. A recent study by Luo et al. investigating HCC (n = 22) and FNHs (n = 5) demonstrated that ADC, *D*, and *D** were significantly lower in the HCC group than in the FNH group and that the AUC for *D* was 0.897, indicating high efficacy for accurate lesion distinction [42]. Contrary to these finding are the results from Klauss et al., in which there was no difference in *D** values for HCC and FNH [58]. Lastly, *D* (AUC 0.961) has also shown superior performance compared to ADC (AUC 0.919) for distinction of hypervascular malignant lesions from hypervascular benign lesions ($P < 0.0005$) [57].

Table 11.2 Ranges of reported values (mean ± SD) for IVIM parameters for benign and malignant liver lesions

	ADC	*D*	*D**	PF (%)
Benign (All)	(1.72–2.32) ± (0.37–0.87)	(1.61–1.70) ± (0.34–0.55)	(21.7–97.89) ± (9.9–78.82)	(26.00–33.5) ± (11.00–14.9)
Hemangioma	(2.00–2.94) ± (0.45–0.81)	(1.70–1.97) ± (0.32–0.79)	(38.96–119.80) ± (27.90–72.32)	(24.00–28.00) ± (10.00–16.02)
FNH	(1.57–2.30) ± (0.28–0.94)	(1.11–1.42) ± (0.14–0.35)	(39.9–166.64) ± (47.2–114.47)	(14.4–27.00) ± (5.8–10.00)
HCA	(1.41–1.86) ± (0.28–0.94)	(1.02–1.32) ± (0.12–0.34)	92.72 ± 54.06	22 ± 12
Malignant (All)	(1.14–1.64) ± (0.24–0.51)	(0.95–1.14) ± (0.19–0.28)	(16.5–102.10) ± (7.7–56.37)	(19.21–23.3) ± (7.38–9.5)
HCC	(1.10–1.76) ± (0.17–0.56)	(0.94–1.13) ± (0.18–0.34)	(21.17–107.23) ± (8.34–79.07)	(13.6–26.43) ± (6.50–9.00)
ICC		1.19 ± 0.35	15.68 ± 4.11	16.98 ± 9.9
Metastasis	(1.06–1.53) ± (0.31–0.43)	(0.93–1.29) ± 0.27–0.39)	(12.22–124.70) ± 3.71–88.68)	(11.16–24.00) ± (4.00–12.00)

Source: [41–43, 49–51, 55, 57, 58]

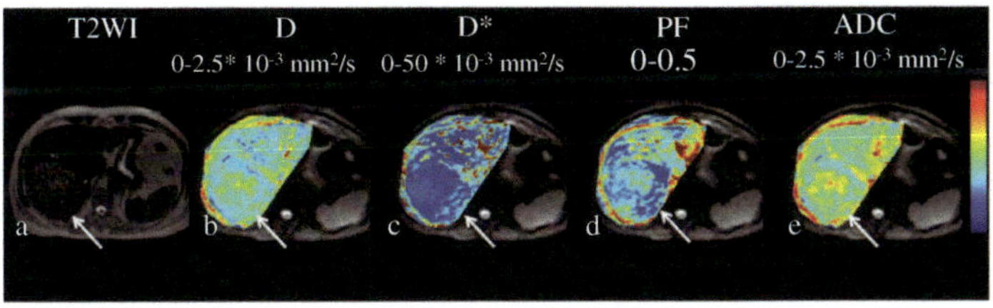

Figure 11.3 A 67-year-old male with a history of abdominal pain found to have a liver mass. The patient underwent MRI with T2 and IVIM DWI, demonstrating a 10.7 cm mass in the right lobe (arrows, a–e) with *D*/*D**/PF/ADC parameter values of 1.1/9.9/0.26/1.2, respectively. The ADC, *D*, and *D** values were expressed as 10^{-3} mm^2/s, and the PF is expressed as a fraction. A biopsy of the lesion revealed high-grade neuroendocrine tumor metastasis.

IVIM parameters have also been investigated for the evaluation of the HCC tumor grade. A recent study by Shan et al. in 106 patients with chronic HBV and HCC found that ADC, *D*, and PF values were significantly different among well-, moderately, and poorly differentiated HCCs. The AUCs of ADC, *D*, and PF for the distinction of well-differentiated HCCs were 0.903, 0.84, and 0.782, respectively, and for poorly differentiated HCCs were 0.787, 0.726, and 0.624, respectively [48]. Similar results were found in a separate study in 40 patients with 42 surgically confirmed HCC lesions, in which *D* ($r = -0.604$; $P < 0.0001$) and ADC ($r = -0.448$, $P = 0.002$) values were both inversely correlated with the HCC grade [56]. However, in this study the receiver operating characteristic (ROC) analysis revealed a higher area under the ROC (AUROC) curve for *D* compared to ADC (0.838 vs. 0.728, $P = 0.026$) for distinguishing poorly differentiated from well-differentiated HCC, contrary to Shan et al. [56].

11.5.2 Potential Role of IVIM as a Surrogate Marker for Perfusion and Enhancement

Malignant liver lesions tend to be highly aggressive and can cause perfusion alterations due to a variety of mechanisms, including invasion of native liver vessels and the development of tumor neoangiogenesis. While both *D** and PF provide perfusion information, they are believed to capture separate and complementary biologic information. *D** is believed to represent the length and velocity of the capillary network, and PF is believed to represent the fractional blood volume of microcirculation [68]. PF is also influenced by other bulk flow phenomena, including glandular secretion and the blood flow pattern. In the study by Woo et al., the percentage of arterial enhancement within HCC was significantly correlated with PF ($r = 0.621$, $P < 0.0001$) [56]. In a study comparing IVIM parameters to dynamic contrast-enhanced (DCE) MRI in 25 patients (23 treatment naïve HCC patients and 2 patients status post LRT), multiple significant correlations were found for the DCE MRI arterial fraction (ART) and IVIM D^* ($r = -0.443$, $P = 0.028$), PF ($r = -0.536$, $P = 0.006$), and PF × D^* ($r = -0.655$, $P < 0.001$) and for DCE MRI arterial flow (F_a) and IVIM PF ($r = -0.455$, $P = 0.023$) and PF × D^* ($r = -0.475$, $P = 0.018$) in liver parenchyma, while no correlations between DCE MRI and IVIM parameters were found for HCCs [40]. Kim et al. found significant positive correlations of D^* and PF with DCE MRI perfusion parameter K^{trans} ($r = 0.519$, $P < 0.023$ and $r = 0.590$, $P = 0.008$, respectively) in a study of 19 patients with hepatic metastases from colorectal cancer [54].

11.5.3 Assessment of Post-Therapy Response

IVIM has been investigated as a noninvasive imaging biomarker for predicting response to therapy for primary and secondary hepatic malignancies, with promising early results. The potential added value in IVIM lies in its ability to demonstrate early changes in functional measurements, reflecting post-treatment alterations in tumor perfusion and vascularity that precede changes in lesion size, thus providing early predictive information regarding treatment efficacy and informing future treatment decisions.

HCC

IVIM has been investigated in HCC patients undergoing LRT. ADC, *D*, and PF all correlated with tumor necrosis assessed at postcontrast subtraction imaging (for *D*, $r = 0.452$ and $P < 0.001$). The D parameter yielded the highest AUC, of 0.811, for predicting complete tumor necrosis; however, it was outperformed by enhancement ratios (ERs) for the prediction of complete tumor necrosis (AUC > 0.95, $P < 0.002$) [69]. In a study of 25 patients with 31 HCC lesions, it was found that ADC and D^* increased by ~30% and ~42%, respectively, while PF decreased by ~37% in responders to LRT, while no significant parameter changes were found in nonresponders. Responders and nonresponders were better differentiated by changes in D^* than by changes in ADC (AUC = 0.878 vs. 0.819) [70]. In a study of 30 HCC patients, it was found that the ratio of ADC and D between baseline and 24–48 h after transarterial chemoembolization were independent significant predictors for 99-day progression free survival ($P = 0.025$, $P = 0.036$) [71]. Pretreatment D^* was found to be significantly higher in HCCs that demonstrated good lipiodol uptake following transarterial chemoembolization compared to HCCs with poor uptake (48.10 ± 15.33 and 26.75 ± 9.55, respectively; $P = 0.001$), a finding which could inform treatment efficacy [44]. IVIM has also been investigated for patients with advanced HCC undergoing systemic therapy with antiangiogenic-targeted agents, such as sorafenib. In a small study of 9 patients, D was found to be significantly higher in patients who responded to sorafenib at four weeks, and using a threshold D cutoff value above 0.8×10^3 mm^2/s was 100% sensitive and 67% specific for identifying responders [59]. A statistically significant increase in PF at a two-week follow-up exam (PF = 0.22 ± 0.06 compared to a baseline value of PF = 0.16 ± 0.04; $P = 0.005$) was found in HCCs that responded to sorafenib compared to nonresponders, whereas ADC and D did not show differences at the follow-up [72].

Liver metastases

In a small study of 19 patients with colorectal cancer liver metastasis assessed with IVIM and DCE MRI, ADC, D, and PF all showed significant changes after chemotherapy compared to the baseline in the patients who showed response ($n = 8$) using response evaluation criteria in solid tumors (RECIST) 1.1, whereas no significant changes were found for DCE MRI parameters for either responders or nonresponders [54]. IVIM has also been used in colorectal liver metastasis patients treated with combined standard chemotherapy and bevacizumab, a novel targeted antibody against the vascular endothelial growth factor with the mechanisms of action that include inhibition of new vessel growth and regression of newly formed tumor vasculature. In a study of 12 patients with 36 metastases scanned prior to and two weeks after initiation of therapy, only PF showed a statistical difference between responder and nonresponder lesions ($P = 0.02$) based on RECIST criteria, thus showing that IVIM perfusion parameters are sensitive to early changes in lesion vascularization [52]. In a recent study of 21 patients with 45 breast cancer metastases treated with Y90 radioembolization, lesions with a higher pretreatment PF showed a greater decrease in size at the six-week follow-up ($P = 0.001$). There was also a greater increase in the six-week post-treatment ADC and D and a decrease in the PF for patients who responded to therapy [46]. In this study, D and PF had a high accuracy (AUC 0.879 and 0.867, respectively) for the prediction of RECIST response. In a separate study by the same authors, pretreatment PF was found to be lower in patients who developed early blood flow stasis intraprocedurally during Y90 administration for the treatment of hepatic breast cancer metastasis, thereby preventing full Y90 dose administration—information that may be valuable at the time of intervention to optimize the safety of microsphere administration [47].

11.5.4 Summary

IVIM parameters have shown promise in the distinction of benign and malignant liver lesions for the assessment of hypervascular lesions/perfusion and for the evaluation of tumor grade and post-treatment response, although results have been mixed. Further work is warranted to assess dynamic changes in IVIM parameters at various time points following therapy, as the measures appear to reflect several concurrent and nonredundant physiologic processes. IVIM parameters are promising for these applications, although the added value over standard ADC measurement remains unclear.

11.6 Limitations

The major limitation of both IVIM and ADC is the nonstandardization of scanning parameters, the acquisition technique, and the b values selected, although reasonable results have been demonstrated using a variety of methods. An insufficient number of smaller b values could result in the underestimation of the perfusion parameters [73]. Furthermore, measurements obtained in the left lobe of the liver could be affected by cardiac or respiratory motion and bowel peristalsis [74–76].

Some studies have indicated that the overall performance of IVIM is inferior to ADC, being more complex and more prone to errors in the calculation process, resulting in reduced efficacy in liver lesion differentiation [50, 51, 58]. In particular, the parameter D^* appears especially prone to error (see Section 11.4.3).

11.7 Future Directions

While promising results have been reported on the use of IVIM DWI for the characterization of liver lesions, the limited repeatability and reproducibility of IVIM parameters in the liver and the requirement of advanced postprocessing limit the application of IVIM DWI in large-scale multicenter studies or in longitudinal evaluation of the treatment response.

Random variability among IVIM parameters may be due to several factors, including image noise and suboptimal fitting of the biexponential diffusion behavior (see Section 11.4). Random errors in IVIM parameter estimation may be reduced by increasing the SNR of the acquisition by choosing a higher number of averages for each b value at the expense of a longer acquisition time. Substantial improvement in the accuracy of IVIM parameters may also be obtained by the application of denoising algorithms during postprocessing of the IVIM DWI images [77]. Further improvement of IVIM DWI parameter accuracy may also be obtained by using a Bayesian fitting algorithm, as described in Section 11.4. Ideally, user-friendly open-source software would need to be developed that incorporates optimal postprocessing of IVIM data using denoising and Bayesian fitting algorithms, to be performed in a timely fashion such that IVIM could be incorporated into routine clinical protocols.

Systematic bias in IVIM parameters among different MR scanners may be introduced by differences in coil configurations, field inhomogeneities, or artifacts related to susceptibility or eddy currents [62]. This bias may be addressed by calibration of MR scanners with the help of hardware phantoms [62].

PF and D^* parameters can be combined (PF × D^*) to provide an estimate of blood flow (please see Chapter 1). Early studies have demonstrated that this measurement may be more stable than PF or D^* alone [40, 78, 79].

In summary, future directions of IVIM DWI for imaging of liver lesions include optimization of acquisition and postprocessing taking into account the recommendations summarized in Table 11.1. Implementation of an optimized and standardized IVIM DWI protocol across different imaging centers would enable large-scale multicenter studies to validate the utility of IVIM DWI for the characterization of liver lesions as well as assessment of the treatment response. Such extensive validation is necessary for the potential implementation of IVIM DWI in standard clinical care liver MRI protocol.

11.8 Conclusions

IVIM DWI can simultaneously probe concurrent physiologic processes, including microvascular perfusion and true cellular diffusion restriction, and has a wide range of potential applications for noninvasively evaluating FLL, including lesion characterization, assessment of tumor grade, and evaluation of response to therapy. Early studies have shown mixed results of IVIM parameters compared to standard ADC measurements for these purposes, which could in part be due to the fact that IVIM parameter quantification is influenced by several factors, including the *b* values selected, the acquisition technique, the field strength, and the processing methods. Furthermore, perfusion-related parameters D^* and PF have shown poor measurement repeatability and reproducibility. The use of newly developed denoising algorithms and the development of optimized and standardized protocols may prove to be of value for improving the accuracy of parameter estimation. In conclusion, IVIM DWI is a promising technique for assessing FLL and future work is warranted to investigate its added value over standard ADC measurement.

References

1. Kaewlai R., Abujudeh H. Nephrogenic systemic fibrosis. *AJR Am. J. Roentgenol.* 199(1), W17–W23, 2012.
2. Gulani V., et al. Gadolinium deposition in the brain: summary of evidence and recommendations. *Lancet Neurol.* 16(7), 564–570, 2017.

3. Kaltenbach T. E., et al. Prevalence of benign focal liver lesions: ultrasound investigation of 45, 319 hospital patients. *Abdom. Radiol. (NY)*, 41(1), 25–32, 2016.
4. Massarweh N. N., El-Serag H. B., Epidemiology of hepatocellular carcinoma and intrahepatic cholangiocarcinoma. *Cancer Control* 24(3), 1073274817729245, 2017.
5. Razumilava N., Gores G. J. Cholangiocarcinoma. *Lancet* 383(9935), 2168–2179, 2014.
6. Weber S. M., et al. Intrahepatic cholangiocarcinoma: expert consensus statement. *HPB (Oxford)* 17(8) 669–680, 2015.
7. Ros P. R., Taylor H. M., Malignant tumors of the liver, in Textbook of Gastrointestinal Radiology. 2nd Ed, Gore, R. M., Levine, M. S., Editor., Saunders: Philadelphia, PA, 1523–1568, 2000.
8. Thampanitchawong P., Piratvisuth T., Liver biopsy: complications and risk factors. *World J. Gastroenterol.* 5(4), 301–304, 1999.
9. Padia S. A., et al. Safety and efficacy of sonographic-guided random real-time core needle biopsy of the liver. *J. Clin. Ultrasound* 37(3), 138–143, 2009.
10. Forner A., Reig M., Bruix J., Hepatocellular carcinoma. *Lancet* 391(10127), 1301–1314, 2018.
11. European Association for the Study of the Liver, European Association for the Study of Diabetes, and European Association for the Study of Obesity, EASL-EASD-EASO Clinical Practice Guidelines for the management of non-alcoholic fatty liver disease. *J. Hepatol.* 64(6), 1388–1402, 2016.
12. Llovet J. M., Burroughs A., Bruix J. Hepatocellular carcinoma. *Lancet* 362(9399) 1907–1917, 2003.
13. Shriki J. E., et al. CT of atypical and uncommon presentations of hepatocellular carcinoma. *AJR Am J Roentgenol.* 205(4), W411–W423, 2015.
14. Bruix J., Reig M., Sherman M. Evidence-based diagnosis, staging, and treatment of patients with hepatocellular carcinoma. *Gastroenterology* 150(4), 835–853, 2016.
15. Jarnagin W. R., et al. Combined hepatocellular and cholangiocarcinoma: demographic, clinical, and prognostic factors. *Cancer* 94(7), 2040–2046, 2002.
16. Lopez P. M., Villanueva A., Llovet J. M., Systematic review: evidence-based management of hepatocellular carcinoma—an updated analysis

of randomized controlled trials. *Aliment Pharmacol. Ther.* 23(11), 1535–1547, 2006.

17. Coenegrachts K., et al. Improved focal liver lesion detection: comparison of single-shot diffusion-weighted echoplanar and single-shot T2 weighted turbo spin echo techniques. *Br. J. Radiol.* 80(955), 524–531, 2007.
18. Bruegel M., et al. Diagnosis of hepatic metastasis: comparison of respiration-triggered diffusion-weighted echo-planar MRI and five T2-weighted turbo spin-echo sequences. *AJR Am. J. Roentgenol.* 191(5), 1421–1429, 2008.
19. Parikh T., et al. Focal liver lesion detection and characterization with diffusion-weighted MR imaging: comparison with standard breath-hold T2-weighted imaging. *Radiology*. 246(3), 812–822, 2008.
20. Soyer P., et al. Preoperative detection of hepatic metastases: comparison of diffusion-weighted, T2-weighted fast spin echo and gadolinium-enhanced MR imaging using surgical and histopathologic findings as standard of reference. *Eur. J. Radiol.* 80(2), 245–252, 2011.
21. Vilgrain V., et al. A meta-analysis of diffusion-weighted and gadoxetic acid-enhanced MR imaging for the detection of liver metastases. *Eur. Radiol.* 26(12), 4595–4615, 2016.
22. Piana G., et al. New MR imaging criteria with a diffusion-weighted sequence for the diagnosis of hepatocellular carcinoma in chronic liver diseases. *J. Hepatol.* 55(1), 126–132, 2011.
23. Park M. S., et al. Hepatocellular carcinoma: detection with diffusion-weighted versus contrast-enhanced magnetic resonance imaging in pretransplant patients. *Hepatology* 56(1), 140–148, 2012.
24. Park M. J., et al. Small hepatocellular carcinomas: improved sensitivity by combining gadoxetic acid-enhanced and diffusion-weighted MR imaging patterns. *Radiology* 264(3), 761–770, 2012.
25. Lewis S., et al. Diffusion-weighted imaging of the liver: techniques and applications. *Magn. Reson. Imaging Clin. N. Am.* 22(3), 373–395, 2014.
26. Park H. J., et al. Small intrahepatic mass-forming cholangiocarcinoma: target sign on diffusion-weighted imaging for differentiation from hepatocellular carcinoma. *Abdom Imaging* 38(4), 793–801, 2013.
27. Kaya B., Koc Z., Diffusion-weighted MRI and optimal *b*-value for characterization of liver lesions. *Acta Radiol.* 55(5), 532–542, 2014.
28. Miller F. H., et al. Utility of diffusion-weighted MRI in distinguishing benign and malignant hepatic lesions. *J. Magn. Reson. Imaging* 32(1), 138–147, 2010.

29. Taouli B., et al. Evaluation of liver diffusion isotropy and characterization of focal hepatic lesions with two single-shot echo-planar MR imaging sequences: prospective study in 66 patients. *Radiology* 226(1), 71–78, 2003.

30. Nakanishi M., et al. Relationship between diffusion-weighted magnetic resonance imaging and histological tumor grading of hepatocellular carcinoma. *Ann. Surg. Oncol.* 19(4), 1302–1309, 2012.

31. Lewis S., et al. Prediction of the histopathologic findings of intrahepatic cholangiocarcinoma: qualitative and quantitative assessment of diffusion-weighted imaging. *Eur. Radiol.* 28(5), 2047–2057, 2017.

32. Besa C., et al. Neuroendocrine liver metastases: Value of apparent diffusion coefficient and enhancement ratios for characterization of histopathologic grade. *J. Magn. Reson. Imaging* 44(6), 1432–1441, 2016.

33. Dyvorne H., et al. Intravoxel incoherent motion diffusion imaging of the liver: optimal *b*-value subsampling and impact on parameter precision and reproducibility. *Eur. J. Radiol.* 83(12), 2109–2113, 2014.

34. ter Voert E. E., et al. Intravoxel incoherent motion protocol evaluation and data quality in normal and malignant liver tissue and comparison to the literature. *Invest. Radiol.* 51(2), 90–99, 2016.

35. Lemke A., et al. Toward an optimal distribution of *b* values for intravoxel incoherent motion imaging. *Magn. Reson. Imaging* 29(6), 766–776, 2011.

36. Meeus E. M., et al. Evaluation of intravoxel incoherent motion fitting methods in low-perfused tissue. *J. Magn. Reson. Imaging* 45(5), 1325–1334, 2017.

37. Andreou A., et al. Measurement reproducibility of perfusion fraction and pseudodiffusion coefficient derived by intravoxel incoherent motion diffusion-weighted MR imaging in normal liver and metastases. *Eur. Radiol.* 23(2), 428–434, 2013.

38. Chiaradia M., et al. Intravoxel incoherent motion (IVIM) MR imaging of colorectal liver metastases: are we only looking at tumor necrosis? *J. Magn. Reson. Imaging* 39(2), 317–325, 2014.

39. Dijkstra H., et al. Assessment of the link between quantitative biexponential diffusion-weighted imaging and contrast-enhanced MRI in the liver. *Magn. Reson. Imaging* 38, 47–53, 2017.

40. Hectors S. J., et al. Intravoxel incoherent motion diffusion-weighted imaging of hepatocellular carcinoma: Is there a correlation with flow

and perfusion metrics obtained with dynamic contrast-enhanced MRI? *J. Magn. Reson. Imaging* 44(4), 856–864, 2016.

41. Jerjir N., et al. Intravoxel incoherent motion and dynamic contrast-enhanced MRI for differentiation between hepatocellular adenoma and focal nodular hyperplasia. *Br. J. Radiol.* 90(1076), 20170007, 2017.
42. Luo M., et al. Intravoxel incoherent motion: application in differentiation of hepatocellular carcinoma and focal nodular hyperplasia. *Diagn. Interv. Radiol.* 23(4), 263–271, 2017.
43. Luo M., et al. Intravoxel incoherent motion diffusion-weighted imaging: evaluation of the differentiation of solid hepatic lesions. *Transl. Oncol.* 10(5), 831–838, 2017.
44. Park Y. S., et al. Using intravoxel incoherent motion (IVIM) MR imaging to predict lipiodol uptake in patients with hepatocellular carcinoma following transcatheter arterial chemoembolization: a preliminary result. *Magn. Reson. Imaging* 32(6), 638–646, 2014.
45. Penner A. H., et al. Intravoxel incoherent motion model-based liver lesion characterisation from three *b*-value diffusion-weighted MRI. *Eur. Radiol.* 23(10), 2773–2783, 2013.
46. Pieper C. C., et al. Evaluation of a simplified intravoxel incoherent motion (IVIM) analysis of diffusion-weighted imaging for prediction of tumor size changes and imaging response in breast cancer liver metastases undergoing radioembolization: a retrospective single center analysis. *Medicine (Baltimore)* 95(14), e3275, 2016.
47. Pieper C. C., et al. Intravoxel incoherent motion diffusion-weighted MR imaging for prediction of early arterial blood flow stasis in radioembolization of breast cancer liver metastases. *J. Vasc. Interv. Radiol.* 27(9), 1320–1328, 2016.
48. Shan Q., et al. Evaluating histologic differentiation of hepatitis B virus-related hepatocellular carcinoma using intravoxel incoherent motion and AFP levels alone and in combination. *Abdom. Radiol. (NY)* 42(8), 2079–2088, 2017.
49. Wang M., et al. Evaluation of hepatic tumors using intravoxel incoherent motion diffusion-weighted MRI. *Med. Sci. Monit.* 22, 702–709, 2016.
50. Zhu L., et al. A comparative study of apparent diffusion coefficient and intravoxel incoherent motion-derived parameters for the characterization of common solid hepatic tumors. *Acta Radiol.* 56(12), 1411–1418, 2015.
51. Doblas S., et al. Determination of malignancy and characterization of hepatic tumor type with diffusion-weighted magnetic resonance

imaging: comparison of apparent diffusion coefficient and intravoxel incoherent motion-derived measurements. *Invest. Radiol.* 48(10), 722–728, 2013.

52. Granata V., et al. Early assessment of colorectal cancer patients with liver metastases treated with antiangiogenic drugs: the role of intravoxel incoherent motion in diffusion-weighted imaging. *PLoS One* 10(11), e0142876, 2015.

53. Kakite S., et al. Hepatocellular carcinoma: short-term reproducibility of apparent diffusion coefficient and intravoxel incoherent motion parameters at 3.0T. *J. Magn. Reson. Imaging* 41(1), 149–156, 2015.

54. Kim J. H., et al. Diffusion-related MRI parameters for assessing early treatment response of liver metastases to cytotoxic therapy in colorectal cancer. *AJR Am. J. Roentgenol.* 207(3), W26–W32, 2016.

55. Watanabe H., et al. Characterizing focal hepatic lesions by free-breathing intravoxel incoherent motion MRI at 3.0 T. *Acta Radiol.* 55(10), 1166–1173, 2014.

56. Woo S., et al. Intravoxel incoherent motion diffusion-weighted MR imaging of hepatocellular carcinoma: correlation with enhancement degree and histologic grade. *Radiology* 270(3), 758–767, 2014.

57. Yoon J. H., et al. Evaluation of hepatic focal lesions using diffusion-weighted MR imaging: comparison of apparent diffusion coefficient and intravoxel incoherent motion-derived parameters. *J. Magn. Reson. Imaging* 39(2), 276–285, 2014.

58. Klauss M., et al. IVIM-diffusion-MRI for the differentiation of solid benign and malign hypervascular liver lesions—evaluation with two different MR scanners. *Eur. J. Radiol.* 85(7), 1289–1294, 2016.

59. Shirota N., et al. Intravoxel incoherent motion MRI as a biomarker of sorafenib treatment for advanced hepatocellular carcinoma: a pilot study. *Cancer Imaging* 16, 1, 2016.

60. Yamada I., et al. Diffusion coefficients in abdominal organs and hepatic lesions: evaluation with intravoxel incoherent motion echo-planar MR imaging. *Radiology* 210(3), 617–623, 1999.

61. Shan Y., et al. Comparison of free-breathing with navigator-triggered technique in diffusion weighted imaging for evaluation of small hepatocellular carcinoma: effect on image quality and intravoxel incoherent motion parameters. *J. Comput. Assist. Tomogr.* 39(5), 709–715, 2015.

62. Barbieri S., et al. Comparison of intravoxel incoherent motion parameters across MR imagers and field strengths: evaluation in upper abdominal organs. *Radiology* 279(3), 784–794, 2016.

63. Cui Y., et al. IVIM Diffusion-weighted imaging of the liver at 3.0T: comparison with 1.5T. *Eur. J. Radiol. Open* 2, 123–128, 2015.

64. Chang K. J., et al. 3.0-T MR imaging of the abdomen: comparison with 1.5 T. *Radiographics* 28(7), 1983–1998, 2008.

65. Orton M. R., et al. Improved intravoxel incoherent motion analysis of diffusion weighted imaging by data driven Bayesian modeling. *Magn. Reson. Med.* 71(1), 411–420, 2014.

66. Neil J. J., Bretthorst G. L., On the use of bayesian probability-theory for analysis of exponential decay data - an example taken from intravoxel incoherent motion experiments. *Magn. Reson. Med.* 29(5), 642–647, 1993.

67. Joo I., et al. Monitoring vascular disrupting therapy in a rabbit liver tumor model: relationship between tumor perfusion parameters at IVIM diffusion-weighted MR imaging and those at dynamic contrast-enhanced MR imaging. *Radiology* 278(1), 104–113, 2016.

68. Le Bihan D. Intravoxel incoherent motion perfusion MR imaging: a wake-up call. *Radiology* 249(3), 748–752, 2008.

69. Kakite S., et al. Hepatocellular carcinoma: IVIM diffusion quantification for prediction of tumor necrosis compared to enhancement ratios. *Eur. J. Radiol. Open* 3, 1–7, 2016.

70. Murtz P., et al. Intravoxel incoherent motion model-based analysis of diffusion-weighted magnetic resonance imaging with 3 *b*-values for response assessment in locoregional therapy of hepatocellular carcinoma. *OncoTargets Ther.* 9, 6425–6433, 2016.

71. Wu L., et al. ADC total ratio and D ratio derived from intravoxel incoherent motion early after TACE are independent predictors for survival in hepatocellular carcinoma. *J. Magn. Reson. Imaging* 46(3), 820–830, 2017.

72. Lewin M., et al. The diffusion-weighted imaging perfusion fraction f is a potential marker of sorafenib treatment in advanced hepatocellular carcinoma: a pilot study. *Eur. Radiol.* 21(2), 281–290, 2011.

73. Cohen A. D., et al. The effect of low *b*-values on the intravoxel incoherent motion derived pseudodiffusion parameter in liver. *Magn. Reson. Med.* 73(1), 306–311, 2015.

74. Schmid-Tannwald C., et al. Diffusion-weighted MR imaging of focal liver lesions in the left and right lobes: is there a difference in ADC values? *Acad. Radiol.* 20(4), 440–445, 2013.

75. Kwee T. C., et al. Influence of cardiac motion on diffusion-weighted magnetic resonance imaging of the liver. *MAGMA* 22(5), 319–325, 2009.

76. Lee Y., et al. Intravoxel incoherent motion diffusion-weighted MR imaging of the liver: effect of triggering methods on regional variability and measurement repeatability of quantitative parameters. *Radiology* 274(2), 405–415, 2015.

77. Reischauer C., Gutzeit A., Image denoising substantially improves accuracy and precision of intravoxel incoherent motion parameter estimates. *PLoS One* 12(4), e0175106, 2017.

78. Yu X. P., et al. Intravoxel incoherent motion diffusion weighted magnetic resonance imaging for differentiation between nasopharyngeal carcinoma and lymphoma at the primary site. *J. Comput. Assist. Tomogr.* 40(3), 413–418, 2016.

79. Shen N., et al. Intravoxel incoherent motion diffusion-weighted imaging analysis of diffusion and microperfusion in grading gliomas and comparison with arterial spin labeling for evaluation of tumor perfusion. *J. Magn. Reson. Imaging* 44(3), 620–632, 2016.

Chapter 12

IVIM MRI of the Pancreas

Miriam Klauß, Philipp Mayer, and Bram Stieltjes
Diagnostic and Interventional Radiology, University of Heidelberg, Im Neuenheimer Feld 110, Heidelberg, 69120, Germany
miriam.klauss@med.uni-heidelberg.de

12.1 Introduction

Healthy pancreatic parenchyma is known to be a well perfused. Both inflammatory and neoplastic conditions of the pancreas are characterized by alterations of microstructure, cellularity, and microvascularity.

Since the intravoxel incoherent motion (IVIM) model allows for separate quantification of molecular movement of water (pure diffusion) and microcirculation of blood in capillaries (perfusion) the above-mentioned alterations of tissue architecture are well reflected by the IVIM-derived parameters. IVIM imaging could be a superior method for the characterization and differentiation of different

Intravoxel Incoherent Motion (IVIM) MRI: Principles and Applications
Edited by Denis Le Bihan, Mami Iima, Christian Federau, and Eric E. Sigmund

ISBN 978-981-4800-19-8 (Hardcover), 978-0-429-42727-5 (eBook)
www.panstanford.com

pancreatic diseases compared to the classic monoexponential apparent diffusion coefficient (ADC) model. In the following section, we will address the application of IVIM in different pancreatic lesions and diseases.

12.2 Common Pancreatic Lesions

Pancreatic ductal adenocarcinomas (PDACs), which are the most frequent malignant pancreatic tumors, often appear hypovascular compared to the healthy pancreatic parenchyma in conventional contrast-enhanced computed tomography (CT) and magnetic resonance imaging (MRI). PDAC is the fourth-most-frequent cause of death from cancer worldwide. The prognosis is poor at the time of diagnosis and is usually made at late stages of the disease due to its unspecific clinical signs and symptoms. In contrast, pancreatic neuroendocrine tumors (PNETs) represent the second-most-common solid pancreatic malignancy and characteristically appear hypervascular compared to normal pancreatic tissue in contrast-enhanced cross-sectional imaging. Chronic pancreatitis and autoimmune pancreatitis are benign pancreatic diseases, which can be difficult to differentiate from malignant adenocarcinomas because of the at-times mass-forming aspect and the often hypovascular appearance compared to the healthy pancreatic parenchyma in conventional CT and MRI.

12.3 Pancreas IVIM Imaging/Acquisition Protocol

Since the pancreas is known to have a well-perfused parenchyma and the first studies using IVIM in pancreas imaging reported high perfusion fractions in healthy pancreas (>25%), the pancreas is a good experimental model for the investigation of the nonmonoexponential signal decay in diffusion-weighted (DW) sequences [1]. Moreover, the dependence on the echo time of f is most important for tissues whose transversal relaxation time is significantly shorter than that of blood. This effect can be expected to be strong for IVIM imaging of organs with short T2 times, like the pancreas (46 ms at 1.5 T [2]). It is classically hypothesized that *f* is primarily related to the blood flow in the capillary network, which connects the arterial and venous systems [3]. However, animal experiments by Duong and Kim [4] strongly suggest that the fast decaying component at low *b* values should be attributed mainly to the arterial blood. They reported that the signal contribution from venous blood and capillary blood was minor. Thus, they proposed that *f* can be described as "apparent arterial fraction."

Lemke et al. measured the signal in the healthy pancreas as a function of the *b* values with and without suppression of the vascular component and under varying echo times (TE = 50, 70, and 100 ms) [1]. They found that the perfusion fraction *f* in the blood-suppressed pancreatic tissue decreased significantly whereas the diffusion coefficient *D* did not change with the suppression. On the other hand, the perfusion fraction *f* increased significantly with increasing TE whereas the relaxation time–compensated perfusion fraction *f* showed no significant dependence on TE. The conclusion was that the steep signal decay at low *b* values observed in diffusion-weighted imaging (DWI) of the healthy pancreas can be attributed to signal arising from the arterial vasculature. These results make a vascular contribution to the DWI measurement in the pancreas at low *b* values plausible and support the IVIM theory.

Besides the importance of the applied TE, the number and levels of *b* values are crucial for IVIM imaging. It is well known that a large number of *b* values allows for a more stable estimation of IVIM-derived parameters, though at the expense of a prolonged examination time. Examination times of up to 12 min. were reported. Some groups focused on that issue to find the optimal protocol for a reasonable compromise between acquisition time and high reproducibility. The minimum number of required *b* values is possibly dependent on the fitting method used. Some authors suggested that three-parameter fitting methods require more *b* values for a reliable derivation of the IVIM parameters than two-parameter fitting methods in which one parameter (mostly D^*) is fixed. Koh et al. and Lemke et al. recommended that for three-parameter fitting methods, a minimum of 8 to 10 *b* values be acquired at 1.5 T for an acceptable variance in IVIM parameter estimates [3, 5].

Recently, Gurney et al. [6] determined the combination of *b* values for DWI acquisitions at 3.0 T that renders the minimum acquisition time necessary to obtain values of IVIM parameters in the pancreas with acceptable reproducibility. They found that when applying a two-parameter fitting method with fixed D^*, 7 *b* values were sufficient for reproducible IVIM modeling with a low bias. However, their data suggest the use of at least 12 *b* values when using a three-parameter fitting method (D^* not fixed).

To date, there is still no standardized IVIM protocol for the examination of the pancreas across different institutions. Therefore, one should keep in mind that the absolute values of IVIM-derived parameters are difficult to compare between IVIM studies of pancreatic lesions with differing acquisition protocols and different MRI scanners (Table 12.1). The protocols, for instance, differ in terms of the number and levels of *b* values, TE values, and the use of a motion compensation method (breath-hold vs. free-breathing/ respiratory-triggered sequences). Type and field strength of the MRI scanner also potentially affect IVIM-derived parameters. The number of *b* values measured in IVIM studies on the pancreas varies from 3 to 11 [5, 7–12]. Also, there is no uniform consent on the absolute values of the applied *b* values. Therefore, absolute values of IVIM-derived parameters from the different studies are comparable to a limited extent only.

For example, Lemke et al. proposed the use of 11 *b* values between 0 and 800 s/mm^2 to reduce the overall variance in IVIM parameter estimation [5]. *b* values were separated into blocks (b_0, b_{25}), (b_0, b_{50}) . . . (b_0, b_{800}), and the acquisition was performed using a breath-hold technique. Using this method, they showed that *f* maps are superior to ADC maps for the visual depiction of pancreatic carcinoma. In contrast to the previous published data of Lee et al. [13] and their own results when estimating the perfusion fraction *f* using only 3 *b* values (0, 400, and 800 s/mm^2) they found almost no overlap for *f* between healthy pancreatic parenchyma and PDAC when using 11 *b* values.

Table 12.1 IVIM-derived parameters *f* and *D* in healthy/normal pancreatic parenchyma

	Number of *b* values	*f* (%) mean	f_{min} (%)	f_{max} (%)	D_{mean} (μm²/ms)	D_{min} (μm²/ms)	D_{max} (μm²/ms)
Lee [13]	3	32.6 ± 14.7	9.69	54.6	1.17 ± 0.39	0.56	1.65
Lemke [5]	3	28.7 ± 9.6	10.1	44.0	1.08 ± 0.20	0.83	1.49
Lemke [5]	11	25.0 ± 6.2	18.5	40.4	1.13 ± 0.15	0.94	1.28
Concia [2]	3	31.2 ± 12.8			1.45 ± 0.40		
Kang [8]	10	24.8	16.6	31.9	1.19	0.81	1.51
Hwang [14]	10	35.3 ± 14.5			1.19 ± 0.22		
Ma [15]	9	37.2 ± 0.06			0.90 ± 0.16		
Kim [9]	10	24	15	36	1.14	0.89	1.52

12.4 Pancreatic Adenocarcinoma

Histologically, PDAC is characterized by a complex microarchitecture with abundant desmoplastic stroma, variable microvascularity, and cellularity. The degree of fibrosis, the microvessel density (MVD), and the cell density are known to influence the prognosis of PDAC. Conventional morphological radiological imaging methods are incapable of adequately assessing these histopathological parameters. However, multiple studies have shown that DWI, particularly using IVIM, reflects differences in the microarchitectural properties of PDAC.

An early study focused on the correlation of ADC derived from a monoexponential diffusion model with a histopathology of PDAC and found that the degree of fibrosis rather than tumor cellularity affects ADC in PDAC [16]. However, a recent study by Heid et al. reported a strong negative correlation between tumor cellularity and the ADC [17].

It appears likely that the biexponential IVIM model is superior to a monoexponential diffusion model for assessing the complex microarchitecture of PDAC. One of the first studies investigating IVIM in PDAC was published in 2008 [13]. It showed that *D* (calculated from b_0, b_{500}, and b_{1000} values) was significantly lower in mass-forming pancreatitis than in pancreatic cancer. The mean perfusion fraction *f* was useful for differentiating PDAC from mass-forming chronic pancreatitis and normal pancreas, with *f* values being the lowest in mass-forming chronic pancreatitis and the highest in normal pancreas. These results indicate that the extraction of perfusion effects from DWI measurements by using a biexponential diffusion model may be of additive value for the characterization of solid pancreatic lesions when compared with the use of a monoexponential model of DWI.

Lemke et al. showed *f* to be the best parameter for differentiation between healthy pancreas and adenocarcinoma, while there was no significant difference of *D* between the two groups [5]. They reported that the acquisition of 11 *b* values markedly improved the stability of the IVIM parameter estimation, thus increasing the specificity and sensitivity when compared to the acquisition of only 3 *b* values [5, 13].

In the following studies with application of IVIM approaches to pancreatic pathology used between 8 and 11 *b* values for the estimation of IVIM-derived parameters (Table 12.2). In line with the first two studies mentioned above, other studies showed that the perfusion fraction *f* is reduced in PDAC compared to healthy pancreatic tissue, while *D* showed no significant difference between healthy and carcinoma tissue [8, 9]. Hence, with the use of IVIM, the perfusion fraction *f* appears to be the most promising diffusion parameter to distinguish between normal pancreatic parenchyma and pancreatic neoplasms [5, 7, 13, 18], with higher degrees of accuracy than ADC or *D*.

The following studies evaluating IVIM DWI in PDAC indicated in part that this IVIM-derived information about microcirculation offers the potential for better discrimination between PDAC, chronic pancreatitis, and healthy pancreatic tissue as well as between PDAC and PNET [5, 10, 13, 18].

The differences in the perfusion fraction *f* probably reflect histopathological changes in PDAC. In contrast to normal pancreatic tissue, PDAC is well known for its abundant desmoplastic stroma around tumor cells [19]. In PDAC, activated pancreatic stellate cells produce increasing fibrous stroma in central areas of the tumor, compressing the blood vessels leading to changes in vascularity and perfusion [20]. In a rat animal model, PDAC showed low-density net-like oriented microvessels in contrast to the more highly differentiated architecture of vessels in normal pancreas [21]. This could be explained by a deficient vasculature caused by a dense stromal matrix despite the presence of neoangiogenesis [22–24]. To summarize, PDAC is histologically characterized by a dense desmoplastic reaction around tumor cells, changes in cellularity, and angiogenesis.

Table 12.2 Reported IVIM-derived parameters f and D in pancreatic adenocarcinoma

	Number of b values	f (%) mean	f_{min} (%)	f_{max} (%)	D_{mean} (μm²/ms)	D_{min} (μm²/ms)	D_{max} (μm²/ms)
Lee [13]	3	20.3 ± 6.2	9.2	38.3	1.00 ± 0.19	0.58	1.38
Lemke [5]	3	13.0 ± 11.7	0.8	37.1	1.03 ± 0.25	0.80	1.77
Lemke [5]	11	8.59 ± 4.6	0	20.4	1.15 ± 0.22	0.74	1.60
Klauß [10]	11	8.2 ± 4.0	3.3	17.1	1.45 ± 0.40		
Concia [7]	3	7.0 ± 4.6			1.72 ±0.36		
Kang [8]	10	11.6	4.2	23.0	1.14	0.53	2.07
Klauß [11]	11	9.9 ± 5.4			1.2 ± 0.18		
Kim [9]	10	10	1	31	1.25	0.73	1.96

Few studies have investigated the relationship between IVIM-derived parameters and histological microvascularity quantitated by MVD in abdominal neoplasms [11, 13] and animal models [25].

One study reported a strong correlation between the IVIM-derived flowing blood volume fraction f and the histologically determined MVD both in PDAC and PNET, which represent the two most common solid pancreatic tumors [11]. There was no correlation between *D* and *D** and MVD in these pancreatic tumors. These findings support the assumption that *f* reflects the vascularization in pancreatic tumors. The analysis showed that MVD, microvessel area (MVA), and *f* values in pancreatic adenocarcinoma were lower compared to PNETs, which underlines the match of both histological results as well as previous reports on these parameters in vivo [11].

As mentioned above, stromal reaction with fibrosis is a predominant histopathological feature of both PDAC and chronic pancreatitis [16]. Two studies, both with a comparatively small patient collective, focused on the association of DWI and the degree of fibrosis in PDAC and chronic pancreatitis with somehow contradictory results. Muraoka et al. reported a significantly lower ADC in PDAC with dense fibrosis than in PDAC with loose fibrosis [16]. In contrast, Klauß et al. found that *D* rises from moderate to severe fibrosis in PDAC and mass-forming chronic pancreatitis [26]. Further studies with larger patient collectives could help to eliminate this ambiguity.

12.5 Differential Diagnosis between Pancreatic Cancer and Chronic Pancreatitis

Various studies investigated the potential of IVIM DW MRI to differentiate PDAC from mass-forming chronic pancreatitis, which is a common problem in clinical daily routine [5, 8–10, 13, 18]. Among the IVIM-derived parameters, *f* appears to be the best discriminator between these entities, with *f* being higher in chronic pancreatitis than in PDAC [7, 8, 10] (Table 12.3).

Klauß et al. hypothesized that differences in ADC between the two entities can be attributed primarily to differences in perfusion since *D* was not significantly different between groups in their study [10]. Therefore, ADC seems to be a suboptimal parameter for the differentiation of pancreatic masses because it is strongly biased by perfusion effects. Variability in *f* values can be graphically illustrated by *f* mapping, which often enables a clearer delineation of PDAC and may aid in the differentiation from mass-forming chronic pancreatitis [18].

These findings are in line with a histopathologic study by Rzepko et al., who reported significantly higher MVD in chronic pancreatitis than in PDAC [27].

12.6 PNETs

In PNETs, which are mostly hypervascular compared to normal pancreatic parenchyma, IVIM DWI could be particularly useful to eliminate pseudodiffusion effects from diffusion measurements. Strong pseudodiffusion effects in this frequently hyperperfused tumor entity might lead to overestimation of ADC values [14].

Table 12.3 Reported IVIM-derived parameters *f* and *D* in chronic pancreatitis

	Number of *b* values	*f* (%) mean	f_{min} (%)	f_{max} (%)	D_{mean} (μm²/ms)	D_{min} (μm²/ms)	D_{max} (μm²/ms)
Lee [13]	3	16.1 ± 6.1	5.2	24.3	0.96 ± 0.28	0.69	1.31
Klauß [10]	11	16.3 ± 5.3	8.3	27.3	1.07 ±0.22		
Concia [2]	3	15.1 ± 4.2			1.54 ± 0.42		
Kang [8]	10	18.6	15.2	26.1	1.11	0.83	1.80

The reported *f* values of PNET were significantly higher than those of PDAC [7, 8, 11, 13], which matches the enhancement patterns seen in contrast-enhanced CT and MRI, where PNETs often appear as hyperdense/hyperintense mass in the arterial phase (Table 12.4).

One study evaluating PNETs with IVIM found that the pure diffusion coefficient *D* was significantly lower in WHO grade 2 and 3 PNETs compared to grade 1 PNETs (no significant differences of *f* and *D**) [14]. This could be caused by increased tissue cellularity of the tumors, which may result in decreased volume of extracellular spaces, thus causing restricted diffusion of free water molecules.

Comparing *D* values between PDACs and PNETs, *D* values were significantly higher in PDACs than in PNETs in one study [11] and higher without significant difference in another study [8], whereas *f* was significantly lower in adenocarcinomas than in PNETs in all reported studies [7, 8, 11].

Table 12.4 Reported IVIM-derived parameters *f* and *D* in PNET

	Number of *b* values	*f* (%) mean	f_{min} (%)	f_{max} (%)	D_{mean} (μm²/ms)	D_{min} (μm²/ms)	D_{max} (μm²/ms)
Lee [13]	3	27.2 ± 15.1	15.0	47.8	0.96 ± 0.28	0.69	1.31
Concia [7]	3	17.6 ± 3.8			1.54 ±0.42		
Kang [8]	10	29.5	12.7	50.6	1.11	0.83	1.80
Hwang [14] G1	10	23.4 ± 10.6			1.21 ± 0.32		
Hwang [14] G2/3	10	26.0 ± 11.9			0.95 ± 0.22		
Klauß [11]	11	15.5 ± 5.2			1.03 ± 0.15		
Kim [9]	10	21	5	46	1.08	0.88	1.65

Kang et al. have reported that with the use of IVIM, *f* and D^* are the most valuable diffusion parameters to discriminate between endocrine pancreatic tumors and pancreatic adenocarcinoma with higher degrees of accuracy than ADC or *D* [14].

But overall there are very few IVIM data for PNETs, so further investigations would be beneficial.

12.7 AIP/Therapy Monitoring

Autoimmune pancreatitis (AIP) is a rare disease, and the exact prevalence in unclear. AIP can cause symptoms like painless jaundice, abdominal pain, and diabetes and shares symptoms also occurring in patients with pancreatic cancer. But the therapy is completely different to pancreatic cancer. Patients suspected of having AIP are treated with high-dose steroid therapy, which reduces the symptoms and the radiological signs of AIP [28]. Histological findings of AIP are dense fibrosis of the pancreatic parenchyma associated with periductal inflammation [29]. If fibrosis occupies large areas of pancreatic parenchyma, AIP causes a mass effect mimicking pancreatic adenocarcinoma [30]. Differentiation from pancreatic cancer can be difficult, since patients may present with classical features of pancreatic cancer, such as painless jaundice, gastrointestinal discomfort, weight loss, and pancreatic mass. The only IVIM study in AIP patients under steroid therapy showed a trend toward higher *f* and *D* values in AIP compared to pancreatic cancer but without a significant difference [12]. But interestingly, they found an increase in *f* under steroid treatment, accompanied by a decrease in *D* under treatment. In the follow-up measurement after the steroid treatment the values were nearly the same as for normal pancreatic tissue [12].

In addition to fibrosis generation, the reduced perfusion could be explained by the histopathological feature of AIP with ductal and periductal inflammatory cell infiltration by lymphocytes, plasma cells, and granulocytes. The acinar cell structures are replaced by inflammatory cells and fibrosis, leading to a loss of the lobular architecture and finally a diffuse fibrosis [31]. Therefore, it can be assumed that the density in capillaries is reduced in AIP due to both inflammatory cell infiltration and fibrosis. This pathomechanism could explain the observation of a reduced perfusion fraction *f* in AIP combined with a slightly increased true diffusion coefficient (Table 12.5).

IVIM DWI seems to be a promising tool for evaluating the response of AIP to steroid treatment and could serve as an imaging-based surrogate marker that can be used to avoid surgery in certain patients.

Table 12.5 Reported IVIM-derived parameters *f* and *D* in autoimmune pancreatitis

	Number of *b* values	*f* (%) mean	f_{min} (%)	f_{max} (%)	D_{mean} (μm²/ms)	D_{min} (μm²/ms)	D_{max} (μm²/ms)
Klauß [12]	11	10.5 ± 4.3			1.19 ± 0.28		
Kim [9]	10	13	5	23	1.11	0.91	1.41

12.8 Pancreatic Fibrosis

Besides differentiation of pancreatic lesions, IVIM DWI was used to investigate diffuse parenchymal changes, especially fibrosis, because as mentioned above, fibrosis is a common finding in pancreatic diseases. On the one hand, fibrosis is a characteristic histopathologic feature of both PDAC and mass-forming chronic pancreatitis/autoimmune pancreatitis. On the other hand, absence of fibrosis among other pancreatic glandular factors has been reported to be associated with an increased rate of postoperative pancreatic fistula [32]. IVIM may enable quantitative assessment of diffuse parenchymal disease in the pancreas, such as fibrosis [33]. Yoon et al. showed that f calculated with 10 b values (0, 25, 50, 75, 100, 150, 200, 500, 800, and 1000 s/mm^2) at 3.0 T was significantly associated with postoperative pancreatic fistula [34]. In this study the perfusion-related IVIM DWI parameters (D^* and f) were significantly decreased in patients with advanced pancreatic fibrosis (F2–F3). Decreased f in patients with advanced fibrosis may represent decreased blood volume, which is consistent with previous studies that showed decreased microvascular density in patients with pancreatic fibrosis [35].

In many studies fibrosis was accompanied by pancreatic steatosis: the fat fraction was significantly higher in patients with advanced fibrosis (F2–F3) than in patients with mild or no fibrosis (F0–F1) [34]. It is plausible that the increased extracellular matrix via pancreatic stellate cell activation and fat accumulation in the pancreatic fibrosis may disturb pancreatic perfusion. But it remains unclear why ADC_{tot} and D in this study did not show significant differences between F0–F1 and F2–F3. The inconsistency between ADC_{tot}, D, and pancreatic fibrosis has been reported previously [26]. However, Yoon et al. assume that fat accumulation in patients with no fibrosis as well as that in patients with advanced fibrosis could contribute to diffusion restriction and may counteract the ADC_{tot} or D values as a confounder.

12.9 Outlook/Perspective

Intratumoral MVD has been associated with prognosis in PDAC [36, 37] and PNET [38]; therefore f, which reflects MVD in PDAC and PNET [11], could serve as an imaging biomarker and may aid in identifying patients with an unfavorable prognosis.

As outlined above, tissue fibrosis is a key histological feature of PDAC. Fibrosis of PDAC is further increased during chemoradiotherapy [39], and, therefore, IVIM imaging could possibly be a helpful tool in assessing therapy response.

IVIM imaging allows for the identification and characterization of focal pancreatic masses without the need for contrast media injection or radiation exposure. Hence, IVIM imaging could qualify as a possible screening method for the early detection of PDAC in high-risk patients.

References

1. Lemke A., Laun F. B., Simon D., Stieltjes B., Schad L. R. An in vivo verification of the intravoxel incoherent motion effect in diffusion-weighted imaging of the abdomen. *Magn. Reson. Med.* 64, 1580–1585, 2010.
2. de Bazelaire C. M., Duhamel G. D., Rofsky N. M. MR imaging relaxation times of abdominal and pelvic tissues measured in vivo at 3.0 T: preliminary results. *Radiology* 230, 652–659, 2004.
3. Koh D. M., Collins D. J., Orton M. R. Intravoxel incoherent motion in body diffusion-weighted MRI: reality and challenges in oncology. *Am. J. Roentgenol.* 196, 1351–1361, 2011.
4. Duong T. Q., Kim S. G. In vivo MR measurements of regional arterial and venous blood volume fractions in intact rat brain. *Magn. Reson. Med.* 43, 393–402, 2000.
5. Lemke A., Laun F. B., Klauß M., Re T. J., Simon D., Delorme S., et al. Differentiation of pancreas carcinoma from healthy pancreatic tissue using multiple b-values. Comparison of apparent diffusion coefficient and intravoxel incoherent motion derived parameters. *Invest. Radiol.* 44, 769–775, 2009.
6. Gurney-Champion O. J., Froeling M., Klaassen R., Runge J. H., Bel A., van Laarhoven H. W. M., et al. Minimizing the acquisition time for intravoxel incoherent motion magnetic resonance imaging acquisitions in the liver and pancreas. *Invest. Radiol.* 51, 211–220, 2016.
7. Concia M., Sprinkart A. M., Penner A. H., Brossart P., Gieseke J., Schild H. H., et al. Diffusion-weighted magnetic resonance imaging of the pancreas: diagnostic benefit from an intravoxel incoherent motion model-based 3 b-value analysis. *Invest. Radiol.* 49, 93–100, 2014.

8. Kang, K. M, Lee J. M., Yoon J. H., Kiefer B., Han J. K., Choi B. I. Intravoxel incoherent motion diffusion-weighted MR imaging for characterization of focal pancreatic lesions. *Radiology* 279, 444–453, 2014.
9. Kim B., Lee S. S., Sung Y. S., Cheong H., Byun J. H., Kim H. J., et al. Intravoxel incoherent motion diffusion-weighted imaging of the pancreas: characterizing of benign and malignant pancreatic pathologies. *J. Magn. Reson. Imaging* 45, 260–269, 2017.
10. Klauß M., Lemke A., Grünberg K., Simon D., Re T. J., Wente M. N., et al. Intravoxel incoherent motion MRI for the differentiation between mass forming chronic pancreatitis and pancreatic carcinoma. *Invest. Radiol.* 46, 57–63, 2011.
11. Klauß M., Mayer P., Bergmann F., Maier-Hein K., Hase J., Hackert T., et al. Correlation of histological characteristics and diffusion-weighted imaging intravoxel incoherent motion-derived parameters in pancreatic ductal adenocarcinomas and pancreatic neuroendocrine tumors. *Invest. Radiol.* 50, 792–797, 2015.
12. Klauß M., Maier-Hein K., Tjaden C., Hackert T., Grenacher L., Stieltjes B. IVIM DW-MRI of autoimmune pancreatitis: therapy monitoring and differentiation from pancreatic cancer. *Eur. Radiol.* 26, 2099–2106, 2016.
13. Lee S. S., Byun J. H., Park B. J., Park S. H., Kim N., Park B., et al. Quantitative analysis of diffusion-weighted magnetic resonance imaging of the pancreas: usefulness in characterizing solid pancreatic masses. *Magn. Reson. Imaging* 28, 928–936,2008.
14. Hwang E. J., Lee J. M., Yoon J. H., Kim J. H., Han J. K., Choi B. I., et al. Intravoxel incoherent motion diffusion-weighted imaging of pancreatic neuroendocrine tumors: prediction of the histologic grade using pure diffusion coefficient and tumor size. *Invest. Radiol.* 49, 396–402, 2014.
15. Ma C., Liu L., Li Y.-J., Chen L.-G., Pan C.-S., Zhang Y., et al. Intravoxel incoherent motion MRI of the healthy pancreas: monoexponential and biexponential apparent diffusion parameters of the normal head, body and tail. *J. Magn. Reson. Imaging* 41, 1236–1241, 2014.
16. Muraoka N., Uematsu H., Kimura H., Imamura Y., Fujiwara Y., Murakami M., et al. Apparent diffusion coefficient in pancreatic cancer: characterization and histopathological correlations. *J. Magn. Reson. Imaging* 27, 1302–1308, 2008.
17. Heid I., Steiger K., Trajkovic-Arsic M., Settles M., Eßwein M. R., Erkan M., et al. Co-clinical assessment of tumor cellularity in pancreatic cancer. *Clin. Cancer Res.* 23, 1461–1470, 2017.

18. Re T. J., Lemke A., Klauss M., Laun F. B., Simon D., Grünberg K., et al. Enhancing pancreatic adenocarcinoma delineation in diffusion derived intravoxel incoherent motion f-maps through automatic vessel and duct segmentation. *Magn. Reson. Med.* 66, 1327–1332, 2011.

19. Klimstra D. S., Adsay N. V. Benign and malignant tumors of the pancreas, In: *Surgical Pathology of the GI Tract, Liver, Biliary Tract, and Pancreas*, Odze R. D., Goldblum J. R., (eds.), Elsevier, Philadelphia, USA, 699–736, 2004.

20. Xu Z., Pothula S. P., Wilson J. S., Apte M. V. Pancreatic cancer and its stroma: a conspiracy theory. *World J. Gastroenterol.* 20, 11216–11229, 2014.

21. Schmidt J., Ryschich E., Daniel V., Herzog L., Werner J., Herfarth C., et al. Vascular structure and microcirculation of experimental pancreatic carcinoma in rats. *Eur. J. Surg.* 166, 328–335, 2000.

22. Chu G. C., Kimmelman A. C., Hezel A. F., DePinho, R. A. Stromal biology of pancreatic cancer. *J. Cell Biochem.* 101, 887–907, 2007.

23. Neesse A., Michl P., Frese K. K., Feig C., Cook N., Jacobetz M. A., et al. Stromal biology and therapy in pancreatic cancer. *Gut* 60, 861–868, 2011.

24. Olive K. P., Jacobetz M. A., Davidson C. J., Gopinathan A., McIntyre D., Honess D., et al. Inhibition of Hedgehog signaling enhances delivery of chemotherapy in a mouse model of pancreatic cancer. *Science* 324, 1457–1461, 2009.

25. Lima M., Reynaud O., Tsurugizawa T., Ciobanu L., Li J. R., Geffroy F., et al. Characterization of glioma microcirculation and tissue features using intravoxel incoherent motion magnetic resonance imaging in a rat brain model. *Invest. Radiol.* 149, 485–490, 2014.

26. Klauß M., Gaida M. M., Lemke A., Grünberg K., Simon D., Wente M. N., et al. Fibrosis and pancreatic lesions: counterintuitive behavior of the diffusion imaging-derived structural diffusion coefficient D. *Invest. Radiol.* 48, 129–133, 2013.

27. Rzepko R., Jaśkiewicz K., Klimkowska M., Nałecz A., Izycka-Swieszewska E. Microvascular density in chronic pancreatitis and pancreatic ductal adenocarcinoma. *Folia Histochem. Cytobiol.* 41, 237–239, 2003.

28. Manfredi R., Graziani R., Cicero C. Autoimmune pancreatitis: CT-patterns and changes after steroid treatment. *Radiology* 247, 435–443, 2011.

29. Kloppel G., Sipos B., Zamboni G., Kojima M., Morohoshi T., Autoimmune pancreatitis: histo- and immunopathological features. *J. Gastroenterol.* 42(18), 28–31, 2007.

30. Frulloni L., Scattolini C., Falconi M. Autoimmune pancreatitis: difference between the focal and diffuse forms in 87 patients. *Am. J. Gastroenterol.* 104, 2288–2294, 2009.

31. Kloppel G., Detlefsen S., Feyerabend B. Fibrosis of the pancreas: the initial tissue damage and the resulting pattern. *Virchows Arch.* 445, 1–8, 2004.

32. Kirihara, Y, Takahashi N., Hashimoto, Y. et al. Prediction of pancreatic anastomotic failure after pancreatoduodenectomy: the use of preoperative, quantitative computed tomography to measure remnant pancreatic volume and body composition. *Ann. Surg.* 257, 512–519, 2013.

33. Watanabe H., Kanematsu M., Tanaka K. et al. Fibrosis and postoperative fistula of the pancreas: correlation with MR imaging findings-preliminary results. *Radiology* 270, 791–799, 2014.

34. Yoon J. H., Lee J. M., Lee K. B., Kim S.-W., Kang M. J., Jang J.-Y., et al. Pancreatic steatosis and fibrosis: quantitative assessment with preoperative multiparametric MR imaging. *Radiology* 270, 140–150, 2016.

35. Bali M. A., Metens T., Denolin V., et al. Tumoral and nontumoral pancreas: correlation between quantitative dynamic CE MRI and histopathologic parameters. *Radiology* 261, 456–466, 2011.

36. Fujioka S., Yoshida K., Yanagisawa S., Kawakami M., Aoki T., Yamazaki Y. Angiogenesis in pancreatic carcinoma: thymidine phosphorylase expression in stromal cells and intratumoral microvessel density as independent predictors of overall and relapse-free survival. *Cancer* 92, 1788–1797.

37. Takagi K., Takada T., Amano H. A high peripheral microvessel density count correlates with a poor prognosis in pancreatic cancer. *J. Gastroenterol.* 40, 402–408, 2005.

38. Marion-Audibert A. M., Barel C., Gouysse G., Dumortier J., Pilleul F., Pourreyron C., et al. Low microvessel density is an unfavorable histoprognostic factor in pancreatic endocrine tumors. *Gastroenterology* 125, 1094–1104, 2003.

39. Sasson A. R., Wetherington R. W., Hoffman J. P., Ross E. A., Cooper H., Meropol N. J., et al. Neoadjuvant chemoradiotherapy for adenocarcinoma of the pancreas: analysis of histopathology and outcome. *Int. J. Gastrointest Cancer* 34, 121–128, 2003.

Chapter 13

IVIM MRI in the Kidney

Moritz J. Schneider,[a,b] Mike Notohamiprodjo,[c,d] and Olaf Dietrich[a]

[a]*Department of Radiology, University Hospital, LMU Munich, Marchioninistr. 15, Munich, Germany*
[b]*Comprehensive Pneumology Center, German Center for Lung Research, Munich, Germany*
[c]*Department of Diagnostic and Interventional Radiology, University Hospital Tübingen, Hoppe-Seyler-Str. 3, Tübingen, Germany*
[d]*DIE RADIOLOGIE, Sonnenstr. 17, Munich, Germany*
moritz.schneider@med.uni-muenchen.de

13.1 Introduction

The kidneys are the best perfused organs of the human body. They receive 30% of the circulating blood volume, while weighing <1% of the total body mass. The renal main function is filtration of blood and elimination of substances to maintain hemostasis of the body. Anatomically, the renal parenchyma consists of two major structures: the peripheral, relatively thin renal cortex directly beneath the renal capsule and the inner renal medulla. The functional unit of the kidney is the so-called nephron (spanning both the cortex and the medulla),

Intravoxel Incoherent Motion (IVIM) MRI: Principles and Applications
Edited by Denis Le Bihan, Mami Iima, Christian Federau, and Eric E. Sigmund

ISBN 978-981-4800-19-8 (Hardcover), 978-0-429-42727-5 (eBook)
www.panstanford.com

consisting of a glomerulus with its proximal tubule, loop of Henle, distal tubule, and collecting duct. Glomerular filtration takes place in the cortex, which receives approximately 90% of the renal blood flow. While approximately 20% of the blood volume is extracted (extraction fraction), only a small fraction is ultimately excreted. Resorptive tubular processes take place in the medulla, which is supplied by efferent vessels. Due to its relative hypoperfusion, the medulla works almost under hypoxic conditions and thus oxygen saturation is susceptible to changes in perfusion. Perfusion and filtration are autoregulated and not necessarily proportional.

The glomerular filtration rate (GFR in mL/min./body surface) is regarded as the quantitative metric for kidney function. However, insulin clearance, which is regarded as the ideal quantification method, requires serial blood drawings and is thus not routinely performed. Estimation of GFR with the Cockraft–Gault or the modification-of-diet-in-renal-disease (MDRD) formula is relatively precise in the case of reduced kidney function but not when it is in the normal range. Furthermore, they do not allow for the assessment of single side renal function or changes in perfusion and ultrastructure.

Noninvasive magnetic resonance imaging (MRI) methods, such as diffusion-weighted imaging (DWI), have been proposed to assess renal function and tissue integrity. The apparent diffusion coefficient (ADC) is typically reduced in the case of acute and chronic renal disease, such as acute ischemia-reperfusion, pyelonephritis, or diabetic nephropathy [1].

Intravoxel incoherent motion (IVIM) MRI appears particularly promising for the investigation of renal pathologies as it allows the differentiation between perfusion and tissue integrity on the basis of pseudodiffusion and tissue diffusion, respectively. The pseudodiffusion effect is expected to be particularly strong and relatively easy to probe, as the kidneys are extremely well perfused. Furthermore, assessment of tissue integrity is of clinical concern, as invasive biopsy, with its complications, such as hemorrhage and infection, is the only method to gain insight into renal ultrastructure. IVIM metrics may thus be beneficial in the case of renal transplant rejection as well as acute and chronic kidney disease. However, several challenges have to be overcome. First, the kidneys are the organs that undergo the most geometric changes during respiratory motion, including in- and through-plane motion as well as rotation and deformation [2]. Secondly, diffusion as a three-dimensional process is strongly anisotropic in the renal medulla, so diffusion measurements in a single direction may strongly vary depending on the gradient direction [2].

The most important challenge, as in other organs, is to maximize reproducibility and variability of the IVIM experiments to obtain reliable and robust results, which can be interpreted in a transversal and longitudinal fashion.

13.2 Data Acquisition and Processing

As explained above, IVIM MRI of the kidneys is worthwhile yet challenging. In this section we will describe the most important aspects regarding the design of IVIM sequence protocols for applications in the kidneys and the processing of the acquired data.

13.2.1 Pulse Sequence and Acquisition Parameters

Most often, renal diffusion-weighted MRI (DWMRI) is performed using twice-refocused spin-echo sequences with bipolar diffusion gradient lobes and fat suppression, that is, with the pulse sequence [FatSat] – 90° – G^+ – 180° – G^- – G^+ – 180° – G^- – [EPI readout]. The bipolar gradients reduce image artifacts caused by eddy currents [3] at the expense of a slight loss in the signal-to-noise ratio (SNR) compared to the conventional, once-refocused Stejskal–Tanner [4] sequence. The echo planar imaging (EPI) data readout is utilized in renal IVIM MRI for its speed and robustness against motion artifacts and is generally employed in the single-shot mode. Multishot EPI readouts have been shown to improve image quality in the kidneys (higher spatial resolution and less geometric distortion) [5–7] by shortening the echo train length (ETL), however, they require motion compensation techniques and result in substantially prolonged scan times. Further methods routinely used in renal DWMRI to shorten the ETL and thus reduce magnetic susceptibility artifacts include partial-Fourier [8] and parallel imaging techniques, such as generalized autocalibrating partially parallel acquisition (GRAPPA) [9] and sensitivity encoding (SENSE) [10]. As an alternative to EPI acquisitions, single-shot fast spin-echo (turbo spin-echo) pulse sequences have been proposed for renal IVIM acquisitions [11, 12], resulting in reduced distortion artifacts but increased blurring in comparison to EPI.

The field of view (FOV) is usually extended to the patient's abdominal circumference to avoid folding artifacts. For both coronal and axial image orientations this results in in-slice dimensions between 320 and 400 mm. A coronal orientation allows for a faster full kidney coverage using fewer image slices, thereby saving scan time. However, with the advent of simultaneous multislice MRI, this advantage might be nullified in the future [13]. The resolution chosen should be high enough (approximately 2–3 mm in-slice) to allow for a delineation of the renal cortex and medulla, while yielding adequate SNR to facilitate robust IVIM parameter estimates. The slice thickness may be increased for an improved SNR and faster full kidney coverage; however, an excessive thickness (>6 mm) can lead to undesirable partial-volume effects and image blurring.

As with all IVIM applications, the informative value of the determined parameters depends on the b value set used for imaging. We recommend performing renal IVIM measurements using at least eight b values, with no less than five b values between 0 and 200 s/mm^2. Since the tissue diffusivity D is relatively high in the kidney (see Table 13.1), the largest b value should not exceed 800 s/mm^2 to avoid unwanted noise floor effects [14] and to keep echo times (TEs) short; at the same time, the largest b value should not be substantially lower than 700 s/mm^2 to enable a precise and accurate estimation of the water diffusion coefficient, D. The kidneys, especially in the medulla, have also been shown to exhibit a markedly anisotropic behavior in DWMRI [2, 15]. Renal IVIM measurement should therefore always be performed using three (or more) orthogonal diffusion gradient directions to base the parameter estimation on trace images. Typical acquisition times for IVIM MRI protocols range from 5 to 12 min.

13.2.2 Respiratory Motion

Respiratory motion is abundant in the kidneys, making a suitable compensation strategy key to generating meaningful results. The consequences are most obvious in the coronal orientation, since respiratory motion occurs mainly in the head-foot direction.

Figure 13.1 shows ADC maps calculated from a motion-corrected (left) and an uncorrected (right) free-breathing DW image series.

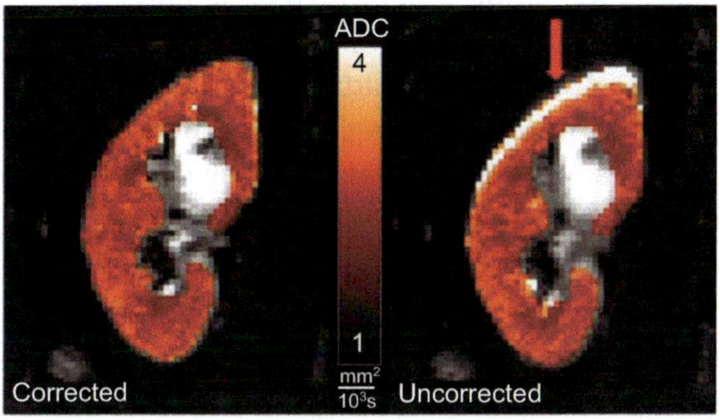

Figure 13.1 Effect of respiratory motion on ADC parameter maps. Voxel-wise ADC calculation using the uncorrected image series (right) leads to pronounced artifacts at the kidney periphery (arrow). Correcting the image series by two-dimensional rigid registration removes the artifact and improves image sharpness.

As the uncorrected kidney moves up and down throughout the image series due to respiration, the voxel-wise signal behavior becomes erratic at the kidney periphery, resulting in artifacts in the calculated ADC maps.

In the presented example, motion was corrected using a two-dimensional (in-plane) image registration algorithm after data acquisition. Image registration may be performed using rigid or affine transformations based on a predefined similarity measure. If multiple diffusion gradient directions and averages have been acquired, images should be registered before averaging and calculation of the trace to improve image sharpness and general data quality. The respiratory motions of the left and right kidneys may not be synchronous, especially if one of the kidneys is transplanted or treated surgically. Therefore, image registration should be performed for each kidney individually.

The effects of respiratory motion can also be diminished during data acquisition by performing breath-hold imaging or triggering of the pulse sequence. However, breath-hold imaging is of limited use in IVIM measurements since it requires patient cooperation and offers only brief intervals for scanning during each breath-hold. For a robust IVIM parameter estimation in the kidneys, it is essential to acquire images at multiple *b* values (>8 preferably), which results in total acquisition times of several minutes, making multiple breath-hold cycles necessary. The resulting scan times offer a negligible advantage over triggered imaging, which provides greater patient comfort. Respiratory triggering uses external devices (abdominal pad, belt transducer, etc.) or the MR signal itself (navigator) to infer the state of the breathing cycle and executes the pulse sequence accordingly. The total scan time is thereby dependent on the breathing pattern and may vary between patients. Similar IVIM results have been reported in a direct comparison of free-breathing and navigator-controlled abdominal acquisitions [16]. Regardless of the chosen compensation strategy, image registration after data acquisition is strongly recommended to remove residual motion.

13.2.3 Data Analysis

IVIM parameters in the kidneys are most often estimated on a voxel-wise basis and subsequently reported as mean or median in manually defined regions of interest (ROIs). The ROIs should be defined to encompass either cortex or medulla solely, as they exhibit different signal behaviors in DWMRI measurements and the determined diffusion parameters may be of a different diagnostic value. Vascular structures and collecting systems should be excluded from analysis, and renal masses are to be investigated separately. To reduce the IVIM parameter variability due to noise, segmented biexponential fitting approaches [17–19] are commonly used for IVIM MRI in the kidneys with a cutoff *b* value of 200 s/mm^2.

13.3 Healthy Kidneys/Peculiarities

To apply and evaluate IVIM measurements related to different pathological changes of the kidneys, the ranges and mean values of the IVIM parameters (tissue [water] diffusion D, pseudodiffusion D^*, and perfusion fraction f) in healthy kidneys of normal subjects must be known. Over the last years, these values have been determined in a relatively large number of renal IVIM studies in healthy subjects. A selection of 13 studies is presented in Table 13.1; included in this overview were studies using at least 10 healthy subjects, data evaluation in the renal cortex or the medulla, and relatively typical IVIM acquisition parameters (e.g., at least eight different b values and a maximum b value between 700 and 1000 s/mm^2). Of these 13 studies, 5 were performed at 1.5 T and 8 at 3 T. Most studies applied diffusion weightings in three orthogonal directions, the TEs of the IVIM acquisition varied between 52 and 93 ms, and acquisitions were performed in breath-hold, during free breathing, or with respiratory triggering. Image orientation was coronal in nine studies, transversal in four studies, and sagittal in one study. All studies determined the tissue diffusion coefficient D, and the perfusion fraction f, at least in the renal cortex; the majority of these studies provided also results for the pseudodiffusion coefficient D^*. The total number of subjects in all included studies is 202.

Compared over all included studies, the evaluated IVIM parameters show a certain variation that is lowest for the tissue diffusion coefficient D and highest for the pseudodiffusion D^*. The weighted mean values of D over all studies are $(1.89 \pm 0.13) \times 10^{-3}$ mm^2/s in the cortex and $(1.78 \pm 0.17) \times 10^{-3}$ mm^2/s in the medulla. In all included studies, D is higher in the cortex than the medulla (in one case, equal values are reported). However, the ranges of the reported mean values over all studies (bottom row of Table 13.1) are quite large, with a substantial overlap of the results in the cortex and the medulla.

The weighted mean values of the perfusion fraction f over all studies are 20.7% ± 7.9% in the cortex and 18.6% ± 7.2% in the medulla. In all but one study, the mean f is reported to be greater in the cortex than in the medulla.

The pseudodiffusion coefficient D^* shows by far the greatest variability over all studies, with study mean values ranging from 12 to 84×10^{-3} mm^2/s. The weighted mean values over all studies are $(28 \pm 14) \times 10^{-3}$ mm^2/s in the cortex and $(27 \pm 21) \times 10^{-3}$ mm^2/s in the medulla. There is no clear tendency whether D^* is greater in the cortex than in the medulla.

Table 13.1 Reported IVIM parameters in healthy subjects[a]

Study	*N*	*b* values (s/mm^2)	D (10^{-3} mm^2/s)		D^* (10^{-3} mm^2/s)		f (%)	
			cortex	medulla	cortex	medulla	cortex	medulla
Liu et al. 2018 [20]	13	10 (0..800)	2.00±0.10	1.95±0.13	24.0± 4.6	25.3± 8.8	19.5±5.1	17.2±4.2
Feng et al. 2018 [21]	20	11 (0..1000)	1.79±0.07	1.69±0.09	13.6± 2.6	14.4± 3.3	24.0±4.6	19.5±5.0
Mao et al. 2018 [22]	20	8 (0..800)	1.77±0.07	1.64±0.08	27.8± 1.4	14.2± 1.4	36.2±2.6	24.7±1.7
Ljimani et al. 2018 [23][b]	10	16 (0..750)	1.65±0.21	1.40±0.29	14.4± 4.7	12.7± 4.9	36.0±7.0	37.0±8.0
Ren et al. 2016 [24][c]	20	11 (0..700)	1.98±0.16	–	42.5± 9.5	–	16.1±3.2	–
Barbieri et al. 2016 [19][d]	10	8 (0..1000)	1.75±0.15	1.75±0.12	58.6±22.4	83.9±21.8	29.7±4.2	26.0±5.1
Seif et al. 2016 [25][e]	20	9 (0..750)	2.07±0.13	1.95±0.13	–	–	10.4±3.1	9.6±2.9
Wurnig et al. 2015 [18][c]	11	10 (0..1000)	1.68±0.05	1.53±0.12	12.4± 2.8	13.4± 5.5	18.5±3.1	18.3±5.6
Jerome et al. 2014 [16][f]	10	9 (0..750)	2.03±0.08	1.94±0.06	33.5± 8.6	42.0± 6.0	15.6±2.5	13.9±1.8
Eisenberger et al. 2014 [26][g]	13	10 (10..700)	1.88±0.12	1.76±0.13	–	–	10.7±3.2	8.8±3.9
Sigmund et al. 2012 [27][h]	10	8 (0..800)	1.96±0.09	1.89±0.11	24.6± 6.1	32.4±11.4	18.7±3.5	17.2±4.3
Rheinheimer et al. 2012 [28]	30	9 (0..800)	1.88±0.11	–	–	–	18.3±2.5	–
Thoeny et al. 2006 [29]	15	10 (0..900)	2.04±0.08	1.97±0.11	–	–	20.0±4.0	18.0±4.0
Combined	**202**		**1.89±0.13**	**1.78±0.17**	**27.7±13.6**	**26.5±20.9**	**20.7±7.9**	**18.6±7.2**
Range			1.65..2.07	1.40..1.97	12.4..58.6	12.7..83.9	10.4..36.2	8.8..37.0

[a](*N*) Number of healthy subjects; (*b* values) Number of *b* values and range (min..max); (–) No data available

[b]Biexponential model

[c]Combined values from left and right kidneys

[d]Only Levenberg–Marquardt (LM) algorithm (from supplemental material)

[e]Combined values from triggered and nontriggered acquisitions with image registration

[f]Combined values from free-breathing and navigator-controlled acquisitions

[g]Combined values from "predonation" and "precept" kidneys (from supplemental material)

[h]"Baseline" values

One potential reason for these large variations in D^* is the influence of the postprocessing strategy and fitting algorithm. This is illustrated, for example, in the study by Barbieri et al. [19] where averaged D^* values between about 15 and >200 × 10^{-3} mm^2/s are calculated for the same data but with different biexponential fitting algorithms. Another reason for these variations may be the existence of a third, very fast diffusion component (>200 × 10^{-3} mm^2/s), as shown by Wurnig et al. [30]; depending on the acquisition parameters (in particular, the number of b values and the distribution of very low b values, <50 s/mm^2), this third component may influence the fitting results to varying degrees.

Several physiological properties are also supposed to influence the IVIM results in healthy subjects, such as the renal hydration status, the respiration, or the pulsatile arterial blood flow. Sigmund et al. demonstrated that the diffusion coefficients D and D^* increase after hydration or a furosemide challenge [27], whereas other groups did not find significant differences in conventional diffusion parameters at different hydration states [31, 32]. To assess the relevance of respiratory motion for IVIM measurements, Jerome et al. compared free-breathing and respiratory-triggered IVIM acquisitions without finding significant differences of f, D, or D^* [16]. The influence of the varying blood flow during the cardiac cycle on IVIM parameters has been analyzed by Wittsack et al. [33]; they show that in particular the perfusion fraction f (in addition to the pseudodiffusion D^*) is substantially increased if the IVIM acquisition is electrocardiogram (ECG)triggered at the time of the maximum pulsatile flow.

A recent development in renal IVIM measurements is the analysis of the anisotropy of the pseudodiffusion D^*, that is, a pseudodiffusion *tensor* imaging approach. This was first proposed by Notohamiprodjo et al., who demonstrated a substantially greater medullary D^* in axial than in radial direction, that is, a significant pseudodiffusion fractional anisotropy FA(D^*) = 0.42 ± 0.02 in the medulla as opposed to a more anisotropic perfusion behavior in the cortex with FA(D^*) = 0.09 ± 0.04 [15]. The remaining IVIM metrics D and f display a directional dependence as well (Fig. 13.2). Similar results were described by Liu et al. [20], Ye et al. [34], and Hilbert et al. [35].

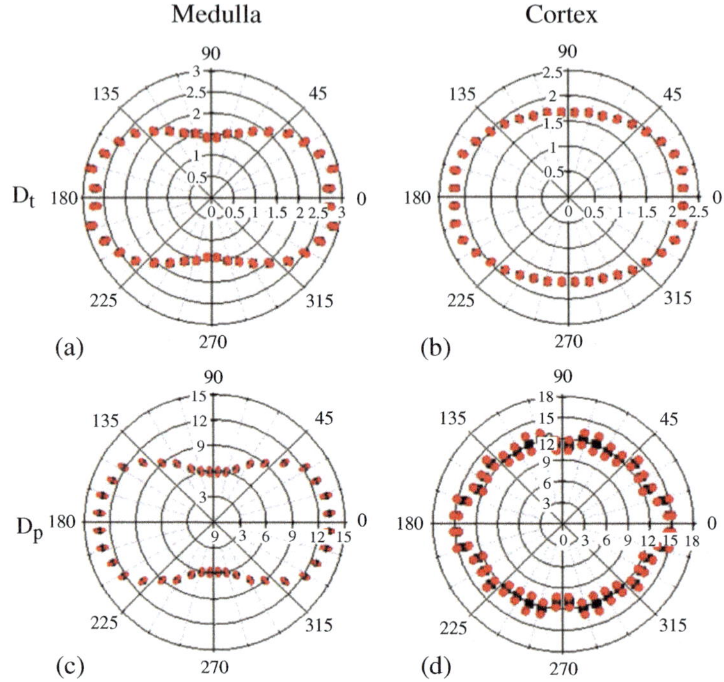

Figure 13.2 Polar plot analysis of *D* (a, b) and *f* (c, d) in the medulla and the cortex, respectively, in a healthy volunteer. The red dots indicate the angular distribution of the mean averaged over multiple regions of interest. The distribution shape indicates a strong anisotropy in the medulla and little anisotropy in the cortex [15].

13.4 Applications in Diseased and Transplanted Kidneys

IVIM MRI holds potential to noninvasively diagnose and characterize acute and chronic parenchymal renal disease. A typical example of acute renal parenchymal disease is ischemia-reperfusion damage, which may be encountered in the case of centralization of blood circulation, for example, in acute shock.

Another reason for acute ischemia-reperfusion is partial nephrectomy (PN), a surgical procedure to treat renal cell carcinoma by removing the renal masses but saving large parts of the diseased kidney [36]. While PN provides good oncological outcome and survival, the function of the treated kidneys has been shown to be impaired after the operation [37]. IVIM MRI is an ideal technique to assess renal function after PN since it provides spatially resolved renal information (and can assess each kidney individually) and bears no risk of nephrogenic systemic fibrosis. In a recent study, the effects of PN in kidneys with solid renal masses on IVIM parameters were investigated [38]. The study included 15 patients who underwent IVIM measurements before and one week after the surgery. Images were acquired on a 3T MRI scanner under free-breathing with 10 diffusion weightings between 0 and 800 s/mm^2 (six diffusion gradient directions each). Rigid registration of the DWMRI series was performed for each kidney individually before the trace-weighted images were calculated. A segmented fitting approach was used to generate maps of the IVIM metrics and the ADC (monoexponential model fit), which were statistically analyzed on the basis of the median inside a multislice cortical ROI. A significant decrease in the partially nephrectomized kidneys was observed for the ADC; however, the IVIM analysis revealed that this change was likely attributed to a reduction in tissue perfusion (Fig. 13.3, Table 13.2). Both perfusion-related IVIM parameters D^* and f decreased significantly in the treated kidneys, while the tissue diffusivity D did not show a clear trend. Conversely, the ADC as well as the product of D^* and f, which can be interpreted as an IVIM "pseudo blood flow" [39], showed a significant increase in the contralateral kidney after surgery, indicating a compensatory upregulation. The post-op IVIM parameter values were also found to correlate significantly with the estimated MDRD-GFR (measured briefly before MRI), with the pseudo blood flow demonstrating the strongest correlation (Fig. 13.4, r^2 = 0.6, p = 0.00075). The study concludes that IVIM measurements have great potential as truly noninvasive biomarkers of renal function.

IVIM MRI also appears particularly interesting for studying chronic renal disease, such as diabetic nephropathy and renal fibrosis, as both changes in perfusion and tissue integrity may occur in the course of the disease.

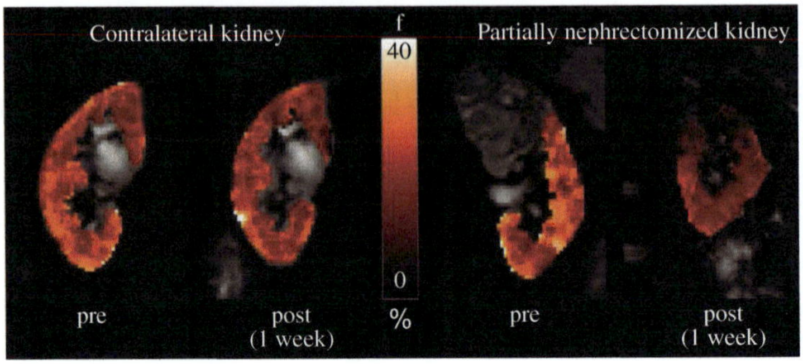

Figure 13.3 Exemplary perfusion fraction (*f*) maps before and after (one week) partial nephrectomy. In this case, no change is discernible in the non-nephrectomized kidney, whereas *f* strongly decreases in the nephrectomized kidney. Note: The shown maps do not represent the volumes of interest used for quantification but cover a larger volume for visualization. Maps have been median-filtered to reduce noise for visual representation. Reprinted from Ref. [38], with permission from Wolters Kluwer Health, Inc.

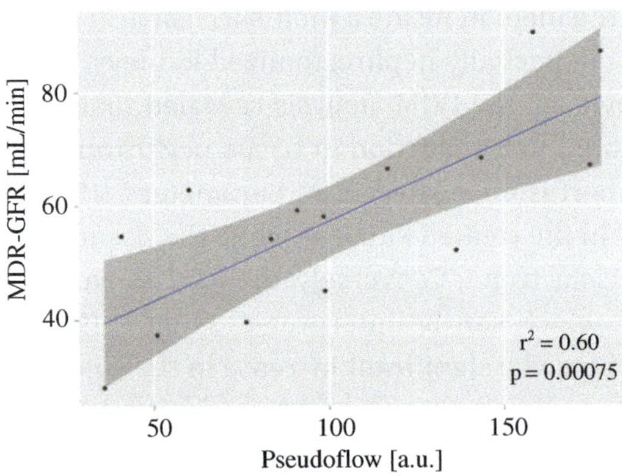

Figure 13.4 Linear (Pearson) correlations of follow-up MDRD-GFR values and IVIM pseudoflow ($D^* \times f$). The blue lines represent the linear regression, and the dark-gray areas are 95% confidence interval. Reprinted from Ref. [38], with permission from Wolters Kluwer Health, Inc.

In the early phase of diabetic nephropathy, hyperperfusion, and hyperfiltration are observed, before fibrosis and diminishing renal function take place [40]. Currently, proteinuria is the first clinical symptom that can be detected noninvasively. However, irreversible microstructural changes may have already taken place so an early noninvasive test is warranted before proteinuria is evident [40].

Table 13.2 Mean values and standard deviations of ADC and IVIM parameters in partially nephrectomized (PN) and contralateral kidneys before and one week after operation

	Baseline	Follow-up	Change
ADC (10^{-3} mm^2/s)			
Contralateral	2.47±0.23†	2.66±0.30*†	+0.19±0.21*
PN	2.50±0.28†	2.29±0.18*†	−0.20±0.26*
***D* (10^{-3} mm^2/s)**			
Contralateral	2.01±0.18	2.11±0.21	+0.09±0.17
PN	2.05±0.23	1.99±0.12	−0.05±0.17
***D** (10^{-3} mm^2/s)**			
Contralateral	8.70±1.62	9.51±2.65*	+0.81±2.27
PN	8.58±1.79†	7.25±1.6*†	−1.33±2.01
***f* (%)**			
Contralateral	19.3±2.7	21.5±4.0*	+2.2±3.4*
PN	19.2±2.9†	13.7±4.4*†	−5.5±4.6*
PF (a.u.)			
Contralateral	169±39†	203±57*†	+34±40*
PN	163±33†	103±47*†	−60±40*
MDRD-GFR (mL/min.)			
-	67.9±15.9†	58.2±17.1†	−9.7±9.3

Source: [38]
*Statistically significant difference between partially nephrectomized and contralateral kidneys
†Statistically significant difference between baseline and follow-up measurement

In a murine model of early fibrosis in streptozocin-induced diabetes, significantly increased ADC and tissue diffusivity *D* were observed, which may correspond to increased water content of the kidney. However fractional anisotropy was significantly reduced in the medulla, indicating either reduced tubular flow or an impaired tubular structure [41]. In patients, renal fibrosis is often associated with advanced diabetic nephropathy. A recent patient study by Deng et al. [42] found reduced tissue diffusivity *D* in cases of diabetic nephropathy but increased perfusion fraction *f*. These results are somewhat deviant from the preclinical findings but similar to findings made by Feng et al. in their clinical study [21], who also detected hyperperfusion, that is, increased *f*, of the renal cortex in their collective of 20 patients with diabetes mellitus 2 in comparison to healthy controls. The tissue diffusivity *D* was also significantly reduced.

Two larger prospective studies by Mao et al. [22, 43] performed in patients with chronic kidney disease observed a significant change in all IVIM metrics (*D*, *D**, and *f*) compared to healthy controls (Fig. 13.5). Furthermore, there was a significant negative correlation between *f* and 24 h urine protein levels as well as histopathologic fibrosis scores.

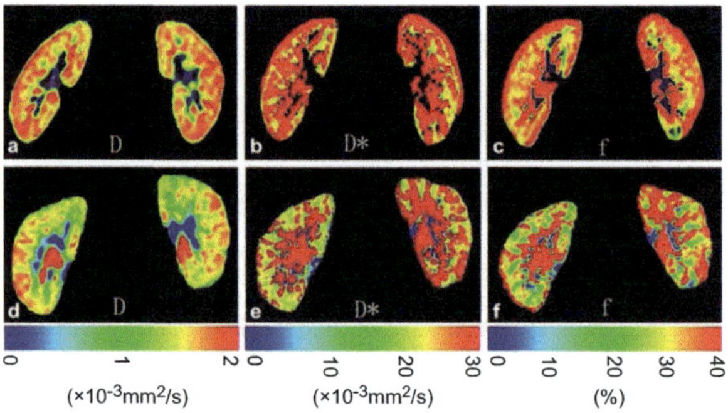

Figure 13.5 Diffusion properties in healthy kidneys of the control group (a–c) and injured kidneys of the study group (d–f, chronic kidney disease). All IVIM metrics are strongly reduced in the study group. Reprinted from Ref. [43], with permission from John Wiley and Sons.

Another disease causing renal fibrosis is chronic urinary obstruction, for example, because of congenital or acquired pathology. In a preclinical animal study, renal fibrosis was induced after unilateral ureter ligation and decreased ADC, tissue diffusivity *D*, and reduced perfusion fraction *f* were detected [44]. Similar findings were observed in another murine model with urinary obstruction by Cai et al. [45], who describe a decrease of IVIM metrics (*D*, *D**, and *f*) over time correlating to histopathological fibrosis marker alpha smooth muscle actin (α-SMA) expression and tumor-infiltrating lymphocyte (TIL) grades.

In pediatric patients, increasing perfusion fraction *f* and pseudodiffusion *D** could be observed in the "reflux" kidney [46]. This is contrary to the preclinical experimental works, which showed decreasing IVIM metrics. However, in animal models the ureter is typically completely ligated, causing rapid interstitial changes. In pediatric reflux patients, a more subtle obstruction without manifest renal fibrosis may occur, so increased water content may be expected.

In adult patients with acute urinary obstruction, changes in ADC were only subtle and detectable in the medulla, whereas analysis of the perfusion fraction *f* was significantly lower in the cortex [47]. These findings suggest that separate analysis of the pseudodiffusion content may improve the diagnostic potential of DWI.

Assessment of renal transplants was one of the first indications for IVIM MRI, as no gross motion artifacts occur in the pelvis. In a study by Thoeny et al. [29], ADC, *D*, and *f* were similar in the cortex and the medulla. In volunteers, values in the medulla were similar to those in the cortex and medulla of patients; however, values in the cortex were higher than those in the medulla ($p < 0.05$). Diffusion and perfusion indexes correlated significantly with serum creatinine concentrations. Another study by the same group [48] allowed reliable determination of diffusion and microcirculation contributions in renal allografts shortly after transplantation. Diffusion parameters in the 10 allografts with stable function early after transplantation demonstrated low variabilities. *f* values were strongly reduced to less than 12% in the cortex and medulla of renal transplants with acute rejection and acute tubular ischemia and correlated with creatinine clearance.

The group performed another study in patients with suspected allograft rejection who underwent biopsy [49]. In this study, biopsy findings were severe in 25 patients and normal or mild in 15 patients. Qualitative DWMRI led to a sensitivity of 44% and a specificity of 93.3%. Combined qualitative and quantitative DWMRI led to an accuracy of 80% for both minimal ADC and minimal perfusion fraction *f*, with a sensitivity of 84% and 92% and a specificity of 73.3% and 60%, respectively.

In a study by Ren et al. performed in 62 allograft recipients and 20 healthy volunteers [24], allografts with normal function showed no significant difference of mean cortical *D*, D^*, and *f* to healthy controls. *D*, D^*, and *f* were significantly lower for allografts with impaired function than those with normal function and showed a positive correlation with eGFR for recipients. The combination of

IVIM MRI with arterial spin labeling (ASL) MRI showed a higher area under the receiver operating characteristic (ROC) curve (0.865) than that of ASL MRI alone.

13.5 Conclusion: Open Questions and Future Directions

Numerous studies have shown the great potential of IVIM MRI to assess kidney function and pathology; however, widespread adoption in the clinical routine is not yet in sight. One relevant reason is the comparably long scan time of typically 5 to 12 min. for a renal IVIM examination. There is also a crucial need for the standardization of imaging protocols as well as data processing to facilitate the comparison between different studies and patient populations. This lack of standardization is reflected in the high variability of reported values in healthy volunteers (Table 13.1).

Respiratory motion of the kidneys is a major concern, and the use of proper compensation techniques is mandatory, resulting in prolonged scan times (triggered acquisition) and demanding image processing steps (image registration).

While IVIM MRI offers a significant improvement compared to the commonly used monoexponential ADC model, there are still open questions regarding the physiological interpretation of the estimated model parameters. Especially in the renal medulla, tubular flow [27, 50] has been shown to affect the signal in DWI MRI and is likely to bias the perfusion-related IVIM parameters f and D^*. Consequently, in the kidneys, it seems appropriate to loosen the original semantic meaning of the IVIM parameters (referring to capillary perfusion) and to regard them as general markers of functionality. Renal IVIM MRI was shown to be sensitive in various diseases, but distinguishing between pathologies and overall specificity may be limited due to this ambiguousness. The recent analysis of more complex models aims to alleviate this issue, for example, by probing the directionality [2, 20, 34, 35] of IVIM parameters akin to diffusion tensor imaging (DTI) or by adding a third exponential [30, 51, 52] to fit the signal decay more closely. At the same time, the accompanied risk of overfitting using high-dimensional models must be addressed by even higher data fidelity requirements.

The results presented in the literature are compelling but mostly based on small sample sizes. Large-scale prospective population studies are necessary to further the understanding and consolidate the role of IVIM imaging in kidneys. Ultimately, it is likely that renal IVIM MRI delivers its potential best in complement to other advanced modalities, such as blood-oxygenation-level-dependent (BOLD) MRI and ASL MRI, to allow for a comprehensive examination of kidneys.

References

1. Notohamiprodjo M., Reiser M. F., Sourbron S. P. Diffusion and perfusion of the kidney. *Eur. J. Radiol.* 76(3), 337–347, 2010.
2. Notohamiprodjo M., et al. Diffusion tensor imaging (DTI) of the kidney at 3 tesla-feasibility, protocol evaluation and comparison to 1.5 Tesla. *Invest. Radiol.* 45(5), 245–254, 2010.
3. Reese T. G., et al. Reduction of eddy-current-induced distortion in diffusion MRI using a twice-refocused spin echo. *Magn. Reson. Med.* 49(1), 177–182, 2003.
4. Stejskal E. O., Tanner J. E. Spin diffusion measurements: Spin echoes in the presence of a time-dependent field gradient. *J. Chem. Phys.* 42(1), 288–292, 1965.
5. Friedli I., et al. New magnetic resonance imaging index for renal fibrosis assessment: A comparison between diffusion-weighted imaging and T1 mapping with histological validation. *Sci. Rep.* 6, 30088, 2016.
6. Friedli I., et al. Comparison of readout-segmented and conventional single-shot for echo-planar diffusion-weighted imaging in the assessment of kidney interstitial fibrosis. *J. Magn. Reson. Imaging,* 46(6), 1631–1640, 2017.
7. Friedli I., et al. Improvement of renal diffusion-weighted magnetic resonance imaging with readout-segmented echo-planar imaging at 3T. *Magn. Reson. Imaging* 33(6), 701–708, 2015.
8. Brown R. W., et al. *Magnetic Resonance Imaging: Physical Principles and Sequence Design*. Wiley, 2014.
9. Griswold M. A., et al. Generalized autocalibrating partially parallel acquisitions (GRAPPA). *Magn. Reson. Med.* 47(6), 1202–1210, 2002.
10. Pruessmann K. P., et al. SENSE: Sensitivity encoding for fast MRI. *Magn. Reson. Med.* 42(5), 952–962, 1999.

11. Jin N., et al. Targeted single-shot methods for diffusion-weighted imaging in the kidneys. *J. Magn. Reson. Imaging* 33(6), 1517–1525, 2011.
12. Hilbert F., et al. Comparison of turbo spin echo and echo planar imaging for intravoxel incoherent motion and diffusion tensor imaging of the kidney at 3 Tesla. *Z. Med. Phys.* 27(3), 193–201, 2017.
13. Kenkel D., et al. Simultaneous multislice diffusion-weighted imaging of the kidney: A systematic analysis of image quality. *Invest. Radiol.* 52(3), 163–169, 2017.
14. Iima M., et al. Quantitative non-Gaussian diffusion and intravoxel incoherent motion magnetic resonance imaging: Differentiation of malignant and benign breast lesions. *Invest. Radiol.* 50(4), 205–211, 2015.
15. Notohamiprodjo M., et al. Combined intravoxel incoherent motion and diffusion tensor imaging of renal diffusion and flow anisotropy. *Magn. Reson. Med.* 73(4), 1526–1532, 2015.
16. Jerome N. P., et al. Comparison of free-breathing with navigator-controlled acquisition regimes in abdominal diffusion-weighted magnetic resonance images: Effect on ADC and IVIM statistics. *J. Magn. Reson. Imaging* 39(1), 235–240, 2014.
17. Cho G. Y., et al. Comparison of fitting methods and *b*-value sampling strategies for intravoxel incoherent motion in breast cancer. *Magn. Reson. Med.* 74(4), 1077–1085, 2015.
18. Wurnig M. C., et al. Systematic analysis of the intravoxel incoherent motion threshold separating perfusion and diffusion effects: Proposal of a standardized algorithm. *Magn. Reson. Med.* 74(5), 1414–1422, 2015.
19. Barbieri S., et al. Impact of the calculation algorithm on biexponential fitting of diffusion-weighted MRI in upper abdominal organs. *Magn. Reson. Med.* 75(5), 2175–2184, 2016.
20. Liu A. L., et al. REnal Flow and Microstructure AnisotroPy (REFMAP) MRI in normal and peritumoral renal tissue. *J. Magn. Reson. Imaging,* 48(1), 188–197, 2018.
21. Feng Y. Z., et al. Intravoxel incoherent motion (IVIM) at 3.0 T: Evaluation of early renal function changes in type 2 diabetic patients. *Abdom. Radiol. (NY)*, 2018, doi: 10.1007/s00261-018-1555-7.
22. Mao W., et al. Intravoxel incoherent motion diffusion-weighted imaging for the assessment of renal fibrosis of chronic kidney disease: A preliminary study. *Magn Reson Imaging* 47, 118–124, 2018.

23. Ljimani A., et al. Non-gaussian diffusion evaluation of the human kidney by Pade exponent model. *J. Magn. Reson. Imaging* 47(1), 160–167, 2018.

24. Ren T., et al. Evaluation of renal allografts function early after transplantation using intravoxel incoherent motion and arterial spin labeling MRI. *Magn Reson Imaging* 34(7), 908–914, 2016.

25. Seif M., et al. Diffusion tensor imaging of the human kidney: Does image registration permit scanning without respiratory triggering? *J. Magn. Reson. Imaging* 44(2), 327–334, 2016.

26. Eisenberger U., et al. Living renal allograft transplantation: Diffusion-weighted MR imaging in longitudinal follow-up of the donated and the remaining kidney. *Radiology* 270(3), 800–808, 2014.

27. Sigmund E. E., et al. Intravoxel incoherent motion and diffusion-tensor imaging in renal tissue under hydration and furosemide flow challenges. *Radiology* 263(3), 758–769, 2012.

28. Rheinheimer S., et al. IVIM-DWI of transplanted kidneys: Reduced diffusion and perfusion dependent on cold ischemia time. *Eur. J. Radiol.* 81(9), e951–e956, 2012.

29. Thoeny H. C., et al. Functional evaluation of transplanted kidneys with diffusion-weighted and BOLD MR imaging: Initial experience. *Radiology* 241(3), 812–821, 2006.

30. Wurnig M. C., Germann M., Boss A. Is there evidence for more than two diffusion components in abdominal organs? A magnetic resonance imaging study in healthy volunteers. *NMR Biomed* 31(1), 2018, doi: 10.1002/nbm.3852.

31. Damasio M. B., et al. Diffusion-weighted MRI sequences (DW-MRI) of the kidney: Normal findings, influence of hydration state and repeatability of results. *Radiol Med* 113(2), 214–224, 2008.

32. Wang W. J., et al. MR diffusion tensor imaging of normal kidneys. *J. Magn. Reson. Imaging* 40(5), 1099–1102, 2014.

33. Wittsack H. J., et al. Temporally resolved electrocardiogram-triggered diffusion-weighted imaging of the human kidney: Correlation between intravoxel incoherent motion parameters and renal blood flow at different time points of the cardiac cycle. *Invest. Radiol.* 47(4), 226–230, 2012.

34. Ye Q., et al. Initial experience of generalized intravoxel incoherent motion imaging and diffusion tensor imaging (GIVIM-DTI) in healthy subjects. *J. Magn. Reson. Imaging* 44(3), 732–738, 2016.

35. Hilbert F., et al. An intravoxel oriented flow model for diffusion-weighted imaging of the kidney. *NMR Biomed.* 29(10), 1403–1413, 2016.

36. Campbell S. C., et al. Guideline for management of the clinical T1 renal mass. *J. Urol.* 182(4), 1271–1279, 2009.

37. Mariusdottir E., et al. Kidney function following partial or radical nephrectomy for renal cell carcinoma: A population-based study. *Scand. J. Urol.* 47(6), 476–482, 2013.

38. Schneider M. J., et al. Intravoxel incoherent motion magnetic resonance imaging in partially nephrectomized kidneys. *Invest. Radiol.* 51(5), 323–330, 2016.

39. Le Bihan D., Turner R. The capillary network: A link between IVIM and classical perfusion. *Magn. Reson. Med.* 27(1), 171–178, 1992.

40. Inoue T., et al. Noninvasive evaluation of kidney hypoxia and fibrosis using magnetic resonance imaging. *J. Am. Soc. Nephrol.* 22(8), 1429–1434, 2011.

41. Yan Y. Y., et al. Intravoxel incoherent motion and diffusion tensor imaging of early renal fibrosis induced in a murine model of streptozotocin induced diabetes. *Magn. Reson. Imaging* 38, 71–76, 2017.

42. Deng Y., et al. Use of intravoxel incoherent motion diffusion-weighted imaging to detect early changes in diabetic kidneys. *Abdom. Radiol.* (NY) 43(10), 2728–2733, 2018.

43. Mao W., et al. Chronic kidney disease: Pathological and functional evaluation with intravoxel incoherent motion diffusion-weighted imaging. *J. Magn. Reson. Imaging* 47(5), 1251–1259, 2017.

44. Hennedige T., et al. Intravoxel incoherent imaging of renal fibrosis induced in a murine model of unilateral ureteral obstruction. *Magn. Reson. Imaging* 33(10), 1324–1328, 2015.

45. Cai X. R., et al. Use of intravoxel incoherent motion MRI to assess renal fibrosis in a rat model of unilateral ureteral obstruction. *J. Magn. Reson. Imaging* 44(3), 698–706, 2016.

46. Kim J. W., et al. Intravoxel incoherent motion magnetic resonance imaging to predict vesicoureteral reflux in children with urinary tract infection. *Eur. Radiol.* 26(6), 1670–1677, 2016.

47. Thoeny H. C., et al. Noninvasive assessment of acute ureteral obstruction with diffusion-weighted MR imaging: A prospective study. *Radiology* 252(3), 721–728, 2009.

48. Eisenberger U., et al. Evaluation of renal allograft function early after transplantation with diffusion-weighted MR imaging. *Eur. Radiol.* 20(6), 1374–1383, 2010.

49. Steiger P., et al. Selection for biopsy of kidney transplant patients by diffusion-weighted MRI. *Eur. Radiol.* 27(10), 4336–4344, 2017.

50. Gaudiano C., et al. Renal diffusion tensor imaging: Is it possible to define the tubular pathway? A case report. *Magn. Reson. Imaging* 29(7), 1030–1033, 2011.

51. van Baalen S., et al. Intravoxel incoherent motion modeling in the kidneys: Comparison of mono-, bi-, and triexponential fit. *J. Magn. Reson. Imaging* 46(1), 228–239, 2017.

52. van der Bel R., et al. A tri-exponential model for intravoxel incoherent motion analysis of the human kidney: In silico and during pharmacological renal perfusion modulation. *Eur. J. Radiol.* 91, 168–174, 2017.

Chapter 14

IVIM Diffusion Model in Prostate Cancer

Baris Turkbey, Stephanie Harmon, Marcin Czarniecki, and Peter L. Choyke
Molecular Imaging Program, National Cancer Institute, NIH, Bethesda, MD, USA
pchoyke@mail.nih.gov

14.1 Introduction

Prostate cancer is the most common noncutaneous cancer type among men [1]. While the mortality rates have decreased as a result of serum prostate-specific antigen (PSA) screening in the last two decades, overdiagnosis of indolent cancer and underdiagnosis of lethal cancers remain a significant problem. Prostate magnetic resonance imaging (MRI) has been utilized to address this issue, and in large-scale studies it has been shown to improve diagnosis of lethal cancers without increasing the overdiagnosis of indolent disease [2, 3]. Widespread adoption of prostate MRI for cancer detection and staging in recent years has resulted in increasing calls for standardization in the acquisition and reporting [4]. Diffusion-weighted MRI (DW MRI) is an integral part of prostate MRI since it has been documented to improve lesion diagnosis and risk stratification.

Intravoxel Incoherent Motion (IVIM) MRI: Principles and Applications
Edited by Denis Le Bihan, Mami Iima, Christian Federau, and Eric E. Sigmund

ISBN 978-981-4800-19-8 (Hardcover), 978-0-429-42727-5 (eBook)
www.panstanford.com

Multiple studies [5, 6] have shown a negative correlation between the mean apparent diffusion coefficient (ADC) of tumors and their Gleason scores. The majority of the experience in prostate DW MRI literature is based on the use of ADC maps derived from the conventional monoexponential signal decay model. However, it is documented that the use of this relatively simplistic approach may not necessarily depict the diffusion characteristics of biological tissues, especially when a strong perfusion component is present in the diffusion signal. To account for these effects, the intravoxel incoherent motion (IVIM) model was proposed by Le Bihan et al. in the late 1980s [7, 8]. This biexponential model proposes that the microscopic translational motion of water in biological tissues has two components, molecular diffusion of water and microcirculation of blood in the capillary network, which is subsequently referred to as perfusion [7]. The IVIM model has been shown to better describe cancer biology in various applications, including prostate cancer, compared with the monoexponential approach [9–17]. Herein, we will discuss the clinical use of IVIM in prostate cancer diagnosis.

14.2 Prostate Cancer Detection Using the IVIM Model

The IVIM model aims to explore DW signal decay at low b values, where both diffusion and perfusion effects are observed and may impact quantitative accuracy of ADC maps on which DW MRI relies heavily for prostate cancer detection and characterization [7, 18]. Different from conventional monoexponential signal decay DW modeling, the IVIM model can compartmentalize diffusion characteristics into quantitative metrics, such as molecular diffusion (D), microcirculation-related diffusion (pseudodiffusion, D^*), and perfusion fraction (f). Several studies have explored the IVIM model and its parameters in prostate cancer detection (Fig.14.1).

In early studies, the IVIM model was reported to be useful in differentiating prostate cancer from normal and benign prostatic hyperplasia (BPH) tissues. A study of 26 patients evaluated IVIM acquired with 10 b values between 0 and 1000 s/mm^2. The results indicated that the ADC and D were significantly lower in cancer than in normal prostate and BPH and f derived from IVIM was also significantly lower in cancer than in normal prostate but not significantly different from BPH. Finally, D^* was found to be similar in cancers, normal prostate, and BPH in that study. The authors indicated that a decrease in the perfusion fraction value may play a role in observed reductions of ADC values in prostate cancer, as well as decreased tissue diffusivity. Although they did not perform a stringent lesion-detection-based analysis, they observed that the IVIM model may offer additional information for tissue characterization in the prostate gland [15]. Shortly after that study another group studied the utility of perfusion fraction in prostate cancer diagnosis and compared the IVIM-derived perfusion fraction and diffusion coefficients with quantitative DCE parameters in 33 patients who underwent DW MRI acquired with five evenly spaced b values (0–750 s/mm^2) followed by a targeted biopsy. They reported significant differences between normal tissue and tumor for IVIM-derived parameters, including perfusion fraction (3.7% vs. 7.2%) and diffusion coefficient (1.76 vs. 0.99), as well as DCE-derived parameters, including volume transfer constant (K^{trans}) (0.18 min.$^{-1}$ vs. 0.39 min.$^{-1}$), fractional volume of extravascular-extracellular space (Ve) (26% vs. 32%), and plasma fractional volume (Vp) (3.4% vs. 8.4%). Given the moderately high correlation between IVIM perfusion fraction with K^{trans} and Ve (r = 0.51 and = 0.46, respectively), the authors proposed that the perfusion fraction can be used to estimate the degree of tumor angiogenesis–related changes in the tissue and DCE MRI, with its requirement for intravenous gadolinium, could be eliminated; however, this is yet to be investigated by an independent study [16].

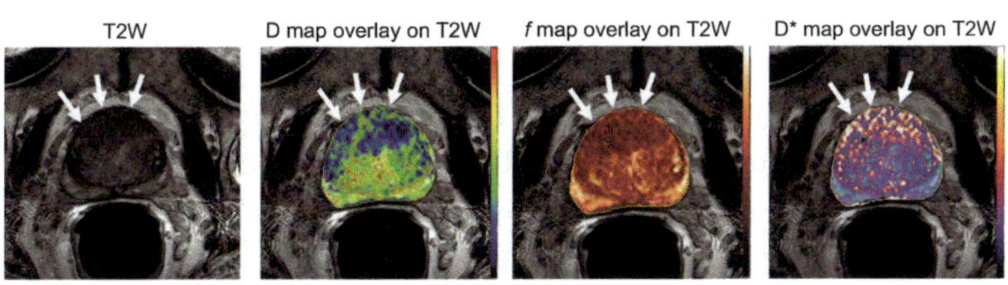

Figure 14.1 A 60-year-old man with a serum PSA of 44.81 ng/mL. An axial T2W MRI shows a large lesion in the anterior transition zone (arrows). Diffusion (D), perfusion fraction (f), and pseudodiffusion (D^*) maps derived from the IVIM model (the included b values were 0, 188, 375, 563, 750, 1000, and 2000 s/mm^2) confirm the presence of a large lesion in the anterior transition zone (arrows). A guided biopsy revealed a Gleason 4+4 prostate cancer within this large lesion.

Several studies have compared ADC values derived from the standard monoexponential decay model with IVIM parameters. In one study with 53 patients, ADC values from monoexponential model were compared with anatomic T2-weighted (T2W) MRI and IVIM parameters (*D*, *D**, and *f*) to distinguish prostate cancer from healthy tissue in the peripheral zone [19]. Authors reported that the T2, ADC, and *D* values were significantly lower in prostate cancers compared to healthy tissue whereas *D** was increased in cancers compared to healthy tissue. The study reported very high sensitivity (100%), specificity (96%), and accuracy (98%) when using quantitative metrics from combined T2W imaging/DWI and IVIM parameters (T2, ADC, *D*, *D**, and *f*) for discriminating cancerous from normal regions. Although the results were promising, the study was limited to the peripheral zone with a small sample size [19]. In a study with 63 patients who underwent DW MRI ($b = 0–1000$ s/mm^2) and subsequent transrectal ultrasound (TRUS)/MRI fusion-guided biopsy, association of diffusion MR metrics within prostate cancer versus BPH, as well as correlation to tumor Gleason grade, was compared using the monoexponential model (ADC) and IVIM model (*f*, *D*, and *D**). The results revealed that the mean ADC and mean *D* achieved areas under the curve (AUCs) of 0.84 and 0.81, respectively, for the distinction of tumor versus BPH, whereas there was a moderate negative correlation of the Gleason score with the mean ADC ($r = -0.522$) and mean *D* ($r = -0.407$). The results of this study indicated that the IVIM-model-derived quantitative parameters did not provide additive utility to already existing monoexponential-model-derived ADC metrics [20].

A high-*b*-value DW MRI is frequently acquired to assist in prostate MRI interpretation. PI-RADS v2 guidelines proposed that a minimum *b* value of 1400 s/mm^2 be obtained for lesion detection and scoring. The guidelines state that this high-*b*-value DW MRI can be either acquired directly or calculated on the basis of lower *b* values [4]. While a number of studies have compared the diagnostic utility of acquired versus calculated high-*b*-value DW MRI in retrospective series, very few have looked into whether a monoexponential or IVIM model should be used to calculate the high-*b*-value DW MRI. In a study of 106 patients who underwent two different sets of DW

MRI protocols on the same day, protocol 1 consisted of five evenly spaced *b* values (0–750 s/mm^2) and protocol 2 had three evenly spaced *b* values (0–1000–2000 s/mm^2). Calculated high *b* values (b = 1000 and 2000 s/mm^2) were derived from protocol 1 using IVIM and kurtosis models. The calculated high-*b*-value DW MRIs were compared with acquired b = 1000 and b = 2000 s/mm^2 DW MRI for lesion visibility. Results indicated that high-*b*-value DW MRI derived from the IVIM model demonstrated lesion visibility comparable to the acquired high-*b*-value DW MRI, whereas the high-*b*-value DW MRI derived from the kurtosis model had a poorer reader detection performance. This large-scale study indicated that the IVIM-model-derived calculated high-*b*-value DW MRI can be used to detect lesions in place of the acquired DW MRI, which takes longer to acquire [21]. Subsequent independent work additionally confirmed that calculated high-*b*-value DW MRI using IVIM or monoexponential models can provide equivalent or better-quality high-*b*-value DW MRI compared to acquired images [11].

Recently, the repeatability of IVIM-based quantitative metrics was evaluated across various fitting methods using the IVIM decay model in a cohort of 81 patients who underwent two repeated 3 TDW MRI using 14 *b* values in the 0–500 s/mm^2 range [22]. Mean signal intensities of regions of interest were fitted using five different fitting methods for IVIM as well as monoexponential, kurtosis, and stretched exponential models. The results demonstrate a higher quality of fit using the monoexponential model compared to the IVIM based on Akaike information criteria. The "pseudodiffusion" parameters demonstrated low repeatability and clinical value. Moreover, none of the IVIM-derived parameters or their combinations outperformed the monoexponential-model-derived ADC values for the prediction of Gleason scores at pathology. The results of this detailed study reveal that proper use of conventional monoexponential DW MRI is sufficient to detect and risk-stratify prostate cancers [22].

A limited number of additional studies have implemented IVIM-derived quantitative parameters in decision support systems. In a pilot study of 10 patients who underwent DW MRI with 16 evenly spaced *b* values and subsequent prostatectomy, the metrics of an IVIM model were used in conjunction with those of a kurtosis model to create an unsupervised cancer detection workflow. The study included index cancers (14/14) in 10 patients, whereas standard

MRI reads could detect only 12/14 of all cancers. This preliminary work suggested possible benefits in sensitivity of IVIM-model-based metrics [23]. However, no further work followed these initial findings and the study is too small to be clinically meaningful.

14.3 Conclusion

In conclusion, DW MRI is a key component of prostate MRI, as documented in current imaging guidelines. The most commonly used signal decay model is the monoexponential model for cancer detection and histopathology estimation. The IVIM model aims to incorporate perfusion-related effects to more accurately estimate diffusion and offers new quantitative metrics that have been shown to be useful for the identification and characterization of prostate cancer in limited studies. While the current literature indicates a limited utility of IVIM over the standard monoexponential decay model, further investigation of the IVIM model and its correlation to cancer biology is warranted.

References

1. Siegel R. L., Miller K. D., Jemal A. Cancer statistics, 2018. *CA: Cancer J. Clin.* 68(1), 7–30, 2018.
2. Kasivisvanathan V., Rannikko A. S., Borghi M., Panebianco V., Mynderse L. A., Vaarala M. H., et al. MRI-targeted or standard biopsy for prostate-cancer diagnosis. *N. Engl. J. Med.* 378(19), 1767–1777 2018.
3. Siddiqui M. M., Rais-Bahrami S., Turkbey B., George A. K., Rothwax J., Shakir N., et al. Comparison of MR/ultrasound fusion-guided biopsy with ultrasound-guided biopsy for the diagnosis of prostate cancer. *JAMA* 313(4), 390–397, 2015.
4. Weinreb J. C., Barentsz J. O., Choyke P. L., Cornud F., Haider M. A., Macura K. J., et al. PI-RADS prostate imaging - reporting and data system: 2015, Version 2. *Eur. Urol.* 69(1), 16–40, 2016.
5. Hambrock T., Somford D. M., Huisman H. J., van Oort I. M., Witjes. J.A., Hulsbergen-van de Kaa C.A., et al. Relationship between apparent diffusion coefficients at 3.0-T MR imaging and Gleason grade in peripheral zone prostate cancer. *Radiology* 259(2), 453–461, 2011.
6. Turkbey B., Shah V. P., Pang Y., Bernardo M., Xu S., Kruecker J., et al. Is

apparent diffusion coefficient associated with clinical risk scores for prostate cancers that are visible on 3-T MR images? *Radiology* 258(2), 488–495, 2011.

7. Le Bihan D., Breton E., Lallemand D., Aubin M. L., Vignaud J., Laval-Jeantet M. Separation of diffusion and perfusion in intravoxel incoherent motion MR imaging. *Radiology* 168(2), 497–505,1988.
8. Le Bihan D., Breton E., Lallemand D., Grenier P., Cabanis E., Laval-Jeantet M. MR imaging of intravoxel incoherent motions: application to diffusion and perfusion in neurologic disorders. *Radiology* 161(2), 401–407, 1986.
9. Pesapane F., Patella F., Fumarola E. M., Panella S., Ierardi A. M., Pompili G. G., et al. Intravoxel incoherent motion (IVIM) diffusion weighted imaging (DWI) in the periferic prostate cancer detection and stratification. *Med. Oncol. (Northwood, London, England)* 34(3), 35, 2017.
10. Barbieri S., Bronnimann M., Boxler S., Vermathen P., Thoeny H. C. Differentiation of prostate cancer lesions with high and with low Gleason score by diffusion-weighted MRI. *Eur. Radiol.* 27(4), 1547–1555,2017.
11. Verma S., Sarkar S., Young J., Venkataraman R., Yang X., Bhavsar A., et al. Evaluation of the impact of computed high *b*-value diffusion-weighted imaging on prostate cancer detection. *Abdom. Radiol. (NY)* 41(5), 934–945, 2016.
12. Yang D. M., Kim H. C., Kim S. W., Jahng G. H., Won K. Y., Lim. S.J., et al. Prostate cancer: correlation of intravoxel incoherent motion MR parameters with Gleason score. *Clin. Imaging* 40(3), 445–450, 2016.
13. Panagiotaki E., Chan R. W., Dikaios N., Ahmed H. U., O'Callaghan J., Freeman A., et al. Microstructural characterization of normal and malignant human prostate tissue with vascular, extracellular, and restricted diffusion for cytometry in tumours magnetic resonance imaging. *Invest. Radiol.* 50(4), 218–227, 2015.
14. Kuru T. H., Roethke M. C., Stieltjes B., Maier-Hein K., Schlemmer H. P., Hadaschik B. A., et al. Intravoxel incoherent motion (IVIM) diffusion imaging in prostate cancer - what does it add? *J. Comput. Assist. Tomogr.* 38(4), 558–564, 2014.
15. Shinmoto H., Tamura C., Soga S., Shiomi E., Yoshihara N., Kaji T., et al. An intravoxel incoherent motion diffusion-weighted imaging study of prostate cancer. *AJR Am. J. Roentgenol.* 199(4), W496–W500, 2012.
16. Pang Y., Turkbey B., Bernardo M., Kruecker J., Kadoury S., Merino M. J.,

et al. Intravoxel incoherent motion MR imaging for prostate cancer: an evaluation of perfusion fraction and diffusion coefficient derived from different *b*-value combinations. *Magn. Reson. Med,* 69(2), 553–562, 2013.

17. Iima M., Le Bihan D. Clinical intravoxel incoherent motion and diffusion MR imaging: Past, present, and future. *Radiology* 278(1), 13–32, 2016.
18. Le Bihan D. What can we see with IVIM MRI? *NeuroImage,* 2017, https://doi.org/10.1016/j.neuroimage.2017.12.062
19. Valerio M., Zini C., Fierro D., Giura F., Colarieti A., Giuliani A., et al. 3T multiparametric MRI of the prostate: Does intravoxel incoherent motion diffusion imaging have a role in the detection and stratification of prostate cancer in the peripheral zone? *Eur. J. Radiol.* 85(4), 790–794, 2016.
20. Bao J., Wang X., Hu C., Hou J., Dong F., Guo L. Differentiation of prostate cancer lesions in the transition zone by diffusion-weighted MRI. *Eur. J. Radiol. Open* 4, 123–138, 2017.
21. Grant K. B., Agarwal H. K., Shih J. H., Bernardo M., Pang Y., Daar D., et al. Comparison of calculated and acquired high *b*-value diffusion-weighted imaging in prostate cancer. *Abdom. Imaging* 40(3), 578–586, 2015.
22. Merisaari H., Movahedi P., Perez I. M., Toivonen J., Pesola M., Taimen P., et al. Fitting methods for intravoxel incoherent motion imaging of prostate cancer on region of interest level: Repeatability and gleason score prediction. *Magn. Reson. Med.* 77(3), 1249–1264, 2017.
23. Freidlin R. Z., Agarwal H. K., Sankineni S., Brown A. M., Mertan F., Bernardo M., et al. Application of an unsupervised multi-characteristic framework for intermediate-high risk prostate cancer localization using diffusion-weighted MRI. *Magn. Reson. Imaging* 34(9), 1227–1234, 2016.

Chapter 15

Clinical Application of IVIM in the Female Pelvis

Elaine Y. P. Lee and Pek-Lan Khong
Department of Diagnostic Radiology, Queen Mary Hospital, Li Ka Shing Faculty of Medicine, The University of Hong Kong, Hong Kong
eyplee77@hku.hk

There is growing interest in multiparametric assessment of female pelvic diseases, especially cervical cancer. Intravoxel incoherent motion (IVIM) provides simultaneous information on tissue or tumor cellularity and perfusion; with that it offers promising clinical applications in diagnosis, disease stratification, and treatment response assessment in female pelvic diseases. Most of the evidence is based on studies in cervical cancer, but its use in other areas of the female pelvis is expanding. In this chapter, we will summarize the current literature in this area and discuss the emerging applications of IVIM in the female pelvis, with technical considerations, its position in the roadmap to clinical translation, and directions for future research.

Intravoxel Incoherent Motion (IVIM) MRI: Principles and Applications
Edited by Denis Le Bihan, Mami Iima, Christian Federau, and Eric E. Sigmund

ISBN 978-981-4800-19-8 (Hardcover), 978-0-429-42727-5 (eBook)
www.panstanford.com

15.1 Cervical Cancer

Cervical cancer is ranked the fourth-most-common female cancer worldwide, with 85% of the cancer burden in less developed regions of the world, and a lethal cancer with an estimated 266,000 deaths in 2012 [1].

15.1.1 Tissue Differentiation

Magnetic resonance imaging (MRI) is the cornerstone in the evaluation of cervical cancer, in diagnosis, staging, treatment planning, and detection of recurrent disease. The addition of diffusion-weighted imaging (DWI) as part of the MRI examination is useful in disease detection and provides prognostic information through the measurement of the apparent diffusion coefficient (ADC), which is based on the monoexponential signal decay model [2, 3]. With the development of IVIM MRI, we know that ADC not only contains information on water diffusivity but also data from the microcirculation [4, 5].

In the feasibility study that applied IVIM in the female pelvis, the diffusional signal decay in cervical cancer demonstrated biexponential function, giving it a unique IVIM profile [6]. Cervical cancer demonstrated a considerable perfusion fraction (f) of 14.9 ± 2.6%, though it is lower when compared to that of the normal cervix (18.6 ± 2.2%) and leiomyoma (17.3 ± 3.6%) [6]. Subsequent studies observed similar findings and reported a lower f in cervical cancer; the f estimates by Lin et al. were higher than those by Lee et al. and Wu et al., which could be related to the higher b values used in their study [6–8].

As ADC intrinsically includes an IVIM effect, ADC values of cervical cancer are higher than the true diffusion coefficient (D) derived from the IVIM model [6–8]. Hence, ADC overestimates the water diffusivity, leading to inaccurate quantification of diffusion in cervical cancer. Nevertheless, in terms of clinical diagnostic performance, both ADC and D performed equally well in discriminating cancerous tissue from normal cervical tissue [6, 7]. These data were derived from cohort who underwent MRI for primary diagnosis, and there has been no study to date that evaluates the value of IVIM in the detection of cervical recurrence. There was no additional benefit of dynamic contrast–enhanced (DCE) MRI over DWI in the detection of cervical recurrence [9, 10]. Therefore, it remains unclear whether the perfusion parameters from IVIM will add value and have a role in cervical recurrence detection; further research is required to clarify the value of the perfusion parameters derived from IVIM in this setting.

15.1.2 Relationship with Dynamic Contrast–Enhanced MRI

The lower *f* in cervical cancer seems counterintuitive to what had been observed in DCE MRI, where rapid and intense contrast uptake was observed in cervical cancer compared to normal cervix [11, 12]. The relationship between IVIM-derived perfusion parameters and the "classical" perfusion parameters, mainly from DCE MRI, is dependent on the tissue under investigation, leading to mixed results in the published literature [13–20].

In a cohort of 25 patients with newly diagnosed cervical cancer (FIGO IB2-IVB), Lee et al. found that the flow-related parameter (fD^*, where D^* represents the pseudodiffusion coefficient derived from IVIM) was positively related to quantitative DCE MRI, that is, the estimated volume transfer constant between blood plasma and the extravascular extracellular space (${}_{est}K^{trans}$ with $r = 0.42$, $p = 0.038$) and the amplitude factor (A with $r = 0.50$, $p = 0.011$), which represented the degree of MRI signal enhancement. Furthermore, fD^* was also moderately correlated with semiquantitative DCE MRI, namely the maximum relative enhancement (maximum relative enhancement [MaxRE], $r = 0.52$, $p = 0.008$). The f was also associated with the area under the signal-time curve on DCE MRI (AUC, $r = 0.58$, $p = 0.003$) (Fig. 15.1) [21].

The measured fD^* is dependent on the complex interplay among different factors that influence tumor microcirculation, for example, the capillaries geometry, the endothelial permeability, the exchange surface areas, the interstitial volume, and flow dynamics. Therefore, fD^* could provide surrogate assessment of the endothelial leakiness and blood flow in cervical cancer; and its positive relationships with DCE MRI parameters support this notion. The signal attenuation that contributed to the IVIM-derived perfusion parameters in cervical cancer is likely related to the increased microvessel density due to tumor angiogenesis [22, 23]. Similarly, the positive correlation between *f* and the area under the signal-time curve or area under the curve (AUC) could be explained by the fact that both measurements are related to quantification of the blood volume. A separate study also found correlations between semiquantitative DCE MRI parameters and *f* in cervical cancer, namely the maximum slope of contrast uptake, the contrast enhancement ratio, and the AUC within the initial 90s of DCE MRI [24].

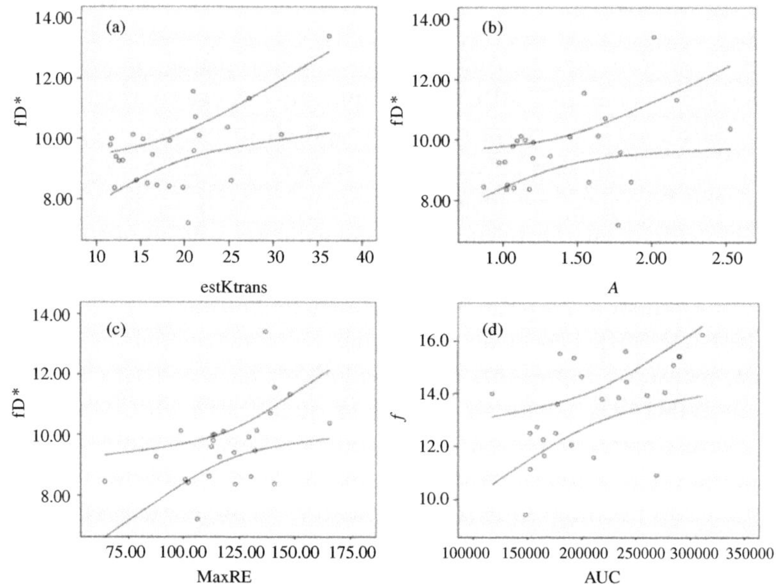

Figure 15.1 Scatterplots of IVIM perfusion parameters against DCE MRI perfusion parameters (a–d). The curved lines represent the 95% confidence intervals. (a) Moderate positive correlation between *fD** ($\times 10^{-3}$ mm^2/s) and $_{est}K^{trans}$ (s^{-1}) (r = 0.42, p= 0.038). (b) Moderate positive correlation between *fD**($\times 10^{-3}$ mm^2/s) and amplitude factor *A* (r = 0.50, p = 0.011). (c) Moderate positive correlation between *fD** ($\times 10^{-3}$ mm^2/s) and MaxRE (%) (r = 0.52, p = 0.008). (d) Moderate to good positive correlation between *f* (%) and AUC (r = 0.58, p = 0.003). Reprinted from Ref. [21], with permission from John Wiley and Sons, copyright 2014.

Despite these positive relationships, the degrees of agreement were only weak to moderate, suggesting that both methods are measuring different aspects of tumor microcirculation in cervical cancer. There are fundamental differences in the model assumptions of both methods, with IVIM investigating the microvessels network, while DCE MRI relies on the intravascular and extravascular distribution of exogenous contrast agent, in this case, gadolinium. Furthermore, the IVIM-derived perfusion parameters are affected not only by microcirculation but also by other physiological processes in cervical cancer, for example, glandular secretion [25].

The perfusion characteristic of cervical cancer affects the sensitivity to radiotherapy and has been a target for antiangiogenic therapy [23, 26]. Understanding the tumor microcirculation is important, given its influence on treatment response to radiation and disease prognosis. Poorly perfused cervical cancer is hypoxic, and hypoxia is a biological determinant of poor outcome to radiation [27]. MRI-derived perfusion parameters are promising surrogates for hypoxic imaging, which may have potential in guiding radiation dose escalation to hypoxic regions of cervical cancer, therefore offering personalized treatment. Although DCE MRI provides prognostic information on cervical cancer outcome, there are associated risks of toxicities related to the use of gadolinium [28]. IVIM-derived perfusion parameters have the advantages of being more sensitive to incoherent motion in the capillaries feeding the tumor and less sensitive to adjacent large vessel signal contamination, as in DCE MRI [14]. Therefore, IVIM-derived perfusion assessment may pose as an alternative to DCE MRI.

15.1.3 Tumor Differentiation

Approximately 85% of cervical cancers are squamous cell carcinoma (SCC) and the remaining 15% are adenocarcinoma (ACA).

Cervical SCC exhibited lower *D* compared to cervical ACA [7, 29] and substantiated by similar findings in our study that utilized histogram-based analysis [30]. In one of the studies, the authors suggested that a possible explanation for this is that SCC contains more tumor but less stroma than ACA, resulting in a higher restriction of water diffusion in SCC [29].

A lower *f* was observed in cervical SCC [7, 29, 31], in agreement with findings on immunostaining where lower microvessel density and lower intensity of vascular endothelial growth factor expression were observed in cervical SCC than in cervical ACA [32]. It is probable that the vascular endothelial organization and tumor architecture are more important in histological subtype differentiation, having a more profound effect on IVIM parameters like *D*, *f*, and *D** [31].

Apart from histological subtype differentiation, *D* is promising in tumor grading. Poorly differentiated cervical cancer was more restricted with a lower *D* [7, 29, 31]. Tumor grading relies on the nuclear polymorphism and frequency of mitotic figures, affecting the cell density, explaining the observed lower *D* in poorly differentiated cervical cancer. Although Wu et al. did not find a significant statistical difference, they observed a similar trend in that poorly differentiated cervical cancer tended to have a lower *D* [8]. *D* remained lower in poorly differentiated tumor when histological subtypes were considered [7, 24].

None of the perfusion-related IVIM parameters could be used to differentiate tumor grading when whole-tumor analysis was performed [7, 8, 31]. Interestingly, when only the periphery of the tumor was considered, *f* was useful in discriminating well/moderately differentiated versus poorly differentiated cervical SCC with a higher *f* in a poorly differentiated tumor [24]. This relates to tumor heterogeneity, especially in a large tumor where tumor growth exceeds neoangiogenesis, resulting in a poorly perfused tumor center [23, 33]. Whole-tumor analysis has the disadvantage of not taking tumor heterogeneity into consideration. With histogram analysis, we observed higher percentiles of *f* in poorly differentiated cervical SCC (Fig. 15.2), in agreement with Zhou et al. [24, 30]. Hence, histogram analysis provides more global assessment of cervical cancer, taking into account of tumor heterogeneity.

With histogram analysis, we were able to demonstrate that locally advanced cervical cancer (FIGO IIB-IVA, high FIGO) had lower values of skewness and kurtosis but higher percentile values in *f* than early cervical cancer (FIGO IB-IIA, low FIGO) (Fig. 15.3) [34]. Only a few of the histogram parameters of *D* were significantly different between the two groups, suggesting that the effect of cellular heterogeneity was not as dominant as the perfusion heterogeneity in the two different FIGO groups.

In recent years, there has been growing interest in the quantity and quality of tumor stroma that impact tumor progression. In cervical cancer, the tumor–stroma ratio (TSR) has a prognostic value in that stroma-rich tumor has a poorer prognosis and outcome [35]. Given the ability of DWI to characterize tumor microenvironment, the correlation between IVIM and TSR was investigated. *D* and *f* were significantly lower in a stroma-poor tumor with moderate negative correlations with TSR [35]. The lower *D* in the stroma-poor tumor could be explained by the higher proportion of tumor cells resulting in more water restriction in the tumor, but the mechanism of the lower *f* remains unclear and will need further exploration.

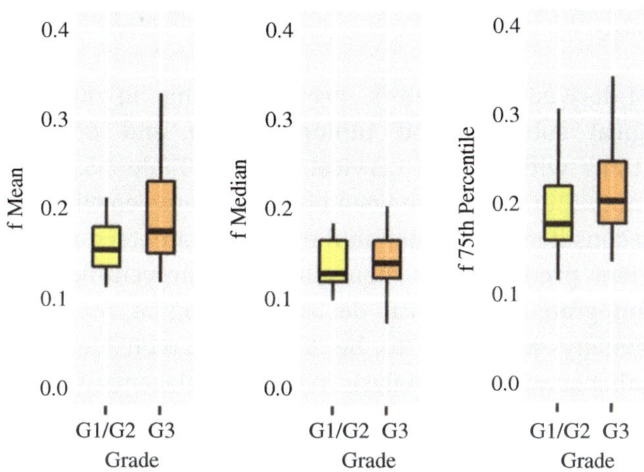

Figure 15.2 Boxplots of mean, median, and 75th percentile of *f* between well-/moderately (G1/2) and poorly differentiated (G3) cervical cancer showing statistical differences.

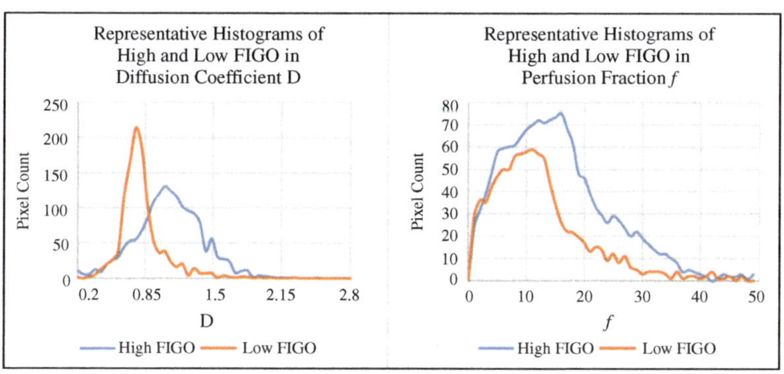

Figure 15.3 Smooth curve renderings of representative histogram distributions of *D* and *f* from high and low FIGO groups.

Table 15.1 Summary of the changes in *D* and *f* in relation to different cervical cancer characteristics

Cervical cancer	*D*	*f*
Cancer vs. normal	Low in cancer	Low in cancer
SCC vs. ACA	Low in SCC	Low in SCC
G1/2 vs. G3*	Low in G3	High in G3

ACA: adenocarcinoma; SCC: squamous cell carcinoma; G: tumor grade.
*only in tumor periphery and on histogram analysis, likely due to tumor heterogeneity

IVIM-derived parameters are promising in differentiating histological subtypes and tumor grading and possibly their correlations with TSR in cervical cancer (Table 15.1). Although significant differences have been observed between clinical groups, there is considerable overlap in the IVIM parameters, making them insufficient predictors by themselves and preventing them from being integrated in clinical decision-making at present. Tumor heterogeneity will need to be taken into consideration when performing quantitative analysis in terms of placement of the region of interest (ROI).

15.1.4 Treatment Response Assessment and Disease Prognostication

The standard treatment regimen for locally advanced cervical cancer is concurrent chemoradiotherapy (CCRT). This usually takes the form of four to five weeks of external beam radiotherapy to the whole pelvis and weekly cisplatin-based chemotherapy. Given the role of MRI in the pretreatment evaluation of cervical cancer, it is increasingly used in treatment response assessment during and following CCRT. However, assessment based on morphological and T2 signal changes is challenging and inaccurate [36, 37]. The addition of DWI and DCE MRI is useful in monitoring the treatment response by observing the cellular and perfusion modulation in the tumor microenvironment following CCRT [38, 39].

The first experience in treatment response assessment with IVIM in cervical cancer was reported in 21 patients who underwent CCRT [40]. Serial MRI examinations, which included IVIM, were performed before, throughout (Week 2 and Week 4 of CCRT), and after CCRT. *D*, *f*, and *D** increased in the early stage of CCRT; *D* continued to increase after CCRT, but the perfusion-related parameters started to decrease after the initial rise [40]. The trends in IVIM-derived perfusion parameters are compatible with those shown on DCE MRI, both semiquantitatively and quantitatively [41]. Herein, the increase in perfusion during CCRT is related to the modulation in the microvasculature of the tumor by radiation resulting in damage of the vascular endothelium and changes in the vascular density [41, 42]. However, subsequently the same group of authors observed a different trend in *D** in that it continued to rise after CCRT [43]. The discordant results are likely the consequence of instability of *D**, given its huge standard deviation and dependence on the signal-to-noise ratio (SNR), therefore limiting its use as a clinical parameter within the constraint of the current clinical MRI systems [44].

Histogram analysis provided an additional dimension to treatment response assessment by taking tumor heterogeneity into consideration. In an exploratory study, we observed that the histogram parameters generated from IVIM metrics significantly changed after CCRT in that both skewness and kurtosis were lower after treatment while other percentile values increased, both in *D* and *f*; and these changes were independent of changes in the tumor volume (Fig. 15.4) [45]. Our results concurred with the trends observed in head and neck SCC that had undergone CCRT [46]. This suggests that histogram analysis of IVIM parameters is able to quantify the spatial variations of *D* and *f* before and after CCRT.

The pretreatment *f* was found to be useful in discriminating complete response from partial response and predicting both, with a higher *f* observed in the former group [43]. The authors went on to say that with a cutoff value of 9.85%, *f* was able to predict the response with a sensitivity of 72% and a specificity of 75% with the area under the receiver operating characteristic (ROC) curve of 0.768. Moreover, the results from the pretreatment *f* were comparable to those achieved on the basis of unidimensional tumor regression between Week 2 MRI and Week 4 MRI (sensitivity 75%, specificity 72%, and the area under ROC curve 0.763) [43]. Pretreatment *f* is advantageous over the serial tumor regression by providing early and timely assessment and prediction without the reliance of the Week 4 MRI, in which by then the impact on treatment is likely going to be small toward the end of the CCRT. Nevertheless, the cohort was small in this study and results will require further validation.

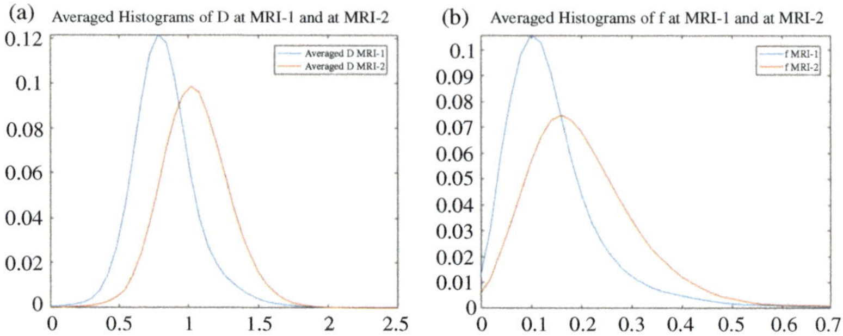

Figure 15.4 From left to right, averaged histogram curves (a) *D* and (b) *f* at baseline (MRI-1) and four weeks after CCRT (MRI-2). The decreasing skewness can be geometrically interpreted as a rightward shift in the histogram mass, while the decreasing kurtosis can be similarly interpreted as a flattening of the peak and lighter tails.

Contrary to this, we did not find *f* predictive of treatment response but *D* was when histogram analysis was applied [47]. We found that the skewness of *D* at baseline MRI was predictive of the treatment response, in addition to the increment in the 90th percentile of *D* following CCRT. The discrepancy between the two studies could be related to the differences in patient dichotomization, in which volume reduction was used as a reference in our study instead of unidimensional measurement in Zhu et al. and the differences in the method of analysis (histogram versus mean values) [43, 47]. Similarly, *D* was found useful in predicting response to neoadjuvant chemotherapy (areas under ROC curves: 0.763–0.823) whereas *f* and D^* were not [48].

A group of researchers studied the prognostic imaging markers from serial IVIM in a cohort of 30 patients who underwent CCRT with a median follow-up of 24 months (range 10–34 months) [49]. In this study, the authors found that some of the imaging parameters were good in predicting prognosis following CCRT, namely the ADC at Week 2 of CCRT and ADC and *f* at Week 3 of CCRT with areas under the ROC curves of 0.767, 0.857, and 0.820, respectively. In particular, the Week 3 imaging parameters performed better than the tumor regression rate, which only achieved an area under the ROC curve of

0.75 [49]. The lack of significance in D suggested that the dominant prognostic effect could be coming from the perfusion component of IVIM. The pattern of f in patients with a good prognosis was concordant with prior studies based on DCE MRI; a higher-perfusion tumor responded better to CCRT, being less hypoxic and less resistant to radiation therapy [23, 39]. These early results are encouraging, but the sample size was small in this study. A larger cohort and external validation are likely going to address the significance of these findings.

15.2 Technical Consideration

Thus far, the number and range of b values were variable among studies that had applied IVIM in the female pelvis described in this chapter, ranging from 9 b values to 14 b values, with the maximum b value reaching 2000 s/mm^2. Furthermore, the number of low b values (<200 s/mm^2 when the "pseudodiffusion" is significant and the perfusion effect of IVIM could be observed) included was variable ranging from 5 to 9. Therefore, we need to identify the optimal number and range of b values to avoid acquisition heterogeneity when applying pelvic IVIM. This will allow standardization of the imaging protocol for subsequent validation in multicenter studies.

Wu et al. tried to address this important question by using different ranges of b values (0–1000 s/mm^2 versus 0–2000 s/mm^2) to fit the IVIM model and assessed the diagnostic performance of the IVIM-derived parameters in differentiating cervical cancer from normal cervix [8]. They found that the IVIM parameters derived from the higher-range b values (0–2000 s/mm^2) performed better than their counterparts but both were able to distinguish cervical cancer from normal tissue, making no clinical impact in diagnosis [8]. However, the range of low b values remained the same in the two groups and the authors did not address the effect of choice of low b values that could significantly affect the f and D^* estimations. In other organs, like the liver and pancreas, a simplified IVIM model based on three b values showed promising results in lesion characterization [50, 51]. If this could be transferrable to the female pelvis and results are reproducible as those in the upper abdomen, it will greatly reduce IVIM acquisition time and potentially allow integration of IVIM into clinical practice.

It is increasingly recognized that the water diffusion in biological tissues derived from DWI does not always follow a Gaussian process [5, 52–54]. As alluded earlier, the signal attenuation on DWI was better ascribed by IVIM in cervical cancer [6]. Apart from IVIM, there are other nonmonoexponential models that can be applied in female pelvic imaging and potentially provide different aspects of tumor biology and microstructures.

In the exploratory study by Winfield et al., the authors fitted the signal attenuation of DWI in cervical cancer with different models, namely the monoexponential, the stretched exponential, kurtosis, statistical, and IVIM [31]. They found that the preferred models were IVIM and stretched exponential in 43% and 36% of the cervical cancers evaluated ($n = 42$), respectively. Furthermore, it was found that f and D^* from IVIM and α from the stretched exponential model (water diffusion heterogeneity index) were significantly different between histological subtypes whereas D from IVIM was significantly different between tumor grades [31]. The results were reproducible in a larger cohort ($n = 71$) except for α, for which there was no statistical difference between SCC and ACA subtypes [7]. Both studies agreed and suggested that parameters from these models provided different and additional information on tumor properties, other than that provided by ADC in the monoexponential model [7, 31].

Clinically useful parameters have to be robust and reliable. Previous studies have shown that repeatability of IVIM parameters is generally poor, especially with f and D^*, having a coefficient of variation (CV) larger than 20% [44, 55–57]. Reliable estimates of f and D^* are dependent on a high SNR and this is higher for D^* than for f [58]. In the presence of a high level of noise, f and D^* were overestimated whereas D was underestimated [58]. These limitations potentially hinder the clinical application of IVIM in the female pelvis. There are suggested methods to improve the estimation certainty of IVIM by averaging over the ROI [58], using the Bayesian probability approach in model fitting [59], applying fusion bootstrap moves [60], and using image denoising [61]. Future research work is required for improving the estimation of IVIM parameters and data reproducibility, specifically in female pelvic diseases. Furthermore, there is also the unresolved challenge of standardization across different MRI platforms.

15.3 Other Applications of IVIM in the Female Pelvis

The application of IVIM in other female pelvic diseases is very limited, but there is emerging evidence that IVIM may have a role in other malignant and benign diseases affecting the female reproductive organs.

15.3.1 Malignant Diseases

In ovarian cancer, lower D and f values were associated with high-grade epithelial ovarian cancer, while D showed a high performance on ROC analysis in differentiating high-grade from low-grade ovarian tumors (AUC > 0.900) [62]. The lower D in high-grade epithelial ovarian cancer is conceivable as D is commonly a surrogate measure of tumor aggressiveness. In the same study, the authors fitted the data using the stretched exponential model and found that both f and α performed less well than D (f and α, AUC ranging from 0.667 to 0.774) but suggested that both parameters provided information other than information on water diffusion [62]. Nevertheless, an earlier study suggested that the stretched exponential model provided a better fit of the diffusional signal from ovarian cancer and its metastases and IVIM was not a suitable fit for the data due to poor repeatability, hence the unreliability as clinically useful quantitative parameters [57].

An exploratory study applying IVIM in endometrial pathology showed that f was lower in the endometrial malignancy compared to normal endometrium, but surprisingly malignancy had a higher D than normal endometrium [63]. The latter finding was not concordant with previous studies that showed lower ADC in endometrial malignancy compared to normal endometrium [64–66]. One potential explanation for this discrepancy could be related to the age of the normal subjects, in which the menopausal status may affect the endometrial DWI signal.

Other than primary pelvic female malignancy, researchers attempted to evaluate the value of IVIM in determining metastatic pelvic nodal disease in cervical cancer but failed to demonstrate its superiority [67]. In this recent study, 157 lymph nodes with high DWI signals were mapped with the surgical specimens to determine their malignant status. Although the authors found that metastatic pelvic lymph nodes had higher D and lower f values, the IVIM parameters did not perform better than size criteria, only achieving areas under the ROC curves in-between 0.610 and 0.633, whereas the short-axis measurement could achieve a higher diagnostic performance (area under ROC curve 0.844). Therefore, on the basis of this study, no additional benefit of IVIM was found in the assessment of pelvic nodal disease.

15.3.2 Benign Disease

With the use of MRI-guided high-intensity focused ultrasound (HIFU) as a nonsurgical therapeutic option for uterine leiomyoma, there is a need for optimal patient selection and to monitor treatment efficacy. To select suitable patients for MRI-guided HIFU, Funaki classification is commonly used, which is based on the T2-weighted signal of the uterine leiomyoma (Type I signal, similar to that of the skeletal muscle; Type II signal, between the signals of the skeletal muscle and the myometrium; and Type III signal, greater than that of the myometrium) and correlates with treatment outcome, whereby response is poor in Type III leiomyoma [68]. Type III uterine leiomyoma tends to enhance avidly and is thought to be highly perfused, in which MRI-guided HIFU has not been shown to be effective [69]. The f was found to be significantly higher in Type II uterine leiomyoma compared to Type I after correction of the T2-weighted effect on the image [70]. This indicates that the potential of IVIM is tissue characterization of uterine leiomyoma, providing quantitative biometrics in patient selection for MRI-guided HIFU, more objective than the qualitative Funaki classification. However, the study was limited by the lack of Type III uterine leiomyoma, and whether the findings can be translated to clinical use is yet to be examined.

The treatment response assessment of MRI-guided HIFU is usually done through contrast-enhanced MRI or DCE MRI [69]. Ikink et al. showed that the ADC derived from low *b* values (≤200 s/mm^2) decreased significantly in treated uterine leiomyoma following MRI-guided HIFU but the value increased if high *b* values were used (≥400 s/mm^2) [71]. The former observation was likely due to the reduced perfusion in the ablated tissue, and this concurred with the visual assessment on contrast-enhanced MRI. The increase in ADC derived from the set of high *b* values could be explained by the expansion of the extracellular volume following treatment [71]. Potentially, IVIM can be used to monitor treatment efficacy following MRI-guided HIFU in uterine leiomyoma, without the dependence on gadolinium-based MRI contrast agent.

15.3.3 Treatment-Related Changes in the Pelvis

Pelvic radiotherapy is commonly used in treating gynecological malignancy, and it is well known that radiation induces injury to the pelvic marrow, manifesting as hematological toxicity (HT) and skeletal complications [72, 73]. In a cohort of locally advanced cervical cancer patients who underwent CCRT, we observed the IVIM signal changes in the pelvic marrow during CCRT [74]. In patients who suffered from HT, that is, those who required blood transfusion or interruptions to their treatment due to thrombocytopenia or neutropenia, had an associated rise in *D* after four weeks of CCRT compared to baseline measurement (Fig. 15.5). Although *f* increased from the baseline, there was no difference in the pattern observed between patients who suffered from HT and those who did not (Fig. 15.6) [74]. IVIM parameters appear to be able to monitor the microenvironmental changes in the pelvic marrow induced by radiation, offering a way to identify the subregion of the pelvis more susceptible to irradiation damage and allowing more precise radiation planning. Nevertheless, its clinical application will require prospective research and a larger study cohort with a longer follow-up to understand the long-term implications of these parametric changes in IVIM.

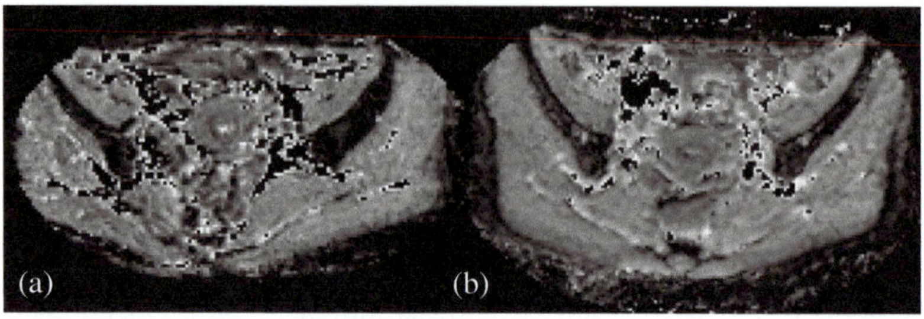

Figure 15.5 *D* maps at the level of the ilium before (a, baseline MRI) and after (b, Week4 MRI) CCRT in a patient who suffered from HT. Note the increase in the ilium marrow signal at MRI-2. Reprinted from Ref. [74], with permission from John Wiley and Sons, copyright 2017.

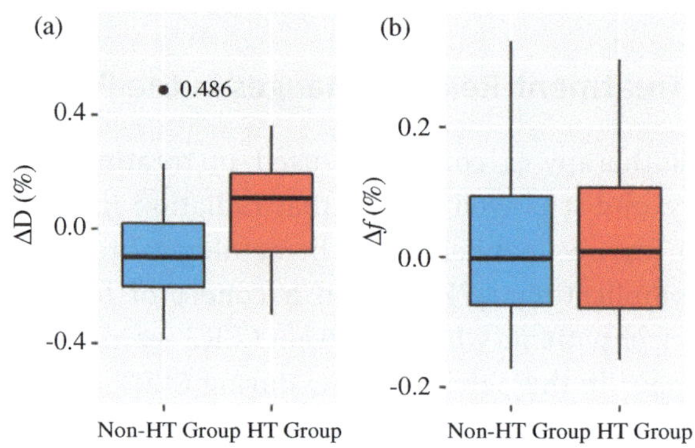

Figure 15.6 Boxplots showing the changes in *D* and *f* in the pelvic marrow in relation to hematological toxicity (HT). Δ*D* represents the changes in *D* between baseline and Week 4 MRI following CCRT, and Δ*f* represents the changes in *f* between baseline and Week 4 MRI following CCRT. There was statistical difference in *D* between HT and non-HT groups, but not in *f*. Adapted from Ref. [74], with permission from John Wiley and Sons, copyright 2017.

15.4 Roadmap to Clinical Translation

There is now evidence of IVIM imaging-pathology correlation in cervical cancer, but this is only based on cervical biopsy specimens; whole-tumor 3D mapping will be preferable given the presence of tumor heterogeneity, which is well known in cervical cancer both spatially and temporally, allowing accurate biological validation of the IVIM parameters at different treatment time points [75]. Robust imaging-pathology correlation will provide insight into the true biophysical meaning of IVIM in cervical cancer, not just based on tumor cellularity and vascularity, but also based on its relationship with tumor hypoxia, which plays an integral role in the response to CCRT. This is likely better achieved through animal study as locally advanced cervical cancer is treated by CCRT, making whole-tumor analysis impossible, whereas surgically resected early-staged cervical cancer maybe too small to permit reliable and accurate quantification of IVIM, especially as a proof-of-concept design.

Despite promising results in diagnosis and tissue differentiation, there is a lack of standardization in IVIM imaging acquisition and quality assurance, with substantial heterogeneity in the published data. By not passing the domain of qualification in technical validation, it will be difficult for IVIM to proceed further into the next “translational gap” in the clinical decision-making tool in the management of gynecological cancers, especially in cervical cancer [76].

An unmet clinical need in cervical cancer is a robust imaging biomarker to monitor the treatment response to CCRT, with the potential of treatment escalation and radiation dose painting to target vulnerable regions. IVIM is superior than currently used imaging biomarkers, like ADC or DCE MRI, as it simultaneously offers both pieces of information with one acquisition, without the need for exogenous intravenous contrast. Early evidence is promising in this area, but the limiting step for clinical translation and qualification is the precision of IVIM parameters to monitor treatment-related changes. Although we do not have data on repeatability of IVIM parameters specific to cervical cancer, the reported low repeatability in other organs is likely applicable in the female pelvis. From our experience, f and D^* are highly variable, especially D^* in which the standard deviation is huge, making it unsuitable as a clinical imaging biomarker at present. With f, this is less but still substantial, and further work in improving the estimation is really needed to move forward IVIM research and its clinical application.

Determination of the nodal status in locally advanced cervical cancer is always challenging on the basis of morphological imaging like computer tomography and MRI predominantly based on the size criteria. However, it is an important clinical question that will affect not only treatment planning but also disease prognostication. Although the only study that applied IVIM in determining the pelvic nodal status in cervical cancer did not show superiority to size criteria, it is perhaps too early to disregard IVIM in the nodal staging of cervical cancer on the basis of the observation of one study. A challenge with this type of study is providing an accurate surgical-imaging-pathology mapping for all resected lymph nodes. Moreover, the results could only be inferred from early-staged disease that will undergo surgery and pelvic lymphadenectomy; this type of study could not be performed in locally advanced cervical cancer, in which CCRT is the recommended treatment regimen, and will not undergo pelvic lymphadenectomy.

15.5 Conclusion

In the clinical application of IVIM in the female pelvis, most work has concentrated on the evaluation of cervical cancer, with promising results in terms of differentiating normal from malignant tissue, histological subtyping, and tumor grading. There is also emerging data to support its use in treatment response assessment in cervical cancer, but the majority of these studies had small cohorts of patients and results have not been externally validated. Therefore, more research is required in this area before IVIM can be applied in clinical practice. Very limited work is present in the current literature on the use of IVIM in other gynecological malignancy or benign female pelvic diseases; hence this could potentially be an area of further exploration. While researchers are keen to apply IVIM in clinical conditions and attempt to use these parameters in diagnosis, disease prognostication, and treatment response assessment, care should be taken in performing IVIM and analyzing the data from IVIM, as there are technical challenges at present, especially with the poor repeatability of f and D^*. We hope that with future improvement in MRI hardware and software and consensus on standardization and validation across different imaging systems, IVIM will be able to provide added value and relevant clinical information for improved patient care and management in the female pelvis.

References

1. Ferlay J. S. I., Ervik M., Dikshit R., Eser S., Mathers C., et al. GLOBOCAN 2012 v1.0. *Cancer Incidence and Mortality Worldwide: IARC CancerBase No. 11*. 2013 [Available from: http://globocan.iarc.fr/].
2. Kuang F., Ren J., Zhong Q., Liyuan F., Huan Y., Chen Z. The value of apparent diffusion coefficient in the assessment of cervical cancer. *Eur. Radiol.* 23(4), 1050–1058, 2013.
3. Nakamura K., Joja I., Nagasaka T., Fukushima C., Kusumoto T., Seki N., et al. The mean apparent diffusion coefficient value (ADC mean) on primary cervical cancer is a predictive marker for disease recurrence. *Gynecol. Oncol.* 127(3), 478–483, 2012.
4. Le Bihan D. Intravoxel incoherent motion imaging using steady-state free precession. *Magn. Reson. Med.* 7(3), 346–351, 1988.
5. Le Bihan D., Breton E., Lallemand D., Aubin M. L., Vignaud J., Laval-Jeantet M. Separation of diffusion and perfusion in intravoxel incoherent motion MR imaging. *Radiology* 168(2), 497–505, 1988.
6. Lee E. Y., Yu X., Chu M. M., Ngan H. Y., Siu S. W., Soong I. S., et al. Perfusion and diffusion characteristics of cervical cancer based on intraxovel incoherent motion MR imaging-a pilot study. *Eur. Radiol.* 24(7), 1506–1513, 2014.
7. Lin M., Yu X., Chen Y., Ouyang H., Wu B., Zheng D., et al. Contribution of mono-exponential, bi-exponential and stretched exponential model-based diffusion-weighted MR imaging in the diagnosis and differentiation of uterine cervical carcinoma. *Eur. Radiol.* 27(6), 2400–2410, 2017.
8. Wu Q., Wang Y., Shi L., Dong L., Liu M., Dou S., et al. Intravoxel incoherent motion diffusion-weighted magnetic resonance imaging of cervical cancer with different *b*-values. *J. Comput. Assist. Tomogr.* 41(4), 592–598, 2017.
9. Kitajima K., Tanaka U., Ueno Y., Maeda T., Suenaga Y., Takahashi S., et al. Role of diffusion weighted imaging and contrast-enhanced MRI in the evaluation of intrapelvic recurrence of gynecological malignant tumor. *PloS One* 10(1), e0117411, 2015.
10. Lucas R., Lopes Dias J., Cunha T. M. Added value of diffusion-weighted MRI in detection of cervical cancer recurrence: comparison with morphologic and dynamic contrast-enhanced MRI sequences. *Diagn. Interv. Radiol.* 21(5), 368–375, 2015.

11. Van Vierzen P. B., Massuger L. F., Ruys S. H., Barentsz J. O. Fast dynamic contrast enhanced MR imaging of cervical carcinoma. *Clin. Radiol.* 53(3), 183–192, 1998.

12. Yamashita Y., Takahashi M., Sawada T., Miyazaki K., Okamura H. Carcinoma of the cervix: dynamic MR imaging. *Radiology* 182(3), 643–648,1992.

13. Bisdas S., Braun C., Skardelly M., Schittenhelm J., Teo T. H., Thng C. H., et al. Correlative assessment of tumor microcirculation using contrast-enhanced perfusion MRI and intravoxel incoherent motion diffusion-weighted MRI: is there a link between them? *NMR Biomed.* 27(10), 1184–1191, 2014.

14. Federau C., O'Brien K., Meuli R., Hagmann P., Maeder P. Measuring brain perfusion with intravoxel incoherent motion (IVIM): Initial clinical experience. *J. Magn. Reson. Imaging* 39(3), 624–632, 2014.

15. Fujima N., Yoshida D., Sakashita T., Homma A., Tsukahara A., Tha K. K., et al. Intravoxel incoherent motion diffusion-weighted imaging in head and neck squamous cell carcinoma: Assessment of perfusion-related parameters compared to dynamic contrast-enhanced MRI. *Magn. Reson. Imaging* 32(10), 1206–1213, 2014.

16. Patel J., Sigmund E. E., Rusinek H., Oei M., Babb J. S., Taouli B. Diagnosis of cirrhosis with intravoxel incoherent motion diffusion MRI and dynamic contrast-enhanced MRI alone and in combination: preliminary experience. *J. Magn. Reson. Imaging* 31(3), 589–600, 2010.

17. Sumi M., Nakamura T. Head and neck tumours: combined MRI assessment based on IVIM and TIC analyses for the differentiation of tumors of different histological types. *Eur. Radiol.* 24(1), 223–231, 2014.

18. Wang L. L., Lin J., Liu K., Chen C. Z., Liu H., Lv P., et al. Intravoxel incoherent motion diffusion-weighted MR imaging in differentiation of lung cancer from obstructive lung consolidation: comparison and correlation with pharmacokinetic analysis from dynamic contrast-enhanced MR imaging. *Eur. Radiol.* 24(8), 1914–1922, 2014.

19. Woo S., Lee J. M., Yoon J. H., Joo I., Han J. K., Choi B. I. Intravoxel incoherent motion diffusion-weighted MR imaging of hepatocellular carcinoma: Correlation with enhancement degree and histologic grade. *Radiology* 270(3), 758–767, 2014.

20. Pang Y., Turkbey B., Bernardo M., Kruecker J., Kadoury S., Merino M. J., et al. Intravoxel incoherent motion MR imaging for prostate cancer: an evaluation of perfusion fraction and diffusion coefficient derived from

different *b*-value combinations. *Magn. Reson. Med.* 69(2), 553–562, 2013.

21. Lee E. Y., Hui E. S., Chan K. K., Tse K. Y., Kwong W. K., Chang T. Y., et al. Relationship between intravoxel incoherent motion diffusion-weighted MRI and dynamic contrast-enhanced MRI in tissue perfusion of cervical cancers. *J. Magn. Reson. Imaging* 42(2), 454–459, 2015.
22. Hawighorst H., Weikel W., Knapstein P. G., Knopp M. V., Zuna I., Schonberg S. O., et al. Angiogenic activity of cervical carcinoma: assessment by functional magnetic resonance imaging-based parameters and a histomorphological approach in correlation with disease outcome. *Clin. Cancer Res.* 4(10), 2305–2312, 1998.
23. Yamashita Y., Baba T., Baba Y., Nishimura R., Ikeda S., Takahashi M., et al. Dynamic contrast-enhanced MR imaging of uterine cervical cancer: pharmacokinetic analysis with histopathologic correlation and its importance in predicting the outcome of radiation therapy. *Radiology* 216(3), 803–809, 2000.
24. Zhou Y., Liu J., Liu C., Jia J., Li N., Xie L., et al. Intravoxel incoherent motion diffusion weighted MRI of cervical cancer—Correlated with tumor differentiation and perfusion. *Magn. Reson. Imaging* 34(8), 1050–1056, 2016.
25. Zhang L., Murata Y., Ishida R., Ohashi I., Yoshimura R., Shibuya H. Functional evaluation with intravoxel incoherent motion echo-planar MRI in irradiated salivary glands: a correlative study with salivary gland scintigraphy. *J. Magn. Reson. Imaging* 14(3), 223–229, 2001.
26. Tewari K. S., Sill M. W., Penson R. T., Huang H., Ramondetta L. M., Landrum L. M., et al. Bevacizumab for advanced cervical cancer: final overall survival and adverse event analysis of a randomised, controlled, open-label, phase 3 trial (Gynecologic Oncology Group 240). *Lancet* 390(10103), 1654–1663, 2017.
27. Zahra M. A., Hollingsworth K. G., Sala E., Lomas D. J., Tan L. T. Dynamic contrast-enhanced MRI as a predictor of tumour response to radiotherapy. *Lancet Oncol.* 8(1), 63–74, 2007.
28. Pasquini L., Napolitano A., Visconti E., Longo D., Romano A., Toma P., et al. Gadolinium-based contrast agent-related toxicities. *CNS Drugs,* 32(3), 229–240, 2018.
29. Li X., Wang P., Li D., Zhu H., Meng L., Song Y., et al. Intravoxel incoherent motion MR imaging of early cervical carcinoma: correlation between imaging parameters and tumor-stroma ratio. *Eur. Radiol.* 28(5), 1875–1883, 2018.

30. Perucho J. A. U., Lee E. Y. P., Tse, K.Y., P Ip. Histogram analysis of intravoxel incoherent motion MRI and associations with histologic features in cervical cancer. *The British Society for Colposcopy and Cervical Pathology Annual Scientific Meeting 2018*; Manchester, United Kingdom 2018.

31. Winfield J. M., Orton M. R., Collins D. J., Ind T. E., Attygalle A., Hazell S., et al. Separation of type and grade in cervical tumours using non-mono-exponential models of diffusion-weighted MRI. *Eur. Radiol.* 27(2), 627–636, 2017.

32. Tokumo K., Kodama J., Seki N., Nakanishi Y., Miyagi Y., Kamimura S., et al. Different angiogenic pathways in human cervical cancers. *Gynecol. Oncol.* 68(1), 38–44, 1998.

33. Hawighorst H., Knapstein P. G., Knopp M. V., Weikel W., Brix G., Zuna I., et al. Uterine cervical carcinoma: comparison of standard and pharmacokinetic analysis of time-intensity curves for assessment of tumor angiogenesis and patient survival. *Cancer Res.* 58(16), 3598–3602, 1998.

34. Perucho J. A. U., Lee E. Y. P., Chan Q. (eds.) Tumour heterogeneity assessment using histogram analysis of IVIM-based diffusion and perfusion characteristics of cervical cancer. *24th Annual Meeting and Exhibition ISMRM*, 2016, Singapore.

35. Liu J., Liu J., Li J., Chen Y., Guan X., Wu X., et al. Tumor-stroma ratio is an independent predictor for survival in early cervical carcinoma. *Gynecol. Oncol.* 132(1), 81–86, 2014.

36. Mayr N. A., Yuh W. T., Taoka T., Wang J. Z., Wu D. H., Montebello J. F., et al. Serial therapy-induced changes in tumor shape in cervical cancer and their impact on assessing tumor volume and treatment response. *Am. J. Roentgenol.* 187(1), 65–72, 2006.

37. Vincens E., Balleyguier C., Rey A., Uzan C., Zareski E., Gouy S., et al. Accuracy of magnetic resonance imaging in predicting residual disease in patients treated for stage IB2/II cervical carcinoma with chemoradiation therapy: correlation of radiologic findings with surgicopathologic results. *Cancer* 113(8), 2158–2165, 2008.

38. Schreuder S. M., Lensing R., Stoker J., Bipat S. Monitoring treatment response in patients undergoing chemoradiotherapy for locally advanced uterine cervical cancer by additional diffusion-weighted imaging: A systematic review. *J. Magn. Reson. Imaging* 42(3), 572–594, 2015.

39. Yuh W. T., Mayr N. A., Jarjoura D., Wu D., Grecula J. C., Lo S. S., et al. Predicting control of primary tumor and survival by DCE MRI during early therapy in cervical cancer. *Invest. Radiol.* 44(6), 343–350, 2009.

40. Zhu L., Zhu L., Shi H., Wang H., Yan J., Liu B., et al. Evaluating early response of cervical cancer under concurrent chemo-radiotherapy by intravoxel incoherent motion MR imaging. *BMC Cancer* 16, 79, 2016.

41. Zahra M. A., Tan L. T., Priest A. N., Graves M. J., Arends M., Crawford R. A., et al. Semiquantitative and quantitative dynamic contrast-enhanced magnetic resonance imaging measurements predict radiation response in cervix cancer. *Int. J. Radiat. Oncol. Biol. Phys.* 74(3), 766–773, 2009.

42. Fajardo L. F. The pathology of ionizing radiation as defined by morphologic patterns. *Acta Oncol.* 44(1), 13–22, 2005.

43. Zhu L., Zhu L., Wang H., Yan J., Liu B., Chen W., et al. Predicting and early monitoring treatment efficiency of cervical cancer under concurrent chemoradiotherapy by intravoxel incoherent motion magnetic resonance imaging. *J. Comput. Assist. Tomogr.* 41(3), 422–429, 2017.

44. Andreou A., Koh D. M., Collins D. J., Blackledge M., Wallace T., Leach M. O., et al. Measurement reproducibility of perfusion fraction and pseudodiffusion coefficient derived by intravoxel incoherent motion diffusion-weighted MR imaging in normal liver and metastases. *Eur. Radiol.* 23(2), 428–434, 2013.

45. Perucho J. A. U., Lee E., Chan W. C., Gong N., Chan Q. (eds.) Histogram analysis of intravoxel incoherent motion parameters in assessing tumour diffusion and perfusion heterogeneity in cervical cancer before and after chemoradiotherapy. *25th Annual Meeting and Exhibition ISMRM*, 2017, Honolulu, Hawaii, USA.

46. King A. D., Chow K. K., Yu K. H., Mo F. K., Yeung D. K., Yuan J., et al. Head and neck squamous cell carcinoma: diagnostic performance of diffusion-weighted MR imaging for the prediction of treatment response. *Radiology* 266(2), 531–538, 2013.

47. Perucho J. A. U., Lee E., Chan W. C., Gong N., Chan Q. (eds.) Histogram analysis of intravoxel incoherent motion MRI in predicting chemoradiotherapy response in cervical cancer. *25th Annual Meeting and Exhibition ISMRM*, 2017, *Honolulu, Hawaii*, USA.

48. Wang Y. C., Hu D. Y., Hu X. M., Shen Y. Q., Meng X. Y., Tang H., et al. Assessing the early response of advanced cervical cancer to neoadjuvant chemotherapy using intravoxel incoherent motion diffusion-weighted magnetic resonance imaging: A pilot study. *Chin. Med. J. (Engl.)* 129(6), 665–671, 2016.

49. Zhu L., Wang H., Zhu L., Meng J., Xu Y., Liu B., et al. Predictive and prognostic value of intravoxel incoherent motion (IVIM) MR imaging in patients with advanced cervical cancers undergoing concurrent chemo-radiotherapy. *Sci. Rep.* 7(1), 11635, 2017.

50. Concia M., Sprinkart A. M., Penner A. H., Brossart P., Gieseke J., Schild H. H., et al. Diffusion-weighted magnetic resonance imaging of the pancreas: Diagnostic benefit from an intravoxel incoherent motion model-based 3 *b*-value analysis. *Invest. Radiol.* 49(2), 93–100, 2014.

51. Penner A. H., Sprinkart A. M., Kukuk G. M., Gutgemann I., Gieseke J., Schild H. H., et al. Intravoxel incoherent motion model-based liver lesion characterisation from three *b*-value diffusion-weighted MRI. *Eur. Radiol.* 23(10), 2773–2783, 2013.

52. Bennett K. M., Schmainda K. M., Bennett R. T., Rowe D. B., Lu H., Hyde J. S. Characterization of continuously distributed cortical water diffusion rates with a stretched-exponential model. *Magn. Reson. Med.* 50(4), 727–734, 2003.

53. Jensen J. H., Helpern J. A., Ramani A., Lu H., Kaczynski K. Diffusional kurtosis imaging: the quantification of non-gaussian water diffusion by means of magnetic resonance imaging. *Magn. Reson. Med.* 53(6), 1432–1440, 2005.

54. Yablonskiy D. A., Bretthorst G. L., Ackerman J. J. Statistical model for diffusion attenuated MR signal. *Magn. Reson. Med.* 50(4), 664–669, 2003.

55. Mazaheri Y., Afaq A., Rowe D. B., Lu Y., Shukla-Dave A., Grover J. Diffusion-weighted magnetic resonance imaging of the prostate: improved robustness with stretched exponential modeling. *J. Comput. Assist. Tomogr.* 36(6), 695–703, 2012.

56. Orton M. R., Messiou C., Collins D., Morgan V. A., Tessier. J., Young H., et al. Diffusion-weighted MR imaging of metastatic abdominal and pelvic tumours is sensitive to early changes induced by a VEGF inhibitor using alternative diffusion attenuation models. *Eur. Radiol.* 26(5), 1412–1419, 2016.

57. Winfield J. M., deSouza N. M., Priest A. N., Wakefield J. C., Hodgkin C., Freeman S., et al. Modelling DW-MRI data from primary and metastatic ovarian tumours. *Eur. Radiol.* 25(7), 2033–2040, 2015.

58. Pekar J., Moonen C. T., van Zijl P. C. On the precision of diffusion/perfusion imaging by gradient sensitization. *Magn. Reson. Med.* 23(1), 122–129, 1992.

59. Orton M. R., Collins D. J., Koh D. M., Leach M. O. Improved intravoxel incoherent motion analysis of diffusion weighted imaging by data driven Bayesian modeling. *Magn. Reson. Med.* 71(1), 411–420, 2014.

60. Freiman M., Perez-Rossello J. M., Callahan M. J., Voss S. D., Ecklund K., Mulkern R. V., et al. Reliable estimation of incoherent motion parametric maps from diffusion-weighted MRI using fusion bootstrap moves. *Med. Image Anal.* 17(3), 325–336, 2013.

61. Reischauer C, Gutzeit A. Image denoising substantially improves accuracy and precision of intravoxel incoherent motion parameter estimates. *Plos One* 12(4), e0175106, 2017.

62. Wang F., Wang Y., Zhou Y., Liu C., Xie L., Zhou Z., et al. Comparison between types I and II epithelial ovarian cancer using histogram analysis of monoexponential, biexponential, and stretched-exponential diffusion models. *J. Magn. Reson. Imaging* 46(6), 1797–1809, 2017.

63. Liu J., Wan Y., Wang Z., Qi Y., Qu P., Liu Y. Perfusion and diffusion characteristics of endometrial malignancy based on intravoxel incoherent motion MRI at 3.0 T: comparison with normal endometrium. *Acta Radiol.* 57(9), 1140–1148, 2016.

64. Inada Y., Matsuki M., Nakai G., Tatsugami F., Tanikake M., Narabayashi I., et al. Body diffusion-weighted MR imaging of uterine endometrial cancer: is it helpful in the detection of cancer in nonenhanced MR imaging? *Eur. J. Radiol.* 70(1), 122–127, 2009.

65. Tamai K., Koyama T., Saga T., Umeoka S., Mikami Y., Fujii S., et al. Diffusion-weighted MR imaging of uterine endometrial cancer. *J. Magn. Reson. Imaging* 26(3), 682–687, 2007.

66. Wang J., Yu T., Bai R., Sun H., Zhao X., Li Y. The value of the apparent diffusion coefficient in differentiating stage IA endometrial carcinoma from normal endometrium and benign diseases of the endometrium: initial study at 3-T magnetic resonance scanner. *J. Comput. Assist. Tomogr.* 34(3), 332–337, 2010.

67. Wu Q., Zheng D., Shi L., Liu M., Wang M., Shi D. Differentiating metastatic from nonmetastatic lymph nodes in cervical cancer patients using monoexponential, biexponential, and stretched exponential diffusion-weighted MR imaging. *Eur. Radiol.* 27(12), 5272–5279, 2017.

68. Funaki K., Fukunishi H., Funaki T., Sawada K., Kaji Y., Maruo T. Magnetic resonance-guided focused ultrasound surgery for uterine fibroids: relationship between the therapeutic effects and signal intensity of preexisting T2-weighted magnetic resonance images. *Am. J. Obstet. Gynecol.* 196(2), 184 e1–e6, 2007.

69. Kim Y. S., Lim H. K., Kim J. H., Rhim H., Park B. K., Keserci B., et al. Dynamic contrast-enhanced magnetic resonance imaging predicts immediate therapeutic response of magnetic resonance-guided high-intensity focused ultrasound ablation of symptomatic uterine fibroids. *Invest. Radiol.* 46(10), 639–647, 2011.

70. Qu F., Hor P. H., Fischer J., Muthupillai R. Tissue characterization of uterine fibroids with an intravoxel incoherent motion model: The need for T2 correction. *J. Magn. Reson. Imaging* 2018.

71. Ikink M. E., Voogt M. J., van den Bosch M. A., Nijenhuis R. J., Keserci B., Kim Y. S., et al. Diffusion-weighted magnetic resonance imaging using different *b*-value combinations for the evaluation of treatment results after volumetric MR-guided high-intensity focused ultrasound ablation of uterine fibroids. *Eur. Radiol.* 24(9), 2118–2127, 2014.

72. Green J. A., Kirwan J. M., Tierney J. F., Symonds P., Fresco L., Collingwood M, et al. Survival and recurrence after concomitant chemotherapy and radiotherapy for cancer of the uterine cervix: a systematic review and meta-analysis. *Lancet* 358(9284), 781–786, 2001.

73. Kwon J. W., Huh S. J., Yoon Y. C., Choi S. H., Jung J. Y., Oh D., et al. Pelvic bone complications after radiation therapy of uterine cervical cancer: evaluation with MRI. *Am. J. Roentgenol.* 191(4), 987–994, 2008.

74. Lee E. Y. P., Perucho J. A. U., Vardhanabhuti V., He J., Siu S. W. K., Ngu S. F., et al. Intravoxel incoherent motion MRI assessment of chemoradiation-induced pelvic bone marrow changes in cervical cancer and correlation with hematological toxicity. *J. Magn. Reson. Imaging* 46(5), 1491–1498, 2017.

75. Cooke S. L., Temple J., Macarthur S., Zahra M. A., Tan L. T., Crawford R. A., et al. Intra-tumour genetic heterogeneity and poor chemoradiotherapy response in cervical cancer. *Br. J. Cancer* 104(2), 361–368, 2011.

76. O'Connor J. P., Aboagye E. O., Adams J. E., Aerts H. J., Barrington S. F., Beer A. J., et al. Imaging biomarker roadmap for cancer studies. *Nat. Rev. Clin. Oncol.* 14(3), 169–186, 2017.

Chapter 16

IVIM MRI of the Placenta

Paddy J. Slator,[a] Jana Hutter,[b,c] Eleftheria Panagiotaki,[a] Mary A. Rutherford,[b] Joseph V. Hajnal,[b,c] and Daniel C. Alexander[a,d]

[a]*Centre for Medical Image Computing and Department of Computer Science, University College London, London, UK*
[b]*Centre for the Developing Brain, King's College London, London, UK*
[c]*Biomedical Engineering Department, King's College London, London, UK*
[d]*Clinical Imaging Research Centre, National University of Singapore, Singapore*
p.slator@ucl.ac.uk

16.1 Introduction

The placenta enables the transfer of oxygen and nutrients to the growing fetus and is vital to the lifelong health of both mother and child [1, 2]. It is highly vascular, contains large volumes of maternal and fetal blood, and undergoes major structural and functional changes across the 40 weeks of gestation. It therefore presents unique challenges and opportunities for intravoxel incoherent motion magnetic resonance imagery (IVIM MRI).

Intravoxel Incoherent Motion (IVIM) MRI: Principles and Applications
Edited by Denis Le Bihan, Mami Iima, Christian Federau, and Eric E. Sigmund

ISBN 978-981-4800-19-8 (Hardcover), 978-0-429-42727-5 (eBook)
www.panstanford.com

16.1.1 Placental Markers of Pregnancy Complications

Many major pregnancy complications are associated with placental malfunction [3]. Deviations in blood flow can disrupt the transfer of oxygen and nutrients to the developing fetus, eventually leading to complications such as fetal growth restriction [4–6] (FGR, defined as growth below the genetic potential of the fetus) and pre-eclampsia [7, 8] (PE, a disease characterized by elevated maternal blood pressure and proteinuria). Despite these underlying placental etiologies, both FGR and PE are difficult to detect before the onset of symptoms. In other words, at the point of FGR or PE diagnosis there has already been substantial inhibition of placental function. Biomarkers that quantify placental development—with their potential for prediction, earlier diagnosis, and better management of high-risk pregnancies—are therefore of great importance.

16.1.2 Imaging Markers of Pregnancy Complications

Ultrasound is currently the main modality for pregnancy monitoring. A wide range of ultrasound-derived biomarkers are currently used in the clinic, such as fetal biometry, heart rate, amniotic fluid volume, and Doppler ultrasound of the umbilical cord and uterine arteries. FGR is generally diagnosed by a combination of Doppler ultrasound of the umbilical cord and uterine arteries and fetal biometry abnormalities [9–11]. However, there are many limitations to placental ultrasound: it has a small field of view limiting whole-organ assessment, especially later in gestation; low contrast; and provides limited functional information [12].

16.1.3 Challenges and Unique Potential of Placental MRI

MRI can probe both structure (what tissue is present and its configuration) and function (e.g., blood flow, oxygenation, and nutrient exchange). It therefore offers a unique perspective on the placenta and has the potential to address the limitations of ultrasound. MRI has been recently shown to offer improvements in sensitivity and specificity; for example, mean placental T2* is a stronger predictor of low birth weight than Doppler ultrasound [13]. However, there are a number of factors that limit the utility of placental MRI. These include maternal and fetal motion, uterine contractions, and magnetic field inhomogeneity. It is likely that the uniqueness of the placenta means that bespoke solutions to these problems are required. Recent work has made significant progress toward these goals [14–17], hence increasing the clinical viability of placenta MRI.

16.1.4 Diffusion MRI of the Placenta

In particular, diffusion MRI (dMRI)—with its potential for noninvasive assessment of tissue microstructure and microcirculation—is emerging as a promising tool for placental assessment. There are a small, but growing, number of in vivo human placenta dMRI studies in the literature. A majority of these studies have utilized IVIM MRI (we review these later in the chapter). In addition, placenta dMRI studies have been performed using apparent diffusion coefficient (ADC) [18–21] and diffusion tensor imaging (DTI) [22] models.

16.1.5 Placenta Structure

The placenta gets attached to the maternal uterine wall and connected to the fetus via the umbilical cord. It is typically around 20 cm across and 2 cm thick and consists of 30–40 lobules (also known as cotyledons). Each lobule contains one or two functional units containing a paired maternal spiral artery and fetal villous tree. Figure 16.1 is a schematic of the placenta structure and outlines the principal blood flow routes. A fetal villous tree consists of a large stem villous attached to the chorionic plate; this stem subsequently branches into a network of smaller intermediate villi, which further divide into a network of capillarized terminal villi. Maternal spiral arteries and decidual veins are located immediately adjacent to the placenta in the uterine wall, which consists of various fibrous cell types and trophoblastic cells.

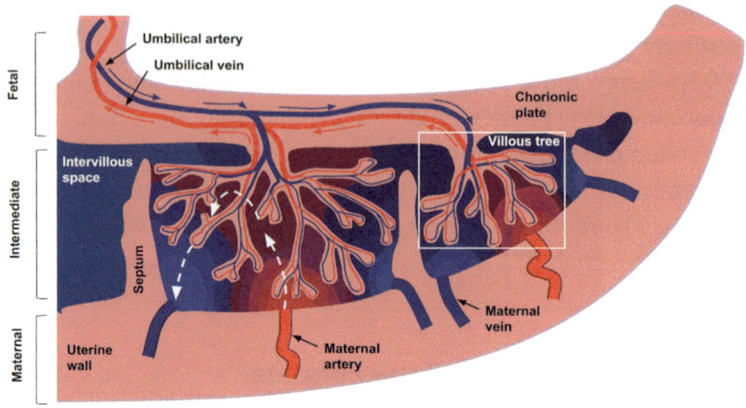

Figure 16.1 Schematic representation of blood flow through the placenta and surrounding tissue. The blue and red arrows show the flow directions of oxygenated (red) and deoxygenated (blue) fetal blood through the placental vasculature. For clarity, only the largest villi are included. The dashed white arrows show idealized flow lines through the intervillous space for maternal blood. Idealized oxygenation states are represented by the color gradient from red to blue. Figure and caption from Ref. [23], used under the CC BY license.

16.1.5.1 Movement of blood

There are two nonmixing blood types in the placenta—fetal and maternal—both of which have very different flow characteristics. Fetal blood resides in the fetal vasculature and perfuses at high pressure through the convoluted villous network. On the other hand, and quite uniquely, maternal blood doesn't flow within vasculature. Instead, it flows at low pressure through spiral arteries into the intervillous space, submerging the fetal villous trees and thereby facilitating oxygen exchange with fetal blood across the villous tree surface.

16.1.5.2 Development across gestational age

The placenta undergoes major functional and structural changes across the 40 weeks of gestation in order to support the developing fetus. For example terminal villi—the principal location of oxygen exchange—develop mainly after 20 weeks [24]. Additionally, calcification generally begins from Week 37 onward, and premature onset has been linked to adverse maternal and fetal outcomes [25–27]. These changes offer both challenges and unique opportunities. Quantitative methods need to be sensitive to the full range that parameters can take over gestation. If such methods could accurately characterize these physiological and pathological developments this would be of great interest clinically.

IVIM MRI provides a unique tool for working toward this goal.

16.1.5.3 How the placenta structure affects the dMRI signal

Due to the unique circulatory structures, it is not immediately clear how the placental dMRI signal will be attenuated at different *b* values. Our thoughts on how placental structure, microstructure, and microcirculation may affect the dMRI signal are as follows. We expect that blood flowing incoherently within fetal vasculature exhibits a pseudodiffusive effect at the voxel scale and hence contributes a fast-attenuating dMRI signal component. We also expect a slow-attenuating dMRI signal component due to water in tissue, such as fetal villous tree walls. It is far from clear how maternal blood flow will impact the dMRI signal. It may exhibit fast incoherent flow on the voxel scale when within vasculature, for example, spiral arteries and decidual veins. Therefore, a fast-attenuating component to the dMRI signal is likely within the uterine wall. However, once it has entered intervillous space, its behavior is very different. Any coherent flow of maternal blood should cause little signal attenuation. However, diffusion within this flow should cause some signal attenuation—with a diffusivity comparable to water at body temperature (3×10^{-2} mm^2 s^{-1}). Additionally, percolation of maternal blood through highly convoluted spaces proximal to fetal villi (in order to facilitate oxygen exchange) may appear incoherent at the voxel scale. If this is the case, it is very difficult to know the speed at which this blood would be percolating and hence what dMRI signal component (fast attenuating, slow attenuating, or otherwise) this would affect. Previous work in mouse placentas by Solomon et al. sheds some light on the problem [28]. They found that maternal blood had near-free diffusion behavior, whereas fetal blood flows 2 orders of magnitude quicker. However, whether this observation translates to human placentas remains unclear.

16.2 IVIM in the Placenta

The first in vivo measurements of IVIM MRI parameter values (in fact, the first applications of dMRI) in the human placenta were presented in two publications in 2000 [29, 30]. The first [29] presents IVIM results from 11 healthy pregnant subjects to give an idea of the ranges and trends over gestation of all three IVIM parameters: the perfusion fraction, pseudodiffusivity, and diffusivity. FGR cases were scanned in the second article, and an IVIM-derived parameter was identified—the difference in perfusion fraction values between outer and inner placental regions of interest (ROIs)—that was lower in FGR pregnancies [30].

In subsequent placental studies, IVIM has remained the most common model for interpreting dMRI data. These papers have generally followed one of the approaches in these first two papers: try to characterize the trajectory of IVIM parameters across gestational age, or try to identify an IVIM parameter that is significantly altered due to pathology. Table 16.1 gives a summary of the published studies of IVIM MRI applied to the in vivo human placenta.

16.2.1 Trends across the Gestational Age

There are two main reasons for characterizing biomarker trends across gestation. Since many change significantly throughout normal gestational aging, knowledge of typical biomarker trends is a requirement to identify deviation. Additionally, we know that the placenta undergoes dramatic microstructural changes across gestation. If we can identify the dMRI-derived parameters that best capture these changes, it follows that these will be good candidates for detecting pathological microstructural changes.

There is variability in the reported trends for IVIM MRI parameters across gestational age. Three studies, all of which began scanning at 22 weeks, have shown a clear decrease in perfusion fraction across gestation [29, 33, 35]. Siauve et al. scanned at earlier gestations (starting at 16 weeks) and found an increase in perfusion fraction between 16 and 22 weeks of GA, stability between 22 and 28 weeks, and then a decrease [36]. On the other hand, two recent papers have shown an apparent increase in perfusion fraction across gestation [31, 37].

Table 16.1 Reported diffusion MRI parameters in the placenta for in vivo human pregnancies

Reference	*b* values (smm^{-2})	No. of subjects	Pseudodiffusivity (10^{-3} mm^{2}s^{-1})	Diffusivity (10^{-3} mm^{2}s^{-1})	Perfusion fraction (%)
Moore et al. [29]	0, 0.2, 3, 15, 47, 80, 115, 206, 246, 346, 463	11	57 ± 41	1.7 ± 0.5	26 ± 6
Moore et al. [30]	0, 0.2, 3, 15, 47, 80, 115, 206, 246, 346, 468	20		1.7 ± 0.9 (inner ROI) 1.4 ± 0.8 (outer ROI)	25 ± 8 (inner ROI) 35 ± 11 (outer ROI)
Derwig et al. [34]	0, 0.7, 3, 9, 18, 32,54, 88, 147, 252, 500	37			36.2 (9.6)
Sohlberg et al. [33]	0, 200, 400, 600, 800	32			29 (8)
You et al. [35]	0, 25, 50, 114, 243,500, 543, 800, 900	16			58 ± 11 (fetal ROI) 56 ± 13 (maternal ROI)
Capuani et al. [31]	0, 50, 100, 150, 400, 700, 1000	30	13 ± 1	1.5 ± 0.15	34 ± 3
Siauve et al. [36]	0, 15, 47, 80, 115, 206, 246, 346, 468, 700, 1000	23	21.22 ± 11.1	1.74 ± 0.30	39.37 ± 10.9
Jakab et al. [37]	0, 10, 20, 30, 40, 60, 80, 100, 150, 200, 300, 400, 500, 600, 700, 800, 900	33	4.77 ± 3.33		29 ± 8

Note: Values are reported as either mean ± SD, or median (IQR). All studies were performed at 1.5 T, excluding both studies by Moore et al. (0.5 T) and some of the subjects in Jakab et al. (3 T). Each study includes a variety of subjects, either with or without disease; we refer the reader to the original studies for full details. Capuani et al. [31] did not report parameter values in the text; the values we present were read from the figures. We have not included a second paper by Sohlberg et al. [32] as it contains the same subjects as those in Ref. [33].

There are a number of factors that could cause this interstudy variability. These include the lack of a common protocol, variability in ROI selection, different gestational age (GA) ranges, and variation in the types of pregnancy included. For example, Capuani et al. used small ROIs within the placenta, rather than a whole-organ average, to calculate perfusion fraction values. Compared to other studies, Jakab et al. have a much larger range in perfusion fraction values, which may reflect differences in the dMRI protocol or model fitting procedure. Clearly further studies are necessary in order to account for these discrepancies. How these factors specifically affect the observed trend in IVIM perfusion fraction across gestation is an important area for future work and of crucial importance for any future use of the perfusion fraction as a biomarker.

16.2.2 Parameter Variation with Pathology

The ultimate aim of IVIM MRI in the placenta is to identify parameters, or combinations thereof, that are sensitive to the presence or severity of pathology. Thus far, although we should emphasize the small number of studies, IVIM-derived parameters have shown reasonable discrimination between normal and pathological placentas. For example, the perfusion fraction appears significantly lower in placentas associated with FGR [30, 32, 34] and early onset PE [33]. Additionally two studies show that ADC, which averages over IVIM effects, was decreased in FGR [19, 21]. However, it should be noted that the choice of *b* values heavily affects the inferred ADC values [18].

16.3 Anisotropic IVIM in the Placenta

While standard models for analyzing dMRI data, such as IVIM, ADC, and DTI, have shown promise in the placenta, it has been shown in other tissues that advanced microstructural models can extract more specific biophysically linked parameters from the signal. We recently undertook a study to assess which microstructural models best explain dMRI data in the placenta [23].

16.3.1 dMRI Scans

We scanned 9 healthy pregnant subjects with a rich, multishell, multidirectional dMRI protocol. The three principal gradient directions were scanned at b = 15, 25, 80, 115, 206, 246, and 346 s mm^{-2}; eight directions were obtained at b = 40, 400, 1000, and 2000 s mm^{-2}; and there were six b = 0 images. We used this acquisition, which is much richer than would typically be available, in order to assess the most expressive models that the placental dMRI signal potentially supports.

16.3.2 Modeling

The models we fit to the data were motivated by our predictions of how placental structure and microstructure will attenuate the dMRI signal (i.e., Section 16.1.5.2). We chose a set of 14 microstructural models, the majority of which consist of two compartments separately modeling the fast-attenuating (primarily associated with perfusion) and slow-attenuating (primarily associated with diffusion) signal components.

In “standard” IVIM MRI, perfusion and diffusion compartments are both considered to be isotropic. This may not hold in the placenta, for example, in areas with fibrous cells or where vasculature has a coherent orientation. We therefore included models that allow anisotropy in perfusion and diffusion compartments and can therefore be considered anisotropic extensions to IVIM. We found it informative to categorize our models depending on the anisotropy of these two compartments. For example, “anisotropic–isotropic” refers to models with anisotropic perfusion compartment and isotropic diffusion compartment.

All models were combinations of compartments as described in Ref. [38], such as ball, stick, zeppelin, and tensor. “Ball” represents an isotropic diffusion compartment (i.e., an ADC model). A “tensor” compartment models the signal using a full diffusion tensor, and “zeppelin” is a cylindrically symmetric tensor. A “stick” is maximally anisotropic, assuming that water only diffuses in a single direction. We built models using combinations of these compartments, again following the terminology in Ref. [38]; for example, the standard IVIM model is referred to as “ball–ball.”

An example of an anisotropic IVIM model is stick–zeppelin, a two-compartment model that contains anisotropic perfusion and diffusion compartments. The signal is given by

$$S(b) = f\exp(-bd_p(-\mathbf{n}_p \cdot \mathbf{G})^2) + (1 - f)\exp(-b\mathbf{G}^T\mathbf{D}\mathbf{G}),$$

where f is the perfusion fraction, b is the b value, d_p is the diffusivity in the stick principle direction, $\mathbf{n}_p$ is the stick principle direction, $\mathbf{G}$ is the gradient direction, and $\mathbf{D}$ is a cylindrically symmetric tensor (i.e., "zeppelin"). The first term in the signal equation therefore models perfusion effects using a stick compartment, and the second term models diffusion effects using a zeppelin compartment.

To see which model best explained the placenta dMRI signal, we calculated a model selection statistic (the Bayesian information criterion) for all 14 models voxel-by-voxel across all 9 subjects.

16.3.3 Results

Figure 16.2 shows voxel-wise model selection results. Clearly, anisotropic IVIM models best explain the dMRI signal in a majority of voxels across all subjects, with the best model categories being anisotropic–anisotropic and anisotropic–isotropic. In other words, each of the best models has an anisotropic perfusion compartment and either an isotropic or an anisotropic diffusion compartment. Figure 16.3 reveals the spatial pattern of the anisotropy of the diffusion compartment. This pattern is consistent with the underlying physiology: there is generally isotropy within the placenta—which may be due to large maternal blood pools—and anisotropy within the uterine wall and chorionic plate, potentially reflecting fibrous cell structures.

Figure 16.4 displays DTI and IVIM parameter maps for four subjects. We see similar patterns in maps across all subjects, and these are consistent with the physiology of the placenta and surrounding tissue. For example, we saw consistently high diffusivity in the uterine wall (e.g., Fig. 16.4, first column). These areas also had a high IVIM perfusion fraction (Fig. 16.4, fourth column), suggesting they reflect areas with high volumes of perfusing blood. Fractional anisotropy (FA) and direction-encoded color (DEC) maps show high anisotropy in the areas around the placenta (Fig. 16.4, columns 2 and 3)—likely due to the prevalence of fibrous cells in the uterine wall and chorionic plate.

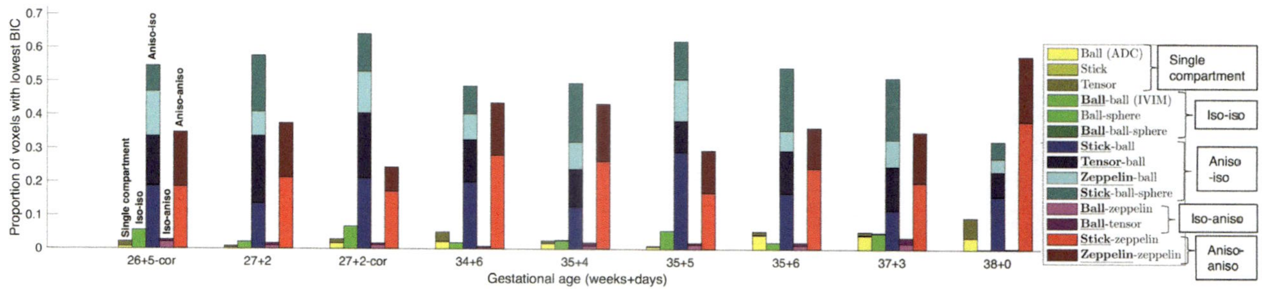

Figure 16.2 Model selection results over nine placenta dMRI scans. Bar plots show the proportion of voxels within a placental ROI where each model has the lowest Bayesian information criterion. Subjects are labeled by gestational age, with "-cor" indicating that the placenta was scanned coronally. The perfusion model compartment is emphasized in the legend text. Image adapted from Ref. [23], used under the CC BY license.

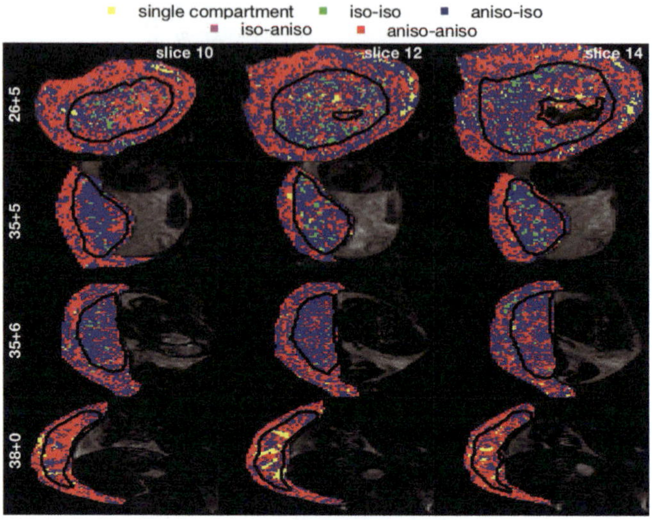

Figure 16.3 Mapping the spatial pattern of model selection results. Each row displays three slices for a single subject, labeled by gestational age (weeks+days). Voxels are colored according to the category of model with the lowest BIC in that voxel. Models are grouped according to the isotropy of the perfusion and diffusion compartments, respectively. For example, "aniso-iso" refers to models with anisotropic perfusion compartments and isotropic diffusion compartments. From Ref. [23], used under the CC BY license.

We display stick–zeppelin, which performed consistently well in model selection, parameter maps in Fig. 16.5. These maps reveal more information than can be accessed with the standard IVIM model (i.e., ball–ball in our terminology). In particular, column 4 maps show the anisotropy of the slow-attenuating dMRI signal component, revealing high anisotropy in the uterine wall and chorionic plate. These models also provide zeppelin diffusivity, stick diffusivity, and stick volume fraction maps (columns 1–3), analogous to diffusivity, pseudodiffusivity, and perfusion fraction, respectively, in the isotropic IVIM model.

Finally, although we emphasize the small number of samples and the lack of longitudinal measurements from individual subjects, our study shows a decrease in the perfusion fraction across gestational age (supporting information in Ref. [23]). This is in agreement with the information in Refs. [29, 33, 35] but disagrees with that in Refs. [31, 37].

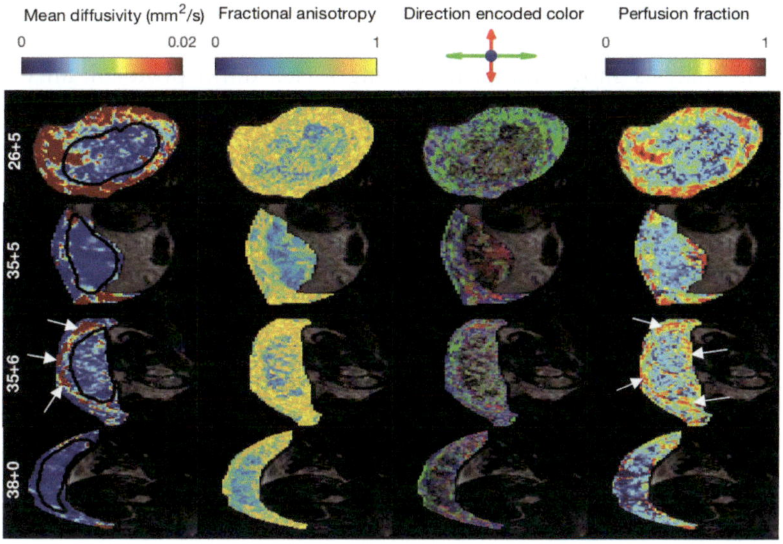

Figure 16.4 Parameter maps derived from DTI and isotropic IVIM model fits. Each row displays maps for a single slice from one subject, labeled by gestational age (weeks + days). Arrows in row 3 highlight areas of high diffusivity and high perfusion at the boundary of the placenta. From Ref. [23], used under the CC BY license.

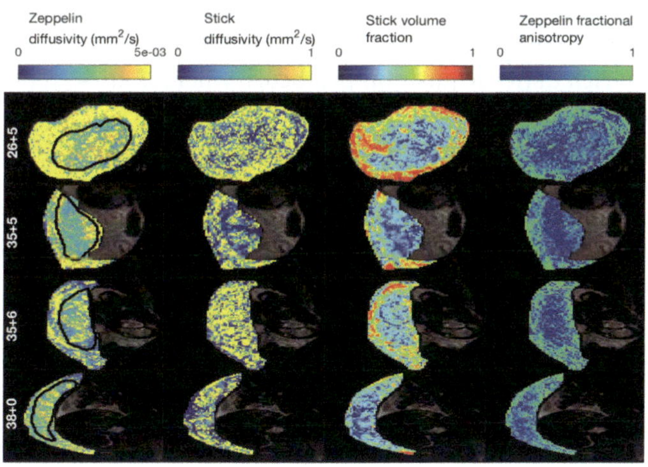

Figure 16.5 Parameter maps derived from the stick–zeppelin model fit. Each row displays maps for a single axial slice from one subject, labeled by gestational age (weeks + days). From Ref. [23], used under the CC BY license.

16.3.4 Discussion

Our analysis shows that when using a rich dMRI protocol, anisotropic IVIM models explain the in vivo human placenta dMRI signal better than ADC, IVIM, and DTI models. We found that the fast-attenuating signal component was anisotropic in nearly all voxels, which matches the interpretation that vasculature has a coherent structure. This orientation may be necessary to facilitate the transport of large volumes of blood—both maternal and fetal—into and out of the placenta. We also observed that the slow-attenuating signal component tended to be isotropic within the placenta, consistent with the lack of coherent tissue structure, and anisotropic in the areas surrounding the placenta, potentially reflecting the prevalence of fibrous tissue in the uterine wall and chorionic plate.

In future work, we will concentrate on the anisotropic IVIM models that best quantify placental microstructure and microcirculation. Stick–zeppelin and zeppelin–zeppelin had consistently high model selection ranking across the placenta and uterine wall and hence show a lot of promise. Zeppelin–zeppelin is the more general model as, unlike a stick compartment, a zeppelin can model isotropic diffusion (when axial and radial tensor diffusivities are equal). However, stick–zeppelin has three fewer parameters and is hence easier to fit to the data. Both models therefore have advantages in certain situations; our view is that zeppelin–zeppelin is preferable for very rich dMRI acquisition protocols, whereas stick–zeppelin is best for sparser acquisitions.

These observations naturally lead to another area for future development: designing dMRI protocols specifically to support these anisotropic IVIM models. The rich dMRI acquisition protocol utilized in this study is for discovery of the models that best explain the placental dMRI signal. Once these models have been identified, we can construct much more economical protocols suitable for clinical application.

16.4 Discussion and Future Directions

IVIM MRI—and anisotropic extensions—show promise as quantitative imaging methods in the placenta. However, there is much further work required to achieve the ultimate goal of translation into biomedical applications.

The IVIM perfusion fraction shows promise as a biomarker for FGR [30, 32, 34] and PE [33], and the ADC is decreased in FGR [19, 21]. A limitation of these studies is that they use parameter values averaged over the whole organ. Future development should harness the increased statistical power available by considering the distribution of quantitative measures across the whole organ rather than averaging to a single descriptive statistic. Future work should also focus not only on whether dMRI-derived biomarkers are significantly different between control and disease groups but also on whether biomarkers can be used for diagnosis and prediction.

Another important topic is the effect of gestational age on dMRI-derived parameters. Previous work has shown that these parameters are highly sensitive to microstructural changes during normal placental development, but there is fundamental disagreement in the literature over the trends [29, 31, 33, 35–37]. If we do not have a good idea of the normal trajectories of these parameters, then we cannot accurately detect pathological changes. Future work should therefore aim to disentangle how pathology and gestational age affect biomarker values. This is likely to require development of analytical approaches that jointly consider these effects.

16.4.1 Protocol Optimization

The utility of dMRI data depends on the choice of b values and gradient directions. Given the observations from an initial cohort of nine placental dMRI scans ([23], as outlined earlier in the chapter) we optimized the choice of gradient table [39]. Our approach was to separately optimize b values and gradient directions in order to best assess the anisotropy in both perfusion and diffusion regimes. The optimization pipeline can be adjusted to comply with clinically limited scanning times.

Improvements in image processing are also important for IVIM MRI in the placenta. The majority of existing studies perform no motion correction, assuming alignment across dMRI volumes. This affects the visual quality of IVIM MRI parameter maps [40] and is presumably a major reason why most studies have focused on whole-organ averages of parameter values. Placental MRI motion correction is a difficult problem and requires correction of nonrigid motion[15]. Continued improvement of motion correction algorithms should increase the utility of placental dMRI data.

16.4.2 It's Not Just about the Placenta!

The placenta is a unique organ that contains both maternal and fetal tissue, and the exact nature of the maternal–placental boundary is debated [41]. Thus far dMRI and IVIM studies have tended to focus exclusively on the placenta, usually ignoring tissue immediately surrounding the organ. It seems likely that useful information can be extracted from measurements in these surrounding areas. In particular, maternal tissue in the uterine wall provides a rich source of information that should not be ignored, since the transport of maternal blood into the placenta through spiral arteries is critical to the health of the fetus. This view is supported a previous IVIM study that showed reduced perfusion fraction in spiral arteries in pregnancies complicated by PE [42]. Fortunately, these surrounding areas are usually within the field of view of a placental scan, so the additional information comes for free.

16.4.3 Joint Diffusion-Relaxometry

The T2* signal strength in MRI depends (to some extent, [43]) on the concentration of oxygen in blood. This has been exploited in a number of placental studies [13, 14, 44, 45]. There are also studies that have quantified T1 and T2 values in the placenta [46–49]. These studies demonstrated that T1, T2, and T2* values decreased across gestational age. An exciting avenue for future development is to combine diffusivity and relaxometry information to improve placental microstructure and microcirculation characterization, as previously demonstrated with T2 and diffusivity [50].

16.4.4 Histological Validation

The placenta is delivered at birth; there are hence unique opportunities to compare in vivo dMRI measurements to histological observations. However, there are a number of practical issues that first need to be addressed. The placenta is highly deformable, so matching the orientation and positioning of the placenta between MRI and histology would be challenging. Another issue relating to IVIM MRI is that there is no perfusion in the delivered placenta, so validation would have to focus on structural, rather than functional, properties. Despite these difficulties, there is clear scope for making initial progress in this area. A first goal might be to match dMRI measurements in cases with gross pathology—such as large infarctions or hemorrhage—with histological observations.

16.5 Conclusion

IVIM MRI shows much promise for studying microstructure and microcirculation in the human placenta and surrounding tissue structures. IVIM parameters are sensitive to both normal placental development and pathological changes. Future work combining dMRI-derived parameters with data from other MRI modalities has the potential to increase the overall sensitivity of MRI to placental viability. The ultimate aim is to develop quantitative imaging methods that can improve prediction, diagnosis, and monitoring of pregnancy complications.

Acknowledgment

We acknowledge the help of all involved radiologists, midwives, obstetricians, and administrators. We would also like to thank all participating mothers for volunteering their time. This work received funding from the NIH Human Placenta Project (grant 1U01HD087202-01), the Wellcome Trust (Sir Henry Wellcome Fellowship, 201374/Z/16/Z), and the EPSRC (grants N018702 and M020533).

References

1. Nelson D. M. How the placenta affects your life, from womb to tomb. *Am. J. Obstet. Gynecol.* 2015, 213, S12–S13. doi:10.1016/j.ajog.2015.08.015.
2. Thornburg K. L., Marshall N. The placenta is the center of the chronic disease universe. *Am. J. Obstet. Gynecol.* 2015, 213, S14–S20. doi:10.1016/j.ajog.2015.08.030.

3. Latendresse G., Founds S. The fascinating and complex role of the placenta in pregnancy and fetal well-being. *J. Midwifery Women's Health* 2015, 60, 360–370. doi:10.1111/jmwh.12344.
4. Vedmedovska N., Rezeberga D., Teibe U., Melderis I., Donders G. G. G. Placental pathology in fetal growth restriction. *Eur. J. Obstet. Gynecol. Reprod. Biol.* 2011, 155, 36–40. doi:10.1016/j.ejogrb.2010.11.017.
5. Mifsud W., Sebire N. J. Placental pathology in early-onset and late-onset fetal growth restriction. *Fetal Diagn. Ther.* 2014, 36, 117–128. doi:10.1159/000359969.
6. Veerbeek J. H. W., Nikkels P. G. J., Torrance H. L., Gravesteijn J., Post Uiterweer E. D., Derks J. B., et al. Placental pathology in early intrauterine growth restriction associated with maternal hypertension. *Placenta* 2014, 35, 696–701. doi:10.1016/j.placenta.2014.06.375.
7. Myatt L. Role of placenta in preeclampsia. *Endocrine*. 2002, 19, 103–111. doi:10.1385/ENDO:19:1:103.
8. Roberts J. M., Escudero C. The placenta in preeclampsia. *Pregnancy Hypertens.* 2012, 2, 72–83. doi:10.1016/j.preghy.2012.01.001.
9. Kaponis A., Harada T., Makrydimas G., Kiyama T., Arata K., Adonakis G., et al. The importance of venous Doppler velocimetry for evaluation of intrauterine growth restriction. *J. Ultrasound. Med.* 30, 529–545, 2011.
10. Figueras F., Gratacós E. Update on the diagnosis and classification of fetal growth restriction and proposal of a stage-based management protocol. *Fetal Diagn. Ther.*, 2014, 86–98. doi:10.1159/000357592.
11. Alfirevic Z., Stampalija T., Dowswell T. Fetal and umbilical Doppler ultrasound in high-risk pregnancies. *Cochrane Database of Systematic Reviews*. John Wiley & Sons, Ltd, 2017. doi:10.1002/14651858.CD007529.pub4.
12. Andescavage N. N., du Plessis A., Limperopoulos C. Advanced MR imaging of the placenta: Exploring the in utero placenta–brain connection. *Semin Perinatol.* 2015, 39, 113–123. Available: http://linkinghub.elsevier.com/retrieve/pii/S0146000515000051.
13. Sinding M., Peters D. A., Frøkjær J. B., Christiansen O. B., Petersen A., Uldbjerg N., et al. Prediction of low birth weight: Comparison of placental T2* estimated by MRI and uterine artery pulsatility index. *Placenta* 2017, 49, 48–54. doi:10.1016/j.placenta.2016.11.009.
14. Schabel M. C., Roberts V. H. J., Lo J. O., Platt S., Grant K. A., Frias A. E., et al. Functional imaging of the nonhuman primate Placenta with endogenous blood oxygen level-dependent contrast. *Magn. Reson. Med.* 2016, 76, 1551–1562. doi:10.1002/mrm.26052.

15. Turk E. A., Luo J., Gagoski B., Pascau J., Bibbo C., Robinson J. N., et al. Spatiotemporal alignment of in utero BOLD-MRI series. *J. Magn. Reson. Imaging* 2017, doi:10.1002/jmri.25585.

16. Hutter J., Christiaens D., Deprez M., Cordero-Grande L., Slator P. J., Price A. N., et al. Dynamic field mapping and motion correction using interleaved double spin-echo diffusion MRI. Descoteaux M., Maier-Hein L., Franz A., Jannin P., Collins D. L., Duchesne S., (eds.) *MICCAI 2017*. Cham: Springer International Publishing, 2017. doi:10.1007/978-3-319-66182-7.

17. Zun Z., Limperopoulos C. Placental perfusion imaging using velocity-selective arterial spin labeling. *Magn. Reson. Med.* 2018, doi:10.1002/mrm.27100.

18. Manganaro L., Fierro F., Tomei A., La Barbera L., Savelli S., Sollazzo P., et al. MRI and DWI: feasibility of DWI and ADC maps in the evaluation of placental changes during gestation. *Prenat. Diagn.* 2010, 30, 1178–1184. Available: http://doi.wiley.com/10.1002/pd.2641.

19. Bonel H. M., Stolz B., Diedrichsen L., Frei K., Saar B., Tutschek B., et al. Diffusion-weighted MR imaging of the placenta in fetuses with placental insufficiency. *Radiology* 2010, 257, 810–819. doi:10.1148/radiol.10092283.

20. Sivrioglu A. K., Ozcan U. A., Turk A., Ulus S., Yildiz M. E., Sonmez G., et al. Evaluation of placenta with relative apparent diffusion coefficient and relative T2 signal intensity analysis. *Diagn. Interv. Radiol.* 2013, 19, 495–500. doi:10.5152/dir.2013.13106.

21. Song F., Wu W., Qian Z., Zhang G., Cheng Y. Assessment of the placenta in intrauterine growth restriction by diffusion-weighted imaging and proton magnetic resonance spectroscopy. *Reprod. Sci.* 2017, 24, 575–581. doi:10.1177/1933719116667219.

22. Javor D., Nasel C., Schweim T., Dekan S., Chalubinski K., Prayera D. In vivo assessment of putative functional placental tissue volume in placental intrauterine growth restriction (IUGR) in human fetuses using diffusion tensor magnetic resonance imaging. *Placenta* 2013, 34, 676–680. doi:10.1016/j.placenta.2013.04.018.

23. Slator P. J., Hutter J., McCabe L., Gomes A. D. S., Price A. N., Panagiotaki E., et al. Placenta microstructure and microcirculation imaging with diffusion MRI. *Magn. Reson. Med.* 2017, doi:10.1002/mrm.27036.

24. Kingdom J., Huppertz B., Seaward G., Kaufmann P. Development of the placental villous tree and its consequences for fetal growth. *Eur. J. Obstet. Gynecol. Reprod. Biol.* 2000, 92, 35–43. doi:10.1016/S0301-2115(00)00423-1.

25. McKenna D., Tharmaratnam S., Mahsud S., Dornan J. Ultrasonic evidence of placental calcification at 36 weeks' gestation: Maternal and fetal outcomes. *Acta Obstet. Gynecol. Scand.* 2005, 84, 7–10. doi:10.1111/j.0001-6349.2005.00563.x.

26. Chen K. H., Chen L. R., Lee Y. H. Exploring the relationship between preterm placental calcification and adverse maternal and fetal outcome. *Ultrasound Obstet. Gynecol.* 2011, 37, 328–334. doi:10.1002/uog.7733.

27. Chen K. H., Chen L. R., Lee Y. H. The role of preterm placental calcification in high-risk pregnancy as a predictor of poor uteroplacental blood flow and adverse pregnancy outcome. *Ultrasound Med. Biol.* 2012, 38, 1011–1018. doi:10.1016/j.ultrasmedbio.2012.02.004.

28. Solomon E., Avni R., Hadas R., Raz T., Garbow J. R., Bendel P., et al. Major mouse placental compartments revealed by diffusion-weighted MRI, contrast-enhanced MRI, and fluorescence imaging. *Proc. Natl. Acad. Sci.* 2014, 111, 10353–8. doi:10.1073/pnas.1401695111.

29. Moore R. J., Issa B., Tokarczuk P., Duncan K. R., Boulby P., Baker P. N., et al. In vivo intravoxel incoherent motion measurements in the human placenta using echo-planar imaging at 0.5 T. *Magn. Reson. Med.* 2000, 43, 295–302.

30. Moore R. J., Strachan B. K., Tyler D. J., Duncan K. R., Baker P. N., Worthington B. S., et al. In utero perfusing fraction maps in normal and growth restricted pregnancy measured using IVIM echo-planar MRI. *Placenta* 2000, 21, 726–732. doi:10.1053/plac.2000.0567.

31. Capuani S., Guerreri M., Antonelli A., Bernardo S., Porpora M. G., Giancotti A., et al. Diffusion and perfusion quantified by magnetic resonance imaging are markers of human placenta development in normal pregnancy. *Placenta* 2017, 58, 33–39. doi:10.1016/j.placenta.2017.08.003.

32. Sohlberg S., Mulic-Lutvica A., Olovsson M., Weis J., Axelsson O., Wikström J., et al. Magnetic resonance imaging-estimated placental perfusion in fetal growth assessment. *Ultrasound Obstet. Gynecol.* 2015, 46, 700–705. doi:10.1002/uog.14786.

33. Sohlberg S., Mulic-Lutvica A., Lindgren P., Ortiz-Nieto F., Wikström A. K., Wikström J. Placental perfusion in normal pregnancy and early and late preeclampsia: A magnetic resonance imaging study. *Placenta* 2014, 35, 202–206. doi:10.1016/j.placenta.2014.01.008.

34. Derwig I., Lythgoe D. J., Barker G. J., Poon L., Gowland P., Yeung R., et al. Association of placental perfusion, as assessed by magnetic resonance imaging and uterine artery Doppler ultrasound, and its relationship

to pregnancy outcome. *Placenta* 2013, 34, 885–891. doi:10.1016/j.placenta.2013.07.006.

35. You W., Andescavage N., Zun Z., Limperopoulos C. Semi-automatic segmentation of the placenta into fetal and maternal compartments using intravoxel incoherent motion MRI. *Proc SPIE Int Soc Opt Eng.* 2017, 10137. doi:10.1117/12.2254610.

36. Siauve N., Hayot P. H., Deloison B., Chalouhi G. E., Alison M., Balvay D., et al. Assessment of human placental perfusion by intravoxel incoherent motion MR imaging. *J. Matern. Neonatal. Med.* 2017, 0, 1–8. doi:10.1080/14767058.2017.1378334.

37. Jakab A., Tuura R. L., Kottke R., Ochsenbein-Kölble N., Natalucci G., Nguyen T. D., et al. Microvascular perfusion of the placenta, developing fetal liver, and lungs assessed with intravoxel incoherent motion imaging. *J. Magn. Reson. Imaging* 2017, doi:10.1002/jmri.25933.

38. Panagiotaki E., Schneider T., Siow B., Hall M. G., Lythgoe M. F., Alexander DC. Compartment models of the diffusion MR signal in brain white matter: A taxonomy and comparison. *Neuroimage* 2012, 59, 2241–2254. doi:10.1016/j.neuroimage.2011.09.081.

39. Slator P. J., Hutter J., Panagiotaki E., Jackson L., Dos Santos Gomes A., Ho A., et al. Optimised b-values & gradient directions for placental diffusion MRI. *ISMRM Workshop on MRI of the Placenta* 2018.

40. Guyader J. M., Bernardin L., Douglas N. H. M., Poot D. H. J., Niessen W. J., Klein S. Influence of image registration on apparent diffusion coefficient images computed from free-breathing diffusion MR images of the abdomen. *J. Magn. Reson. Imaging* 2015, 42, 315–330. doi:10.1002/jmri.24792.

41. Burton G. J., Jauniaux E. What is the placenta? *Am. J. Obstet. Gynecol.* 2015, 213, S6.e1–S6.e4. doi:10.1016/j.ajog.2015.07.050.

42. Moore R. J., Ong S. S., Tyler D. J., Duckett R., Baker P. N., Dunn W. R., et al. Spiral artery blood volume in normal pregnancies and those compromised by pre-eclampsia. *NMR Biomed.* 2008, 21, 376–380. doi:10.1002/nbm.1199.

43. Christen T., Lemasson B., Pannetier N., Farion R., Remy C., Zaharchuk G., et al. Is T2* Enough to assess oxygenation? Quantitative blood oxygen level–dependent analysis in brain tumor. *Radiology* 2012, 262, 495–502. doi:10.1148/radiol.11110518.

44. Sinding M., Peters D. A., Frøkjaer J. B., Christiansen O. B., Petersen A., Uldbjerg N., et al. Placental magnetic resonance imaging T2* measurements in normal pregnancies and in those complicated by

fetal growth restriction. *Ultrasound Obstet. Gynecol.* 2016, 47, 748–754. doi:10.1002/uog.14917.

45. Lo J. O., Roberts V. H. J., Schabel M. C., Wang X., Morgan T. K., Liu Z., et al. Novel detection of placental insufficiency by magnetic resonance imaging in the nonhuman primate. *Reprod. Sci.* 2017, 25, 64–73. doi:10.1177/1933719117699704.
46. Duncan K. R., Gowland P., Francis S., Moore R., Baker P. N., Johnson IR. The investigation of placental relaxation and estimation of placental perfusion using echo-planar magnetic resonance imaging. *Placenta* 1998, 19, 539–543. doi:10.1016/S0143-4004(98)91048-7.
47. Wright C., Morris D. M., Baker P. N., Crocker I. P., Gowland P. A., Parker G. J., et al. Magnetic resonance imaging relaxation time measurements of the placenta at 1.5 T. *Placenta* 2011, 32, 1010–1015. doi:10.1016/j.placenta.2011.07.008.
48. Derwig I., Barker G. J., Poon L., Zelaya F., Gowland P., Lythgoe D. J., et al. Association of placental T2 relaxation times and uterine artery Doppler ultrasound measures of placental blood flow. *Placenta* 2013, 34, 474–479. doi:10.1016/j.placenta.2013.03.005.
49. Ingram E., Hawkins L., Morris D. M., Myers J., Sibley C. P., Johnstone E. D., et al. R1 changes in the human placenta at 3 T in response to a maternal oxygen challenge protocol. *Placenta* 2016, 39, 151–153. doi:10.1016/j.placenta.2016.01.016.
50. Melbourne A., Pratt R., Owen D., Sokolska M., Bainbridge A., Atkinson D., et al. DECIDE: Diffusion-rElaxation combined imaging for detailed placental evaluation. *Proc. Intl. Soc. Mag. Reson. Med.* 2017, 25, 4800.

Chapter 17

Fetal IVIM MRI

András Jakab,[a] Raimund Kottke,[b] Ianina Scheer,[b] and Ruth Tuura[a]
[a]*Center for MR Research, University Children's Hospital Zürich, Steinwiesstrasse 75, Zürich, CH-8032, Switzerland*
[b]*Department of Diagnostic Imaging, University Children's Hospital Zürich, Steinwiesstrasse 75, Zürich, CH-8032, Switzerland*
andras.jakab@kispi.uzh.ch

Until the mid-1970s, obstetricians could "image" the anatomy and pathophysiology of the living fetus by relying on their senses: manual palpation and auscultation were common practice apart from the rather exceptional cases where the use of conventional radiography or invasive methods was justified. The emergence of clinically feasible ultrasonography (US) complemented the diagnostic armamentarium with a method that directly visualized the developing fetus in vivo, in utero. US remains an indispensable and ubiquitous part of prenatal care and management, whereas the technically more complicated, time-consuming, and more expensive magnetic resonance imaging (MRI) has established itself as a valuable second line of investigation, especially for the evaluation of

Intravoxel Incoherent Motion (IVIM) MRI: Principles and Applications
Edited by Denis Le Bihan, Mami Iima, Christian Federau, and Eric E. Sigmund

ISBN 978-981-4800-19-8 (Hardcover), 978-0-429-42727-5 (eBook)
www.panstanford.com

intracranial structures. Undoubtedly, the greatest advantages of fetal MRI are a larger field of view, independence of fetal position, and excellent tissue contrast, allowing detailed assessment of different aspects of human anatomy and pathology. We start this chapter with a short introduction to fetal MRI. MRI safety and the challenges and possible solutions of image acquisition and postprocessing options are discussed with particular attention. We then review the surprisingly few studies that have utilized the IVIM technique for prenatal diagnostics to date, concentrating on feasibility and reproducibility. By reviewing the literature regarding fetal motion correction studies, we outline a possible framework for acquiring and analyzing clinically usable fetal intravoxel incoherent motion (IVIM) MRI. We illustrate potential pathologies where IVIM MRI could be useful and discuss their relevance in the context of postnatal follow-up.

17.1 Fetal Magnetic Resonance Imaging

Today, fetal MRI is used in specialized diagnostic centers, and clinical research using fetal MRI has gained increasing attention since the 2000s. The most important enabling factor of this technique is perhaps the possibility to radically shorten imaging time, as for example by using single-shot fast spin-echo or half-Fourier acquisition single-shot turbospin-echo (HASTE) sequences [1–3]. Using a series of short scans, fetal MRI can be performed within the time constraints of a typical clinical imaging session without maternal or fetal sedation, with a total scan time that typically varies between 30 and 60 min. [1, 4, 5]. Fetal MRI is a helpful and safe secondary modality for confirmation and further characterization of fetal malformations suspected on US, as well as the detection or exclusion of additional pathology. It is most commonly performed for abnormalities of the central nervous system, diaphragmatic herniation, or neural tube defects [6, 7]. While the T2-weighted fast MRI sequence is considered to be the workhorse of fetal MRI, more and more sequences are being applied to fetal MRI that reflect development beyond pure morphology. Some of the techniques that have been adapted to in utero imaging include diffusion-weighted MRI [8], diffusion tensor MRI [9], susceptibility-weighted imaging

[10], functional MRI based on the blood-oxygen level–dependent contrast [11], proton spectroscopy [12], and musculoskeletal imaging techniques [13].

The precise assessment of feto-maternal circulation, fetal viability, and the stage of functional maturity of fetal organs has central importance for decision making in obstetric practice. The depiction of the fine vasculature in fetuses is challenging, and therefore tissue viability is often assessed on the basis of indirect markers of tissue perfusion. Perfusion—the measure of blood circulation in the vascular bed per unit volume—can be characterized by the transit of various tracer compounds across living tissues, using either intravascular contrast agents or metabolic tracers. Perfusion computed tomography, nuclear medicine techniques, and contrast-enhanced MRI are nevertheless contraindicated for most pregnancies, and therefore, other noninvasive approaches are required to map tissue perfusion prenatally.

IVIM captures the randomized intrinsic displacements of fluids in tissues, which arise as a consequence of blood flow at the level of capillaries and short arterioles in living tissues [14]. Prenatal IVIM MRI is a particularly appealing method for assessing organ viability and the development of vasculature or other fluid spaces, and placental IVIM MRI in particular has recently gained popularity. The first studies in the early 2000s to utilize fetal IVIM MRI exclusively assessed placental development [15] and its pathologies, such as intrauterine growth retardation of placental origin [16–18]. The signal from the placenta remains mostly unaffected by the unpredictable movements of the fetus, and its volume is large enough to acquire reliable region of interest (ROI)-based IVIM estimates or even IVIM parametric maps. Placental IVIM MRI is discussed in a separate chapter of this book. In contrast to the placenta, several problems must be addressed before the imaging of the organs of the freely moving fetus with IVIM becomes clinically feasible.

To date, two studies have been published reporting nonplacental fetal IVIM MRI [19, 20], and our work group has conducted preliminary studies to estimate the repeatability and signal-to-noise ratio (SNR) of such data. Further works comprise that by Moore et al. [21], in which the biexponential model was fitted to multi-*b*-value fetal diffusion MRI data of the lung, but they concluded that the data were too noisy to resolve two diffusion components within the lung.

17.2 Fetal IVIM Acquisition

Due to the scarcity of studies utilizing low *b* values during prenatal diffusion-weighted imaging (DWI) or IVIM, there are no clear protocol recommendations. In this section we give an example on how to optimize IVIM MRI for fetal applications. We start by suggesting how to find the optimal *b*-value range and then propose ways of shortening the acquisition time to combat fetal motion.

It is crucial to consider the *b* value that separates the pure diffusion from the microvascular perfusion part of the signal. Unfortunately, we currently lack information about how this separation should be performed for the IVIM signal of developing organs. The brains of neonates and young infants have higher water content than adults, which is associated with longer T2- and higher apparent diffusion coefficient (ADC) values. It is safe to assume that the water content of fetal organs is higher than that of the infant or adult organs and so lower maximal *b* values might be sufficient. It is typical to use 600–700 s/mm^2 during DWI of the fetal brain [22], which may also mark the meaningful maximum *b* value for fetal IVIM. Data dropout is considerable, and according to our experience, up to 25%–50% of the image frames may have to be removed due to motion-induced artifacts. In our current practice, corrupted images are marked manually and are removed together with the corresponding entry from the *b* matrix. We suggest avoiding signal averaging during the acquisition (i.e., by using a higher number of averages/excitations) and propose acquiring multiple images with partial k-space sampling and averaging during postprocessing after corrupted images have been removed.

These considerations lead us to the conclusion that it is worth using multiple repetitions for each set of *b* values such that sufficient data remain after removing up to 50% of the frames. In recent works by Jakab et al. [19, 20], the following acquisition parameters were used for fetal IVIM MRI, which were implemented for 1.5 T and 3 T scanners.

- **MR coil:** A 32-channel phased array cardiac coil or 8-channel body flex coil according to maternal body habitus. The coil is positioned according to the expected location of the relevant fetal structures.

- **Sequence**: Dual spin-echo echo-planar sequence, TE/TR: 2200/75 ms.
- **Diffusion-weighting scheme:** Tetrahedral gradient encoding scheme, one b_0 image, *b*-value range: 10, 20, 30, 40, 60, 80, 100, 150, 200, 300, 400, 500, 600, 700, 800, and 900 s/mm^2.
- **Positioning and image dimensions:** Image matrix, 80 * 100; resampled to an in-plane voxel size of 0.5 * 0.5 mm; number of slices, 8–14; slice thickness, 3 or 4 mm; and slice gap, 0.5 mm. Slice orientation and positioning are adjusted to cover the relevant fetal organ with the fewest possible slices.
- **Imaging time:** 1 min. 40 s to 3 min. 20 s.

17.3 Motion Correction

Fetal IVIM is particularly affected by two different types of dynamic signal changes within the images. First, spatial artifacts are induced due to fetal motion, maternal breathing, and physiological pulsations. The fetus is not sedated during the MRI. Therefore, fetal motion cannot be controlled. Second, image contrast is dynamically changing with the increasing *b* values. When correcting for motion, both processes have to be taken into consideration. The problem of the changing image contrast as a function of the *b* value might be resolved by using normalized gradient fields during nonlinear motion correction or with the progressive principal component registration method [23, 24]. One way to counteract motion is to shorten the effective acquisition time by using the fewest possible slices.

17.3.1 Motion Correction and Image Reconstruction Methods

The retrospective correction of motion by image processing appears to be more challenging for fetal IVIM than for other fetal imaging modalities. IVIM most commonly uses echo-planar imaging, which acquires several 2D slices, each in a single shot, over a 3D imaging volume. Fetal movement can occur in the direction that is perpendicular to the imaging plane before the complete acquisition of all slices. This means that there is fetal motion present between the slice acquisitions, leading to a distortion in the anatomy of the fetus.

The latter problem is addressed by reconstruction approaches that are commonly used to generate higher resolution images from a series of lower-resolution 2D acquisitions (= "super-resolution" [25]). A further complication of fetal movement is the spin history artifact, which can partially be tackled by outlier rejection methods during the image reconstruction [26]. Slice-to-volume (SVR) approaches inject individual 2D slices into the image registration process to tackle between-slice movements and to achieve a higher resolution [27]. The most common application of fetal imaging using SVR is the brain, as this method can only be used for correcting motion of rigid objects.

Surprisingly, in fetal DWI, diffusion tensor imaging (DTI), and IVIM, the brain appears to undergo nonlinear spatial distortions as well as linear distortions due to the complex chemical environment that leads to unpredictable susceptibility-related shifts in the image. Other organs may be shifted relative to each other, and they are not encaged by rigid skeletal structures. It was suggested that patch-to-volume reconstruction (PVR) methods can potentially tackle such nonlinear distortions in nonbrain fetal imaging [28]. PVR is a more recent super-resolution method that is able to reconstruct a large field of view of nonrigidly deforming structures using a parallelized patchwork optimization (patch-to-volume registration is used instead of slice-to-volume registration) and automatic outlier rejection. In both approaches, robust statistics are used to identify improperly registered data or data that are heavily corrupted by artifacts [8]. The use of such advanced postprocessing methods has been suggested for fetal diffusion MRI [29, 30]. However, to the best of our knowledge, no study exists that has applied SVR or PVR for IVIM data sets. With the currently clinically available scan times it is an unrealistic expectation to acquire multiplane, thin-slice IVIM of the whole fetal body for SR reconstruction. A realistic compromise is to have thicker slices and choose an acquisition plane that depicts the anatomy of the pathology with fewest possible slices, such as coronal imaging for fetal body pathologies. The nonlinear distortion could be tackled by frame-by-frame image registration using elastic or fluid registration approaches, as has been suggested for compensating the breathing motion in different imaging modalities

[31, 32]. However, it might become necessary to regularize the deformation fields to allow for physically realistic organ motion in the human body [33]. We utilized a free-form deformation algorithm for nonrigid registration, which was implemented as the reg_f3d command in the NiftyReg software [34] and which was found to be able to compensate for smaller shifts of thoracic and abdominal fetal organs.

17.3.2 Tracking Organ Motion Using Image Registration Methods and Artificial Intelligence

IVIM benefits from a higher SNR, which, depending on the clinical question, is feasibly achieved by fitting the model to intensity values that have been averaged over larger volumes of interest (VOIs). An example of fetal IVIM MRI acquisition is shown in Fig. 17.1, and the mean signal over a VOI is demonstrate in Fig. 17.1(e). The precise segmentation of whole fetal organs is important for this VOI-based approach. As discussed in this chapter, images are affected by nonlinear shifts, which necessitate the delineation of the VOI for each image frame, as motion compensation with postprocessing might not be perfect. The outlines of organs on medical images can be segmented using machine learning approaches, and this can be used to track the trajectory of organs in the presence of motion. For the fetal brain, the deep convolutional neural network method was suggested to overcome the object detection and tracking problem [35]. Image registration using the optical flow approach may also be useful for this purpose: here, motion is estimated by assuming that image pixels conserve their intensity along their trajectory, to which a spatial regularity constraint of the estimated motion is added [36].

17.4 Quality of Fetal IVIM MRI

In a reproducibility study [20], we found that 6.1 ± 7.4 out of 64 image frames with excessive motion had to be removed before the analysis. The reproducibility of the f, d, and D^* over the repeated scans were given as the test-retest variability (VAR%). We found that the reproducibility of the diffusion coefficient was the highest for all the investigated fetal structures and the placenta (VAR%; frontal cortex, 4.8%; placenta, 12.2%), as estimated by the monoexponential decay of signal intensities corresponding to image frames with a b factor >250 s/mm^2. In contrast, f and D^* values were twice as variable across repeated scans as the diffusion coefficient. Only three organs, namely the placenta, the fetal liver, and the fetal lungs, were found to show moderately reproducible perfusion fractions and pseudodiffusion coefficients, while the f and D^* of the investigated brain area and kidneys showed poor reproducibility, which was defined as a test-retest variability of over 25%.

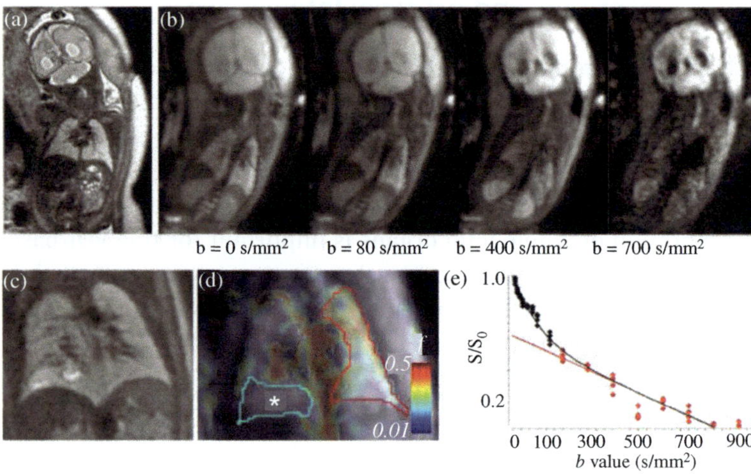

Figure 17.1 A fetal IVIM MRI. (a) Acoronal whole-body acquisition, T2-weighted image, (b) four frames of the IVIM imaging sequence illustrated with increasing b values, (c) a T2-weighted image of the lung of a fetus at the 30th week of gestation, diagnosed with congenital pulmonary airway malformation (CPAM), (d) a microvascular perfusion fraction (f) map (*: CPAM showing decreased f values), and (e) IVIM signal characteristic over the contralateral, unaffected lung, corresponding to the averaged values inside the red outlines.

IVIM is particularly sensitive to noise, and a high SNR is required for the reliable estimation of the microvascular perfusion fraction. Noise is particularly prominent at higher b values for which the SNR becomes low. We estimated the SNR of IVIM MRI acquisitions for the placenta of five fetuses between the 22nd and 36th week of gestation. For these subjects, the same IVIM sequence was repeated twice in consecutive scans. The SNR was measured for four different b values (b = 0, 150, 700, and 900 s/mm^2) using the National Electrical Manufacturers Association (NEMA) subtraction method applied to within-subject repeated IVIM scans [37]. We found the following SNR values: b = 0 s/mm^2 images, 15.0 ± 7.0 (10.2–27.2); b = 150 s/mm^2 images, 10.5 ± 3.2 (8.0–16.0); b = 700 s/mm^2 images, 6.4 ± 1.3 (4.6–7.8), and for the b = 900 s/mm^2 images, 4.5 ± 2.0 (2.4–7.7).

17.5 IVIM MRI of Fetal Organ Maturation

Fetal MRI is typically indicated and performed during the second and third trimesters of gestation. During this period, organs undergo a rapid maturation process. In addition to their apparent quantitative change—volume growth—crucial events take place that enable physiological function after birth and greatly determine the viability of the fetus in the case of premature birth.

Fetal lungs undergo significant microstructural development during mid- and late gestation, marking the maturation of the airways and vasculature. The surfactant producing and storing ability of type II alveolar cells of the lungs has long been known to determine not only survival but also any urgent need for medical intervention. Fetal airways contain no air, and imaging by MRI, especially diffusion-weighted MRI, is technically feasible [38]. A currently accepted marker of maturity and predictor of outcome in certain diseases, such as in congenital diaphragmatic hernia, is lung volume, which is relatively easy to measure in T2-weighted MRI [39]. In contrast, the signal intensity in T2-weighted imaging or ADC values showed only weak or no correlation to surfactant levels [40, 41].

The fetal lungs demonstrate rapid changes of the diffusion coefficient with development [42]. Fetal IVIM MRI can potentially shed light on this maturation process. We found increasing microvascular perfusion fraction of the fetal lungs during gestation [19], and fetuses older than the 32nd gestational week demonstrated a 72% higher f than those between the 17th and 31st weeks. To better understand how ADC and f values change over gestation, multiple coexisting compartments in the lungs have to be considered. The IVIM signal is likely to be influenced by vascular development. The ingrowth and proliferation of capillaries in the lung parenchyma begins in the canalicular phase (until the 26th week), and the development of the vasculature and increase in arterial blood flow parallels the arborization of the airways. After the 26th week, the saccular phase begins, arborization continues, and surfactant production takes place. The airways are filled with free-diffusing and actively secreted fluid, and the diameter and apparent segment lengths of these airways also change dynamically. Due to the relatively large volume of the fetal lungs, especially at the critical period of fetal lung development at the beginning of the third trimester, fetal IVIM MRI may play an important role in the diagnostic workup.

The fetal liver is easily recognized in an MRI, and its large relative volume makes it a good candidate to be examined with IVIM MRI. The liver also undergoes rapid gestational change, and the fetal liver and its complex network of vessels play an important role in fetal circulation, which gradually adapts to the growing body mass. The proportion of arterial blood that is shunted away from the liver via the ductus venosus gradually decreases as the fetus grows. We revealed a significantly decreasing microvascular perfusion fraction in the fetal liver with an increasing gestational age [19], which may reflect a vascular process, which is a consequence of the reduction of weight-normalized blood supply and venous drainage through the umbilical vessels. This assumption is supported by the large blood content of the liver: blood volume accounts for one-third of the water content in liver, and the greatest contributor to blood flow is the small vessel content.

17.6 Clinical Cases

Fetal IVIM MRI has not yet reached clinical maturity due to different factors. First, we lack normative data on how the IVIM metrics change during gestation and how they reflect the maturation of tissue microstructure. Data dropout and the need for complicated post processing may also delay clinical translation and render fetal IVIM to be a specialist method that is performed for select cases only. Here we demonstrate possible applications for fetal IVIM in selected pathologies.

17.6.1 Vein of Galen Aneurysmal Malformations

Vein of Galen aneurismal malformations are the most frequent arteriovenous malformations in fetuses. Fetal MRI of the brain may provide novel information in addition to the US: first, to depict the 3D anatomy of the dilated vessels that are supported by arteriovenous fistulas, and second, to demonstrate early complications, such as hydrocephalus, cerebral ischemia, or hemorrhage. The turbulent flow within the aneurysm may mimic incoherent intravoxel dephasing, which leads to a distribution of velocities and an isotropic IVIM signal attenuation that is similar to, or even larger than, the perfusion-driven component of the IVIM signal (Fig. 17.2). This way IVIM angiograms could be generated without the use of contrast agents and voxels can be identified with excessive flow compared to their environment, which is expected in the presence of feeding vessels.

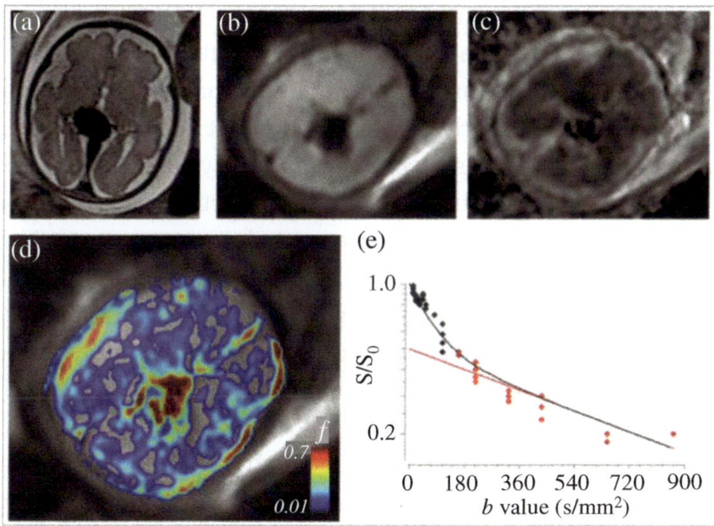

Figure 17.2 A fetus at the 31st week of gestation, diagnosed with aneurysmal malformation of the vein of Galen. (a) An axial T2-weighted MRI showing the aneurysmatically dilated veins, (b) an axial DWI at the level of the aneurysm, (c) an ADC map, (d) a microvascular perfusion fraction (*f*) map, calculated from IVIM MRI, overlaid after masking with the b_0 image, and (e) the IVIM signal from a single voxel in the center of the vein Galen aneurysm; the calculated *f* is 0.6.

17.6.2 Neoplasms

While in the pediatric and adult population, IVIM MRI has recently gained increasing popularity for oncological applications, congenital tumors are relatively rare, with a prevalence of 1 in 12,500 to 1 in 27,500 live births [43]. Extracranial teratomas with sacrococcygeal occurrence are the most common. Sacrococcygeal teratomas are diagnosed on the basis of morphological imaging (MRI or US) with high confidence; nevertheless, IVIM MRI may capture the heterogeneity of the solid tumor parts and highlight the highly perfused and highly vascularized areas within the tumor mass or could possibly differentiate highly perfused tumors from other masses.

17.6.3 Lung Malformations

Congenital pulmonary airway malformation (CPAM), pulmonary sequestrations, and congenital lobar overinflation form part of the heterogeneous group of congenital lung masses [44]. They are developmental lesions that are now thought to share bronchial obstruction or atresia as a common pathophysiologic component [45]. These malformations may be detected using prenatal ultrasound as an echogenic mass or only become apparent in the neonatal period with respiratory distress due to mass effect [46].

CPAM is the most common congenital lung malformation (30%–40%). It consists of hamartomatous tissue with varying degrees of cystic components, the spectrum ranging from microcystic changes that may appear solid on imaging to large macrocystic lesions without an apparent solid component. It has a communication with the bronchial tree. Pulmonary sequestrations are the second-most-common congenital lung malformation. Congenital lobar overinflation represents an overdistended lung segment, an entire pulmonary lobe, or a part of a lobe. When filled with fluid, as in the prenatal period and the first days of life, it will give the impression of a mass lesion on imaging. In the following illustrated clinical case, fetal IVIM MRI has been used to demarcate the pulmonary sequestration, which had lower perfusion fraction values compared to the unaffected lung parts (Fig. 17.3). Postnatally, this region was not ventilated, and it was characterized by T2 hyperintensity and delayed contrast enhancement.

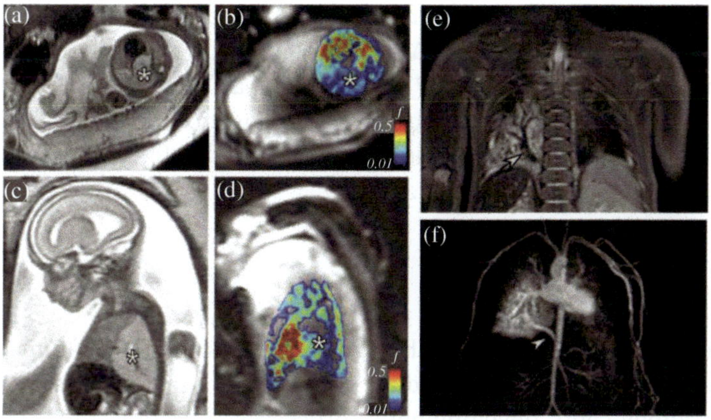

Figure 17.3 A right-sided pulmonary sequestration and overinflated lung in a fetus at the 23rd week of gestation. (a) A T2-weighted coronal MRI, (b) a microvascular perfusion fraction map, calculated from IVIM MRI, (c) a sagittal T2-weighted MRI, (d) a sagittal microvascular perfusion fraction map, (e) a STIR (short tau inversion recovery) coronal image showing the supplying vessel (arrow), and (f) an MR angiography demonstrating the abdominal aortic origin of the supplying vessel.

17.7 Fetal IVIM MRI: Safety Considerations

The clinical studies conducted to assess the biological effects of MRI during pregnancy showed no evidence of injury or harm to the fetus. There has been on-going concern that the acoustic noise generated in an MRI system may be cause of damage to the fetus, which is particularly important for DWI and IVIM sequences, where the electromagnetic gradient fields are rapidly changing and the scans are relatively loud (the FDA limits sound intensity to 140 dB in the MRI room). However, follow-up studies on human subjects show that exposure of the fetus to MRI at 1.5 T in the second and third trimester was not associated with hearing abnormality [47]. It seems that some level of sound attenuation does occur in utero, especially at higher frequencies [48].

According to simulations, specific absorption rates (SAR) above the recommended range should be avoided to prevent heating of fetal tissues [49] and even more rigorous limits should be imposed in cases of intrauterine growth retardation, when heat stress can impair placental function. In our initial experience with the first 30 data sets acquired, the SAR value of a fetal IVIM sequence in the clinical population was 0.37 ± 0.08 W/kg at 1.5T and 1.51 ± 0.34 W/kg at 3T, which are well below the absorption rates that caused a potentially harmful temperature rise in the fetus in previous simulation experiments [49].

17.8 Conclusions

Normal gestational and pathological changes of IVIM parameters can improve our understanding of the underlying microstructure, physiology, and developmental processes. Cerebral blood flow and cerebral blood volume can be estimated from IVIM using experimentally determined features of the underlying vascular microanatomy, such as the MRI-visible water fraction (78% in the adult human brain), the total capillary length, and the mean capillary segment length. However, these parameters may change significantly during development as a consequence of qualitative maturation of the tissue vasculature, changes in the tortuosity and geometry of extracellular water spaces, and changes in the MRI-visible water content. Therefore, IVIM measurements may reflect a possible, unknown mixture of the above-mentioned physiological phenomena and may necessitate multiple compartment models. Quality and data dropout remain a significant issue in fetal IVIM MRI. We anticipate that more advanced image postprocessing approaches, such as SVR reconstruction of IVIM data, may result in more reproducible results. Manual quality checking and rejection of corrupted image frames or parts may still be required in the future.

Here we summarize the specific challenges related to fetal IVIM and suggested solutions:

Corrupted image frames by unpredictable, large fetal motion

- "Oversampling," multiple repetitions of each *b* value
- Frame removal—manual or automatic (outlier-based)
- Preferable to image larger fetuses where space is more constrained for whole-body movements
- Low-frequency motion, such as maternal respiration of slow fetal motion

- Motion correction by nonlinear image registration
- Tracking of location of individual fetal organs
- SVR or PVR as part of the motion correction

Lower SNR

- "Oversampling" by multiple repetitions of each *b* value
- Calculation of IVIM parameters over ROI or VOI

Field inhomogeneities

- Imaging at 1.5 T rather than 3 T
- Bias field correction using image postprocessing

References

1. Yamashita Y., Namimoto T., Abe Y., Takahashi M., Iwamasa J., Miyazaki K. et al. MR imaging of the fetus by a HASTE sequence. *AJR Am. J. Roentgenol.* 168, 513–519, 1997.
2. Levine D., Barnes P. D., Sher S., Semelka R. C., Li W., McArdle C. R., et al. Fetal fast MR imaging: reproducibility, technical quality, and conspicuity of anatomy. *Radiology* 206, 549–554, 1998.
3. Chung H. W., Chen C. Y., Zimmerman R. A., Lee K. W., Lee C. C., Chin S. C. T2-Weighted fast MR imaging with true FISP versus HASTE: comparative efficacy in the evaluation of normal fetal brain maturation. *AJR Am. J. Roentgenol.* 175, 1375–1380, 2000.
4. Levine D., Barnes P. D., Madsen J. R., Li W., Edelman R. R. Fetal central nervous system anomalies: MR imaging augments sonographic diagnosis. *Radiology* 204, 635–642, 1997.
5. Coakley F. V., Glenn O. A., Qayyum A., Barkovich A. J., Goldstein R., Filly R. A. Fetal MRI: a developing technique for the developing patient. *AJR Am. J. Roentgenol.* 182, 243–252, 2004.
6. Bulas D., Egloff A. Benefits and risks of MRI in pregnancy. *Semin. Perinatol.* 37, 301–304, 2013.
7. Prayer D., Malinger G., Brugger P. C., Cassady C., De Catte L., De Keersmaecker B., et al. ISUOG Practice Guidelines: performance of fetal magnetic resonance imaging. *Ultrasound Obstet. Gynecol.* 49, 671–680, 2017.
8. Righini A., Bianchini E., Parazzini C., Gementi P., Ramenghi L., Baldoli C., et al. Apparent diffusion coefficient determination in normal fetal

brain: a prenatal MR imaging study. *AJNR Am. J. Neuroradiol.* 24, 799–804, 2003.

9. Jakab A., Tuura R., Kellenberger C., Scheer I. In utero diffusion tensor imaging of the fetal brain: A reproducibility study. *Neuroimage Clin.* 15, 601–612, 2017.
10. Neelavalli J., Mody S., Yeo L., Jella P. K., Korzeniewski S. J., Saleem S., et al. MR venography of the fetal brain using susceptibility weighted imaging. *J. Magn. Reson. Imaging* 40, 949–957, 2014.
11. Schopf V., Kasprian G., Brugger P. C., Prayer D. Watching the fetal brain at 'rest'. *Int. J. Dev. Neurosci.* 30, 11–17, 2012.
12. Pugash D., Krssak M., Kulemann V., Prayer D. Magnetic resonance spectroscopy of the fetal brain. *Prenat. Diagn.* 29, 434–441, 2009.
13. Robinson A. J., Blaser S., Vladimirov A., Drossman D., Chitayat D., Ryan G. Foetal "black bone" MRI: utility in assessment of the foetal spine. *Br. J. Radiol.* 88, 20140496, 2015.
14. Le Bihan D., Turner R. The capillary network: a link between IVIM and classical perfusion. *Magn. Reson. Med.* 27, 171–178, 1992.
15. Moore R. J., Issa B., Tokarczuk P., Duncan K. R., Boulby P., Baker P. N., et al. In vivo intravoxel incoherent motion measurements in the human placenta using echo-planar imaging at 0.5 T. *Magn. Reson. Med.* 43, 295–302, 2000.
16. Alison M., Chalouhi G. E., Autret G., Balvay D., Thiam R., Salomon L. J., et al. Use of intravoxel incoherent motion MR imaging to assess placental perfusion in a murine model of placental insufficiency. *Invest. Radiol.* 48, 17–23, 2013.
17. Derwig I., Lythgoe D. J., Barker G. J., Poon L., Gowland P., Yeung R., et al. Association of placental perfusion, as assessed by magnetic resonance imaging and uterine artery Doppler ultrasound, and its relationship to pregnancy outcome. *Placenta* 34, 885–891, 2013.
18. Siauve N., Chalouhi G. E., Deloison B., Alison M., Clement O., Ville Y. et al. Functional imaging of the human placenta with magnetic resonance. *Am. J. Obstet. Gynecol.* 213, S103–S114, 2015.
19. Jakab A., Tuura R. L., Kottke R., Ochsenbein-Kolble N., Natalucci G., Nguyen T. D., et al. Microvascular perfusion of the placenta, developing fetal liver, and lungs assessed with intravoxel incoherent motion imaging. *J. Magn. Reson. Imaging* 2017
20. Jakab A., Tuura R., Kottke R., Kellenberger C. J., Scheer I. Intra-voxel incoherent motion MRI of the living human foetus: technique and test-retest repeatability. *Eur. Radiol. Exp.* 1, 26, 2017.

21. Moore R. J., Strachan B., Tyler D. J., Baker P. N., Gowland P. A. In vivo diffusion measurements as an indication of fetal lung maturation using echo planar imaging at 0.5 T. *Magn. Reson. Med.* 45, 247–253, 2001.

22. Kim D. H., Chung S., Vigneron D. B., Barkovich A. J., Glenn O. A. Diffusion-weighted imaging of the fetal brain in vivo. *Magn. Reson. Med.* 59, 216–220, 2008.

23. Melbourne A., Atkinson D., White M. J., Collins D., Leach M., Hawkes D. Registration of dynamic contrast-enhanced MRI using a progressive principal component registration (PPCR). *Phys. Med. Biol.* 52, 5147–5156, 2007.

24. Hodneland E., Lundervold A., Rorvik J., Munthe-Kaas A. Z. Normalized gradient fields for nonlinear motion correction of DCE-MRI time series. *Comput. Med. Imaging Graph* 38, 202–210, 2014.

25. Rousseau F., Kim K., Studholme C., Koob M., Dietemann J. L. On super-resolution for fetal brain MRI. *Med. Image Comput. Comput. Assist. Interv.* 13, 355–362, 2010.

26. Kuklisova-Murgasova M., Quaghebeur G., Rutherford M. A., Hajnal J. V., Schnabel J. A. Reconstruction of fetal brain MRI with intensity matching and complete outlier removal. *Med. Image Anal.* 16, 1550–1564, 2012.

27. Gholipour A., Estroff J. A., Warfield S. K. Robust super-resolution volume reconstruction from slice acquisitions: application to fetal brain MRI. *IEEE Trans. Med. Imaging* 29, 1739–1758, 2010.

28. Alansary A., Rajchl M., McDonagh S. G., Murgasova M., Damodaram M., Lloyd D. F. A., et al. PVR: Patch-to-volume reconstruction for large area motion correction of fetal MRI. *IEEE Trans. Med. Imaging* 36, 2031–2044, 2017.

29. Marami B., Mohseni Salehi S. S., Afacan O., Scherrer B., Rollins C. K., Yang E., et al. Temporal slice registration and robust diffusion-tensor reconstruction for improved fetal brain structural connectivity analysis. *Neuroimage* 156, 475–488, 2017.

30. Kuklisova-Murgasova M., Lockwood Estrin G., Nunes R. G., Malik S. J., Rutherford M. A., Rueckert D., et al. Distortion correction in fetal EPI using non-rigid registration with a Laplacian constraint. *IEEE Trans. Med. Imaging* 37, 12–19, 2018.

31. Fayad H., Schmidt H., Wuerslin C., Visvikis D. Non rigid respiratory motion correction in whole body PET/MR imaging. *EJNMMI Phys.* 1, A73, 2014.

32. Royuela-del-Val J., Cordero-Grande L., Simmross-Wattenberg F., Martin-Fernandez M., Alberola-Lopez C. Nonrigid groupwise registration

for motion estimation and compensation in compressed sensing reconstruction of breath-hold cardiac cine MRI. *Magn. Reson. Med.* 75, 1525–1536, 2016.

33. Vishnevskiy V., Gass T., Szekely G., Tanner C., Goksel O. Isotropic total variation regularization of displacements in parametric image registration. *IEEE Trans. Med. Imaging* 36, 385–395, 2017.

34. Modat M., Ridgway G. R., Taylor Z. A. Fast free-form deformation using graphics processing units. *Comput. Methods Programs Biomed.* 98, 2010.

35. Salehi S. S. M., Hashemi S. R., Velasco-Annis C., Ouaalam A., Estroff J. A., Erdogmus D., et al. Real-time automatic fetal brain extraction in fetal MRI by deep learning, arXiv:1710.09338 [cs.CV], 2017.

36. Zachiu C., Papadakis N., Ries M., Moonen C., Denis de Senneville B. An improved optical flow tracking technique for real-time MR-guided beam therapies in moving organs. *Phys. Med. Biol.* 60, 9003–9029, 2015.

37. Goerner F. L., Clarke G. D. Measuring signal-to-noise ratio in partially parallel imaging MRI. *Med. Phys.* 38, 5049–5057, 2011.

38. Balassy C., Kasprian G., Brugger P. C., Csapo B., Weber M., Hormann M., et al. Diffusion-weighted MR imaging of the normal fetal lung. *Eur. Radiol.* 18, 700–706, 2008.

39. Benachi A., Cordier A. G., Cannie M., Jani J. Advances in prenatal diagnosis of congenital diaphragmatic hernia. *Semin. Fetal Neonatal Med.* 19, 331–337, 2014.

40. Moore R. J., Strachan B., Tyler D. J., Baker P. N., Gowland P. A. In vivo diffusion measurements as an indication of fetal lung maturation using echo planar imaging at 0.5 T. *Magn. Reson. Med.* 45, 247–253, 2001.

41. Mills M., Winter T. C., Kennedy A. M., Woodward P. J. Determination of fetal lung maturity using magnetic resonance imaging signal intensity measurements. *Ultrasound Q.*, 30, 61–67, 2014.

42. Afacan O., Gholipour A., Mulkern R. V., Barnewolt C. E., Estroff J. A., Connolly S. A., et al. Fetal lung apparent diffusion coefficient measurement using diffusion-weighted MRI at 3 Tesla: Correlation with gestational age. *J. Magn. Reson. Imaging* 44, 1650–1655, 2016.

43. Moore S. W., Satge D., Sasco A. J., Zimmermann A. Plaschkes J. The epidemiology of neonatal tumours. Report of an international working group. *Pediatr. Surg. Int.* 19, 509–519, 2003.

44. Berrocal T., Madrid C., Novo S., Gutierrez J., Arjonilla A., Gomez-Leon N. Congenital anomalies of the tracheobronchial tree, lung, and

mediastinum: embryology, radiology, and pathology. *Radiographics* 24, e17, 2004.

45. Fowler D. J., Gould S. J. The pathology of congenital lung lesions. *Semin. Pediatr. Surg.*, 24, 176–182, 2015.
46. Chowdhury M. M., Chakraborty S. Imaging of congenital lung malformations. *Semin. Pediatr. Surg.* 24, 168–175, 2015.
47. Strizek B., Jani J. C., Mucyo E., De Keyzer F., Pauwels I., Ziane S., et al. Safety of MR imaging at 1.5 T in fetuses: A retrospective case-control study of birth weights and the effects of acoustic noise. *Radiology* 275, 530–537, 2015.
48. Reeves M. J., Brandreth M., Whitby E. H., Hart A. R., Paley M. N. J., Griffiths P. D., et al. Neonatal cochlear function: Measurement after exposure to acoustic noise during in utero MR imaging. *Radiology* 257, 802–809, 2010.
49. Gowland P. A., De Wilde J. Temperature increase in the fetus due to radio frequency exposure during magnetic resonance scanning. *Phys. Med. Biol.* 53, L15–L18, 2008.

Chapter 18

IVIM MRI and Bone Marrow

Robert Burns, Sébastien Mulé, Pierre Zerbib, Alexandre Vignaud, Emmanuel Itti, Alain Rahmouni, and Alain Luciani
Departments of Medical Imaging and Nuclear Medicine, Henri Mondor University Hospital, 51 Ave Mal de Lattre de Tassigny, 94010 Créteil, France
CEA\DRF\JOLIOT\NeuroSpin & Paris-Saclay University, Gif-Sur-Yvette, France
alain.luciani@aphp.fr

Bone marrow is one of the largest organs in humans, accounting for approximately 4%–5% of the total body weight [1]. It ensures the continuous generation of red blood cells, platelets, and white blood cells. Bone marrow is found within the central cavities of bones and is surrounded by a network of trabecular bone. It is composed of both hematopoietic tissue and adipocytes, together with supportive vascular sinuses, collagen fibers, reticular cells, macrophages, and lymphocytes. Two types of bone marrow can be distinguished macroscopically on the basis of their color: The red bone marrow is mainly responsible for hematopoiesis and shows a higher proportion of hematopoietic cells (60%) over that of adipocytes (40%). On

Intravoxel Incoherent Motion (IVIM) MRI: Principles and Applications
Edited by Denis Le Bihan, Mami Iima, Christian Federau, and Eric E. Sigmund

ISBN 978-981-4800-19-8 (Hardcover), 978-0-429-42727-5 (eBook)
www.panstanford.com

the contrary, the yellow bone marrow is primarily composed of adipocytes (80%). Both aging and hematopoietic needs influence the relative balance of red and yellow marrow across lifetime [2, 3]. In addition, osteoporosis, metabolic diseases, focal benign or malignant tumors, fractures, and hematological disorders can directly involve the bone marrow.

Imaging plays a key role in the evaluation of the bone marrow. X-rays and CT are capable of visualizing the "container," that is, the trabecular bone and the cortical bone. Hence, both CT and conventional X-ray techniques indirectly detect bone marrow lesions on the basis of their impact on bone mineralization, represented either by osteocondensation (triggered by osteoblasts or the inhibition of osteoclasts) or by osteolysis (triggered by osteoclasts). In addition, both CT and X-rays can show normal bone marrow aging (demonstrated by the progressive decrease of the bone marrow density over time) as well as bone marrow infiltration (demonstrated by an increase in the bone marrow density, especially in the medullary part of the diaphysis of long bones, in itself linked to yellow bone marrow replacement) [4–6]. However, the sensitivity of X-rays and CT techniques for bone marrow disease detection and follow-up remains insufficient.

Radiolabeled compounds such as ^{99m}Tc-nanocolloid, ^{99m}Tc-sulfur colloid, ^{111}In-chloride, and radiolabeled white blood cells allow the recognition of three separate compartments within the bone marrow: the reticuloendothelial system, the erythroid compartment, and the myeloid compartment. Positron emission tomography (PET) tracers have in addition allowed the analysis of the cellular metabolism and of the proliferative activity within the bone marrow with the use of 18F-fluorodeoxyglucose or 18F-fluorothymidine. These techniques are available now in clinical practice or in research [7].

MRI is now recognized as the key imaging modality for the assessment of bone marrow owing to its rich soft-tissue contrast. Conventional anatomical MRI—T1-weighted, T2-weighted, and contrast-enhanced imaging—is now used in routine clinical practice to diagnose bone marrow lesions and monitor treatment response in patients [8, 9].

Diffusion-weighted imaging (DWI) can provide additional information at the tissular and cellular level within the bone marrow. DWI is used for both detection and characterization of focal lesions within the bone marrow. However, bone marrow is a highly vascularized organ with a rich capillary network [10]. As a result, the fast movement of the water molecules within the bone marrow, induced by its rich vascularized stroma, directly impacts the signal observed in DWI, especially when low *b* values are selected for sequence design [11]. Because of its ability to separate both perfusion-related diffusion and true molecular diffusion components at the cellular level, intravoxel incoherent motion (IVIM) DWI, using a dual exponential analysis and multiple *b* values—encompassing both low *b* values (< 200 s/mm^2) and high *b* values (> 200 s/mm^2)—has been recently adapted for bone marrow analysis, with promising clinical applications [12].

18.1 Technical Aspects of IVIM in Bone Marrow

Single-shot spin-echo echo-planar imaging (SSSE-EPI) is the most frequently used sequence design for optimal IVIM imaging owing to its inherent ability to reduce motion artifacts. But the anatomical specificities of the bone marrow still yield technical challenges that must be overcome.

Even though bone marrow is one of the largest organs in the body, it is contained within a relatively small-sized bone medullar cavity, surrounded by cortical bone and spread out over the entire skeleton. To distinguish the bone marrow signal from that of the adjacent cortical bone, a high spatial resolution is required. As a result, the off-resonance effects, linked to the magnetic susceptibility difference between the bone marrow and the cortical bone, are increased, leading to artifacts such as spatial distortion or blurring. In addition, a higher spatial resolution further reduces the signal-to-noise ratio (SNR) of DWI. To reduce off-resonance artifacts, parallel imaging can be used. Reducing the train of gradient echoes in the echo-planar imaging (EPI)-readout in combination with a faster k-space traversal increases the bandwidth per pixel in the phase-encoding direction, thereby improving the image quality [13]. An alternative technique, mostly used in spinal cord imaging, is to reduce the field of view, which increases the bandwidth, thus reducing off-resonance effects. Outer volume suppression pulses or 2D radiofrequency excitation pulses can also be used. Although reduced fields of view can be used to characterize focal lesions of the bone marrow, this strategy is not capable of covering the entire axial skeleton [14, 15]. To maintain a sufficient SNR, diffusion gradient settings are particularly important. The number of excitations per b gradient can be increased, and if possible there should be more excitations for the highest b value to compensate for the loss of signal on high b values. In our experience, very high b values do not bring additional clinical information or allow a significant increase in the quality of true molecular diffusion (D) maps. As a result, we limit the highest b values to 800 s/mm^2 to keep the time echo (TE) as short as possible, preferably under 60 ms (Figs. 18.1 and 18.2). In other organs of the body, such as in the liver, it has been shown that perfusion-related diffusion effects are underestimated when very low b values ($0 < b < 50$ s/mm^2) are excluded from the distribution [16]. It has also been shown that perfusion-related diffusion effects do not contribute significantly to the DWI signal for b values above 200 s/mm^2 [11, 17].

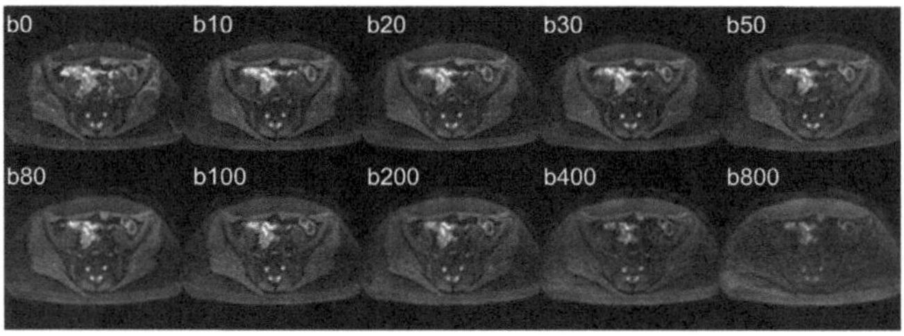

Figure 18.1 Axial pelvic IVIM acquisition obtained in a healthy volunteer on a 1.5 T MR scanner with 10 increasing b values, using a SSSE-EPI sequence, TR = 1900 ms, TE = 58 ms, matrix size of 208 × 256, three directional b gradients, and parallel imaging factor 2.

Many bone marrow diseases are diffuse, making whole-body IVIM protocols potentially interesting but difficult to apply to the bone marrow. Filli et al. proposed in 2014 a whole-body IVIM protocol allowing the computation of parametric maps with good to fair image quality, using a 3 T MR scanner [18]. The images were acquired using an SSSE-EPI sequence in the transverse plane with three to six stacks of axial slices acquired with free breathing. A total of eight b values (0, 10, 20, 50, 150, 300, 500, and 800 s/mm^2) were selected, combined with fat suppression using spectral selection attenuated inversion recovery (SPAIR). Even though this study showed that whole-body IVIM images of fair quality could be obtained, the sequence design was neither tested nor adapted for bone marrow imaging.

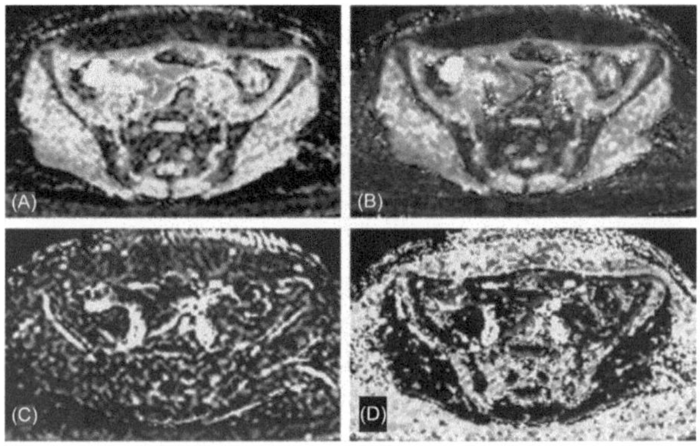

Figure 18.2 An ADC map (A), a true molecular diffusion coefficient map (B), a perfusion-related diffusion coefficient map (C), and a perfusion fraction map (D) from axial IVIM images of Fig. 18.1. The respective mean values in the bone marrow were $0.25 \pm 0.18 \times 10^{-3}$ mm^2/s, $0.35 \pm 0.14 \times 10^{-3}$ mm^2/s, $49 \pm 18 \times 10^{-3}$ mm^2/s, and 9 ± 12%.

18.2 Present and Future Clinical Applications of IVIM MRI in Bone Marrow

18.2.1 IVIM and Normal Bone Marrow Evaluation

Literature data regarding normal quantitative IVIM parameters observed within the bone marrow remain scarce to date.

In 2004, Yeung et al. [11] studied the bone marrow of 20 healthy subjects—mean age 28 y/o—with IVIM on a 1.5 T MR scanner. They acquired a single transverse slice at the L3 level using an SSSE-EPI sequence (TR/TE of 2000/105, four excitations, and a matrix size of 128 × 120) and 10 *b* values (0, 20, 40, 60, 80, 100, 200, 300, 400, and 500 s/mm^2). They reported a normal ADC value of $0.43 \pm 0.08 \times 10^{-3}$ mm^2/s and a normal D value of $0.44 \pm 0.11 \times 10^{-3}$ mm^2/s within the bone marrow. Perfusion-related diffusion coefficient (D^*) and perfusion fraction (f) were not quantified.

In 2014, Marchand et al. [19] reported the normal bone marrow ADC, D, D^*, and f values observed at 1.5 T in a group of 15 healthy women volunteers in the age range between 18 and 30 years. They used a transverse SSSE-EPI sequence acquired across L1 (TR of 10900 ms, TE of 75 ms, matrix size of 269 × 384, and 40 slices of 4 mm thickness), with five different b values (0, 50, 100, 200, and 600 s/mm^2) for a total acquisition time of 6 min. and 22 s. Data analyses were carried out using the non-negative least-squares (NNLS) method. The authors reported D values of $0.45 \pm 0.27 \times 10^{-3}$ mm^2/s, D^* values of $63 \pm 145 \times 10^{-3}$ mm^2/s, and f values of 27 ± 17%.

More recently, Ohno et al. studied IVIM values in 11 healthy volunteers (7 men and 4 women) with a mean age of 25.8 years [20]. Their protocol comprised an SSSE-EPI sequence with 16 b values (0, 10, 20, 30, 50, 80, 120, 180, 250, 350, 500, 800, 1200, 1800, 2200, and 2600 s/mm^2) on a 1.5 T MR scanner. They reported much lower values than those by Marchand et al., with D values ranging between 0.1 and 0.3×10^{-3} mm^2/s, D^* values ranging between 3 and 8×10^{-3} mm^2/s, and f values ranging between 10% and 20%. They also compared IVIM parameters to the bone mineral density obtained with dual-energy X-ray absorptiometry and to the fat fraction derived from double-gradient echo images with and without spectral adiabatic inversion recovery. The authors reported a significant positive correlation between the bone mineral density and D^* and a negative correlation between D or ADC and the fat fraction.

Many differences between the two studies could explain the observed differences in IVIM parameters. The study by Marchand et al. included only women with regular menstruations. These subjects could bear a higher proportion of red bone marrow than the more predominantly masculine population reported in the study by Ohno et al., where most of the red marrow could already have been replaced by adipose tissue. The protocol parameters were also different in the two studies. Furthermore, f and D^* seem to be poorly reproducible even when using the same MR scanner and protocol [21–23].

Further studies are still necessary, first to optimize IVIM protocols but also to better understand and identify the factors potentially impacting the quantitative parameters obtained from IVIM, especially the physiological factors, such as age, gender, and the fat content of the bone marrow.

18.2.2 IVIM Parameters and Osteoporosis

IVIM sequences have been seldom tested in osteoporotic patients. Yeung et al. [11] reported a population of 44 consecutive women (mean age of 70 years) and 20 normal subjects (mean age of 28 years) imaged using IVIM. Both ADC and D values tended to decrease with decreasing bone marrow density measured using dual energy X-ray absorptiometry (T-score) suggesting that a decrease in true molecular diffusion could accompany the progressive fatty replacement of bone marrow observed in elderly patients.

18.2.3 IVIM and Diffuse Bone Marrow Infiltration

Shah et al. examined 31 patients with monoclonal plasma cell diseases who underwent IVIM MRI of the pelvis. These imaging findings were correlated to the pathological results of targeted bone marrow biopsies [24]. The 1.5 T MR protocol was based on a transverse SSSE-EPI sequence (TR/TE 2800/56 ms, slice thickness of 5 mm, and 100 × 100 matrix size) with 11 b values (0, 25, 50, 100, 150, 200, 250, 300, 600, 800, and 1000 s/mm^2). ADC, D, and f values were extracted. The authors reported a positive association of ADC and D with the pathologically observed plasma cell infiltration (slope = 0.46, p = 0.01 and slope = 0.43, p = 0.02, respectively) and a borderline positive association of ADC and D with the bone marrow microvessel density (slope = 0.37, p = 0.04 and slope = 0.35, p = 0.05, respectively). The perfusion fraction f correlated neither with the pathologically documented plasma cell infiltration nor with microcirculation parameters. The authors suggested that this could be linked to residual fat signal insufficiently suppressed in the DWI protocol.

Bourillon et al. [25] studied the correlation of quantitative IVIM parameters with that of Gd-enhanced perfusion parameters derived from dynamic contrast–enhanced (DCE) curves observed in a population of 27 multiple myeloma (MM) patients imaged at 1.5 T. The IVIM sequence was an SSSE-EPI sequence (TR of 1500 ms, TE of 59 ms, 5 mm slice thickness, and matrix size of 106 × 132) acquired with 10 b values (0, 10, 20, 30, 50, 80, 100, 200, 400, and 800 s/mm^2). All IVIM acquisitions were centered on MM focal lesions larger than 20 mm. ADC and D values positively correlated with maximal bone marrow enhancement (r = 0.7, p < 0.001 and r = 0.455, p = 0.435, respectively) and were significantly higher in patients with an increased maximal bone marrow enhancement than in those with normal maximal bone marrow enhancement (ADC, 0.67×10^{-3} mm^2/s vs. 0.54×10^{-3} mm^2/s, $p = 0.03$; D, 0.58×10^{-3} mm^2/s vs. 0.42×10^{-3} mm^2/s, $p < 0.01$). D^* and f were not correlated to bone marrow enhancement parameters. An example of IVIM acquisition in a patient with plasma cell bone marrow infiltration linked to MM is shown in Figs. 18.3 and 18.4.

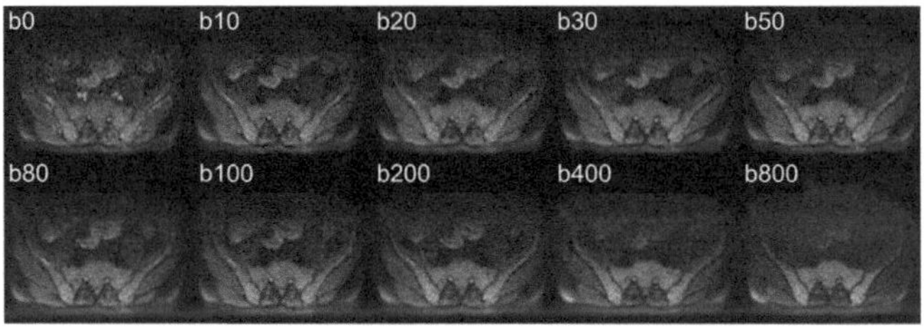

Figure 18.3 Axial pelvic IVIM acquisition obtained in a patient with severe plasmocytic diffuse bone marrow infiltration on a 1.5 T MR with 10 increasing b values, using a SSSE-EPI sequence, TR = 1900 ms, TE = 58 ms, matrix size of 208 × 256, three directional b gradients, and factor 2 parallel imaging. Both ADC and D values are significantly increased. The standard deviation of D^* and f values remain too high to date to be used in daily routine to evaluate bone marrow infiltration.

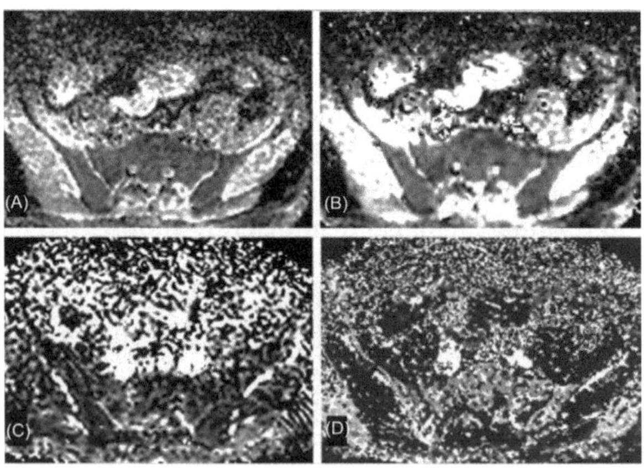

Figure 18.4 An ADC map (A), a true molecular diffusion coefficient map (B), a perfusion-related diffusion coefficient map (C), and a perfusion fraction map (D) from axial IVIM images of Fig. 18.3. The respective mean values of ADC, D, D^*, and f in the infiltrated bone marrow were $0.66 \pm 0.64 \times 10^{-3}$ mm^2/s, $0.63 \pm 0.60 \times 10^{-3}$ mm^2/s, $35.7 \pm 25.2 \times 10^{-3}$ mm^2/s, and 7 ± 5%. The ADC and D values are significantly increased. The standard deviations of D^* and f values remain too high to allow a robust interpretation of diffuse bone marrow infiltration.

Niu et al. [26] studied whether IVIM parameters could predict a patient's complete remission in 53 patients with acute myeloid leukemia (AML) undergoing standard chemotherapy. They used a 1.5 T MR scanner with an SSSE-EPI sequence (TR of 2000 ms, TE of 91 ms) and 11 *b* values (50, 10, 25, 50, 100, 200, 400, 600, 800, 1000, and 1200 s/mm^2) acquired in the sagittal plane. The *D* values were significantly higher and *f* values were significantly lower in the complete responders. ADC and *D** did not differ significantly between the two groups. Overall, increased *D* and reduced *f* values appeared as independent predictors of complete response in AML.

18.2.4 IVIM and Focal Bone Lesions

Baik et al. [27] retrospectively reviewed 42 patients who underwent a musculoskeletal MRI with an IVIM MR sequence and corresponding computed tomography (CT) or PET/CT scans. IVIM was performed at 3 T using an SSSE-EPI sequence (TR > 4000 ms, TE between 54 and 65 ms, echo train length of 108, section thickness of 5 mm, three orthogonal diffusion-sensitizing gradients, and matrix size of 128 × 108) and 9 *b* values (0, 25, 50, 75, 100, 200, 300, 500, and 800 s/mm^2). Among the 42 patients, 14 benign proven nodular hyperplastic hematopoietic bone marrow (HHBM) and 28 malignant focal marrow abnormalities (hematological malignancies and solid tumor metastases) were identified. Both ADC and *D* were significantly lower in benign lesions with respective ADC and *D* values of 0.436 × 10^{-3} mm^2/s and 0.415 × 10^{-3} mm^2/s for benign lesions and of 0.965 × 10^{-3} mm^2/s and 0.925 × 10^{-3} mm^2/s for malignant lesions. In this study, perfusion-related parameters as well as DCE-derived parameters were not significantly different between HHBM and malignant focal marrow abnormalities.

Park et al. retrospectively reviewed 1356 patients who had undergone thoracolumbar or lumbar MRI for back pain or malignant vertebral bone marrow lesions [28]. In 33 patients, there were 58 vertebral bone marrow lesions (39 metastases, 10 multiple myelomas, and 9 nodular HHBM). All images were acquired on a 3 T MR scanner using an SSSE-EPI sequence (TR of 2500 ms, TE of 70 ms, 5 mm slice thickness, and matrix size of 256 × 254) and 11 *b* values (0, 10, 15, 20, 25, 50, 80, 120, 200, 300, and 800 s/mm^2) in the sagittal plane. Both ADC and *D* values of nodular HHBM were significantly lower than those of malignant vertebral bone marrow lesions ($0.5 \pm 0.19 \times 10^{-3}$ mm²/s vs. $0.93 \pm 0.3 \times 10^{-3}$ mm²/s, $p <$ 0.001; and $0.22 \pm 0.08 \times 10^{-3}$ mm²/s vs. $0.79 \pm 0.29 \times 10^{-3}$ mm²/s, p < 0.001, respectively). The f value was significantly higher in HHBM than malignant lesions (19.8 ± 8.72% vs. 10.21 ± 4.59%, $p < 0.001$). The D^* values showed no significant differences between HHBM and malignant lesions.

Lim et al. [29] retrospectively reviewed 65 patients presenting 47 malignant and 23 benign lesions on a 3 T MRI with IVIM using an SSSE-EPI sequence (TR of 5000–8700 ms, TE of 71–85 ms, slice thickness of 2–5 mm, and matrix size of 64 × 45 to 120 × 128) and 9 b values (0, 25, 50, 75, 100, 200, 300, 500, and 800 s/mm²). The D and ADC values were significantly lower in malignant tumors (respective values of $0.923 \pm 0.360 \times 10^{-3}$ mm²/s and $0.965 \pm 0.353 \times 10^{-3}$ mm²/s respectively) than in benign tumors (respective values of $1.668 \pm 0.546 \times 10^{-3}$ mm²/s and $1.689 \pm 0.526 \times 10^{-3}$ mm²/s, p < 0.001). The f values of malignant tumors were significantly higher than those of benign tumors (9.6% and 7.2%, respectively; $p = 0.021$), whereas the D^* values showed no significant difference ($p > 0.05$). The authors proposed a cutoff value for D and ADC of 1.2×10^{-3} mm²/s to distinguish benign from malignant tumors, with a sensitivity, specificity, and accuracy of 92, 83, 89%, 92, 87, and 90% respectively.

In the study by Bourillon et al. on multiple myeloma patients, f was maximum in lesions showing enhancement followed by washout [25]. An example of IVIM acquisition in a patient with focal nodular lesions in MM is shown in Figs. 18.5 and 18.6.

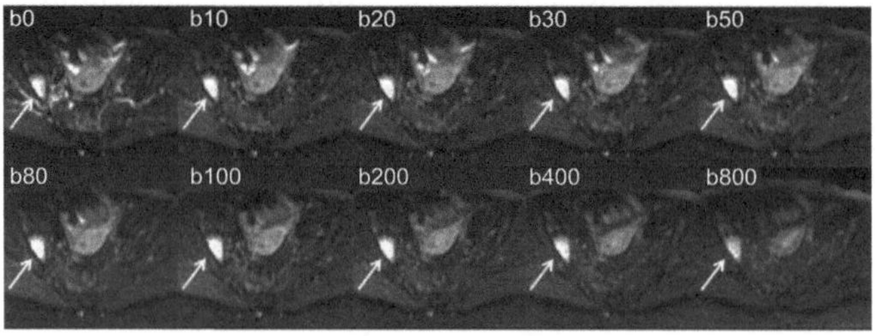

Figure 18.5 Axial pelvic IVIM acquisition obtained in a patient with multiple myeloma and focal bone lesions on a 1.5 T MR with 10 increasing b values, using a SSSE-EPI sequence, TR = 1900 ms, TE = 58 ms, matrix size of 208 × 256, 3 directional b gradients, and factor 2 parallel imaging. The diffusion-weighted signal intensity of the focal lesions is increased compared to the rest of the bone marrow even at high b values.

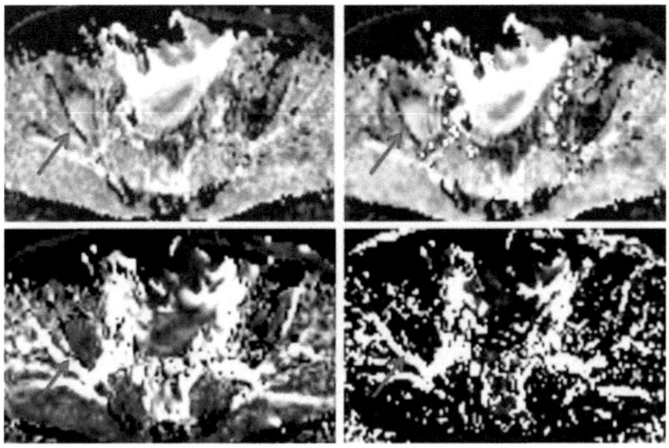

Figure 18.6 An ADC map (A), a true molecular diffusion coefficient map (B), a perfusion-related diffusion coefficient map (C), and a perfusion fraction map (D) from axial IVIM images of Fig. 18.5. The respective mean values of ADC, D, D^*, and f in the infiltrated bone marrow were $1.1 \pm 0.72 \times 10^{-3}$ mm^2/s, $1.09 \pm 0.9 \times 10^{-3}$ mm^2/s, $31.1 \pm 40.6 \times 10^{-3}$ mm^2/s, and 8 ± 3%. The ADC and D values are significantly increased compared to those of the bone marrow outside of focal lesions. The standard deviations of D^* and f remain, to date, too high to be robust in clinical practice.

18.2.5 IVIM and Therapeutic Response Evaluation

Bourillon et al. tested the role of IVIM in treatment monitoring of MM under chemotherapy [25]. The authors compared the changes observed in Gd-enhanced perfusion parameters with the IVIM parameters. The authors reported that in good responders, the significant decrease of the maximal enhancement value observed in focal lesions (baseline vs. after treatment, 213.9% ± 78.8 vs. 131% ± 53.6, respectively; $p < 0.001$) was accompanied by a significant decrease in f (baseline vs. after treatment, 11% ± 3.8% vs. 5.8% ± 4.7%, respectively; $p < 0.001$) and a nonsignificant increase in D and ADC.

Reischauer et al. studied 34 prostate cancer metastases in 12 treatment-naïve patients. They reported that a non-monoexponential diffusion model better matched the changes in prostate-specific antigen levels observed in clinically responding patients than that of monoexponential DWI [30].

More recently, Lee et al. reported that D could detect the early cellular environment changes observed within the bone marrow after combined radiotherapy and chemotherapy in cervical cancer and might have a role in identifying the patients potentially at risk of hematological toxicity [31].

18.3 Conclusion

IVIM is a promising technique for bone marrow imaging. IVIM can better reflect at the tissular and cellular level the changes observed within the bone marrow during aging. IVIM could also better match the changes of perfusion observed in cases of bone marrow infiltration and could hence be integrated as a novel biomarker helping clinicians to better adapt treatment regimens. Technical challenges still have to be overcome in order to reduce off-resonance effects and increase the bone marrow SNR. To date, however, IVIM robustness and scan times are still insufficient for it to be fully integrated in daily routine practice.

References

1. Vogler J. B. 3rd, Murphy W. A. Bone marrow imaging. *Radiology* 168, 679–693, 1988.
2. Custer R. P., Ahlfeldt A. F. Studies on the structure and function of bone marrow. II. Variations in cellularity in various bones with advancing years of life and their relative response to stimuli. *J. Lab. Clin. Med.* 17, 960–962, 1932.
3. Dunnill M. S., Anderson J. A., Whitehead R. Quantitative histologic studies on age changes in bone. *J. Pathol. Bacteriol.* 94, 275–291, 1937.
4. Raza S., Leng S., Lentzsch S. The critical role of imaging in the management of multiple myeloma. *Curr. Hematol. Malig. Rep.* 12, 168–175, 2017.
5. Lecouvet F. E., Vande Berg B. C., Malghem J., Maldague B. E. Magnetic resonance and computed tomography imaging in multiple myeloma. *Semin. Musculoskelet. Radiol.* 5, 43–55, 2001.
6. Caers J. et al. Diagnosis, treatment, and response assessment in solitary plasmacytoma: Updated recommendations from a European Expert Panel. *J. Hematol. Oncol.* 11, 10–19, 2018.
7. Agool A.et al. Radionuclide imaging of bone marrow disorders. *Eur. J. Nucl. Med. Mol. Imaging* 38, 166–178, 2011.

8. Morone M. et al. Whole-body MRI: Current applications in oncology. *Am. J. Roentgenol.* 209, 336–349, 2017.

9. Luciani A., Rahmouni A. *IRM en pratique clinique: imagerie neuroradiologique, musculosquelettique, abdominopelvienne, oncologique, hématologique, corps entier, et cardiovasculaire*, 1st Ed. (Elsevier Masson, France)., 2017

10. Nombela-Arrieta C., Manz M. G. Quantification and three-dimensional microanatomical organization of the bone marrow. *Blood Adv.* 1, 407–416, 2017.

11. Yeung D. K., Wong S. Y., Griffith J. F., Lau E. M. Bone marrow diffusion in osteoporosis: Evaluation with quantitative MR diffusion imaging. *J. Magn. Reson. Imaging* 19, 222–228, 2004.

12. Karampinos D. C. et al. Quantitative MRI and spectroscopy of bone marrow. *J. Magn. Reson. Imaging* 47, 332–353, 2018.

13. Bammer R. Basic principles of diffusion-weighted imaging. *Eur. J. Radiol.* 45, 169–184, 2003.

14. Finsterbusch J. High-resolution diffusion tensor imaging with inner field-of-view EPI. *J. Magn. Reson. Imaging* 29, 987–993, 2009.

15. Sapkota N. et al. Two-dimensional single-shot diffusion-weighted stimulated EPI with reduced FOV for ultrahigh-b radial diffusion-weighted imaging of spinal cord. *Magn. Reson. Med.* 77, 2167–2173, 2017.

16. Cohen A. D., Schiecke M. C., Hohenwalter M. D., Schmainda K. M. The effect of low b-values on the intravoxel incoherent motion derived pseudodiffusion parameter in liver. *Magn. Reson. Med.* 73, 306–311, 2009.

17. Freiman M. et al. In vivo assessment of optimal b-value range for perfusion-insensitive apparent diffusion coefficient imaging. *Med. Phys.* 39, 4832–4839, 2012.

18. Filli L., Wurnig M. C., Luechinger R., Eberhardt C., Guggenberger R., Boss A. Whole-body intravoxel incoherent motion imaging. *Eur Radiol.* 25, 2049–2058, 2015.

19. Marchand A. J. et al. MRI quantification of diffusion and perfusion in bone marrow by intravoxel incoherent motion (IVIM) and non-negative least square (NNLS) analysis. *Magn. Reson. Imaging* 32, 1091–1096, 2014.

20. Ohno N. et al. Evaluation of perfusion-related and true diffusion in vertebral bone marrow: a preliminary study. *Radiol. Phys. Technol.* 8, 135–140, 2015.

21. Dyvorne H., Jajamovich G., Kakite S., Kuehn B., Taouli B. Intravoxel incoherent motion diffusion imaging of the liver: Optimal b-value subsampling and impact on parameter precision and reproducibility. *Eur. J. Radiol.* 83, 2109–2113, 2014.

22. Jiang J. et al. Lung cancer: Short-term reproducibility of intravoxel incoherent motion parameters and apparent diffusion coefficient at 3T. *J. Magn. Reson. Imaging* 47, 1003–1012, 2018.

23. Lecler A. et al. Repeatability of apparent diffusion coefficient and intravoxel incoherent motion parameters at 3.0 Tesla in orbital lesions. *Eur. Radiol.* 27, 5094–5103, 2017.

24. Shah R. et al. Intravoxel incoherent motion imaging for assessment of bone marrow infiltration of monoclonal plasma cell diseases. *Ann. Hematol. J.* 92, 1553–1557, 2013.

25. Bourillon C. et al. Intravoxel incoherent motion diffusion-weighted imaging of multiple myeloma lesions: Correlation with whole-body dynamic contrast agent-enhanced MR imaging. *Radiology* 277, 773–783, 2015.

26. Niu J. et al. Intravoxel incoherent motion diffusion-weighted imaging of bone marrow in patients with acute myeloid leukemia: a pilot study of prognostic value. *J. Magn. Reson. Imaging* 46, 476–482, 2017.

27. Baik J. S. et al. Differentiation of focal indeterminate marrow abnormalities with multiparametric MRI. *J. Magn. Reson. Imaging* 46, 49–60, 2017.

28. Park S., Kwack K. S., Chung N. S., Hwang J., Lee H. Y., Kim J. H. Intravoxel incoherent motion diffusion-weighted magnetic resonance imaging of focal vertebral bone marrow lesions: initial experience of the differentiation of nodular hyperplastic hematopoietic bone marrow from malignant lesions. *Skeletal Radiol.* 46, 675–683, 2017.

29. Lim H. K. et al. Intravoxel incoherent motion diffusion-weighted MR imaging for differentiation of benign and malignant musculoskeletal tumours at 3 T. *Br. J. Radiol.* 91, 20170636, 2018, Epub 2017 Dec 15.

30. Reischauer C., Patzwahl R., Koh D. M., Froehlich J. M., Gutzeit A. Non-mono-exponential analysis of diffusion-weighted imaging for treatment monitoring in prostate cancer bone metastases. *Sci Rep.* 7, 5809, 2017.

31. Lee E. Y. P. et al. Intravoxel incoherent motion MRI assessment of chemoradiation-induced pelvic bone marrow changes in cervical cancer and correlation with hematological toxicity. *J. Magn. Reson. Imaging* 46, 1491–1498, 2017.

Section IV

NEXT FRONTIERS OF IVIM MRI

Chapter 19

IVIM Models: Advantages, Disadvantages, and Analysis Pitfalls

Gabrielle Fournet, Luisa Ciobanu, and Denis Le Bihan
NeuroSpin/Joliot/CEA Saclay, Bat 145, 91191 Gif-sur-Yvette, France
denis.lebihan@gmail.com

Since its introduction by Le Bihan et al. in 1988 [1], the perfusion-driven monoexponential intravoxel incoherent motion (IVIM) model has been widely used, especially for medical applications. However, over the years, other models have emerged. This chapter aims to describe the evolution of IVIM models and present their respective advantages and disadvantages. The quality of the analysis method used together with the IVIM model is also essential. The second part of this chapter gives a review of the possible analysis methods, and, finally, the third part covers some of the analysis pitfalls.

Intravoxel Incoherent Motion (IVIM) MRI: Principles and Applications
Edited by Denis Le Bihan, Mami Iima, Christian Federau, and Eric E. Sigmund

ISBN 978-981-4800-19-8 (Hardcover), 978-0-429-42727-5 (eBook)
www.panstanford.com

19.1 IVIM Models

For notation purposes, the diffusion component will be labeled F_{Diff} and the IVIM component F_{IVIM} so that the total signal acquired with a diffusion-weighted (DW) sequence, S, can be expressed as

$$S(b) = (1 - f_{\text{IVIM}}) \cdot F_{\text{Diff}}(b) + f_{\text{IVIM}} \cdot F_{\text{IVIM}}(b), \tag{19.1}$$

where b is the diffusion weighting, also called the b value, and f_{IVIM} the flowing blood volume fraction.

In this section, we will focus on IVIM models. First, we will present the two models originally introduced by Le Bihan et al. [1] Then, considerations leading to the emergence of other types of models, intermediate and multicompartment models, are presented. Finally, we show how the T_1/T_2 dependence of the blood and tissue compartments can be incorporated into the IVIM model.

19.1.1 The Two Original Models

Making the hypothesis that the microvascular network can be modeled by a series of straight segments randomly oriented in space and uniformly distributed over 4π within each voxel in the 3D space, the expression for the IVIM signal as a function of diffusion weighting $F_{\text{IVIM}}(b)$ depends on the mean vessel segment length l, the mean blood flow velocity V, and the diffusion encoding time. Two limit cases can be defined.

19.1.1.1 The exponential model

The original IVIM model assumes that blood flow changes directions several times during the diffusion time, as shown in Fig. 19.1a. In this case, the isochromat trajectories can be modeled as random walks, thereby adding up to a process that resembles diffusion and is commonly called "pseudodiffusion." In this case, $F_{\text{IVIM}}(b)$ can be expressed as

$$F_{\text{IVIM}}(b) = e^{-b(D_{\text{b}}+D^*)}, \tag{19.2}$$

where D_{b} is the diffusion coefficient of water in blood and D^* the pseudodiffusion coefficient.

The expression for D^* can be found by going back to Einstein's equation [2]

$$D^* = \frac{lV}{6}, \tag{19.3}$$

where l is the mean vessel segment length instead of the mean intermolecular distance and V the mean blood velocity (in three dimensions).

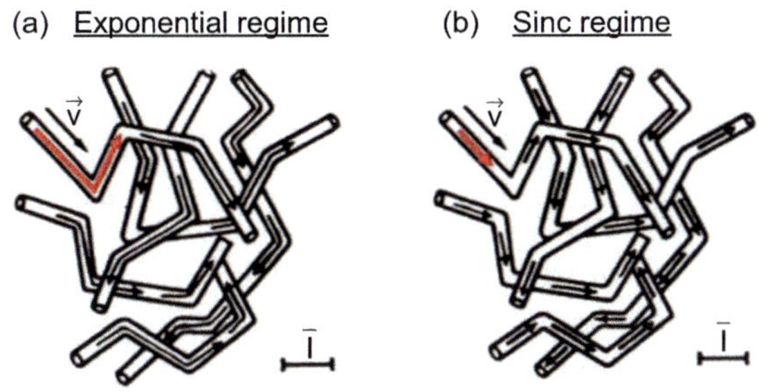

Figure 19.1 Representation of isochromats flowing in a capillary network. Each arrow corresponds to one isochromat trajectory in the capillary network during the diffusion encoding time. In the case of the exponential regime (a), the arrows and thus trajectories consist of two or more segments. The isochromats see several vessel segments during the diffusion time. On the contrary, in the sinc regime (b), the arrows always appear in a single segment; therefore, isochromats stay in the same capillary segment during the diffusion encoding time. The scale bar represents the mean capillary segment length. Adapted from Ref. [1].

This model represents one of the two limit cases, namely, it is valid when the measurement time ("diffusion time") is long, the blood flow velocity is fast, or the vessel segments are short.

19.1.1.2 The sinc model

The second model is valid when blood never changes vessel segments during the measurement time, that is, when segments are long, the blood flow velocity is slow or the diffusion time is short, as shown in Fig. 19.1b.

The phase shift Φ of the transverse magnetization due to spin motion between $t = 0$ and $t = \mathrm{TE}$ (echo time) for a spin-echo sequence can be expressed as

$$\Phi = \gamma \left[\int_{0}^{\frac{\mathrm{TE}}{2}} -\vec{V} \cdot \vec{G} \cdot t \cdot dt + \int_{\frac{\mathrm{TE}}{2}}^{\mathrm{TE}} \vec{V} \cdot \vec{G} \cdot t \cdot dt \right], \tag{19.4}$$

where γ is the proton gyromagnetic ratio, $\vec{V}$ the instantaneous velocity vector, and $\vec{G}$ the instantaneous magnetic field gradient.

Introducing the angle between the direction of a capillary segment and the gradient direction θ, Eq. 19.4 can be simplified to

$$\Phi = c \cdot V \cdot \cos(\theta), \tag{19.5}$$

with

$$c = \gamma \left[\int_0^{\frac{TE}{2}} -G \cdot t \cdot dt + \int_{\frac{TE}{2}}^{TE} G \cdot t \cdot dt \right]. \tag{19.6}$$

To obtain the expression for F_{IVIM}, Eq. 19.5 needs to be generalized for a distribution of capillary orientations ρ(θ, ξ) in the voxel in 3D and a velocity distribution p(*V*):

$$F_{\text{IVIM}} = \left| \int_0^{\infty} \int_0^{2\pi} \int_0^{\pi} e^{i \cdot c \cdot V \cdot \cos(\theta)} \cdot \rho(\theta, \xi) p(V) \sin(\theta) d\theta d\xi dV \right|. \tag{19.7}$$

In this regime and if the blood flow velocity is assumed to be constant, F_{IVIM} becomes a sinc function

$$F_{\text{IVIM}}(c) = e^{-bD_b} \cdot \text{sinc}(cV). \tag{19.8}$$

A pseudodiffusion coefficient D^*_{sinc} can also be defined in this regime by calculating the Taylor expansion limited to the first orders of $F_{\text{IVIM}}(c)$ (neglecting D_b)

$$F_{\text{IVIM}}(c) = 1 - \frac{(cv)^2}{3!} + o\left((cv)^4\right), \tag{19.9}$$

and comparing it to the Taylor expansion limited to the first orders of F_{IVIM} in Eq. 19.2 (neglecting D_b),

$$F_{\text{IVIM}}(b) = 1 - bD^* + o\left((bD^*)^2\right). \tag{19.10}$$

This gives

$$D^*_{\text{sinc}} \sim \frac{c^2 v^2}{6b}. \tag{19.11}$$

For a basic pulsed-gradient spin-echo (PGSE) sequence (with δ and Δ = gradient pulse duration and separation interval, respectively),

$$c = \gamma G \delta \Delta. \tag{19.12}$$

In the short pulse approximation, $\delta \ll \Delta$, $b \cong \gamma^2 G^2 \delta^2 \Delta$, and D^*_{sinc} simplifies to

$$D^*_{\text{sinc}} \sim \frac{v^2 \Delta}{6}. \tag{19.13}$$

It can be noticed that D^*_{sinc} is independent of l as spins never get to probe the entire capillary segment.

As often, the real situation probably lies between these two extreme models. The transition between the sinc and exponential regimes can be studied both analytically and numerically, and several approaches have been proposed to handle this intermediate case (see Section 19.1.2). Without considering the exponential term for the dependence of $F_{\text{IVIM}}(c)$ on D_{b} and using the short pulse approximation ($\Delta+\delta\sim\Delta$), the magnetic resonance imaging (MRI) signal corresponding to an isochromat that sees an N number of segments during the diffusion encoding time Δ, $S_{\text{IC}}(b)$, can be expressed as a product of sinc functions:

$$S_{\text{IC}}(b)=\left(\text{sinc}\left(\frac{v\sqrt{b\Delta}}{N}\right)\right)^N. \tag{19.14}$$

As N goes to infinity, the equation for $S_{\text{IC}}(b)$ becomes exponential and the expression for D^* in the exponential regime can be recovered:

$$\lim_{N\to\infty} S_{\text{IC}}(b)=e^{-\frac{bv^2\Delta}{6N}}=e^{-\frac{bvl}{6}}. \tag{19.15}$$

Using numerical simulations of a random walk of molecules in a network of a varying number N of randomly oriented capillary segments, Fig. 19.2 illustrates the transition from the sinc to the exponential regime. The signal attenuation becomes monoexponential for $N \geq 5$ capillaries for the example shown.

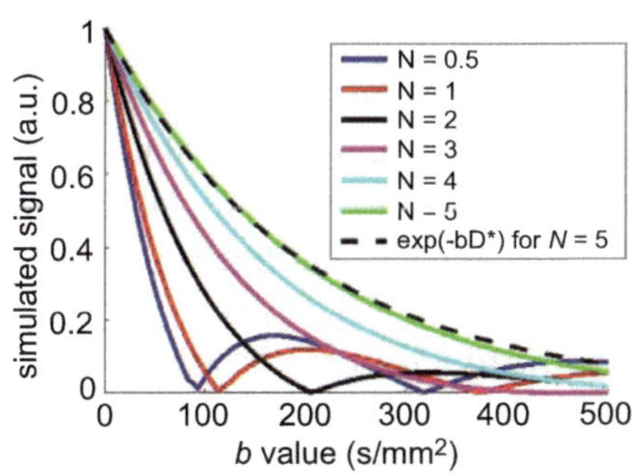

Figure 19.2 Evolution of the simulated signal versus b value with $N = V(\Delta+\delta)/l$, the number of segments seen by an isochromat during $\Delta+\delta$. N is varied by changing the segment length l and keeping the blood flow velocity V at 3 mm/s, δ = 3 ms, and Δ = 14 ms. For N = 5, exp($-bD^*$) with $D^* = lV/6$ has been added to show that the simulated signal becomes exponential for this N value (difference between the two curves <3%).

Performing numerical simulations of a random walk of molecules in a network of randomly oriented capillary segments [3], it is possible to show that, when considering a Gaussian distribution of blood flow velocities instead of a constant blood flow velocity, the IVIM signal plotted against the *b* value looks "exponential" even though isochromats do not change direction many times (sinc regime). Figure 19.3 displays this phenomenon, which is coherent with results from the literature [4, 5].

Therefore, in practice, if there is a Gaussian distribution of the blood flow velocity in the vessel network, it is not possible to distinguish between a sinc and an exponential curve. This likely explains why the sinc model has never been observed experimentally.

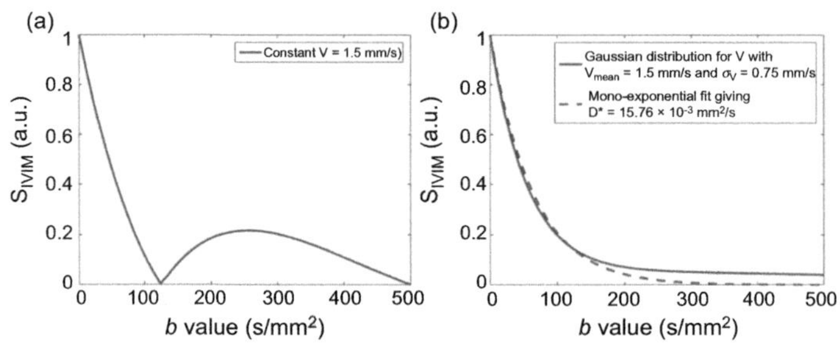

Figure 19.3 Plot of the IVIM signal in the sinc regime for δ = 3 ms, Δ = 34 ms, and (a) a constant V = 1.5 mm/s or (b) a Gaussian distribution for V with V_{mean} = 1.5 mm/s, $s_V = 0.5 \cdot V_{mean}$, and 1000 samples of V. In (b), a monoexponential fit of the IVIM signal was added. It gives $D^* = 15.76 \cdot 10^{-3}$ mm²/s.

But then, in the intermediate regime, the IVIM signal would be in between the true pseudodiffusion model (D^* only depends on the capillary geometry and flow) and the distributed sinc model (D^* also depends on the acquisition parameters, mainly the measurement time). Hence, other intermediate regime models have been proposed.

19.1.2 Intermediate Models

Kennan et al. [6] have presented a model based on a velocity autocorrelation function to cover intermediate situations between the two extreme regimes, exponential and sinc.

Kennan's model uses a velocity autocorrelation function to describe the isochromats' dynamics. The velocity autocorrelation function is a measure of velocity fluctuations in the capillary network and is defined as the average of the scalar product of the velocity of an isochromat evaluated at different times t' and t'': $\langle \overrightarrow{V(t'')} \cdot \overrightarrow{V(t')} \rangle$. For a capillary network with a distribution of segments with different lengths, this product can be expressed as

$$\langle \overrightarrow{V(t'')} \cdot \overrightarrow{V(t')} \rangle = \langle \bar{V}^2 \rangle e^{-\frac{|t''-t'|}{T_0}}, \qquad (19.16)$$

where $\langle \bar{V}^2 \rangle$ is the mean squared blood flow velocity and T_0 the correlation time that corresponds to the average time the isochromats stay in a given segment.

After integrating the expression of the signal attenuation for a PGSE sequence and the assumed velocity autocorrelation function in Eq. 19.16, the IVIM signal becomes

$$F_{\text{IVIM}}(b) = e^{-b\left(\frac{\langle \bar{V}^2 \rangle}{3} T_0 \Omega + D_{\text{b}}\right)}, \qquad (19.17)$$

where Ω is a function of δ, Δ, and T_0.

The parameters extracted from this model are $\langle \bar{V}^2 \rangle$, T_0, and the mean segment length l, which can be estimated by the relation

$$l = 2T_0 \sqrt{\langle \bar{V}^2 \rangle}. \qquad (19.18)$$

This model converges toward the exponential and the sinc regimes at long and very short diffusion times, respectively, and is expected to also cover intermediate regimes. When comparing the standard monoexponential IVIM model to Kennan's model, the models are very similar except that D^* has been replaced by $\langle \bar{V}^2 \rangle$ $T_0\Omega/3$.

The validity of the Gaussian phase approximation used by Kennan et al. has been questioned by Wetscherek et al., who suggested a different model (see Chapter 21). Arguing that the assumption that isochromats change direction enough times during the diffusion encoding time to mimic a diffusion process is invalid in some cases, Wetscherek et al. introduced a model to describe the signal attenuation of the perfusion fraction in-between the two original models based on normalized phase distributions [5]:

$$F_{\text{IVIM}}(b) = F(b, V, T, \tau) e^{-bD_{\text{b}}}, \qquad (19.19)$$

where

$$F(b,V,T,\tau)=\left|\int_{-\infty}^{+\infty}\rho\left(\varphi,\frac{T}{\tau}\right)e^{iV\sqrt{bT}\varphi}d\varphi\right|, \tag{19.20}$$

with $\tau = l/V$, T the total duration of the diffusion gradients, φ the normalized phase, and $\rho(\varphi,T/\tau)$ the phase distributions.

To obtain $F(b,V,T,\tau)$, only the phase distribution for the applied diffusion gradient profile and the number of directional changes $N = T/\tau$ need to be calculated. Since at short and long diffusion encoding times, the sinc and exponential models can be recovered from the proposed model, it is also assumed to describe well the intermediate regime. Wetscherek et al. proposed to estimate τ and V directly, instead of their combination through $D^* = \tau V^2/6$, to obtain a more detailed description of the incoherent motion by combining flow-compensated and non-flow-compensated diffusion gradients, but this method is out of the scope of this chapter and will be discussed in Chapter 21.

The models described so far assume a single IVIM compartment. However, in biological tissues, the existence of multiple compartments must be considered.

19.1.3 Multicompartment Models

Using innovative ways to isolate the signal coming from flowing blood from that coming from static tissue, a number of authors have shown that there might be several vascular compartments to consider instead of just one when describing the IVIM signal.

Neil et al. developed a strategy to directly suppress the diffusion component by injecting a contrast agent intravenously [7]. The IVIM signal they obtained was better fitted to a biexponential model. Their hypothesis for this second exponential in the IVIM signal is that it is associated with an incompletely suppressed signal from nonflowing blood. In a second experiment, the contrast agent was replaced by perfluorocarbon (PFC) to test this hypothesis [8]. Once again, a biexponential model was found to better describe the IVIM signal, invalidating the previous hypothesis and instead suggesting that multiple vascular pools could be observed within the IVIM signal.

On the basis of Neil's findings, Henkelman et al. have suggested an IVIM model that takes into account not only capillaries but all types of vessels, including larger vessels [10]. However, the blood flow estimated with their model is one order of magnitude lower than the one reported in the literature (12 mL/min/100 g compared to 130 ± 50 mL/min/100 g), suggesting that large vessels likely do not contribute to the IVIM effect.

Duong et al. took inspiration from Neil's PFC experiments and exploited the fact that the spin-lattice relaxation rate of the PFC correlates linearly with the dissolved oxygen concentration [11]. This allowed them to link each of the pseudodiffusion coefficients of the biexponential IVIM model to the arterial and venous trees and measure the associated regional arterial and venous blood volume fractions.

Recently, we established that the perfusion-driven IVIM signal could, indeed, be better described by a biexponential model at short diffusion times. This model assumes the coexistence of a slow and a fast flow pool [3]

$$F_{\text{IVIM}}(b) = e^{-bD_{\text{b}}}\left(f_{\text{slow}}e^{-bD^*_{\text{slow}}} + f_{\text{fast}}e^{-bD^*_{\text{fast}}}\right), \tag{19.21}$$

with the constraints $f_{\text{slow}} + f_{\text{fast}} = 1$ and $D^*_{\text{fast}} > D^*_{\text{slow}}$.

This model should not be confused with the biexponential model used to separate diffusion and IVIM effects or the biexponential model that can be used to describe the diffusion component.

In an in vivo rat brain study the biexponential IVIM model was shown to perform better in describing the IVIM model than the standard monoexponential model, Kennan's model, and a triexponential model at short diffusion times (Δ = 14 and 24 ms) but less clearly at longer diffusion times in the left cortex and left thalamus of 11 rats. Figure 19.4 illustrates this result by showing the Akaike weights corresponding to the fits with each model.

The difference in the corrected Akaike information criterion (AICc) between the monoexponential and biexponential models was also calculated [13]. The model with the smallest AICc value is assumed to be the best model to describe the data at hand. This difference in AICc was found to decrease significantly with increasing Δ (p value < 0.001), implying that the two models converge at a long diffusion encoding time and that the biexponential model can only be seen at short diffusion encoding times.

The physical meaning behind this biexponential model is different from that of Henkelman and Duong. We hypothesize that the biexponential behavior reflects the contribution of flow in two distinct vascular pools: a slow-flowing pool corresponding to capillaries and a fast-flowing pool corresponding to medium-sized vessels. T_2 of venous blood being much smaller than T_2 of arterial blood, the vessels contributing the most to the magnetic resonance (MR) signal are mainly coming from the arterial part of the vascular tree.

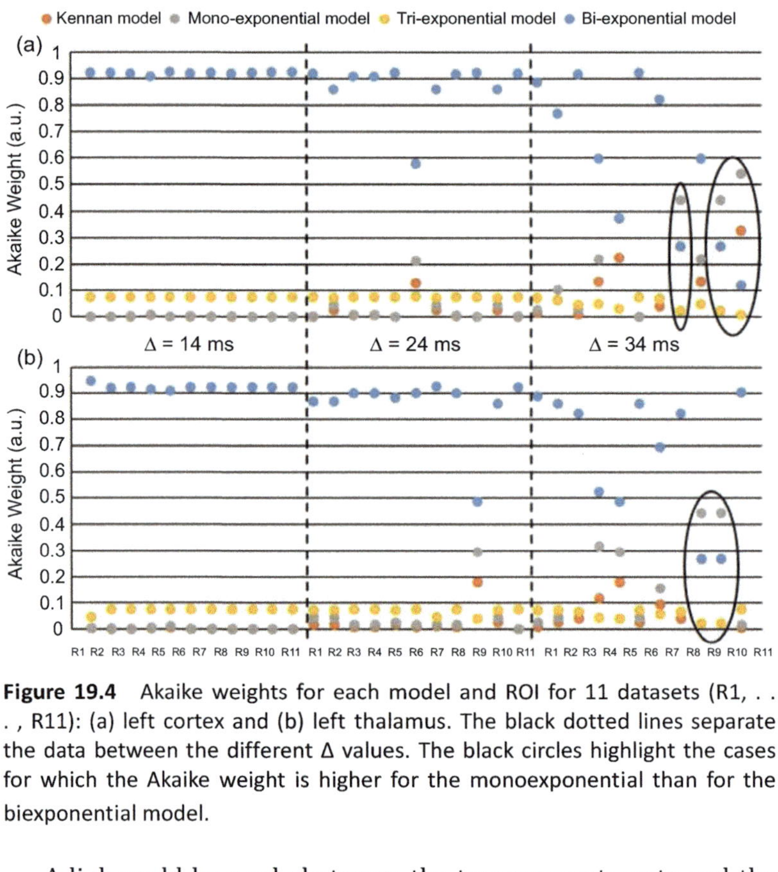

Figure 19.4 Akaike weights for each model and ROI for 11 datasets (R1, . . ., R11): (a) left cortex and (b) left thalamus. The black dotted lines separate the data between the different Δ values. The black circles highlight the cases for which the Akaike weight is higher for the monoexponential than for the biexponential model.

A link could be made between the two compartments and the different regimes. Varying the diffusion encoding time by changing Δ, D^*_{slow} was found to significantly increase with increasing Δ. Figure 19.5 illustrates this result.

This increase in D^*_{slow} with Δ suggests that the slow blood component is likely to be in the sinc regime for which D^* also varies with Δ or in an intermediate regime. As for D^*_{fast}, it was found to decrease between $\Delta = 14$ ms and 24 ms and not significantly vary between $\Delta = 24$ and 34 ms. Therefore, for long diffusion encoding times, the fast component is likely to be in the exponential regime for which D^* does not vary with Δ. The larger D^*_{fast} value observed at a short diffusion encoding time could be explained by an additional phase caused by the laminar flow present in the medium-sized vessels in the fast pool.

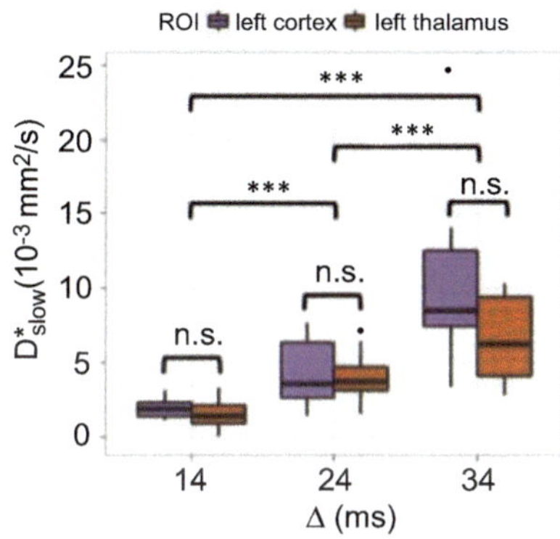

Figure 19.5 Box-and-whisker plot of D^*_{slow} against Δ for two ROIs drawn in the left cortex, in violet, and in the left thalamus, in orange, of a rat. Error bars represent SD (number of rats = 11). A two-way ANOVA test was performed to look for differences between ROIs and Δ values. ***: p values < 0.001; n.s.: nonsignificant p value.

Comparing these results with Neil's, in this study, D^*_{slow} is larger than the one reported by Neil et al. ($2–10 \cdot 10^{-3}$ mm^2/s compared to $1 \cdot 10^{-3}$ mm^2/s) [8], which makes it less likely that this component comes from tissue diffusion signal. D^*_{fast} is on the contrary smaller than in Neil's work, $20 \cdot 10^{-3}$ mm^2/s compared to $82 \cdot 10^{-3}$ mm^2/s.

19.1.4 IVIM Models with T_1 and T_2 Relaxation Effects

An issue that has not yet been raised is the dependence of the IVIM fraction on the relaxation times of tissue and blood. Indeed, as shown in Table 19.1, T_1 and T_2 of tissue and blood can be very different and depend on the magnetic field strength.

In all the diffusion/IVIM models presented above, this difference is not considered. However, depending on the echo time (TE) and the repetition time (TR) used for the acquisitions, relaxation effects can have a high impact on the value of f_{IVIM}.

Table 19.1 T_1 and T_2 relaxation times of different tissues at 1.5 T and 3 T

	T_1 (ms)		T_2 (ms)	
Tissue	**1.5 T**	**3 T**	**1.5 T**	**3 T**
White matter	560	832	82	110
Gray matter	1100	1331	92	80
Liver	570	809	-	34
Pancreas	-	725	-	43
Prostate	-	1597	-	74
Blood	1441	1932	290	275

Data citation: For white and gray matter T_1 at 1.5 T [18] and 3 T [19] for white and gray matter T_2 at 1.5 T [20] and 3 T [19]; for liver T_1 at 1.5 T [21]; for liver, pancreas, and prostate T_1 and T_2 at 3 T [22]; and for blood T_1 and T_2 at 1.5 T and 3 T [23].

Several authors have incorporated the relaxation times directly into the IVIM model. For instance, Lemke et al. have suggested the following model [14]:

$$\frac{S(b)}{S_0}=\frac{(1-f')\cdot\left(1-e^{-\frac{\mathrm{TR}}{T_{1\mathrm{tiss}}}}\right)\cdot e^{-\frac{\mathrm{TE}}{T_{2\mathrm{tiss}}}-bD'}+f'\cdot\left(\left(1-e^{-\frac{\mathrm{TR}}{T_{1\mathrm{bl}}}}\right)\cdot e^{-\frac{\mathrm{TE}}{T_{2\mathrm{bl}}}-b(D'+D^*_{\mathrm{av}})}\right)}{(1-f')\cdot e^{-\frac{\mathrm{TE}}{T_{2\mathrm{tiss}}}}\cdot\left(1-e^{-\frac{\mathrm{TR}}{T_{1\mathrm{tiss}}}}\right)+f'\cdot e^{-\frac{\mathrm{TE}}{T_{2\mathrm{bl}}}}\cdot\left(1-e^{-\frac{\mathrm{TR}}{T_{1\mathrm{bl}}}}\right)}, \tag{19.22}$$

where $T_{1\mathrm{tiss}}$ and $T_{2\mathrm{tiss}}$ are the longitudinal and transversal relaxation times, respectively, of tissue and $T_{1\mathrm{bl}}$ and $T_{2\mathrm{bl}}$ are the longitudinal and transversal relaxation times, respectively, of blood. D^*_{av} is the fixed average pseudodiffusion coefficient, D' is the relaxation-time-compensated diffusion coefficient, and f' is the relaxation-time-compensated perfusion fraction.

In their model, $T_{1\mathrm{tiss}}$, $T_{2\mathrm{tiss}}$, $T_{1\mathrm{bl}}$, and $T_{2\mathrm{bl}}$ are fixed and obtained from the literature. D^*_{av} is fixed and obtained by fitting the averaged signal of a cohort of subjects with

$$\frac{S(b)}{S_0} = (1 - f_{av}) \cdot e^{-bD_{av}} + f_{av} \cdot e^{-b(D^*_{av} + D_{av})}, \tag{19.23}$$

where f_{av} and D_{av} are the average perfusion fraction and diffusion coefficient, respectively.

This equation was designed in the first place to obtain a more reliable estimation of D' and f'. With the proposed model, only two parameters need to be fitted, making this fitting method more stable than the standard three-parameter-fit method. This method has, however, some pitfalls, as T_{1tiss}, T_{2tiss}, T_{1bl}, and T_{2bl} are fixed and only approximated values are known from the literature. A bias is also introduced on fitting D^*_{av} with the standard IVIM equation and using its fixed value with the more complex model.

Jerome et al. focused on correcting for the dependence of the IVIM fraction on T_2 and measured the T_2 values during the same acquisition [15]. Their equation has the form

$$\frac{S(b)}{S_0} = f_{IVIM} \cdot e^{-\frac{TE}{T_{2bl}} - bD^*} + (1 - f_{IVIM}) \cdot e^{-\frac{TE}{T_{2tiss}} - bD}. \tag{19.24}$$

The T_1 dependence of f_{IVIM} is neglected as the authors considered long TRs.

Using this method, the obtained value for f_{IVIM} does not depend on T_2 and the acquisition parameter TE. This method opens the path toward quantitative measurements of the blood volume fraction. The simultaneous measurement of T_2 and the diffusion coefficients of the tissue and blood compartments also shows that T_2 values can be separated for the two compartments and could also be used as disease biomarkers.

A drawback of this method could be a too-extensive scanning time to acquire enough combinations of different TE and b values to have a dataset large enough to yield reliable measurements. To counter this problem, Jerome et al. showed that adding only a few low b-value scans at different TEs might be sufficient and that all TE and b values do not need to be acquired, making this method usable in clinical practice.

A review of the main models proposed for IVIM imaging has been provided in this section. Apart from choosing a suitable model depending on the acquisition parameters and the targeted measurement parameters, the way the analysis is performed is also of great importance.

19.2 IVIM Analysis

The goal of the second section of this chapter is to introduce the main fitting strategies used in the analysis of the IVIM signal. The most commonly used model to fit IVIM data in clinical practice is the biexponential diffusion/IVIM model. To fit the data, two strategies are usually employed—the one-step and two-step approaches—but more sophisticated algorithms can also be used.

19.2.1 Common Fitting Strategies

19.2.1.1 One-step approach

The most simple strategy is to fit the entire signal in one step and to simultaneously extract D, D^*, and f_{IVIM} using a nonlinear least-squares (NLLS) fitting algorithm [16]. Although this kind of fit is much more accurate when bound constraints and initial guesses are imposed [17], the large number of degrees of freedom renders it less stable than the methods described in the following sections. To choose the best values for the initial guesses, Lu et al. have suggested using a multiple-start scheme [18]. For a certain number of iterations, usually around 10, the initial guess for each fitted parameter is varied randomly between the lower and upper boundaries. The final starting values for each parameter are those with which the estimated fitted parameters are obtained with the minimum chi-square value. Also, Wittsack et al. have shown that it is easily influenced by noise in the images and needs a high signal-to-noise ratio (SNR) to be reliable [19].

19.2.1.2 Two-step approaches

To lower the number of degrees of freedom in the model equation and increase the robustness of iterative fitting algorithms, an alternative to the one-step approach is the two-step, also called a "segmented," strategy [16]. Hypothesizing that D^* is significantly greater (at least 10 times) than D, it is assumed that the IVIM component can be neglected at high b values (typically for $b > 200\ \mathrm{s/mm^2}$). The first step consists in a monoexponential fit of the signal at high b values to extract D (assuming a Gaussian diffusion that requires using not-so-large b values; see below):

$$S_{\text{high}}(b) = S_{\text{high0}}e^{-bD}. \tag{19.25}$$

For the second step, many approaches exist. One is to fit the entire signal with D fixed at the value obtained in the first step to get f_{IVIM} and D^*.

Another method is to use the zero intercept, S_{high0}, and the unweighted signal for $b = 0$, S_0, to first calculate f_{IVIM}:

$$f_{\text{IVIM}} = \frac{S_0 - S_{\text{high0}}}{S_0}. \tag{19.26}$$

Then, the signal is fitted with D and f_{IVIM} fixed at the values obtained from the first step to obtain D^*. However, this method requires a good estimation of S_0 to get an accurate value of f_{IVIM}, which is challenging in practice.

Another approach consists in extrapolating the diffusion component part of the signal (estimated from the highest b values) to low b values and subtracting it from the total DW signal [20]. Then, the remaining signal is fitted with the IVIM model to extract f_{IVIM} and D^*. When images are acquired with somewhat high b values (more common for preclinical studies) the monoexponential diffusion model is no longer valid and must be replaced with a non-Gaussian diffusion model, such as the kurtosis model (when b values remain below 2500–3000 s/mm^2) or the biexponential diffusion model to account for the curvature of the DW signal at high b values. With modern clinical MRI scanners equipped with strong gradient hardware high b values can be reached and some clinical studies are now using the kurtosis model [21, 22].

One important issue to consider in the two-step approach is the choice of the b-value threshold to separate the diffusion from the IVIM component. While a threshold of around 200 s/mm^2 has often been considered in the literature, the optimal threshold can be around 200–400 s/mm^2, or even up to 600 s/mm^2 in some cases where f_{IVIM} is large and D^* low. This threshold is expected to vary across organs and pathologic conditions. Wurnig et al. have developed an algorithm to analyze the signal without having to pick the b-value threshold [23]. In an iterative manner, the number of b values used for the diffusion fit is reduced at each step of the algorithm and the b-value threshold is chosen as the one for which the sum of the squared residuals of the fit is the smallest. This method therefore allows for the fit to be independent from the choice of the *b*-value threshold.

19.2.2 More Complex Fitting Algorithms

19.2.2.1 Dictionary-based method

Iima et al. introduced a dictionary-based approach in which the entire MRI signal is compared to a dictionary of model signals with different values for the diffusion and IVIM parameters [24]. The dictionary only needs to be generated once, and then the algorithm runs quickly as it only has to calculate the error between the studied signal and the dictionary signals and minimize it. This approach was found to behave better than NLLS.

19.2.2.2 Non-negative least-squares fitting

As the most commonly used models to fit IVIM data consist in the addition of several exponential functions, a fitting strategy not involving any a priori on the number of exponential functions in the model was suggested: the non-negative least-squares (NNLS) fitting. Inside of the NNLS framework, the DW signal, $S(b_i)$, at b value i, b_i, can be described as:

$$S(b_i)=\sum_j a_j e^{-b_i D_j}=\sum_j a_j A_{ij};\quad i=1,2,\ldots N_b;\quad j=1,2,\ldots,M\,,\qquad(19.27)$$

where a_j is the amplitude of the component with diffusion coefficient D_j, N_b is the number of b values, M is the number of allowed diffusion components, and A is the matrix containing the exponential kernel functions.

This approach assumes a large number of possible diffusion and IVIM components and solves for the amplitudes a_j that minimize the least-squares misfit calculated as:

$$\sum_i\left(\sum_j a_j A_{ij}-S(b_i)\right)^2+\mu\sum_i\left(\sum_j a_j R_{ij}\right)^2,\qquad(19.28)$$

where μ is the regularization parameter and R_{ij} the regularization matrix.

Regularization allows one to obtain more robust outcomes and smoother diffusion distributions. For regularization order 0, R_{ij} is simply the identity matrix.

Figure 19.6a shows an example of the diffusion spectrum obtained using the NNLS algorithm to fit a simulated biexponential diffusion model to which an IVIM monoexponential component was added without noise and regularization. D and D^* correspond to the peaks revealed by the diffusion spectrum with $D^* > D$. f_{IVIM} is then calculated as the normalized amplitude of the faster diffusion component.

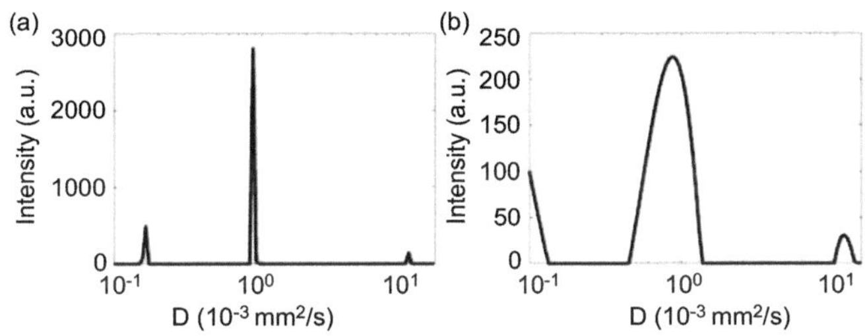

Figure 19.6 NNLS diffusion spectrum obtained from fitting a simulated biexponential diffusion component with $D_{\text{slow}} = 0.17 \cdot 10^{-3}$ mm²/s, $D_{\text{fast}} = 0.88 \cdot 10^{-3}$ mm²/s, and $f_{\text{slow}} = 16\%$ added to a monoexponential IVIM component with $D^* = 10 \cdot 10^{-3}$ mm²/s and $f_{\text{IVIM}} = 5\%$ with a SNR of 400 (a) without and (b) with first-order regularization.

This method is valid only when a multiexponential, multiple-compartment behavior of the DW signal is present. In vivo the demonstration of the contribution of tissue compartments to the DW signal has remained elusive, probably due to the permeability of cell membranes, and the diffusion biexponential model should be seen more as a mathematical way to describe the DW signal than a genuine two-physical-compartment model, precluding the use of the NNLS approach. Moreover, if the diffusion coefficients sought are too close to each other, as the biexponential diffusion coefficients found in vivo in the healthy rat brain [25], for example, applying regularization can also result in a single large peak with a diffusion coefficient value in-between the true diffusion coefficients, as shown in Fig. 19.6.

19.2.2.3 Bayesian fitting

Another approach that has recently gained popularity is the Bayesian method. The Bayesian analysis method does not require initial parameter estimates. Instead, it allows the incorporation of prior probability distributions. Many studies have shown that Bayesian-based methods yield higher accuracy and precision when estimating IVIM parameters compared to NLLS-based algorithms [26, 27]. The Bayesian analysis algorithm used to retrieve the IVIM parameters has an impact on the accuracy and precision of its estimates. However, other biases can also contribute to render these estimations less robust with some IVIM/diffusion parameters combinations, although such biases may be corrected during the IVIM analysis. More details about the Bayesian methods can be found in Chapter 23.

19.3 Potential Sources of Bias in IVIM Data Analysis

The IVIM component of the signal is small, and the diffusion/IVIM analysis can be biased at different levels. These sources of bias must be taken into account and, if possible, corrected to have meaningful estimates of IVIM models' parameters.

19.3.1 Effective *b* Values

When fitting the MRI signal, the quality of the signal is of course very important, but the experimental parameter values against which the signal is fitted must also be accurately known. In IVIM imaging, this parameter is the *b* value.

The *b* value can be expressed as

$$b = \gamma^2 \int_0^{\mathrm{TE}} F^2(t)dt, \tag{19.29}$$

with

$$\vec{F}(t) = \int_0^{t} \vec{G}(t')dt', \tag{19.30}$$

where $\vec{G}(t)$ represents the effective gradient strength and includes all the gradients in the MRI sequence (at t = TE/2 the sign for $\vec{G}$ has to be reversed to take into account the phase reversal produced by the 180° radiofrequency pulse of the spin-echo sequence).

It is of utmost importance to use accurate b values, especially for small b values for which the IVIM effect, which is very small, is present.

Figure 19.7 displays the full sequence diagram of the PGSE sequence with an echo-planar imaging (EPI) readout.

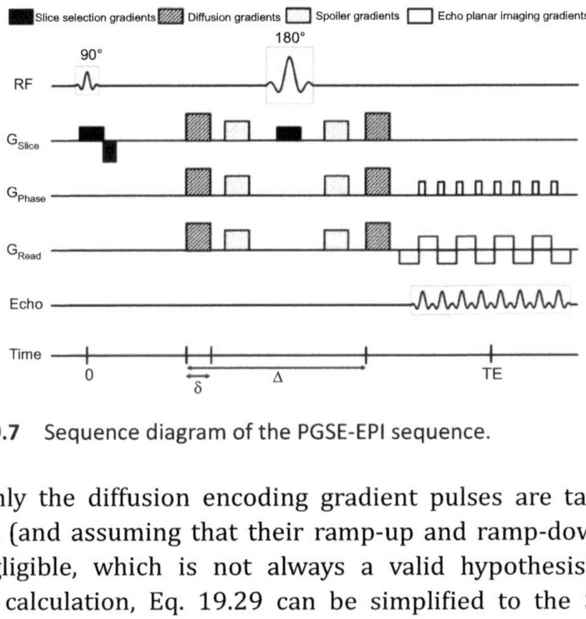

Figure 19.7 Sequence diagram of the PGSE-EPI sequence.

If only the diffusion encoding gradient pulses are taken into account (and assuming that their ramp-up and ramp-down times are negligible, which is not always a valid hypothesis) in the b-value calculation, Eq. 19.29 can be simplified to the Stejskal–Tanner formula:

$$b = \gamma^2 G_D^2 \delta^2 \left(\Delta - \frac{\delta}{3} \right), \quad (19.31)$$

where G_D, δ, and Δ are the diffusion gradient strength, duration, and separation time, respectively.

However, when doing so, the gradient pulses used for imaging (spatial encoding and signal spoiling) and their cross-terms with the diffusion gradient pulses are ignored, although they contribute a great deal to the b value, the very reason why the "b value" was introduced (instead of the Stejskal–Tanner equation) when diffusion

MRI was pioneered [1, 28]. Mattiello et al. have analytically calculated the contributions of all diffusion gradients and imaging gradients and the intra-/interdirectional cross-terms between them, with different pulse shapes (including ramp-up and ramp-down times) in the framework of diffusion tensor imaging [29–31]. It is therefore possible by using simple analytical expressions and knowing the gradient strengths and delays specific to each scanner to calculate the effective b value that takes into account the diffusion gradients and the imaging gradients and the cross-terms between them. With more complex gradient pulse schemes a numerical calculation based on Eq. 19.29 is always possible.

Most vendors of MRI software today take into account these considerations and provide the effective b values, which may differ from the b values programmed at the console, as these values will also depend on the other imaging parameters (e.g., pixel size or slice thickness). Unfortunately, the presence of spoiler gradient pulses in most imaging sequences (to suppress unwanted resonances and clean the images from artifacts) implies that the lowest b values are sometimes larger than 0. Furthermore, gradient amplifiers may not be able to supply low current intensities with good stability. For these technical reasons, b values lower than 50 s/mm^2 are precluded on some MRI scanners, which can pose a problem for IVIM studies.

19.3.2 Gradient Nonlinearity

As one gets further away from the magnet isocenter, gradients become nonlinear. This characteristic of the gradients can have an impact on diffusion/IVIM parameter maps when imaging far from the isocenter. However, as MRI vendors provide information regarding the gradient nonlinearity, it is possible to correct for this bias. Malyarenko et al. show how to build correction factors using the gradient design spherical harmonics coefficients and the nominal b values at the isocenter [32]. These correction factors can be applied either to the b value matrices or directly to the parameter maps. In their study, Malyarenko et al. showed that with the correction, apparent diffusion coefficient (ADC) maps were significantly improved with a reduction in the shift and broadening of the ADC distribution. However, they saw no improvement in the f_{IVIM} maps.

19.3.3 Noise Effects

The fitting algorithms used for IVIM data analysis are very sensitive to noise and measurement errors. In particular, due to the non-Gaussian nature of noise in magnitude reconstructed images usually chosen to process the data, the MRI signal does not go to zero at high *b* values. Not taking into account this effect introduces a bias in the signal analysis: f_{IVIM} is overestimated, as shown in Fig. 19.8.

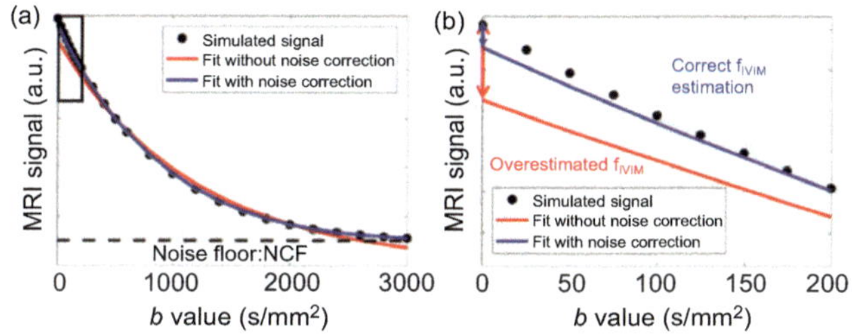

Figure 19.8 (a) Simulated diffusion/IVIM data with a noise floor fitted to the monoexponential ADC model for $b > 200$ s/mm² with and without the noise correction method. (b) Zoom on the 0–200 s/mm² *b*-value range from Fig. 19.8a (corresponds to the area in the black rectangle). The arrows indicate f_{IVIM} estimation.

To overcome this effect, many approaches exist [33–38]. Iima et al. have shown that by slightly adapting the fitting model, it is possible to correct for this bias [21, 39]. The authors introduced a new parameter, called the noise correction factor (NCF), and expressed the noisy acquired signal to be fitted, $S_{\text{corr}}(b)$, as:

$$S_{\text{corr}}(b) = \sqrt{(S(b))^2 + \text{NCF}}\,, \tag{19.32}$$

where $S(b)$ is the signal to be modeled.

NCF is an estimate of the intrinsic noise floor level characterizing the acquired data. NCF can be estimated using a phantom with a diffusion coefficient close to that of the tissues to investigate. The value of the NCF obtained that way is usually a good approximation of the noise effects that will be seen in vivo, provided the acquisition protocol (including the radiofrequency coils) remains unchanged. The method does have the limitation that in vivo noise sources and spatial patterns are not reproduced in the phantom, and the effect of parallel imaging should generally be considered as well. In theory, at a very low SNR, the NCF depends on the SNR but it rapidly becomes constant when the SNR is not extremely low [33, 40]. This method was validated in clinics using *b* values smaller than 3000 s/mm^2.

19.3.4 Diffusion Anisotropy

In almost all of the models presented in the first section, diffusion was supposed to be isotropic as the diffusion coefficient *D* is modeled by a scalar parameter. However, in some tissues, diffusion can be highly anisotropic, that is, in the white matter or the skeletal muscle. To take diffusion anisotropy into account in the diffusion/IVIM model, *D* must be replaced by a tensor in the diffusion part of Eq. 19.1 [41].

Numerous studies perform acquisitions with a limited number of diffusion directions, usually three or six. To fully characterize the diffusion tensor, theoretically at least six directions are needed.

We have shown that diffusion anisotropy, if not handled properly, can induce an artifactual anisotropic IVIM effect [42]. Indeed, when simulating the diffusion signal using a biexponential tensor model and fitting it using the kurtosis model for each direction separately, a direction-dependent nonzero IVIM contribution is obtained.

Mimicking a variation of the tissue orientation by rotating the diffusion tensor eigenvectors about an axis, we also observed differences in the residual IVIM fraction for the different directions with varying tissue orientation. However, we showed that taking the geometric mean of the signal over the diffusion directions considerably reduces the artifactual f_{IVIM}. These results are shown in Fig. 19.9

This artifactual IVIM effect is decreased even more when the number of acquired diffusion directions is increased. The choice of the set of directions also matters. We introduced a new criterion to help choose the optimum set of directions: the absolute normalized sum of the *b*-matrix cross-terms, aNSBC,

$$\mathrm{aNSBC} = \left| \frac{1}{N_{\mathrm{b}} N_{\mathrm{Dir}}} \sum_{i=1}^{N_{\mathrm{Dir}}} \sum_{j=1}^{N_{\mathrm{b}}} \frac{2b_{ij\mathrm{xy}} + 2b_{ij\mathrm{xz}} + 2b_{ij\mathrm{yz}}}{b_{\mathrm{nom}j}} \right|, \tag{19.33}$$

where N_{b} is the number of *b* values, N_{Dir} is the number of diffusion gradient directions, $b_{ij(\mathrm{xy/xz/yz})}$ is the *b*-matrix cross-terms for the *b* value *j* and the direction *i*, and $b_{\mathrm{nom}j}$ is the nominal value of *b* value *j*.

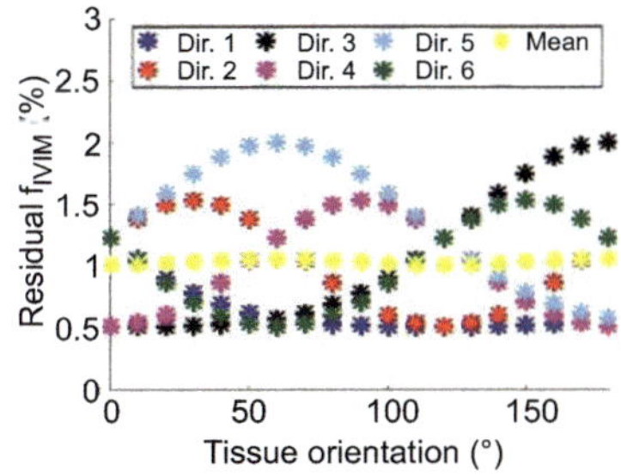

Figure 19.9 Residual f_{IVIM} against the tissue orientation for different diffusion directions of a set of six directions (dual-gradients from Ref. [43]) and the geometric mean over all of the diffusion directions. The simulated biexponential tensor signals ($\text{MD}_{\text{slow/fast}}$ = 0.2/1.1 10^{-3} mm^2/s, f_{slow} = 0.35, and $\text{FA}_{\text{slow/fast}}$ = 0.5/0.28) were fitted to the kurtosis model for diffusion for b = 300–3000 s/mm^2. The diffusion component was then extrapolated for b < 300 s/mm^2 and subtracted from the total signal to look for a residual IVIM component. The tissue orientation variation was mimicked by changing the angle between the diffusion tensor eigenvectors and the laboratory frame in the range 0°–180°.

Sets of directions with a small aNSBC (ideally 0) are the least prone to residual tissue orientation effects after diffusion/IVIM processing. Indeed, Fig. 19.10 displays the standard deviation of the residual f_{IVIM} over the tissue orientation against aNSBC for different sets of six diffusion directions and shows a high correlation between the two parameters, r = 0.98.

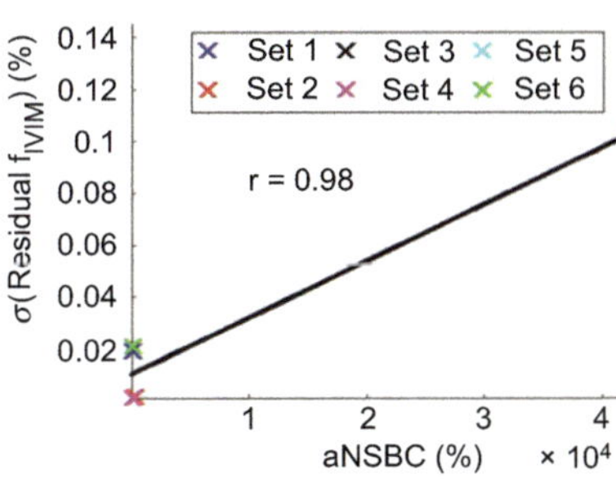

Figure 19.10 Standard deviation, σ, of the residual f_{IVIM} over the tissue orientation against aNSBC for different sets of six diffusion directions; 1, dual-gradients; 2, Jones6; 3, tetrahedral; 4, Muthupallai; 5, cond6; and 6, DSM6 (the name codes for those 6 directions encoding schemes are taken from Refs. [43, 44]). The black line represents a linear regression. The corresponding correlation coefficient, r, has been added.

By adding a simulated monoexponential IVIM component to the simulated diffusion component, we were able to infer that the diffusion anisotropy effect would be more important for low-perfused tissue with small f_{IVIM} and D^* values, that is, for instance in the brain and the prostate.

This anisotropy bias, which is mostly present in low-perfused organs, can be corrected by either modeling the diffusion component using a tensor model or averaging the signal over several diffusion directions, at least six, chosen using the aNSBC value criterion.

In this third section, potential sources of bias that can be corrected during the analysis have been presented. Knowing the advantages and disadvantages of the different models and analysis methods currently in use, new approaches to extract even more information from the IVIM signal can emerge. This is the purpose of the next chapters.

References

1. Le Bihan, D., Breton, E., Lallemand, D., Aubin M. L., Vignaud J., Laval-Jeantet M. Separation of diffusion and perfusion in intravoxel incoherent motion MR imaging. *Radiology* 168, 497–505, 1988.
2. Einstein A. *Investigations on the Theory of the Brownian Movement*, (Courier Corporation), 1956.
3. Fournet G., Li J.-R., Cerjanic A. M., Sutton B. P., Ciobanu L., Le Bihan D. A two-pool model to describe the IVIM cerebral perfusion. *J. Cereb. Blood Flow Metab.* 37, 2987–3000, 2017. https://doi.org/10.1177/0271678X16681310
4. Nevo U., Özarslan E., Komlosh M. E., Koay C. G., Sarlls J. E., Basser P. J. A system and mathematical framework to model shear flow effects in biomedical DW-imaging and spectroscopy. *NMR Biomed.* 23, 734–744, 2010. https://doi.org/10.1002/nbm.1591
5. Wetscherek A., Stieltjes B., Laun F. B. Flow-compensated intravoxel incoherent motion diffusion imaging. *Magn. Reson. Med.* 74, 410–9, 2015. https://doi.org/10.1002/mrm.25410
6. Kennan R. P., Gao J.-H., Zhong J., Gore J. C. A general model of microcirculatory blood flow effects in gradient sensitized MRI. *Med. Phys.* 21, 539–45, 1994. https://doi.org/10.1118/1.597170.
7. Neil J. J., Scherrer L. A., Ackerman J. J. An approach to solving the

dynamic range problem in measurement of the pseudodilusion coefficient in vivo with spin echoes. *J. Magn. Reson. (1969)*, 95, 607–614, 1991.

8. Neil J. J., Ackerman J. J. Detection of ps eudodiffusion in rat brain following blood substitution with perfluorocarbon. *J. Magn. Reson. (1969)*, 97, 194–201, 1992.
9. Neil J. J., Bosch C. S., Ackerman J. J. An evaluation of the sensitivity of the intravoxel incoherent motion (IVIM) method of blood flow measurement to changes in cerebral blood flow. *Magn. Reson. Med.* 32, 60–65,1994.
10. Henkelman R. M., Neil J. J., Xiang, Q.-S. A quantitative interpretation of IVIM measurements of vascular perfusion in the rat brain. *Magn. Reson. Med.* 32, 464–469, 1994.
11. Duong T. Q., Kim S.-G. In vivo MR measurements of regional arterial and venous blood volume fractions in intact rat brain. *Magn. Reson. Med.* 43, 393–402, 2000. https://doi.org/10.1002/(SICI)1522-2594(200003)43:3<393::AID-MRM11>3.0.CO;2-K.
12. Wagenmakers E.-J., Farrell S. AIC model selection using Akaike weights. *Psychon. Bull. Rev.* 11, 192–196, 2004.
13. Akaike H. Information theory and an extension of the maximum likelihood principle. In: Parzen E., Tanabe K., Kitagawa G. (eds) Selected Papers of Hirotugu Akaike. (1998) Springer Series in Statistics (Perspectives in Statistics). Springer, New York, NY
14. Lemke A., Laun F. B., Simon D., Stieltjes B., Schad L. R. An in vivo verification of the intravoxel incoherent motion effect in diffusion-weighted imaging of the abdomen. *Magn. Reson. Med.* 64, 1580–1585, 2010. https://doi.org/10.1002/mrm.22565
15. Jerome N. P., d'Arcy J. A., Feiweier T., Koh D.-M., Leach M. O., Collins, D.J. et al., Extended T2-IVIM model for correction of TE dependence of pseudo-diffusion volume fraction in clinical diffusion-weighted magnetic resonance imaging. *Phys. Med. Biol.* 61, N667–N680, 2016. https://doi.org/10.1088/1361-6560/61/24/N667
16. Suo S., Lin N., Wang H., Zhang L., Wang R., Zhang S. et al., Intravoxel incoherent motion diffusion-weighted MR imaging of breast cancer at 3.0 tesla: Comparison of different curve-fitting methods. *J. Magn. Reson. Imaging* 42, 362–70, 2015. https://doi.org/10.1002/jmri.24799
17. Dijkstra H., Baron P., Kappert P., Oudkerk M., Sijens P. E. Effects of microperfusion in hepatic diffusion weighted imaging. *Eur. Radiol.* 22, 891–899, 2012. https://doi.org/10.1007/s00330-011-2313-1

18. Lu Y., Jansen J. F. A., Stambuk H. E., Gupta G., Lee N., Gonen M. et al. Comparing primary tumors and metastatic nodes in head and neck cancer using intravoxel incoherent motion imaging: a preliminary experience. *J. Comput. Assist. Tomogr.* 37, 2013. https://doi.org/10.1097/RCT.0b013e318282d935

19. Wittsack H.-J., Lanzman R. S., Mathys C., Janssen H., Mödder U., Blondin D. Statistical evaluation of diffusion-weighted imaging of the human kidney. *Magn. Reson. Med.* 64, 616–22, 2010. https://doi.org/10.1002/mrm.22436

20. Iima M., Reynaud O., Tsurugizawa T., Ciobanu L., Li J.-R., Geffroy F. et al. Characterization of glioma microcirculation and tissue features using intravoxel incoherent motion magnetic resonance imaging in a rat brain model. *Invest. Radiol.* 49, 485–490, 2014.

21. Iima M., Kataoka M., Nakanishi Y., Umehana M., Ito T., Yano K., et al. Computer-aided IVIM/kurtosis diffusion MRI for breast lesions: Comparison with BI-RADS MRI categories, 2014, DOI: 10.1594/ecr2014/C-1494.

22. Lu Y., Jansen J. F. A., Mazaheri Y., Stambuk H. E., Koutcher J. A., Shukla-Dave A. Extension of the intravoxel incoherent motion model to non-gaussian diffusion in head and neck cancer. *J. Magn. Reson. Imaging* 36, 1088–96, 2012. https://doi.org/10.1002/jmri.23770

23. Wurnig M. C., Donati O. F., Ulbrich E., Filli L., Kenkel D., Thoeny, H.C., et al. Systematic analysis of the intravoxel incoherent motion threshold separating perfusion and diffusion effects: Proposal of a standardized algorithm. *Magn. Reson. Med.* 74, 1414–1422, 2015. https://doi.org/10.1002/mrm.25506

24. Iima M., Yano K., Kataoka M., Umehana M., Murata K., Kanao, S., et al. Quantitative non-Gaussian diffusion and intravoxel incoherent motion magnetic resonance imaging: Differentiation of malignant and benign breast lesions. *Invest. Radiol.* 50, 205–211, 2015.

25. Niendorf T., Dijkhuizen R. M., Norris D. G., van Lookeren Campagne M., Nicolay K. Biexponential diffusion attenuation in various states of brain tissue: Implications for diffusion-weighted imaging. *Magn. Reson. Med.* 36, 847–857, 1996.

26. Neil J. J., Bretthorst G. L. On the use of Bayesian probability theory for analysis of exponential decay date: An example taken from intravoxel incoherent motion experiments. *Magn. Reson. Med.* 29, 642–647, 1993. https://doi.org/10.1002/mrm.1910290510

27. Barbieri S., Donati O. F., Froehlich J. M., Thoeny H. C., Impact of the calculation algorithm on biexponential fitting of diffusion-weighted

MRI in upper abdominal organs. *Magn. Reson. Med.* 75, 2175–2184, 2016. https://doi.org/10.1002/mrm.25765

28. Le Bihan D., Breton E., Lallemand D., Grenier P., Cabanis E., Laval-Jeantet M. MR imaging of intravoxel incoherent motions: application to diffusion and perfusion in neurologic disorders. *Radiology* 161, 401–407, 1986.
29. Boujraf S. b matrix errors in echo planar diffusion tensor imaging. *J. Appl. Clin. Med. Phys.* 2, 178, 2001. https://doi.org/10.1120/1.1382710
30. Mattiello J., Basser P. J., Lebihan D. Analytical expressions for the b matrix in NMR diffusion imaging and spectroscopy. *J. Magn. Reson. A* 108, 131–141, 1994. https://doi.org/10.1006/jmra.1994.1103
31. Mattiello J., Basser P. J., Le Bihan D. The b matrix in diffusion tensor echo-planar imaging. *Magn. Reson. Med.* 37, 292–300, 1997.
32. Malyarenko D. I., Pang Y., Senegas J., Ivancevic M. K., Ross B. D., Chenevert T. L. Correction of gradient nonlinearity bias in quantitative diffusion parameters of renal tissue with intravoxel incoherent motion. *Tomography* 1, 145–151, 2015. https://doi.org/10.18383/j.tom.2015.00160
33. Gudbjartsson H., Patz S. The Rician distribution of noisy MRI data. *Magn. Reson. Med.* 34, 910–914, 1995.
34. Sijbers J., den Dekker A. J., Scheunders P., Van Dyck D. Maximum-likelihood estimation of Rician distribution parameters. *IEEE Trans. Med. Imaging* 17, 357–361, 1998. https://doi.org/10.1109/42.712125
35. Brion V., Poupon C., Riff O., Aja-Fernández S., Tristán-Vega A., Mangin, J.-F. et al. Parallel MRI noise correction: An extension of the LMMSE to noncentral χ distributions. In: Fichtinger G., Martel A., Peters T. (eds) *Medical Image Computing and Computer-Assisted Intervention – MICCAI 2011*. Lecture Notes in Computer Science, vol 6892. Springer, Berlin, Heidelberg
36. Constantinides C. D., Atalar E., McVeigh E. R. Signal-to-noise measurements in magnitude images from NMR phased arrays. *Magn. Reson. Med.* 38, 852–857, 1997.
37. Aja-Fernández S., Tristán-Vega A., Hoge W. S., Statistical noise analysis in GRAPPA using a parametrized noncentral Chi approximation model. *Magn. Reson. Med.* 65, 1195–1206, 2011. https://doi.org/10.1002/mrm.22701
38. André E. D., Grinberg F., Farrher E., Maximov I. I., Shah N. J., Meyer C., et al., Influence of noise correction on intra- and inter-subject variability

of quantitative metrics in diffusion kurtosis imaging. *PLOS One*, 9, e94531, 2014. https://doi.org/10.1371/journal.pone.0094531

39. Le Bihan D., Iima M., Kataoka M., Umehana M., Yano K., Togashi K. An empirical phantom-based approach to correct for non-Gaussian noise bias in diffusion MRI., *Proc 23rd ISMRM-ESMRMB Joint Annual Meeting*, (Milan, Italy), 2014.
40. Koay C. G., Basser P. J. Analytically exact correction scheme for signal extraction from noisy magnitude MR signals. *J. Magn. Reson.* 179, 317–22, 2006. https://doi.org/10.1016/j.jmr.2006.01.016
41. Basser P. J., Mattiello J., LeBihan D. MR diffusion tensor spectroscopy and imaging. *Biophys J.* 66, 259–267, 1994. https://doi.org/10.1016/S0006-3495(94)80775-1
42. Fournet G., Ciobanu L., Le Bihan D. Inadequate modeling of diffusion anisotropy can lead to artefactual IVIM effects: evidence from numerical simulations, *Proc 27th ISMRM Annual Meeting*, (Paris, France), 2018.
43. Skare S., Hedehus M., Moseley M.E., Li T-Q. Condition number as a measure of noise performance of diffusion tensor data acquisition schemes with MRI. *J. Magn. Reson.* 147, 340–352, 2000. https://doi.org/10.1006/jmre.2000.2209
44. Muthupallai R., Holder C., Song A., Dixon W. Navigator-aided, multishot EPI diffusion images of brain with complete orientation and anisotropic information. In: *Proceedings of the 7th ISMRM Annual Meeting*, Philadelphia, PA, USA, 1999.

Chapter 20

Flow-Compensated IVIM in the Ballistic Regime: Data Acquisition, Modeling, and Brain Applications

André Ahlgren[a,b] **and Ronnie Wirestam**[a]
[a]*Department of Medical Radiation Physics, Lund University, Lund, Sweden*
[b]*Center for Medical Imaging and Visualization (CMIV), Linköping University, Linköping, Sweden*
andreahlgren@gmail.com

20.1 Introduction

20.1.1 The IVIM Imaging Concept

Intravoxel incoherent motion (IVIM) imaging has been used to obtain diffusion and perfusion information for more than three decades [1, 2]. As magnetic resonance imaging (MRI) hardware and acquisition techniques have improved over the years, the interest in IVIM imaging has increased and the number of applications has grown. The popularity of the method can partially be explained by the elegance in its simplicity; the diffusion MRI signal is modeled as

Intravoxel Incoherent Motion (IVIM) MRI: Principles and Applications
Edited by Denis Le Bihan, Mami Iima, Christian Federau, and Eric E. Sigmund

ISBN 978-981-4800-19-8 (Hardcover), 978-0-429-42727-5 (eBook)
www.panstanford.com

a biexponential function of diffusion-encoding strength, where the two components correspond to the intravoxel signal contributions from diffusing spins and spins flowing through the microvascular network (perfusion):

$$S(b) = S_0[\underbrace{(1-f)e^{-bD_t}}_{\text{diffusion}} + \underbrace{fe^{-bD^*}}_{\text{perfusion}}] \tag{20.1}$$

The independent variable b is the diffusion encoding strength, S_0 is the signal without diffusion weighting, f is the so-called perfusion fraction, and the respective decay rates correspond to the diffusion coefficient in tissue (D_t) and the pseudo-diffusion coefficient related to blood flow (D^*). As such, the flow of blood through the microvascular network is modeled as a signal attenuation similar to a diffusion process, and diffusion and perfusion can be separated and quantified with appropriate data acquisition and analysis strategies. The water self-diffusion in blood, D_b, may also be included, and the last term would then read $fe^{-b(D_b+D^*)}$.

In a majority of the IVIM research studies and applications, this original compact model has been employed and the data acquisition has usually been realized using a standard single diffusion encoding (SDE) MRI sequence, that is, the "Stejskal–Tanner sequence," with varying diffusion encoding strengths. Furthermore, conventional IVIM analysis is based on biexponential least-squares fitting of diffusion-weighted signal data, a method that suffers from an inordinate sensitivity to noise. Although the pseudodiffusion coefficient of the flowing blood (D^*) is approximately an order of magnitude larger than the regular diffusion coefficient, perfused capillaries contribute to the observable signal by only a small fraction (about 4% in the brain), and the IVIM effect is thus very difficult to detect with a high degree of reliability. Imaging and processing methods with a potential to improve the stability of the IVIM analysis would therefore be of considerable importance for the use of IVIM in clinical applications.

Some studies have indeed demonstrated the potential value in expanding the scope of the acquisition and modifying the IVIM model. In particular, the assumption that capillary blood particles flow mainly along straight paths during the encoding time allows for new imaging and processing approaches. This chapter aims to cover the underlying theory of the signal attenuation due to incoherent motion, the corresponding time dependence and temporal regimes, the effect of flow compensation, and examples of applications (primarily in the brain).

20.1.2 Temporal Regimes of Incoherent Motion

In 1907, Einstein noted that it would be "impossible" to measure the instantaneous velocity of a Brownian particle because the velocity and direction of the motion would be rapidly and randomly altered, even during an "extraordinarily short" observation time [3]. Although it took a little more than 100 years for Einstein's statement to be challenged [3], we are still not even close to being able to measure ballistic Brownian motion with magnetic resonance techniques. On the other hand, random and pseudorandom particle motions with longer characteristic time scales of the velocity fluctuations, such as microvascular blood flow, can pertain to the "diffusive," "ballistic," or "intermediate" temporal regime and be probed with motion-/diffusion-encoded MRI [4]. The difference in scale between microscopic Brownian motion and macroscopic motion is enormous; the velocity fluctuations of a Brownian particle (such as a water molecule) at room temperature is of the order of ~10 ps, whereas macroscopic velocity changes of a blood water molecule traversing the human capillary network is believed to be of the order of ~100 ms. The latter time scale is of a similar order of magnitude as the motion encoding time (observation time) of the MRI sequence, which means that the temporal regime of microvascular blood flow is likely to depend on the settings of the pulse sequence protocol.

The characteristic time for velocity fluctuations (i.e., the average time for a particle to change speed and/or direction) can be defined by the velocity autocorrelation time T_0. If the motion encoding time of the MRI sequence is long compared to T_0, the blood particles change directions several times during the encoding, that is, mimic a diffusion process, and hence the motion is approximately diffusive (referred to as pseudodiffusion). It has been suggested that at least 6–10 velocity changes are needed for the diffusive approximation to be valid [4]. In the other limiting case, if the encoding time is short compared to T_0, the blood particles flow mostly along straight lines and this situation corresponds to the ballistic regime. Finally, if the encoding time is close to T_0, the motion pertains to the intermediate regime. It is of particular interest, in this context, to note that flow compensation affects the signal attenuation curves for motion patterns belonging to the intermediate and ballistic regimes and flow compensation can therefore be used to characterize and quantify microvascular blood flow and also to improve IVIM imaging. This chapter will mainly focus on the ballistic regime.

20.1.3 Motion Patterns in the Microvascular Network

Independently of the IVIM concept, Nalcioglu et al. and Ahn et al. developed an alternative method to estimate the relative capillary density [5, 6]. In the corresponding model, it is assumed that the blood flows coherently, on a subvoxel scale, in straight and randomly oriented capillary segments (i.e., the ballistic regime, as previously described). Coherent motion normally leads to a shift in the MR signal phase (see phase contrast MR), but variations in blood particle velocities and/or spatial orientation of capillary vessel segments yield a phase dispersion, resulting in a signal attenuation similar to that of pseudodiffusion. An important difference from diffusive motion is that the phase shift caused by straight flow in an individual segment can be rephased (i.e., the spin magnetization can be refocused) using velocity/flow compensation, and the corresponding signal attenuation caused by the collective effect of a large number of randomly oriented segments can thus be inhibited. Therefore, a combination of noncompensated (NC) and flow-compensated (FC) data was suggested as a way to probe perfusion [6]. In the original IVIM work by Le Bihan et al., it was acknowledged that both the pseudodiffusion model (i.e., the diffusive regime) and the straight-flow model (i.e., the ballistic regime) of microvascular blood flow would lead to much stronger signal attenuation than that of microscopic diffusion in tissue [2]. However, it was the pseudodiffusion interpretation and the corresponding model that primarily became associated with IVIM imaging.

Figure 20.1 displays a simplified illustration of the microvascular network in an MRI voxel, and the two limiting and contrasting cases, that is, diffusive and ballistic motion. As previously inferred, and elegantly described by Kennan et al. [4], the two models correspond to different temporal regimes (or extreme/limiting cases) of a more general description of a random walk, and the transition between them is referred to as the intermediate regime. To accurately describe and exploit random motion in the intermediate regime, even more delicate experiments and models are required, and this will be described in more detail in Chapter 21.

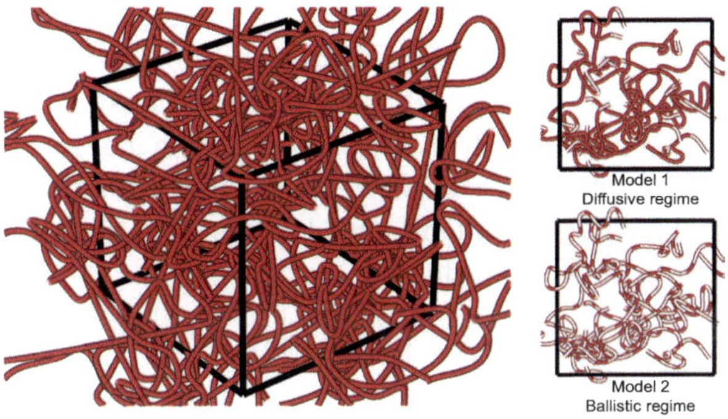

Figure 20.1 Schematic figure (not to scale) of the intricate network of highly tortuous and pseudorandomly oriented microvessels in a voxel (left). The two figures on the right visualize the two most common models for phase dispersion due to incoherent blood flow. In these figures, the red filling in the vessels corresponds to the pathway that a given blood particle has traveled during the motion encoding period. For the diffusive regime (Model 1), the blood particles travel relatively long distances and pass several bends of the capillaries. In contrast, for the ballistic regime (Model 2), the blood particles travel only a short distance and in mostly straight paths.

Since flow compensation, in theory, completely recalls the phase dispersion caused by velocity dispersion, Ahn et al. suggested calculating the signal difference between an FC and an NC acquisition, which would be proportional to the capillary density within the voxel (i.e., similar to the perfusion fraction *f*) [6]. Since then, a few other approaches of perfusion measurement using flow encoding have been proposed, as will be discussed in the following sections.

General flow and motion encoding with MR, that is, outside the field of perfusion MRI, has been described in detail in the past (e.g., Refs. [7–9]), and publications from these neighboring fields of MR are likely to serve as an important source of inspiration also in the future development of IVIM imaging.

20.2 Motion Encoding and Flow Compensation

20.2.1 General Signal Expressions

The normalized MR signal at echo time t_E can be described as

$$\frac{S(t_E)}{S_0} = E(t_E) = \langle e^{-i\phi(t_E)} \rangle , \tag{20.2}$$

where S_0 is the relaxation-weighted signal without motion encoding, ϕ is the spin phase, and $\langle\cdot\rangle$ denotes the ensemble average over the entire spin packet. The sensitivity of the signal to motion is adjusted by varying the magnetic field gradient $G(t)$, that is, motion/diffusion encoding. The field gradient encodes the time-dependent spin position in the phase according to

$$\phi(t) = \gamma \int_0^t G(t')x(t')dt' , \tag{20.3}$$

where γ is the gyromagnetic ratio and x is the spin position. The cumulated phase at the echo time, caused by the combination of the motion encoding and the movement of spins, can also be described in terms of velocity, according to [9]

$$\phi(v) = \gamma \int_0^{t_E} G(t) \int_0^t v(t')dt'dt , \tag{20.4}$$

where v is the spin velocity. Summation over all subensembles according to Eq. 20.2 yields the normalized signal as [9]

$$E(t_E) = \int_{-\infty}^{\infty} f(v)e^{-i\phi(v)}dv , \tag{20.5}$$

where $f(v)$ is the distribution of spin velocities. If the spin velocities are described by a Gaussian distribution, the phase distribution will also be Gaussian, and using Eq. 20.5, the normalized signal can be written as

$$E(t_E) = e^{-i\mu_\phi - \sigma_\phi^2} \tag{20.6}$$

where μ_ϕ and σ_ϕ^2 are the mean and variance of the phase distribution, respectively. This expression can also be obtained by performing a cumulant expansion to the second order of Eq. 20.2. The expression is referred to as the Gaussian phase approximation, and it infers that coherent bulk motion is encoded in the signal phase and incoherent motion and velocity dispersion is encoded in the signal magnitude.

As shown below, at least one model discussed in this chapter is based on this approximation.

Using Eq. 20.4, it is possible to show that the phase shift of a spin or a spin packet with a constant velocity v_c is given by

$$\phi(t_E) = \gamma v_c \int_0^{t_E} tG(t)dt = \alpha v_c, \tag{20.7}$$

where α is the flow weighting factor. Later, velocity and orientation dispersion will be added for derivation of the corresponding signal equations. It can be shown that the flow weighting factor can be calculated in two ways, according to

$$\alpha = \gamma \int_0^{t_E} tG(t)dt = -\int_0^{t_E} q(t)dt, \tag{20.8}$$

where $q(t)$ is the dephasing function given by

$$q(t) = \gamma \int_0^{t} G(t')dt'. \tag{20.9}$$

For an SDE sequence, the flow weighting is given by $\alpha = -\gamma g \delta \Delta$, where g is the gradient amplitude, δ is the duration of each gradient pulse, and Δ is the separation between the gradient pulses (see Fig. 20.2). The accumulated phase due to spins moving with a constant velocity can be nulled using velocity/flow compensation, which is achieved by designing the gradient waveforms so that $\alpha = 0$ (first-order gradient moment nulling). It is also possible to compensate for higher orders of motion (e.g., acceleration). The calculation of α can be compared to the general expression for the diffusion weighting factor (i.e., diffusion encoding strength) according to

$$b = \int_0^{t_E} q(t)^2 dt, \tag{20.10}$$

which yields the well-known b-value expression for an SDE sequence, that is, $b = \gamma^2 g^2 d^2 (\Delta - \delta/3)$.

20.2.2 MRI Pulse Sequence Design

As mentioned above, an FC pulse sequence is designed to null the first-order moment of the magnetic field gradients. There are two common sequence implementations to achieve flow compensation: (i) a single refocused spin-echo sequence, with bipolar gradient pulses on each side of the 180° refocusing radio frequency (RF) pulse, and (ii) a twice refocused spin-echo sequence, with two pairs of gradient pulses (one pair surrounding each refocusing RF pulse). Both of these belong to a class of sequences known as double diffusion encoding (DDE), which means that they encode the spins in two separate instances [10]. A DDE sequence is always less effective in terms of encoding strength per echo time, compared to the classic SDE sequence.

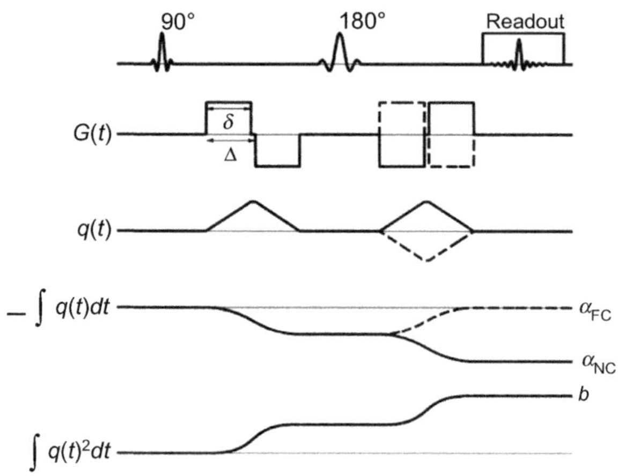

Figure 20.2 Scheme of a pulse sequence capable of acquiring both NC and FC motion-encoded data with otherwise matched settings. The top row shows RF pulses and signal readout, $G(t)$ shows the applied gradient waveforms, $q(t)$ is the dephasing function (see Eq. 20.9), and the two bottom rows show the time integrals that result in the flow weighting α and diffusion weighting b at the time of readout. Solid and dashed lines correspond to the NC and FC acquisitions, respectively.

Figure 20.2 displays how the first type can be implemented and corresponds to the sequence employed in the study by our group [11]. The sequence is designed so that both FC and NC data can be acquired with the same basic sequence (by reversing the polarity of the second gradient block). This also ensures that the diffusion encoding strength and gradient timings are matched between the acquisitions. This matching is important because it ensures that effects unrelated to blood flow are identical in the acquired FC and NC data. Earlier studies often relied on separate pulse sequences, typically an SDE sequence for NC data acquisition and a DDE sequence for FC data acquisition (i.e., unmatched acquisitions). It should be noted that, compared to a standard SDE experiment employing the same gradient settings, the flow and diffusion weighting factors are doubled in a DDE experiment, that is, $\alpha_{NC} = -2\gamma g\delta\Delta$ and $b = 2\gamma^2 g^2 d^2(\Delta - \delta/3)$. We reiterate that the FC acquisition yields zero flow encoding, that is $\alpha_{FC} = 0$ always.

For the NC acquisition, the flow and diffusion weighting factors will vary together with the gradient strengths. More advanced pulse sequence designs can allow for α and b to be varied independently.

20.3 Signal Equations for the Ballistic Regime

20.3.1 The Nalcioglu–Ahn Model

Derivation of signal equations for the straight-flow model (i.e., the ballistic regime) can be approached in at least two different ways. First, the approach proposed by Nalcioglu et al. and Ahn et al. is described [5, 6]. If a single tube (capillary segment) with direction $\hat{k}$ is considered, in which particles flow with a velocity distribution (derived from an assumed flow profile) $f_k(v)$, the signal attenuation due to the flow is given by (see Eq. 5)

$$F = \int_{-\infty}^{\infty} f_k(v) e^{i\hat{\alpha}v\hat{k}} dv , \qquad (20.11)$$

where $\hat{\alpha}$ is the flow weighting factor, with the direction of the applied magnetic field gradient preserved. If θ_k is defined as the angle between $\hat{\alpha}$ and $\hat{k}$, and the velocity distribution is assumed to be identical in all tubes, that is, $f_k(v) = f(v)$, summation over multiple tubes yields

$$F = \sum_k \int_{-\infty}^{\infty} f_k(v) e^{i\alpha v \cos\theta_k} dv = \int f(\theta) \int_{-\infty}^{\infty} f(v) e^{i\alpha v \cos\theta} dv d\theta , \qquad (20.12)$$

where $f(\theta)$ is the orientation distribution. For an isotropic orientation distribution, that is, $f(\theta) = \sin(\theta)/2$ for $\theta \le \pi$, the expression is further simplified to

$$F = \int_{-\infty}^{\infty} f(v) \text{sinc}(\alpha v) dv , \qquad (20.13)$$

where $\text{sinc}(x) = \sin(x)/x$. This is a convenient expression from which signal equations can be derived for different intravascular velocity distributions or flow profiles. For example, plug flow with a mean velocity v_0 yields a signal attenuation according to

$$F_{\text{plug}} = \text{sinc}(av_0) \tag{20.14}$$

and a laminar (parabolic) flow profile with a mean velocity $v_0 = v_{\text{max}}/2$ yields

$$F_{\text{laminar}} = \frac{\text{Si}(2\alpha v_0)}{2\alpha v_0}, \tag{20.15}$$

where Si is the sine integral. Hence, if an appropriate type of flow profile can be established, and the ballistic limit is valid, blood flow can be probed with this type of model.

The oscillating signal patterns inferred from the models have only been observed in controlled phantom experiments. Still, Ahn et al. demonstrated a strong refocusing effect for FC data acquired from a flow phantom using variable encoding strengths, confirming the potential value of flow compensation in perfusion MRI [6]. For practical imaging purposes, Ahn et al. proposed to compute the signal difference between an FC (S_{FC}) acquisition and an NC (S_{NC}) acquisition at a single diffusion encoding strength, rather than to measure and model the in vivo signal at variable flow encoding strengths. This signal difference was theoretically shown to be proportional to the actively perfused capillary density, that is, $\Delta S = S_{\text{FC}} - S_{\text{NC}} \propto f$. In other words, $\Delta S = 0$ ($S_{\text{FC}} = S_{\text{NC}}$) if the capillary density is zero and ΔS increases with increasing capillary density. The derivations indicated, however, that the signal difference was also dependent on relaxation and diffusion effects. The feasibility of this signal difference approach was also demonstrated in vivo (whole body images) in the same study [6].

Fujita et al. were the first to apply the FC/NC signal difference approach to brain perfusion imaging [12]. Figure 20.3 shows the FC, NC, and difference images of a healthy volunteer. The b value was ~40 s/mm^2 for an echo time of 120 ms. They also acquired phantom data at multiple encoding strengths and highlighted the analogy to the perfusion fraction in IVIM imaging (pseudodiffusion). One advantage of the signal difference approach over IVIM imaging, they argued, is that the former can be achieved with only two images, whereas IVIM imaging requires at least three images.

Maki et al. realized that, instead of directly using the signal difference between an NC acquisition and an FC acquisition, relaxation and diffusion effects are better compensated for by using the relative signal difference, that is, $\Delta S/S_{\text{FC}} = 1 - S_{\text{NC}}/S_{\text{FC}}$ [13]. This expression will also be zero for no perfusion effects and tends to 1 as the perfusion increases. Maki et al. also demonstrated a clear signal difference between FC and NC data in phantom and animal experiments.

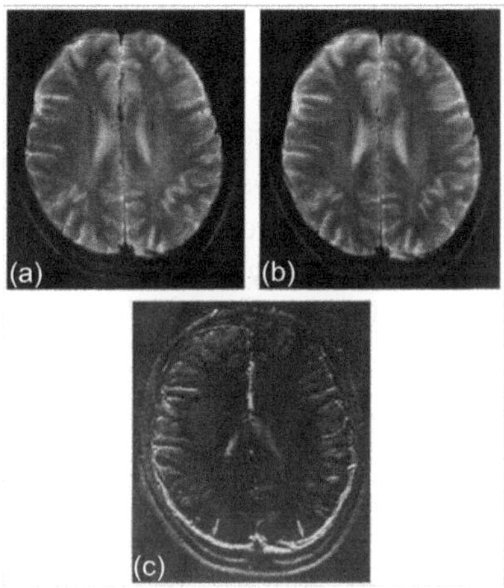

Figure 20.3 Early demonstration of brain perfusion imaging using a combination of FC and NC pulse sequences, by Fujita et al. [12]. The images correspond to (a) NC acquisition, (b) FC acquisition, and (c) difference image ($\Delta S = S_{FC} - S_{NC}$). A clear difference between the acquisitions was demonstrated, as well as a visible gray matter–white matter contrast in the difference image, in agreement with the known higher perfusion and blood volume of gray matter. Reprinted from Ref. [11], with permission from John Wiley and Sons, copyright 2016.

20.3.2 Gaussian Velocity Distribution

The second approach, derived from the same common expressions, is based on identifying velocity distributions on a voxel level. A tube with mean velocity $\bar{v}_k$ contributes to the signal according to $e^{-i\phi_k} = e^{-i\alpha\bar{v}_k}$, where ϕ_k is the cumulative phase for the entire tube. Summation over all tubes yields the signal attenuation according to (see Eq. 20.5)

$$F = \sum_k e^{-i\alpha\bar{v}_k} = \int_{-\infty}^{\infty} f(\bar{v}) e^{-i\alpha\bar{v}} d\bar{v} , \tag{20.16}$$

where $f(\bar{v})$ is the distribution of mean velocity. This expression is convenient since we can choose velocity distributions on a voxel level without defining any velocity profile. Although it is challenging to establish an appropriate velocity distribution for capillary blood flow, a large spread in velocities is likely to be present due to the heterogeneity of microcirculatory properties [14]. If we assume a Gaussian velocity distribution of mean velocities, $f(\overline{v})$, with variance $\langle \overline{v}^2 \rangle$ and zero mean, the signal attenuation is given by

$$F_{\text{gaussian}} = e^{-\alpha^2 \frac{\langle \overline{v}^2 \rangle}{2}}, \tag{20.17}$$

where $\langle \overline{v}^2 \rangle$ is the average mean-squared velocity. This expression was described in the context of perfusion imaging by Kennan et al. [4] and was recently applied in vivo by our group [11]. Note that this model corresponds to the Gaussian phase approximation, as described earlier (Eq. 20.6). It is also clear that, in comparison to the Nalcioglu–Ahn model, this model infers a strict, monotonically decreasing signal as a function of flow encoding strength (i.e., no oscillations), which seems to represent the data better since no oscillating signal behavior has been observed in vivo.

The same results can actually be obtained from the two approaches described above, by acknowledging that the velocity distribution is a combination of random orientation and speed distributions within the tubes. Hence, for example, for a Gaussian velocity distribution on the voxel level, $g(\overline{v})$ the corresponding tube velocity distribution is given by the Maxwell–Boltzmann distribution of speeds, that is, $f(v) = 4\pi v^2 g(v)$.

If the blood flow is only approximately ballistic, or even belongs to the intermediate or diffusive regimes, the models discussed here are inaccurate and corresponding errors in the perfusion parameters can be expected (e.g., an underestimation of f if the FC data are only partially rephased).

20.4 Inclusion of Flow Models in IVIM Imaging

20.4.1 Generalized IVIM Model and Flow Compensation

It may be argued that, if microvascular blood flow in vivo is better described as a ballistic motion pattern, IVIM imaging can be improved by replacing the pseudodiffusion model with a flow model, especially if combined with FC data acquisition. A general

IVIM model, where the perfusion component is described by a flow model, can be written as

$$S(b, \alpha) = S_0[(1 - f)e^{-bD_t} + fe^{-bD_b}F(\alpha)], \tag{20.18}$$

where $F(\alpha)$ is the signal attenuation due to straight flowing blood. It can be seen that the signal equation now includes two independent variables, which can be varied in different ways to improve the quantification. Note that, for FC acquisitions, $\alpha = 0$ and $F(\alpha) = 1$ and for NC acquisitions $\alpha > 0$ and $F(\alpha) < 1$. The incorporation of flow models in the original IVIM model in this way, and the acquisition of data at multiple diffusion and flow encoding strengths, has regained interest in recent years. This can probably partly be explained by improvements in MRI hardware and software, yielding improved signal, improved image quality, and shorter scanning times.

20.4.2 Applications to Cerebral Microcirculation

In a recent study by our group [11], it was suggested that if capillary blood flow can be characterized as ballistic motion, acquisition of NC and FC data at variable flow and diffusion encoding strengths, combined with joint analysis of both data sets, should improve IVIM quantification. The reasoning behind this is that flow compensation increases the contrast between flowing and nonflowing spins and that the joint analysis uses multidimensional data to strengthen the analysis without introducing additional model parameters. Since capillary topography and blood flow are highly variable in vivo, the Gaussian velocity distribution (Eq. 20.17) was employed, or, to be specific, a slight generalization of this attenuation factor according to $F = e^{-\alpha^2 v_d^2}$. Here, v_d is a measure of velocity dispersion, which scales with velocity depending on the particular dispersion model, for example, $v_d^2 = \langle \bar{v}^2 \rangle / 2$ for a Gaussian velocity distribution.

The notion that IVIM imaging may be improved by joint analysis of NC and FC data was confirmed by simulations (Fig. 20.4). The joint analysis of NC and FC data resulted in improved accuracy and precision across all model parameters compared to two conventional IVIM analysis approaches (i.e., nonlinear and segmented fitting of the standard IVIM model to NC data).

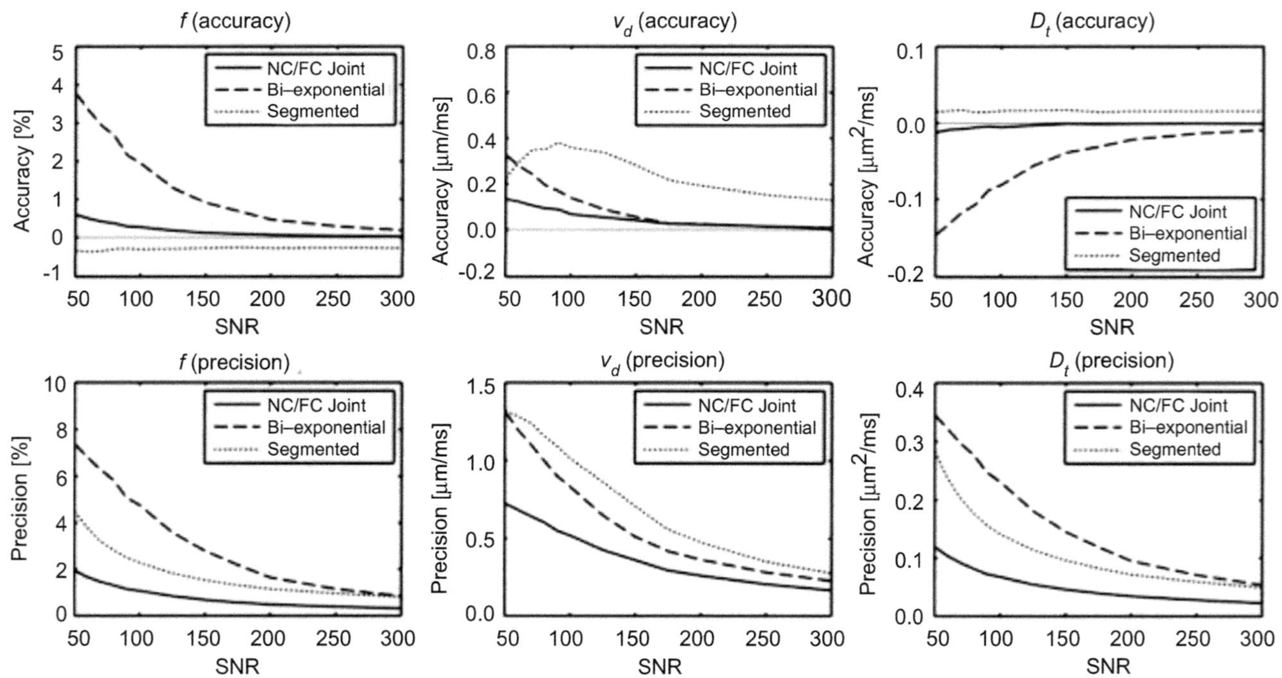

Figure 20.4 Simulation results demonstrating improved accuracy and precision of IVIM parameters when using a joint analysis of FC and NC data, compared to conventional IVIM analysis approaches, that is, nonlinear (biexponential) and segmented fitting. Graphs show accuracy (top row) and precision (bottom row) for f, $\mathbf{v}_d$ and D_t as a function of the SNR. Simulated parameter values were $f = 5\%$, $\mathbf{v}_d = 1.75$ μm/ms, and $D_t = 0.8$ μm^2/ms. Reprinted from Ref. [11] with permission from John Wiley & Sons Ltd., copyright 2016.

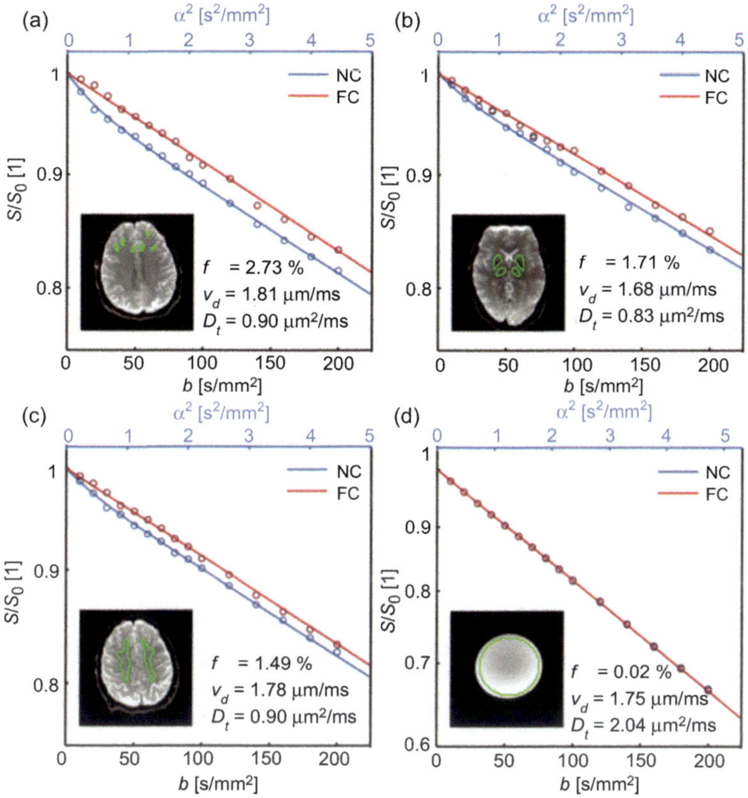

Figure 20.5 Examples of experimental data and model fit for joint diffusion and flow encoding. The different ROIs correspond to (a) frontal gray matter, (b) deep gray matter, and (c) white matter, as well as (d) the stationary water phantom. The insets show the corresponding S_0 images, with the ROIs indicated in green. The graphs show the mean ROI signal magnitude (circles) and the corresponding model fit (solid lines) as a function of diffusion and flow weighting. Note the consistent separation of FC and NC data in vivo and the approximately monoexponential decay of the FC data. Reprinted from Ref. [11] with permission from John Wiley & Sons Ltd., copyright 2016.

In our study, the sequence design shown in Fig. 20.2 was implemented and the total encoding time was kept as short as possible to tilt the capillary blood flow toward the ballistic regime. Hence, the encoding time was 37.7 ms, although this limited the b value to a maximum of 200 s/mm^2. Eight healthy volunteers were investigated, and the data were analyzed using the modified IVIM model (Eq. 20.18). Figure 20.5 displays examples of signal curves from different brain regions as well as from a static water phantom; a clear refocusing effect was observed across the brain, and the 2D model fitted the data well. The phantom experiment confirmed that the NC and FC data acquisitions were well matched with regard to effects unrelated to flow.

Voxel-by-voxel analysis was also accomplished, yielding parametric maps of S_0, D_t, v_d, and f. An example from a single slice is shown in Fig. 20.6. The S_0 and D_t maps looked convincing, whereas the map of v_d was fairly isointense, likely due to regularization of this parameter in the fitting algorithm. The map of f on the other hand showed high tissue contrast and actually resembled a blood volume map.

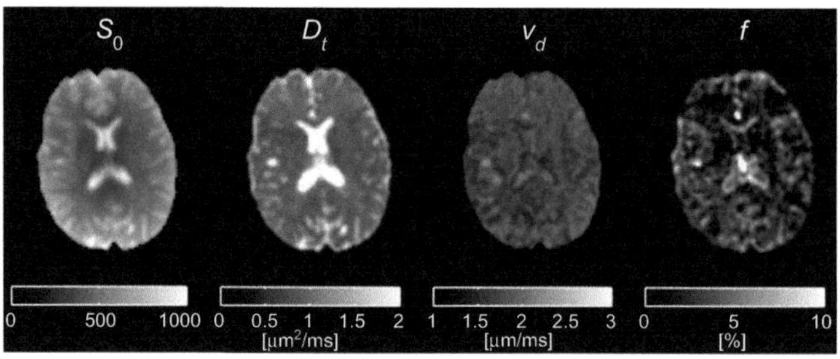

Figure 20.6 Results from a voxel-by-voxel analysis of the joint analysis of NC and FC data at multiple diffusion and flow encoding strengths, taken from one slice in one subject. The images from left to right correspond to parametric maps of S_0, D_t, v_d, and f. Reprinted from Ref. [11] with permission from John Wiley & Sons Ltd., copyright 2016.

In Fig. 20.7, three different suggested approaches for in vivo characterization of perfusion using ballistic modeling and flow compensation are visualized. In particular, the approaches as suggested by Ahn et al. [6], Maki et al. [13], and Ahlgren et al. [11] are compared.

Although straight-flow models work well for ballistic motion, they breakdown if the blood flow pertains to another temporal regime. In this regard, the FC information can, in theory, be used to infer the relevant temporal regime of the blood flow. If the blood flow pertains to the diffusive regime, the flow compensation should have no effect on the signal; if it pertains to the ballistic regime, the flow compensation should yield a complete refocusing of the phase dispersion due to perfusion (so that only the effects of diffusion remain); and if it pertains to the intermediate regime flow compensation, it should yield a partial refocusing. In a recent work, Wetscherek et al. suggested the use of NC/FC acquisitions with variable encoding times to probe blood flow pertaining to the intermediate regime [15]. It was demonstrated that variable encoding times varied the amount of partial refocusing in vivo (liver and pancreas), implying that the blood flow did in fact pertain to the intermediate regime. Although the Gaussian phase approximation works well in the diffusive and ballistic regimes, it is not valid in the intermediate regime, especially at high encoding strengths. Wetscherek et al., therefore, applied a numerical Monte Carlo approach instead of analytical signal models. This approach will be further described in Chapter 21.

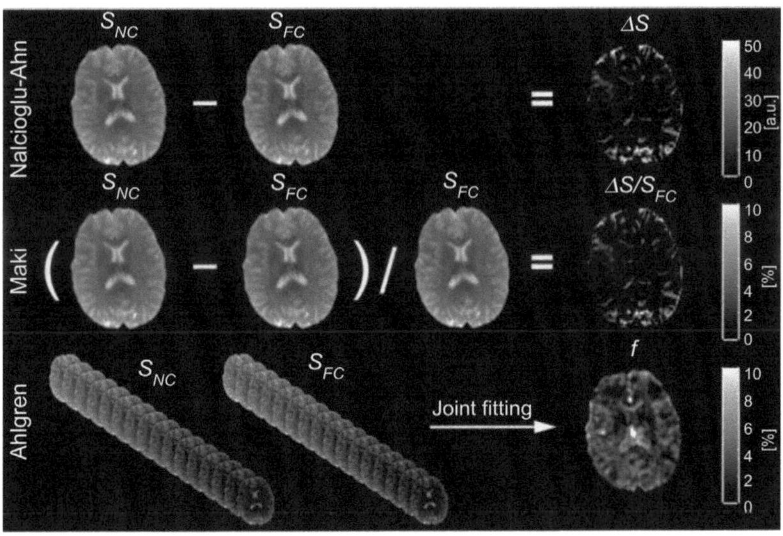

Figure 20.7 Schematic overview of three different approaches used to analyze NC and FC data for characterization of tissue perfusion. (Top row) Calculation of the signal difference between an NC and FC acquisition, that is, the Nalcioglu–Ahn approach [6]. (Middle row) Calculation of the relative signal difference between an NC and FC acquisition, that is, the Maki approach [13]. (Bottom row) Acquisition of NC and FC data at multiple diffusion and flow encoding strengths and subsequent joint analysis of the data sets with a ballistic IVIM model, that is, the Ahlgren approach [11]. Whereas the Nalcioglu–Ahn and Maki approaches tend to generate similar perfusion maps, the Ahlgren approach produces a considerably different contrast pattern.

Acknowledgment

This work was supported by the Swedish Research Council (Grant 2017-00995).

References

1. Le Bihan D., Breton E., Lallemand D., Grenier P., Cabanis E., Laval-Jeantet M. MR imaging of intravoxel incoherent motions: application to diffusion and perfusion in neurologic disorders. *Radiology* 161, 401–407, 1986.
2. Le Bihan D., Breton E., Lallemand D., Aubin M. L., Vignaud J., Laval-Jeantet M. Separation of diffusion and perfusion in intravoxel incoherent motion MR imaging. *Radiology* 168, 497–505, 1988.
3. Li T., Kheifets S., Medellin D., Raizen M. G. Measurement of the instantaneous velocity of a Brownian particle. *Science* 328, 1673–1675, 2010.
4. Kennan R. P., Gao J. H., Zhong J., Gore J. C. A general model of microcirculatory blood flow effects in gradient sensitized MRI. *Med. Phys.* 21, 539–545, 1994.
5. Nalcioglu O., Cho Z. H., Xiang Q. S., Ahn C. B. Incoherent flow imaging. *Proc. SPIE* 671, 285–289, 1986.
6. Ahn C. B., Lee S. Y., Nalcioglu O., Cho Z. H. The effects of random directional distributed flow in nuclear magnetic resonance imaging. *Med. Phys.* 14, 43–48, 1987.
7. Callaghan P. T., Xia Y. Velocity and diffusion imaging in dynamic NMR microscopy. *J. Magn. Reson.* 91, 326–352, 1991.
8. Callaghan P. T., Stepišnik J. Generalized analysis of motion using magnetic field gradients. *Adv. Magn. Opt. Reson.* 19, 325–388, 1996.
9. Caprihan A., Fukushima E. Flow measurements by NMR. *Phys. Rep.*198, 195–235, 1990.
10. Shemesh N., Jespersen S. N., Alexander D. C., Cohen Y., Drobnjak I., Dyrby T. B., et al. Conventions and nomenclature for double diffusion encoding NMR and MRI. *Magn. Reson. Med.* 75, 82–87, 2016.
11. Ahlgren A., Knutsson L., Wirestam R., Nilsson M., Ståhlberg F., Topgaard D., et al. Quantification of microcirculatory parameters by joint analysis of flow-compensated and non-flow-compensated motion-sensitized MRI data. *NMR Biomed.* 29, 640–649, 2016.

12. Fujita N., Harada K., Sakurai K., Akai Y., Kozuka T. Separation of diffusion and slow flow effects by use of flow rephasing and dephasing. *Magn. Reson. Med.* 24, 109–122, 1992.

13. Maki J. H., MacFall J. R., Johnson G. A. The use of gradient flow compensation to separate diffusion and microcirculatory flow in MRI. *Magn. Reson. Med.* 17, 95–107, 1991.

14. Itoh Y., Suzuki N. Control of brain capillary blood flow. *J. Cereb. Blood. Flow. Metab.* 32, 1167–1176, 2012.

15. Wetscherek A., Stieltjes B., Laun F. B. Flow-compensated intravoxel incoherent motion diffusion imaging. *Magn. Reson. Med.* 74, 410–419, 2015.

Chapter 21

Flow Compensation and Modeling of IVIM MRI in the Liver and Pancreas

Andreas Wetscherek
Joint Department of Physics, Institute of Cancer Research, 15 Cotswold Rd, Sutton, Surrey, SM2 5NG, United Kingdom
andreas.wetscherek@icr.ac.uk

The combined use of flow-compensated and non-flow-compensated gradients in diffusion weighted MRI—aiming at separate characterization of diffusion and perfusion—is a natural choice from the perspective of Le Bihan's original work [1]. In this chapter a brief history of flow-compensated IVIM in liver and pancreas is presented and the mathematical theory necessary to measure the characteristic timescale of the incoherent blood motion is derived. Experimental results indicate that the IVIM signal in the strongly perfused organs liver and pancreas cannot be fully understood within the commonly assumed pseudodiffusion limit and is closer to the microcirculatory straight-flow limit discussed in Ref. [2].

Intravoxel Incoherent Motion (IVIM) MRI: Principles and Applications
Edited by Denis Le Bihan, Mami Iima, Christian Federau, and Eric E. Sigmund

ISBN 978-981-4800-19-8 (Hardcover), 978-0-429-42727-5 (eBook)
www.panstanford.com

21.1 Introduction: History and Rationale of Flow-Compensated IVIM in Strongly Perfused Organs

"What is the characteristic timescale of the incoherent blood motion?" was the fundamental research question driving the work on IVIM in the group of Frederik Laun at the German Cancer Research Center (DKFZ) Heidelberg. Inspired by temporal diffusion spectroscopy [3], the first attempt to measure the characteristic timescale τ of the incoherent motion was to probe the perfusion spectrum $D^*(\omega)$ with oscillating gradients. The core idea here is to rewrite the signal attenuation of the perfusion compartment as an integral over the product of gradient spectrum $S(\omega)$ and perfusion spectrum (Eq. 21.1). For details regarding this formalism see Ref. [4].

$$\exp(-bD^*) \rightarrow \exp\left(-\frac{\gamma^2}{2\pi}\int_{-\infty}^{\infty} D^*(\omega)S(\omega)\,d\omega\right) \tag{21.1}$$

On the basis of Kennan's derivation of the IVIM velocity autocorrelation function [5], τ could be characterized by the width of the central peak of $D^*(\omega)$, which can be probed using sine and (flow-compensated) cosine gradients with different oscillation frequencies ω_0 (Fig. 21.1). It becomes apparent that this method is most sensitive for $\tau\omega_0 < 2\pi$, which is equivalent to $T_0 > \tau$, with T_0 denoting the oscillation period. As experimental results shown later in this chapter reveal, the characteristic timescale τ for pancreas and liver is of the order of a typical diffusion experiment, which would make very long echo times necessary to fit in several periods of oscillating diffusion gradients.

The pursued solution was to effectively reduce the number of oscillations to 1 and rectify the waveform for increased diffusion weighting, which yielded the well-known Stejskal–Tanner [6] and the flow-compensated field even-echo refocusing (FEER) [7] waveform as the limits of sine and cosine, respectively. The first flow-compensated in vivo diffusion images of the abdomen must be attributed to Ahn et al., who calculated a difference image between those diffusion weightings, which was "believed to correspond to the capillary density map" [8]. Further analysis was performed by Maki et al., who detected perfusion changes in the rat brain with

10% CO_2 ventilation on the normalized difference image between flow-compensated and Stejskal–Tanner diffusion weighting [9]. Initial results obtained by combining those two diffusion weightings with echo-planar imaging showed a large signal difference in liver and pancreas between flow-compensated and non-flow-compensated gradients [10] but also revealed the susceptibility of the FEER diffusion-weighting scheme for artifacts originating from concomitant fields [11].

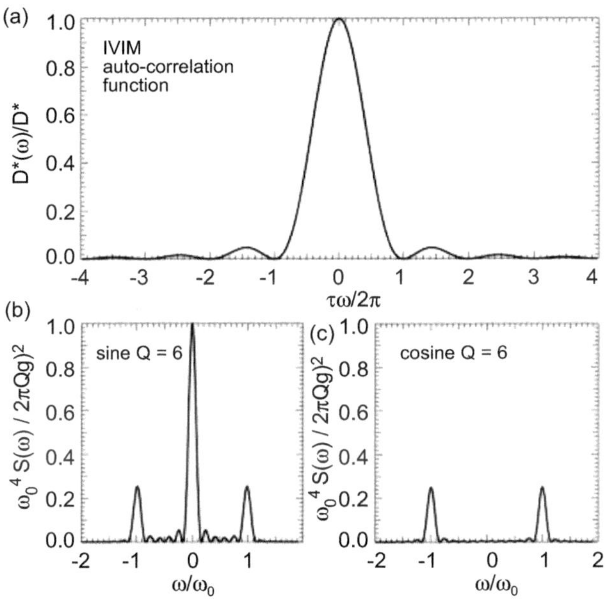

Figure 21.1 (a) IVIM autocorrelation function (perfusion spectrum) according to Ref. [5] and normalized gradient spectrum $S(\omega)$ for (b) sine and (c) cosine diffusion weighting with Q = 6 oscillations, oscillation frequency ω_0, and gradient amplitude g.

By introducing a flow-compensated diffusion weighting, which could be placed symmetrically around a refocusing pulse, concomitant field artifacts were effectively suppressed [12]. Figure 21.2 shows the symmetric monopolar and flow-compensated diffusion-weighting profiles and the definition of the diffusion time T used in this chapter. Being second-order motion compensated, the symmetric flow-compensated profile was adopted in cardiac diffusion tensor imaging [13]. It allows for higher b values within the same preparation time than the M1M2 diffusion preparation introduced by Nguyen et al. [14].

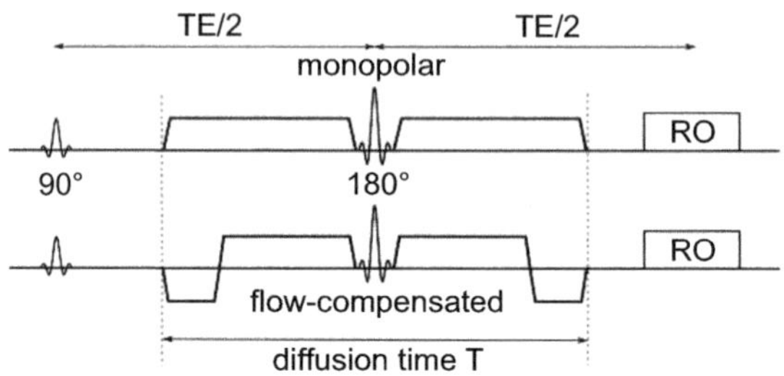

Figure 21.2 Symmetric monopolar and flow-compensated diffusion gradients and definition of the diffusion time *T* used in this chapter.

21.2 Theory

We start from the well-known IVIM signal equation (21.2),

$$S(b) = S_0\left[(1-f)e^{-bD} + fe^{-bD_b}F(b,T,v,\tau)\right], \qquad (21.2)$$

in which the attenuation of the tissue compartment with the fraction $(1 - f)$ is described by the tissue's apparent diffusion coefficient D. The perfusion compartment with the signal fraction f is attenuated both due to self-diffusion with the apparent diffusion coefficient of blood D_b and due to perfusion. While it was recently shown that the measured D_b depends on the hematocrit and the applied gradient waveform (because of a heavy exchange between red blood cells and plasma) [15], the attenuation F caused by blood flow is the focus of this theory section. For a more detailed derivation, the reader is directed to Refs. [12, 16].

In diffusion-weighted MRI, signal attenuation is caused by dephasing due to motion during the diffusion-weighting gradients. The signal attenuation F is therefore given by the phase distribution $\rho(\phi)$:

$$F = \left|\langle e^{i\phi}\rangle\right| = \left|\int_{-\infty}^{\infty}\rho(\phi)e^{i\phi}d\phi\right| = \left|\int_{-\infty}^{\infty}\rho(\vartheta)e^{i\bar{v}\sqrt{bT}\vartheta}d\vartheta\right| \qquad (21.3)$$

Realizing that the accumulated phase ϕ scales with flow speed and gradient amplitude, a "normalized phase" ϑ was introduced

[12], which is related to ϕ via $\phi = \bar{v}\sqrt{bT}\,\vartheta$, where $\bar{v}$ denotes the average blood flow velocity. It is left as an exercise to the reader to show that in this formalism a Gaussian distribution with $N = T/\tau$ corresponding to the number of directional changes during the diffusion experiment recovers the pseudodiffusion limit (Eq. 21.4a) and a uniform distribution with the width $1/\sqrt{3}$ represents straight flow (Eq. 21.4b), as discussed in Ref. [2]:

$$\rho(\vartheta)=\sqrt{\frac{3N}{2\pi}}e^{-3N\vartheta^2/2}\xrightarrow{\text{yields}}F=e^{-b\frac{\tau v^2}{6}}=e^{-bD^*} \tag{21.4a}$$

$$\rho(\vartheta)=\frac{1}{\sqrt{3}}\theta\left(\frac{\sqrt{3}}{2}-|\vartheta|\right)\xrightarrow{\text{yields}}F=\operatorname{sinc}\left(\frac{\sqrt{3}}{2}\sqrt{bT}\cdot\bar{v}\right) \tag{21.4b}$$

In Eq. 21.4b the Heaviside function $\theta(x)$ was employed. For an idealized monopolar (two-lobe) diffusion-weighting profile with a b value = $\gamma^2 g^2 T^3/12$ and a first gradient moment $m_1 = \gamma g T^2/4$, the signal attenuation matches $F = \operatorname{sinc}(m_1 \cdot v)$, reproducing the result of Ref. [2]. In the following an approach to obtain the phase distributions between those limits is described, which enables calculation of the signal attenuation F for arbitrary gradient profiles and any number of directional changes N. We study the phase ϕ_k accumulated by a particular isochromat traveling the path $\mathbf{r}_k(t)$ during application of the gradient $\mathbf{g}(t)$:

$$\phi_k=\gamma\int_0^T \mathbf{r}_k(t)\cdot\mathbf{g}(t)dt=\int_0^T \mathbf{v}_k(t)\cdot\mathbf{m}_0(t)dt \tag{21.5}$$

One way to obtain the distribution of the phase ϕ_k is the Monte Carlo simulation of a large number of particle trajectories. With the computing power available on a workstation, it is straightforward to calculate the signal attenuation F for a particular diffusion gradient profile and particle trajectories $\mathbf{v}_k(t)$, assuming, for example, a certain flow speed $\bar{v}$ and directionality with respect to the orientation of the diffusion gradients. The IVIM case is modeled by directional change of $\mathbf{v}_k(t)$ after the characteristic time τ is passed. However, this method would not be suited to perform pixel-wise fits of the parameters $\bar{v}$ and τ describing the trajectories, because a repetition of the complete Monte Carlo simulation would be required for a change in either of those parameters.

This is where the concept of "normalized phase distributions" shines. Typically, the effective gradient profile $\mathbf{g}^*(t)$ can be expressed as in Eq. 21.6 by a scaled normalized profile $h(s)$, with $s \in (0,1)$ and $|h(s)| \leq 1$ and a fixed axis $\hat{\mathbf{e}}_{\mathrm{g}}$:

$$\mathbf{g}^*(t) = gh\left(\frac{T}{\tau}\right)\hat{\mathbf{e}}_{\mathrm{g}} \tag{21.6}$$

In this case simplifications are possible because the phase acquired along a particular path with the mean velocity $\bar{v}$ and characteristic timescale τ scales according to the scaling Eq. 21.7:

$$\phi_{\mathrm{k}}(b,T,\bar{v},\tau) = \bar{v}\sqrt{bT}\vartheta\left(\frac{T}{\tau}\right) \tag{21.7}$$

This makes the phase distributions for a given temporal gradient profile $h(s)$ and a particular distribution of velocity directions universal, that is, only dependent on the ratio T/τ. Once $\rho(\vartheta,N)$ is known for a sufficient number of different N, calculation of the signal and fitting of the parameters $\bar{v}$ and τ becomes possible. In standard IVIM modeling, no directional preference is assumed. If the flow speed in successive vessel segments is assumed constant and the orientations of the different vessel segments are furthermore assumed uncorrelated, analytical expressions for $\rho(\vartheta,N)$ can be derived for $N \in (0,1)$ [12]. Normalized phase distributions for the gradient profiles shown in Fig. 21.2 are displayed in Fig. 21.3. The phase distributions and volunteer imaging data shown here are available online (https://github.com/awetscherek/ivim_tools).

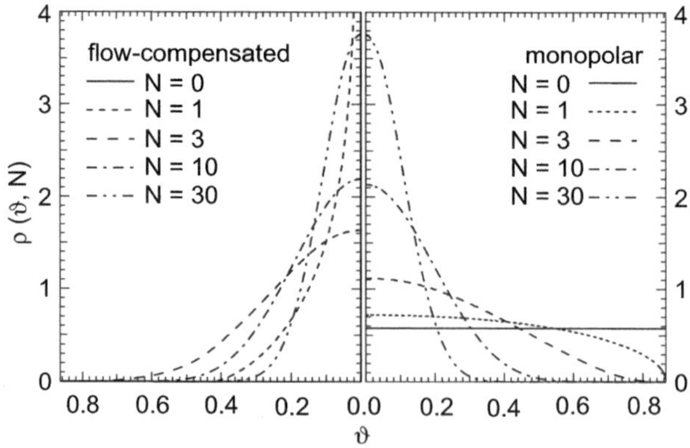

Figure 21.3 Normalized phase distributions for idealized symmetric flow-compensated and monopolar diffusion profiles with different ratios $N = T/\tau$.

21.3 Experimental Results

In Fig. 21.4 typical signal attenuation curves within a region of interest in the healthy human liver are displayed (volunteer no. 6 of the above-mentioned online data set). The data was acquired in a single-shot spin-echo diffusion weighted echo-planar imaging experiment with repeated voluntary breath hold in exhalation. Both monopolar and flow-compensated diffusion weighting were applied with diffusion times T = 40 ms, 70 ms, and 100 ms, while the echo time was kept constant at TE = 120 ms. For more details on the acquisition see Ref. [12]. Flow-compensated diffusion signals were less attenuated than monopolar ones, where the attenuation of the flow-compensated diffusion signal at a fixed b value increased with the diffusion time T. While for each different diffusion weighting, the attenuation curve could be fitted by a biexponential decay, the parameters would be different. Kuai et al. further analyzed this data set and found that the flow-compensated data are described by smaller f and D^* values than the monopolar data and that within the flow-compensated data f and D^* increased with T [17]. This observation would suggest that the pseudodiffusion limit ($N > \sim 7$ according to Ref. [2]) is not reached in liver and pancreas. On the other hand, the straight-flow limit ($N = 0$) doesn't characterize the data well, either, as flow-compensated schemes ($m_1 = 0$) should yield the same signal attenuation for the perfusion compartment according to Eq. 21.4. With the concept of normalized phase distributions, it is possible to fit Eq. 21.2 to the data, with F given by Eq. 21.3. All experimental data points can be described by a four-parameter model (D, f, τ, and v), in which the perfusion compartment is characterized by the two "microscopic" parameters v and τ. After denoising is performed, parameter maps can be obtained via a pixel-wise fit (Fig. 21.5). In addition to the D and f maps, which can also be obtained from a biexponential fit to conventional diffusion-weighted images, the τ and v maps, which contain information on the microvasculature, are only accessible using flow-compensated IVIM imaging.

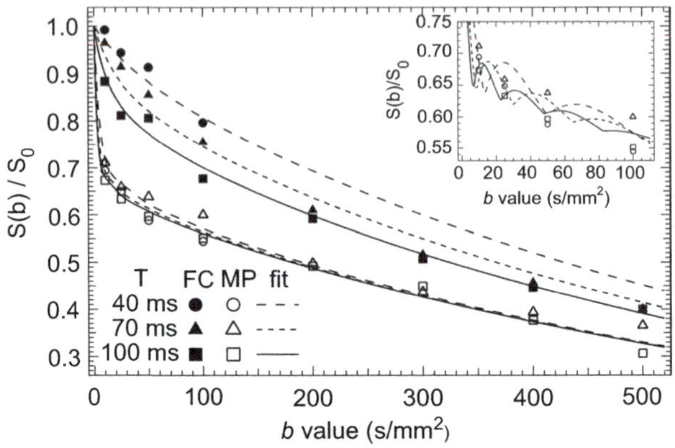

Figure 21.4 Diffusion signal attenuation measured in the liver of a healthy volunteer with monopolar (MP) and flow-compensated (FC) gradient profiles of different duration *T*. If only a single flow velocity is assumed, oscillations in the monopolar signal attenuation increase the amount of local minima of the fit-function (insert). If a velocity distribution is assumed, for example, a parabolic (laminar) flow profile, the characteristic timescale and the mean velocity can be determined. These experimental data are best described by the model parameters $D = 1.34 \pm 0.06$ μm²/ms, $f = 0.36 \pm 0.01$, $\tau = 107 \pm 7$ ms, and $v = 5.3 \pm 0.2$ m/s.

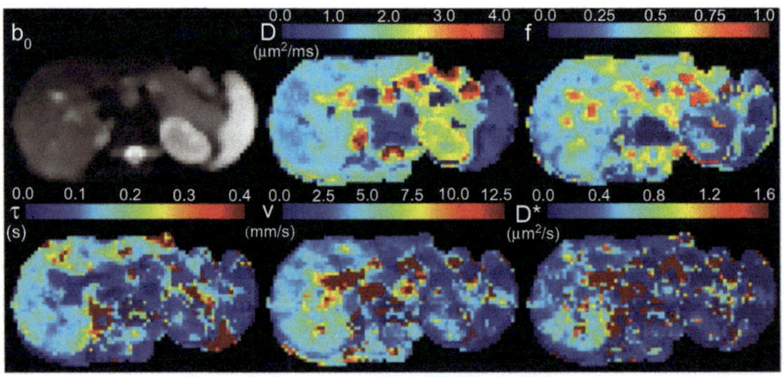

Figure 21.5 Parameter maps obtained by a pixel-wise fit of the flow-compensated IVIM data acquired in a healthy volunteer. Noise was reduced by applying a median filter (see the unweighted b0 image), and regions with a too-low SNR or motion were masked out. "Macroscopic" IVIM parameters (*D* and *f*) can be obtained by a standard biexponential fit, but the microscopic parameters (τ and *v*) are only accessible with flow-compensated diffusion gradients. D^* was calculated using the microscopic definition of $D^* = \tau v^2/6$ explaining the larger values compared to conventional biexponential fits, where the Gaussian phase approximation leads to an underestimation of the product $\tau v^2/6$ by the fitted D^* [12].

21.4 Discussion

The concept of using flow-compensated diffusion-weighted gradients to characterize IVIM has the potential to reveal additional information on microvasculature, which might be of particular interest for applications in oncology. Using standard IVIM diffusion MRI in pancreatic cancer, "the added value of fitting D^* was considered limited" in a recent publication [18] and a least-squares fit with a fixed value of D^*, as already suggested by Lemke et al. [19] performed similarly to a Bayesian fit. Poor reproducibility of f and, in particular, D^* has limited wide clinical application of the biexponential IVIM model fit even in the strongly perfused abdominal organs [20]. Though abdominal diffusion-weighted MRI can reveal early changes induced by antivascular treatment, with a stretched exponential model being found most sensitive, changes in the most descriptive parameters could not be related to particular tissue changes [21]. While the parameters v and τ in the flow-compensated IVIM model are directly related to properties of the microvasculature, the protocol presented in Ref. [12] is challenging to apply clinically because of the long acquisition time and multiple breath holds. Apart from devising a suitable management strategy for respiratory motion, the high coefficients of variation currently still present in abdominal flow-compensated IVIM data might also be related to other sources. The effect of the cardiac cycle, which was shown to affect IVIM measurements in the brain [22], needs to be investigated, as it might compromise the joint evaluation of flow-compensated IVIM data acquired in subsequent breath holds. An interesting approach to characterize IVIM employing (flow-compensated) oscillating gradients was presented by Wu et al. [23], but its application might be restricted to preclinical MRI scanners and might not be suitable for abdominal imaging due to the gradient hardware requirements to achieve sufficient diffusion weighting.

There are still many open research questions to address within the young field of flow-compensated IVIM imaging in pancreas and liver. The additional sensitivity to the circulating blood signal is metaphorically opening Pandora's IVIM box: the exchange between blood compartments, the signal dependence on blood parameters [15], self-diffusion of blood, and contribution from vessels at different branching levels could all potentially affect the measured diffusion-weighted signal. The hope remains that though the higher sensitivity is complicating the problem, it could lead to new insight, which in turn requires appropriate modeling. It is possible that descriptive parameters, which are not directly related to tissue properties, such as diffusional kurtosis or parameters similar to α in the stretched exponential model, need to be employed to robustly characterize the flow-compensated diffusion-weighted signal. Machine learning approaches could help, which have recently been applied successfully to IVIM [24]. To further increase our understanding of abdominal flow-compensated IVIM, studies that include histopathological correlation would be of great value.

References

1. Le Bihan D., Breton E., Lallemand D., Grenier P., Cabanis E., Laval-Jeantet M. MR imaging of intravoxel incoherent motions: application to diffusion and perfusion in neurologic disorders. *Radiology* 161, 401–407, 1986.
2. Le Bihan D., Breton E., Lallemand D., Aubin M. L., Vignaud J., Laval-Jeantet M. Separation of diffusion and perfusion in intravoxel incoherent motion MR imaging. *Radiology* 168, 497–505, 1988.
3. Gore J. C., Xu J., Colvin D. C., Yankeelov T. E., Parsons E. C., Does M. D. Characterization of tissue structures at varying length scales using temporal diffusion spectroscopy. *NMR Biomed.* 23, 745–756, 2010.
4. Stepišnik J. Analysis of NMR self-diffusion measurements by a density matrix calculation. *Physica* 104B, 350–364, 1981.
5. Kennan R. P., Gao J.-H., Zhong J., Gore J. C. A general model of microcirculatory blood flow effects in gradient sensitized MRI. *Med. Phys.* 21, 539–545, 1994.
6. Stejskal E. O., Tanner J. E. Spin diffusion measurements: Spin echoes in the presence of a time-dependent field gradient. *J. Chem. Phys.* 42, 288–292, 1965.
7. Simonetti O. P., Wendt III R. E., Duerk J. L. Significance of the point of expansion in interpretation of gradient moments and motion sensitivity. *J. Magn. Reson. Med.* 1, 569–577, 1991.
8. Ahn C. B., Lee S. Y., Nalcioglu O., Cho Z. H. The effects of random directional distributed flow in nuclear magnetic resonance imaging. *Med. Phys.* 14, 43–48, 1987.

9. Maki J. H., MacFall J. R., Johnson G. A. The use of gradient flow compensation to separate diffusion and microcirculatory flow in MRI. *Magn. Reson. Med.* 17, 95–107, 1991.

10. Wetscherek A., Stieltjes B., Semmler W., Laun F. B. Investigation of the theoretical background of the IVIM model using flow-compensated DWI, *Proc. ISMRM 19th Annual Meeting and Exhibition*, 2991, 2011.

11. Bernstein M. A., Zhou X. J., Polzin J. A., King K. F., Ganin, A. Pelc N. J., et al. Concomitant gradient terms in phase contrast MR: analysis and correction. *Magn. Reson. Med.* 39, 300–308, 1998.

12. Wetscherek A., Stieltjes B., Laun F. B. Flow-compensated intravoxel incoherent motion diffusion imaging. *Magn. Reson. Med.* 74, 410–419, 2015.

13. Stoeck C. T., von Deuster C., Genet M., Atkinson D., Kozerke S. Second-order motion-compensated spin echo diffusion tensor imaging of the human heart. *Magn. Reson. Med.* 75, 1669–1676, 2016.

14. Nguyen C., Fan Z., Sharif B., He Y., Dharmakumar R., Berman D. S., et al. In vivo three-dimensional high resolution cardiac diffusion-weighted MRI: A motion compensated diffusion-prepared balanced steady-state free precession approach. *Magn. Reson. Med.* 72, 1257–1267, 2014.

15. Funck C., Laun F. B., Wetscherek A. Characterization of the diffusion coefficient of blood. *Magn. Reson. Med.* 79, 2752–2758, 2018.

16. Wetscherek A. Magnetic resonance diffusion weighted imaging: Flow compensated intravoxel incoherent motion imaging as a tool to probe microvasculature (doctoral dissertation), German Cancer Research Center (DKFZ) Heidelberg, Germany, 2013, DOI: 10.11588/heidok.00015226.

17. Kuai Z.-X., Liu W.-L., Zhang Y.-L., Zhu Y.-M. Generalization of intravoxel incoherent motion by introducing the notion of continuous pseudodiffusion variable. *Magn. Reson. Med.* 76, 1594–1603, 2016.

18. Gurney-Champion O. J., Klaassen R., Froeling M., Barbieri S., Stoker J., Engelbrecht M. R. W., et al. Comparison of six fit algorithms for the intra-voxel incoherent motion model of diffusion-weighted magnetic resonance imaging data of pancreatic cancer patients. *Plos One* 13, e0194590, 2018.

19. Lemke A., Laun F. B., Klauß M., Re T. J., Simon D., Delorme S., Schad L. R., et al. Differentiation of pancreas carcinoma from healthy pancreatic tissue using multiple b-values: Comparison of apparent diffusion coefficient and intravoxel incoherent motion derived parameters. *Invest. Radiol.* 44, 769–775, 2009.

20. Koh D.-M. Science to practice: Can intravoxel incoherent motion diffusion-weighted MR imaging be used to assess tumor response to antivascular drugs? *Radiology* 272, 307–308, 2014.

21. Orton M. R., Messiou C., Collins D., Morgan V. A., Tessier J., Young H., et al. Diffusion-weighted MR imaging of metastatic abdominal and pelvic tumours is sensitive to early changes induced by a VEGF inhibitor using alternative diffusion attenuation models. *Eur. Radiol.* 26, 1412–1419, 2016.

22. Federau C., Hagman P., Maeder P., Müller M., Meuli R., Stuber M., O'Brien K. Dependence of brain intravoxel incoherent motion perfusion parameters on the cardiac cycle. *Plos One* 8, e72856, 2013.

23. Wu D., Zhang J. The effect of microcirculatory flow on oscillating gradient diffusion MRI and diffusion encoding with dual-frequency orthogonal gradients (DEFOG). *Magn. Reson. Med.* 77, 1583–1592, 2017.

24. Bertleff M., Domsch S., Weingärtner S., Zapp J., O'Brien K., Barth M., et al. Diffusion parameter mapping with the combined intravoxel incoherent motion and kurtosis model using artificial neural networks at 3T. *NMR Biomed.* 30, e3833, 2017.

Chapter 22

Perfusion Marries Diffusion: Arterial Spin Labeling Prepared IVIM

Xingxing Zhang[a] and Matthias J. P. van Osch[b]
[a]*Neusoft Medical Systems, Shanghai, China*
[b]*C. J. Gorter Center for High Field MRI, Dept. of Radiology, Leiden University Medical Center, Leiden, The Netherlands*
x.zhang.radi@gmail.com

22.1 Introduction

Noninvasive perfusion imaging can be achieved by two major magnetic resonance techniques: arterial spin labeling (ASL) [1–3] and intravoxel incoherent motion (IVIM) imaging [4, 5]. Whereas the first has been widely and successfully used in diverse brain applications, studies with IVIM imaging of the brain are scarcer. However, attention to IVIM has regained significant interest during the last decade [6–12]. The fact that application of IVIM in the brain is still lagging behind could be attributed to the small cerebral perfusion fraction, approximately 5% of the whole brain, resulting in a low signal-to-noise ratio (SNR) [8, 13].

Intravoxel Incoherent Motion (IVIM) MRI: Principles and Applications
Edited by Denis Le Bihan, Mami Iima, Christian Federau, and Eric E. Sigmund

ISBN 978-981-4800-19-8 (Hardcover), 978-0-429-42727-5 (eBook)
www.panstanford.com

This chapter will mainly focus on unraveling the signal origin of IVIM using ASL prepared IVIM (ASL-IVIM), and other applications of ASL-IVIM will be also discussed, for instance, water exchange measurement, arterial blood volume measurement, and microvascular flow pattern investigation.

The concept behind ASL-IVIM is relatively easy to understand: the ASL preparation module generates an endogenous tracer by inversion of the magnetization of arterial blood that will first fill up the arterial tree and then subsequently flow into the brain tissue, while the IVIM readout module monitors the diffusion properties of the tissues of interest using various motion-sensitizing gradient strengths. Marrying these two can exclusively limit the influence of the IVIM module to the contribution of the ASL signal, that is, the arterial compartment. By monitoring the ASL signal at multiple timepoints, the IVIM signal can be monitored within different parts of the vascular tree.

22.2 Unravel the Origin of the IVIM Signal

The basic assumption of IVIM is that the blood flow in capillaries, also known as cerebral perfusion, can be considered a pseudodiffusion process due to the random orientations of vessels at the capillary level of the vascular tree [5]. Traditionally, a two-compartment IVIM model is employed to separate the contribution of perfusion from diffusion effects: a slow compartment in which the signal decays slowly as a function of diffusion weighting (i.e., b value) and a fast compartment where the signal drops much faster as a function of the b value due to the faster-moving spins in the pseudorandom capillaries, that is, perfusion instead of diffusion. The main concern regarding the validity of this model is that a distribution of velocities as well as nonrandom orientations could result in a more complex relationship than the simple biexponential assumption. Doubts on the validity of the IVIM approach have arisen, for example, from the reported ratio of gray and white matter cerebral blood flow (CBF) with IVIM, which is frequently much lower compared to values obtained from other techniques (dynamic susceptibility contrast [DSC], ASL, O15-H_2O positron emission tomography [PET]) [7, 11, 14, 15]. To better understand the signal generation mechanisms of

IVIM, it is important to be able to exclusively measure the diffusion properties of the blood pool and to do this for different parts of the vascular tree. By employing ASL-IVIM the contribution of the arterial compartment can be isolated. The blood signal as a function of *b* values can be further investigated while the blood traverses through the different subparts of the vascular tree, by employing ASL at different delay times. Not only is this important for increasing our understanding of cerebral IVIM studies, it can also result in a wealth of information on the cerebral hemodynamics.

To achieve the goal of understanding the origin of the IVIM signal, an ASL-IVIM study was recently performed with T_1-adjusted time-encoded pseudocontinuous ASL (te-pCASL) as an ASL preparation in combination with a conventional IVIM readout (eight *b* values ranging from 0 to 168 s/mm^2 achieved by a 90° excitation pulse followed by a bipolar gradient with different gradient strengths) [16]. T_1-adjusted te-pCASL is a very efficient time method to acquire ASL data at multiple postlabeling delay (PLD) times [17, 18]. In te-pCASL, the traditional long labeling duration is divided into several short blocks (in this study 11; block duration values were adjusted to compensate for a T_1 decay of label for each specific block on the basis of an assumed T_1 of blood of 1650 ms, resulting in approximately similar SNRs for all blocks), whereas the label/control condition of each block is varied according to a Hadamard matrix encoding scheme (Fig. 22.1).

After Hadamard decoding, perfusion images can be reconstructed for all blocks that have similar SNRs to a traditional pCASL experiment, with the labeling duration equal to the duration of the specific labeling block, a PLD equal to the time between the end of the block and the start of the readout (Fig. 22.2), and an equal number of acquisitions (i.e., equal scan time when the repetition time (TR) of the sequence would be the same). The same decoding technique was performed for each of the *b* values.

The value of ASL-IVIM signals averaged over the whole brain gray matter mask was first fitted as a function of *b* value to a monoexponential model:

$$\mathrm{S(PLD}, \tau, b) / \mathrm{S0} = S_{\mathrm{ASL}}(\mathrm{PLD}, \tau) \cdot \exp(-b \cdot D^*)$$

$S_{\mathrm{ASL}}(\mathrm{PLD}, \tau)$ is the amplitude of the ASL signal without any diffusion weighting for a certain PLD and labeling duration of a block (τ). This model assumes that the entire all signal originates from the arterial compartment, that is, it reflects only the perfusion compartment of the IVIM model. However, labeled spins in ASL are known to cross the blood–brain barrier (BBB) almost unrestricted, and therefore one can expect that some of the signal of an ASL-IVIM experiment originates from the extravascular compartment.

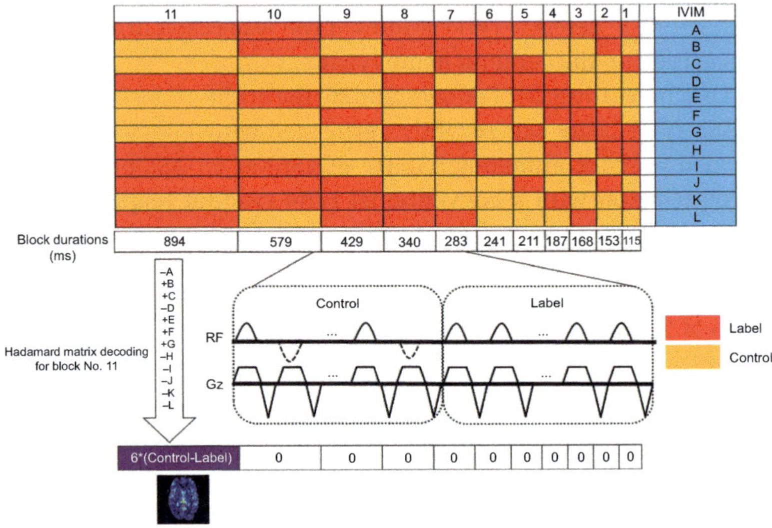

Figure 22.1 Sequence diagram of time-encoded pseudocontinuous arterial spin labeling IVIM (te-pCASL IVIM, order of Hadamard matrix: 12, labeling block duration of 894, 579, 429, 340, 283, 241, 211, 187, 168, 153, and 115 ms resulting in a total labeling duration of 3600 ms) and a Hadamard decoding scheme for a specific block (block number 11). The red and yellow blocks represent the label and control conditions, respectively. When applying this specific decoding scheme, for all blocks except block number 11, the contribution of a specific labeling (control) block is cancelled by the subtraction of the label (control) block of another line from the Hadamard acquisition, resulting in zero net signal. For the 11th block, a proper ASL signal is obtained (6*control–6*label).

To further distinguish the intravascular and extravascular contributions to the ASL signal, an alternative two-compartment, biexponential model can be employed:

$$S(\text{PLD},\tau,b) = S_{\text{ASL\_intra}}(\text{PLD},\tau)\cdot\exp(-b\cdot D_{\text{intra}}) + S_{\text{ASL\_extra}}(\text{PLD},\tau)\cdot\exp(-b\cdot D_{\text{extra}})$$

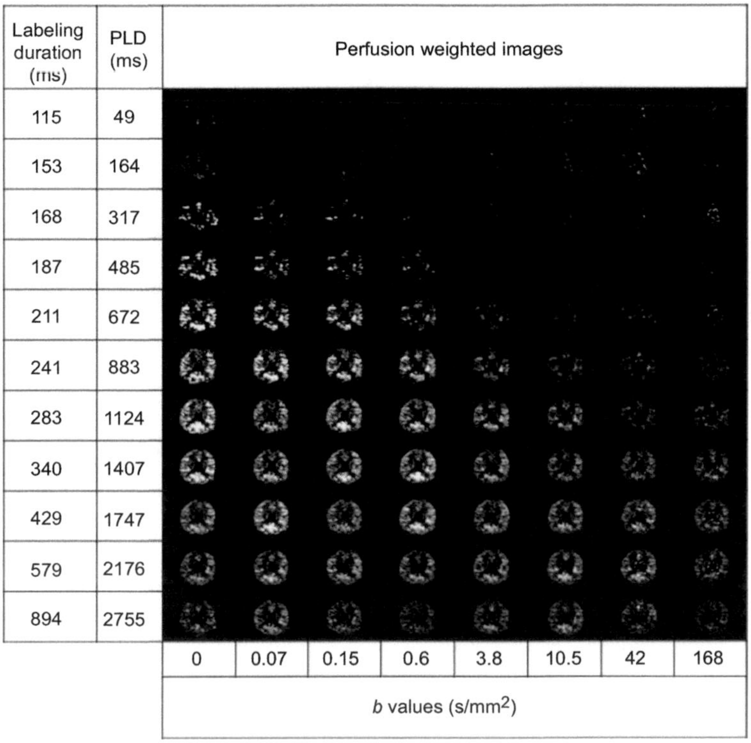

Figure 22.2 Hadamard-decoded, ASL prepared IVIM images for different PLDs and different *b* values. Reprinted from Ref. [16], with permission from John Wiley and Sons, copyright 2017.

Here, $S_{\text{ASL\_intra}}(\text{PLD}, \tau)$ and $S_{\text{ASL\_extra}}(\text{PLD}, \tau)$ are the amplitudes of the intravascular and extravascular ASL signals for a certain PLD and labeling duration (τ) without any diffusion weighting and D_{intra} and D_{extra} are the pseudodiffusion coefficients of the intravascular and extravascular compartments, respectively.

According to the results published by Zhang et al., the pseudodiffusion coefficient D^* as calculated from ASL-IVIM data using the monoexponential model was found to decrease exponentially for 883 ms < PLD < 2176 ms, while it was relatively stable for PLDs > 2176 ms (Fig. 22.3) [16]. The fast compartment of the conventional IVIM experiment showed comparable apparent diffusion values as the ASL signal with PLDs between 1747 ms and 2176 ms. Very high D^* values of 8 ~ 13 mm^2/s were observed for short PLDs, which can be explained by the fact that the ASL signal

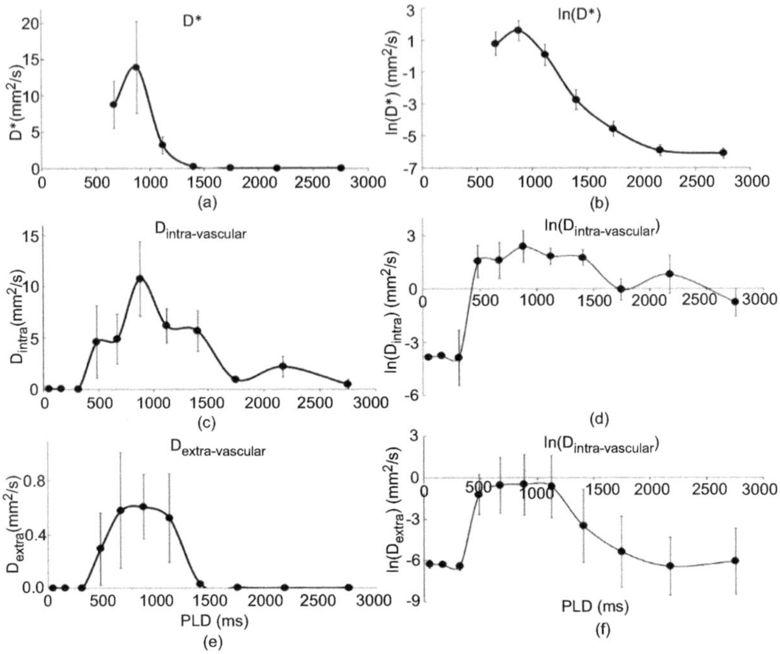

Figure 22.3 Pseudodiffusion coefficient D^* (a) and the natural logarithm of D^* (b) as obtained from the monoexponential fit to the ASL-IVIM data; D_{intra} (c), natural logarithm of $D_{\text{intravascular}}$ (d), $D_{\text{extravascular}}$ (e), and the natural logarithm of $D_{\text{extravascular}}$ (f) for different PLDs as obtained from the biexponential fit. The error bars represent the standard error of the mean values among the subjects. Reprinted from Ref. [16], with permission from John Wiley and Sons, copyright 2017.

was still present in larger arteries for these short PLDs. For longer PLDs the labeled blood travels further down the vascular tree, with D^* decreasing exponentially, suggesting that more and more of the ASL signal originates from the microvasculature or even originates from the extravascular compartment of the brain tissue. Finally, for the longest PLDs, that is, 2176 and 2755 ms, the D^* remains relatively stable, suggesting that the inverted spins have extravasated into the extravascular compartment, reflecting diffusion in tissue. To distinguish the intravascular and extravascular contributions of the ASL signal the two-compartment biexponential model was also applied. In general, the biexponential fitting was found to describe the ASL signal more accurately as a function of the b value. The averaged extravascular D at long PLDs (PLD > 2176 ms) was found to be ~$1.9 \pm 1.4 \times 10^{-3}$ mm^2/s, which is two times lower than the D^* using the monoexponential model (~$4.0 \pm 2.8 \times 10^{-3}$ mm^2/s). This lower value could be explained by the fact that the monoexponential model is indeed too simplified, resulting in a weighted average between diffusion properties of the intravascular and extravascular ASL signal. However, the $D_{extravascular}$ is still two times higher than the diffusion coefficient of the slow compartment ($0.90 \pm 0.05 \times 10^{-3}$ mm^2/s) of the conventional IVIM experiment, which might again indicate that the ASL signal does not exchange with the complete extravascular compartment but with only a subpart.

The comparison between the ASL-IVIM and conventional IVIM showed much more complicated diffusion properties of the vascular signal than the conventionally assumed single D^* of the perfusion compartment in the two-compartment model of IVIM. This should be taken into account when interpreting IVIM studies of the brain.

22.3 Vascular Water Exchange Measurement

More and more studies indicate that the exchange rate of water across the BBB could be a sensitive biomarker of subtle changes in BBB integrity [19–21]. Due to insufficient leakage of the contrast agent into the interstitial space, imaging using an exogenous contrast agent may not be adequate to detect such subtle changes of BBB permeability. Moreover, approaches monitoring the slow enhancement of tissue due to subtle BBB damage are time consuming because they involve dynamic scanning for 25 min. [19]. As illustrated in the previous paragraph, inclusion of motion-sensitizing gradients can provide information on the compartment of the ASL signal. Hence, an approach to ASL-IVIM, commonly referred to as diffusion-weighted ASL (DWASL), was proposed by Silva et al. [22] and subsequently applied by St. Lawrence et al. [23] and Wang et al. [24] to measure vascular water exchange and quantify water permeability both in rats and in humans. DWASL employs an ASL preparation module followed by a spin-echo diffusion-weighted imaging module. The basic assumption is that by combining diffusion and perfusion techniques, ASL contributions from the capillary space and the tissue space can be differentiated due to different sensitivities to the flow velocity of the blood spins.

After analysis of the diffusion characteristics of the arterial blood in the brain, the extraction fraction of arterial blood water or the relative amount of labeled water in the tissue compartment can be estimated. By using, for example, the single-pass approximation model the water permeability can subsequently be estimated on the basis of the derived relative water fractions in the tissue and microvasculature [24–26].

22.4 Arterial Blood Volume Measurement

An approach similar to ASL-IVIM was adopted by Duong and Kim [27], who, instead of using arterial blood as the endogenous tracer, injected perfluorocarbon 19F as an intravascular tracer to measure the diffusion properties of the arterial and venous blood volume compartments in rats. Marrying 19F inversion recovery with the IVIM readout can help resolve regional arterial and venous blood volume on the basis of pseudodiffusion coefficients (high in the fast compartment but low in the slow compartment) or T_1 components (shorter T_1 with high oxygenation in the fast compartment and longer T_1 with low oxygenation in the slow compartment). The ASL-IVIM methods were further employed to measure arterial blood volume in rats by Kim and Kim [28] using the arterial blood as an endogenous tracer. Similar to other studies, their hypothesis is that arterial blood is the major signal source of the fast compartment in ASL-IVIM measurements. Thus, arterial CBV can be measured by incorporating the IVIM diffusion gradient suppressing the signal originating from the arterial vasculature. The arterial CBV measurement by ASL-IVIM was subsequently validated through a comparison with other arterial CBV measurements; for instance, arterial blood signals can be separated from the tissue signals using magnetization transfer (MT) saturation to selectively reduce the tissue signals.

22.5 Cerebral Microvascular Flow Patterns Investigation

A recent study by Wells et al. [29] applied motion-sensitizing gradients in three directions in an ASL-IVIM technique to investigate cerebral microvascular flow patterns in rats ("perfusion tensor imaging"), showing that ASL-IVIM has the ability to capture important information on the architecture of the microvascular bed. The ASL preparation, in combination with multidirectional IVIM readout, was employed to map the microvascular architecture in a way similar to the traditional white matter fiber-tracking technique, except the signal will exclusively arise from the microvasculature.

22.6 Other ASL Techniques Similar to IVIM

Intrinsically, IVIM uses motion-sensitizing gradients to detect moving spins and separates the different compartments on the basis of their mobility. Instead of ASL techniques that label arterial blood spatially below the imaging volume within the feeding arteries, some new ASL techniques have been proposed that label spins globally, that is, also within the imaging volume, on the basis of blood flow velocity (velocity-selective ASL, VSASL [30, 31]) or acceleration (acceleration-selective ASL, AccASL [32, 33]). Because they label on the basis of arterial blood mobility, these spatial nonselective ASL techniques can be considered very similar to IVIM. VSASL preparation is achieved by a 90° pulse followed by a couple of adiabatic 180° refocusing pulses surrounded by gradients with a net zero moment, resulting in dephasing of fast-moving spins above an encoding cutoff velocity. Finally, the magnetization is flipped back by means of a –90° radio frequency (RF) pulse. For the control condition, no motion-sensitizing gradients are used within the VS module. Labeling on the basis of blood velocity tags not only arterial blood but also venous blood. To avoid overestimation of perfusion by the contribution of venous blood, a second VSASL module (with motion encoding gradients for both the label and control acquisition) is applied after a PLD of 1–2 s, right before imaging. Since venous spins will have accelerated between the two velocity-selective preparation modules, they will be suppressed [34]. AccASL uses a similar strategy to label the blood, but by inducing dephasing for spins that are accelerating or decelerating [32]. By setting the cutoff velocities, you can depict the signals from different subparts of the vascular tree. Due to the inconsistent existence of motion-sensitizing gradients for the control and label condition, differences in diffusion can also result in a signal difference between label and control images and therefore lead to a bias in the perfusion quantification. New developments have been proposed to improve the SNR and eliminate the diffusion effects in the VSASL, for instance, by VS inversion ASL that will invert the moving spins instead of saturating these spins by employing a composite pules train [35]. These new developments in VSASL can further enhance our understanding of IVIM and together they could provide a wealth of information on the microvascular blood flow.

22.7 Conclusion

As a future eventuality the development of more complex models for IVIM can be envisioned that take the various velocities and nonrandom directions of blood flow in the different subparts of the capillary tree into account or, even more interestingly, try to extract this information and other information, such as tortuosity, from an ASL-IVIM experiment to provide more information on the microvascular architecture. Furthermore, ASL-IVIM can be used to distinguish between spin compartments by combining the current approach with a TRUST module to measure the T_2 of the ASL signal [36, 37]. Similarly, mirroring the method of diffusion MRI–based fiber tracking [38], directional tracking on the fast diffusion compartment could enable visualizing the microvascular structure in the brain [29]. Therefore, a bold prediction is that ASL prepared tensor imaging may be able to map the structure of the whole vascular tree as well as probe its microvascular characteristics.

References

1. Williams D. S., Detre J. A., Leigh J. S., Koretsky A. P. Magnetic resonance imaging of perfusion using spin inversion of arterial water. *Proc. Natl. Acad. Sci. U. S. A.* 89, 212–216, 1992.

2. Detre J. A., Leigh J. S., Williams D. S., Koretsky A. P. Perfusion imaging. *Magn. Reson. Med.* 23, 37–45, 1992. doi: 10.1002/mrm.1910230106.

3. Alsop D. C., Detre J. A., Golay X., et al. Recommended implementation of arterial spin-labeled perfusion MRI for clinical applications: A consensus of the ISMRM perfusion study group and the European

consortium for ASL in dementia. *Magn. Reson. Med.*, 2014. doi: 10.1002/mrm.25197.

4. Le Bihan D., Breton E., Lallemand D., Grenier P., Cabanis E., Laval-Jeantet M. MR imaging of IVIM: application to diffusion and perfusion in neurologic disorders. *Radiology* 161, 401–407, 1986.
5. Le Bihan D., Breton E., Lallemand D., Aubin M. L., Vignaud J., Laval-Jeantet M. Separation of diffusion and perfusion in intravoxel incoherent motion MR imaging. *Radiology* 168, 497–505, 1988.
6. Federau C., Meuli R., O'Brien K., Maeder P., Hagmann P. Perfusion measurement in brain gliomas with intravoxel incoherent motion MRI. *AJNR. Am. J. Neuroradiol.* 35, 256–262, 2014. doi: 10.3174/ajnr.A3686.
7. Federau C., Sumer S., Becce F., Maeder P., O'Brien K., Meuli R., et al. Intravoxel incoherent motion perfusion imaging in acute stroke: initial clinical experience. *Neuroradiology* 56, 629–635, 2014. doi: 10.1007/s00234-014-1370-y.
8. Federau C., Maeder P, O'Brien K., Browaeys P., Meuli R., Hagmann P. Quantitative measurement of brain perfusion with intravoxel incoherent motion MR imaging. *Radiology* 265, 874–881, 2012.
9. Federau C., Maeder P., Brien K. O., Browaeys P., Klarhoefer M., Meuli R., et al. Validation of quantitative human brain perfusion measurement with intravoxel incoherent motion (IVIM), with a hypercapnia and hyperoxygenation challenge. *Proc. Intl. Soc. Mag. Reson. Med.* 20, 2012.
10. Federau C., O'Brien K. Increased brain perfusion contrast with T_2-prepared intravoxel incoherent motion ($T_{2\text{prep}}$ IVIM) MRI. *NMR Biomed.* 28, 9–16, 2015. doi: 10.1002/nbm.3223.
11. Federau C., O'Brien K., Meuli R., Hagmann P., Maeder P. Measuring brain perfusion with intravoxel incoherent motion (IVIM): initial clinical experience. *J. Magn. Reson. Imaging* 39, 624–632, 2014. doi: 10.1002/jmri.24195.
12. Rydhög A. S., van Osch M. J. P., Lindgren E., Nilsson M., Lätt J., Ståhlberg F., et al. Intravoxel incoherent motion (IVIM) imaging at different magnetic field strengths: what is feasible? *Magn. Reson. Imaging* 32, 1247–1258, 2014. doi: 10.1016/j.mri.2014.07.013.
13. Lu H., Law M., Johnson G., Ge Y., van Zijl P. C. M., Helpern J. A. Novel approach to the measurement of absolute cerebral blood volume using vascular-space-occupancy magnetic resonance imaging. *Magn. Reson. Med.* 54, 1403–1411, 2005. doi: 10.1002/mrm.20705.
14. Wang L., Lin J., Liu K., Chen C., Liu H., Lv P., et al. Intravoxel incoherent motion diffusion-weighted MR imaging in differentiation of lung

cancer from obstructive lung consolidation: comparison and correlation with pharmacokinetic analysis from dynamic contrast-enhanced MR imaging. *Eur. Radiol.* 24, 1914–1922, 2014. doi: 10.1007/s00330-014-3176-z.

15. Wu W.-C., Chen Y.-F., Tseng H.-M., Yang S.-C., My P.-C. Caveat of measuring perfusion indexes using intravoxel incoherent motion magnetic resonance imaging in the human brain. *Eur. Radiol.*, 2015. doi: 10.1007/s00330-015-3655-x.
16. Zhang X., Ingo C., Teeuwisse W. M., Chen Z., van Osch M. J. P. Comparison of perfusion signal acquired by arterial spin labeling–prepared intravoxel incoherent motion (IVIM) MRI and conventional IVIM MRI to unravel the origin of the IVIM signal. *Magn. Reson. Med.* 79, 723–729, 2018. doi: 10.1002/mrm.26723.
17. Gunther M. Highly efficient accelerated acquisition of perfusion inflow series by cycled arterial spin labeling. In: *Proceedings of the 15th Annual Meeting of ISMRM*. Berlin, Germany, 2007.
18. Teeuwisse W. M., Schmid S., Ghariq E., Veer I. M., van Osch M. J. Time-encoded pseudocontinuous arterial spin labeling: Basic properties and timing strategies for human applications. *Magn Reson Med*, 2014. doi: 10.1002/mrm.25083.
19. Kim Y. R., Tejima E., Huang S., Atochin D. N., Dai G., Lo E. H., et al. In vivo quantification of transvascular water exchange during the acute phase of permanent stroke. *Magn. Reson. Med.* 60, 813–821, 2008. doi: 10.1002/mrm.21708.
20. Starr J. M., Farrall A. J., Armitage P., McGurn B., Wardlaw J. Blood-brain barrier permeability in Alzheimer's disease: a case-control MRI study. *Psychiatry Res.* 171, 232–241, 2009. doi: 10.1016/j.pscychresns.2008.04.003.
21. Paulson O. Blood–brain barrier, brain metabolism and cerebral blood flow. *Eur. Neuropsychopharmacol.* 12, 495–501, 2002. doi: 10.1016/S0924-977X(02)00098-6.
22. Silva A. C., Williams D. S., Koretsky A. P. Evidence for the exchange of arterial spin-labeled water with tissue water in rat brain from diffusion-sensitized measurements of perfusion. *Magn. Reson. Med.* 38, 232–237, 1997. doi: 10.1002/mrm.1910380211.
23. St Lawrence K. S., Owen D., Wang D. J. J. A two-stage approach for measuring vascular water exchange and arterial transit time by diffusion-weighted perfusion MRI. *Magn. Reson. Med.* 67, 1275–1284, 2012. doi: 10.1002/mrm.23104.

24. Wang J., Fernández-Seara M. A., Wang S., Lawrence K. S. S. When perfusion meets diffusion: in vivo measurement of water permeability in human brain. *J. Cereb. Blood Flow Metab.* 27, 839–849, 2007. doi: 10.1038/sj.jcbfm.9600398.

25. St Lawrence K. S., Frank J. A., McLaughlin A. C. Effect of restricted water exchange on cerebral blood flow values calculated with arterial spin tagging: A theoretical investigation. *Magn. Reson. Med.* 44, 440–449, 2000. doi: 10.1002/1522-2594(200009)44:3<440::AID-MRM15>3.0.CO;2-6.

26. St. Lawrence K. S., Wang J. Effects of the apparent transverse relaxation time on cerebral blood flow measurements obtained by arterial spin labeling. *Magn. Reson. Med.* 53, 425–433, 2005. doi: 10.1002/mrm.20364.

27. Duong T. Q., Kim S. G. In vivo MR measurements of regional arterial and venous blood volume fractions in intact rat brain. *Magn. Reson. Med.* 43, 393–402, 2000. doi: 10.1002/(SICI)1522-2594(200003)43:3<393::AID-MRM11>3.0.CO;2-K.

28. Kim T., Kim S.-G. Quantification of cerebral arterial blood volume using arterial spin labeling with intravoxel incoherent motion-sensitive gradients. *Magn. Reson. Med.* 55, 1047–1057, 2006. doi: 10.1002/mrm.20867.

29. Wells J. A., Thomas D. L., Saga T., Kershaw J., Aoki I. MRI of cerebral micro-vascular flow patterns : A multi-direction diffusion-weighted ASL approach. *J. Cereb. Blood Flow Metab.* 2016 (Epub). doi: 10.1177/0271678X16660985.

30. Wong E. C., Cronin M., Wu W.-C., Inglis B., Frank L. R., Liu T. T. Velocity-selective arterial spin labeling. *Magn. Reson. Med.* 55, 1334–1341, 2006. doi: 10.1002/mrm.20906.

31. Norris D. G., Schwarzbauer C. Velocity selective radiofrequency pulse trains. *J. Magn. Reson.* 137, 231–236, 1999. doi: 10.1006/jmre.1998.1690.

32. Schmid S., Ghariq E., Teeuwisse W. M., Webb A., Van Osch M. J. P. Acceleration-selective arterial spin labeling. *Magn. Reson. Med.* 71, 191–199, 2014. doi: 10.1002/mrm.24650.

33. Schmid S., Petersen E. T., Van Osch M. J. P. Insight into the labeling mechanism of acceleration selective arterial spin labeling. *Magn. Reson. Mater. Phys. Biol. Med.* 30, 165–174, 2017. doi: 10.1007/s10334-016-0596-6.

34. Duhamel G., De Bazelaire C., Alsop D. C. Evaluation of systematic quantification errors in velocity-selective arterial spin labeling of the brain. *Magn. Reson. Med.* 50, 145–153, 2003. doi: 10.1002/mrm.10510.

35. Qin Q., van Zijl P. C. M.Velocity-selective-inversion prepared arterial spin labeling. *Magn. Reson. Med.* 76, 1136–1148, 2016. doi: 10.1002/mrm.26010.

36. Lu H., Ge Y. Quantitative evaluation of oxygenation in venous vessels using T_2-relaxation-under-spin-tagging MRI. *Magn. Reson. Med.* 2008, 60, 357–363, doi: 10.1002/mrm.21627.

37. Schmid S., Teeuwisse W. M., Lu H., van Osch M. J. P. Time-efficient determination of spin compartments by time-encoded pCASL T_2-relaxation-under-spin-tagging and its application in hemodynamic characterization of the cerebral border zones. *Neuroimage* 2015, 123, 72–79, doi:10.1016/j.neuroimage.2015.08.025.

38. Mori S., Van Zijl P. C. M. Fiber tracking: principles and strategies: A technical review. *NMR Biomed.* 2002, 15, 468–480, doi: 10.1002/nbm.781.

Chapter 23

Advanced Methods for IVIM Parameter Estimation

Peter T. While
Department of Radiology and Nuclear Medicine,
St. Olav's University Hospital, Trondheim, Norway
peter.thomas.while@stolav.no

This chapter reviews the difficult problem of parameter estimation in intravoxel incoherent motion (IVIM) modeling and attempts to summarize the various advanced approaches that have been proposed to improve the precision and accuracy of the pseudodiffusion parameter estimates.

23.1 Introduction

Parameter estimation by fitting a biexponential model to noisy data is a notoriously difficult problem [1–5]. Using synthetic data and nonlinear least squares (NLLS) curve fitting, Bromage [1] showed that estimation error (relative to data error) increases substantially as the amplitudes of the exponential components become

Intravoxel Incoherent Motion (IVIM) MRI: Principles and Applications
Edited by Denis Le Bihan, Mami Iima, Christian Federau, and Eric E. Sigmund

ISBN 978-981-4800-19-8 (Hardcover), 978-0-429-42727-5 (eBook)
www.panstanford.com

increasingly dissimilar. Unfortunately, this is precisely the situation in IVIM imaging studies, where the pseudodiffusion volume fraction, f, is often in the range 5%–10% [6] and is generally lower than 30% [7]. As such, information about the pseudodiffusion component is contained in only a small fraction of the signal, and the measurement is said to have a poor dynamic range [8]. Of course, this situation is exacerbated by the low signal-to-noise ratio (SNR) typically encountered in diffusion-weighted imaging (DWI).

In the majority of cases, IVIM parameter estimation is performed using either NLLS fitting or an asymptotic approach, as described below. Typically NLLS fitting is implemented using either the Levenberg–Marquardt algorithm [9, 10], a trust-region algorithm [11, 12], or occasionally the Nelder–Mead simplex method [13, 14]; all of these are readily available in many data analysis programs. However, if performed on a pixel-wise basis, corresponding estimates for f, and especially the pseudodiffusion coefficient, D^*, generally possess a high degree of variability, such that averaging over entire regions of interest (ROIs) is often required in the pursuit of meaningful results [7, 15, 16]. As such, it is generally accepted that NLLS fitting is inadequate in the pursuit of clinical IVIM imaging.

In this chapter we review the various alternative approaches that have been proposed to date for improving the robustness of IVIM parameter estimation. We begin with a brief overview of asymptotic approaches and the important task of b-value (diffusion weighting) optimization before exploring more advanced methods, focusing in particular on Bayesian inference with a variety of different priors; we also cover non-negative least squares (NNLS), total variation regularization, various noise-based approaches, and machine learning. Note that alternative models [17] and flow-compensated IVIM [18, 19] are discussed in detail elsewhere in this book.

23.2 Asymptotic Approaches

23.2.1 Simplified IVIM

While discussion of simplified IVIM may appear somewhat misplaced in a chapter on advanced methodology, it has been included here for completeness and for historical reasons. Simplified IVIM is based on the assumption that the pseudodiffusion component has essentially decayed to zero for *b* values above a suitably high threshold, and this assumption also forms the basis of the segmented fitting approach, which is described below. In the first exposition of the IVIM model, Le Bihan et al. [20] showed that as few as three *b* values are required to provide estimates of the diffusion coefficient, *D*, and *f* (i.e., D^* is not estimated). Taking the natural logarithm of the data, the slope of the straight line passing through the data at the higher two *b* values provides an estimate of *D*, and after rearranging the expression provided by Le Bihan et al. [20], it can be shown that the difference between the vertical intercept of this straight line (S_{int}) and the datum at $b = 0$ s/mm^2 (S_0) can be used to estimate $f = (S_0 - S_{int})/S_0$.

Acquiring data at only three *b* values is attractive with regard to the scan time and permits pseudodiffusion information to be obtained at little or no cost to existing clinical protocols used for estimating the apparent diffusion coefficient (ADC). Such information has been shown to hold diagnostic value in a number of recent studies [21–23]. Several other metrics have also been proposed that essentially provide alternative weightings of the simplified IVIM parameters [24–28]. Of course, the choice of *b* values has a substantial impact on parameter precision and accuracy (see Fig. 23.1), and the optimal choice also depends on both tissue type and SNR [28–30].

Possibly implicit in the use of simplified IVIM is the belief that the expected uncertainty in D^* does not warrant the additional scan time necessary for its estimation [23]. An alternative approach, therefore, is simply to fix D^* and solve for *f* and *D* using NLLS, which has been shown to provide more robust estimates than simplified IVIM [31]. However, in that study the observed improvement was arguably primarily due to the additional *b* values sampled rather than differences in methodology.

23.2.2 Segmented Fitting

The framework behind simplified IVIM can be extended easily to incorporate multiple *b* values above the assumed threshold, thereby improving the robustness of the estimates for *f* and *D* [32, 33]. This approach has been shown to provide more stable estimates of *f* than

NLLS, even when using the asymptotic estimates as the starting values for NLLS [34]. Note that the fitting can be performed either by applying weighted least squares to the log-transformed data or by applying NLLS with a monoexponential model.

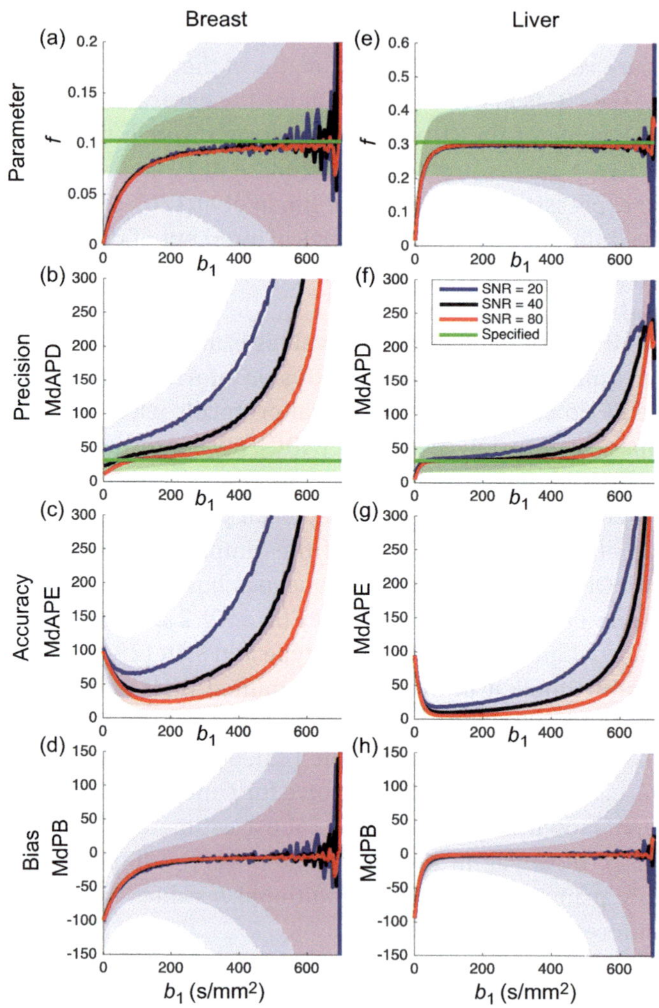

Figure 23.1 Impact of the choice of middle b value and SNR on the estimation of parameter f (shading depicts interquartile range) when applying simplified IVIM to synthetic data appropriate to the breast (a-d) and liver (e-h). Reprinted Ref. [28] with permission from Springer Nature, copyright 2017.

Segmented fitting extends this idea further by also solving for D^* by applying NLLS using the full biexponential model after first fixing f and D to the asymptotic estimates [35]. Alternatively, one can solve for both f and D^* using NLLS after fixing only D [36]. The argument is that the stability of NLLS is improved by reducing the number of parameters to be estimated. Note that a check should be included to ensure that the signal at higher b values has not yet reached the noise floor, which would otherwise heavily bias the estimates of f (increase) and D (decrease) [37].

Segmented fitting has been compared extensively against full NLLS, and while full NLLS by definition should provide a better fit to the data (i.e., lower residual sum of squares), the estimates of the pseudodiffusion coefficients provided by segmented fitting generally contain fewer outliers and have lower coefficients of variation [6, 38–43]. However, when comparing the approaches using median statistics, which are themselves less susceptible to the existence of outliers and therefore arguably more representative of the bulk of the data, studies have shown the full NLLS approach (trust-region) in certain simulations to be slightly superior [44, 45].

The estimates for f and D obtained using segmented fitting are always biased to a certain extent because of the finite pseudodiffusion component that is still present in the signal at the threshold b value, and the influence of the choice of threshold is highly tissue dependent. Rather than fixing the threshold for a given study, Wurnig et al. [46] proposed an automated approach whereby segmented fitting is applied multiple times using every possible threshold from the available set of b values, and the one providing the best fit to the data is used for determining the parameter estimates (see Fig. 23.2). Indeed, this optimal threshold has also been proposed as a possible biomarker in its own right [47].

A number of variants to segmented fitting have been proposed. For example, the second step of solving for D^* using NLLS can be replaced by further linearized least squares fitting using either a Taylor series approximation at low b values [48] or transformed data [45]. A variable projection approach has also been proposed that bears some similarities to segmented fitting in that it reduces the parameter space by first solving a linear equation for f [49]. The algorithm requires initial guesses for D and D^*, followed by iteration involving NLLS at each step.

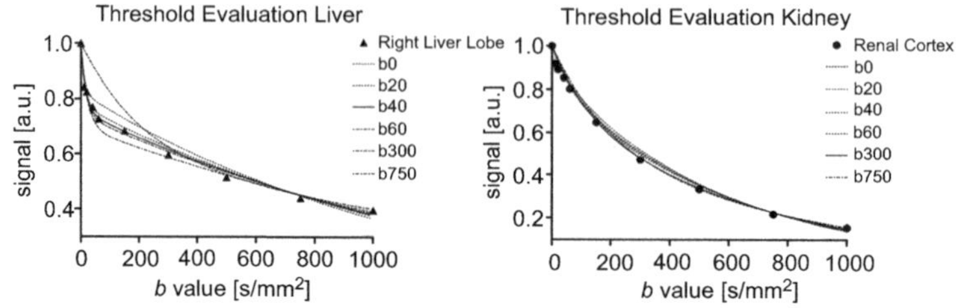

Figure 23.2 Impact of the choice of threshold *b* value on the resulting biexponential curve when applying segmented fitting to liver and kidney data (best fit using thresholds at b = 40 s/mm^2 and b = 300 s/mm^2, respectively). Reprinted from Ref. [46] with permission from John Wiley and Sons, copyright 2014.

23.3 *b*-Value Optimization

Given the sensitivity of the IVIM parameters to both the SNR of the underlying data and the chosen method of estimation, it is reasonable to expect that the number and distribution of *b* values are also important factors. Hence *b*-value optimization has become an important means to improve the robustness of IVIM parameter estimation.

Lemke et al. [7] considered three perfusion regimes corresponding to brain (low), kidney (medium), and liver (high) tissue and used Monte Carlo simulations to generate synthetic noisy data sets. These authors started with three fixed *b* values and successively added *b* values that minimized the relative overall error of the parameter estimates (obtained using the Levenberg–Marquardt algorithm). Thus, an ordered set was presented, and a minimum of ten *b* values was recommended. Histogram analysis showed that optimal *b* values were concentrated within three broad clusters. A similar approach has been applied to the optimization of *b* values for other diffusion models [50].

Zhang et al. [51] derived an error propagation factor equal to the ratio of the relative parameter error to the relative input noise (assuming NLLS fitting). A weighted sum of error propagation factors for each parameter was integrated over parameter ranges appropriate to the kidney and then optimized with respect to 4, 6, 8, and 10 *b* values. The optimal distributions involved repeated sampling at key *b* values and afforded improved precision and accuracy over the use of a uniform distribution of *b* values. Cho et al. [40] tested such an optimal distribution on synthetic and in vivo data of the breast and found that it generally resulted in lower relative error compared to a more conventional distribution, both for NLLS and segmented fitting, with the latter approach being preferred.

Cohen et al. [52] considered a conventional distribution and demonstrated the importance of including at least two additional low *b* values between 0 and 50 s/mm^2 for the estimation of D^* using segmented fitting of liver data, with respect to bias and the number of outliers.

Dyvorne et al. [53] considered a model-free approach by using in vivo liver data sets comprising 16 *b* values along with exhaustive sampling to find the optimal subsets of 4–15 *b* values in terms of a global parameter error (relative to reference estimates obtained using all 16 *b* values). These authors found that as few as four optimal *b* values yielded parameter estimates with deviations lower than the repeatability deviation of the full 16 *b*-value set (using NLLS).

In contrast, ter Voert et al. [54] found that a minimum of 16 *b* values was necessary for reliable results in the liver using NLLS. These authors considered three reference protocols comprising 25 *b* values with which to compare the results of a series of optimized subsets, obtained by considering the error propagation factor introduced by Zhang et al. [51], along with 35 other distributions found in the literature (see Fig. 23.3). A substantial reduction in the average relative error was demonstrated when the number of *b* values was increased from 4 to 16, and especially when using an optimized 16 *b*-value protocol. Errors for the pseudodiffusion parameters were generally higher for inhomogeneous tumors than for normal liver tissue.

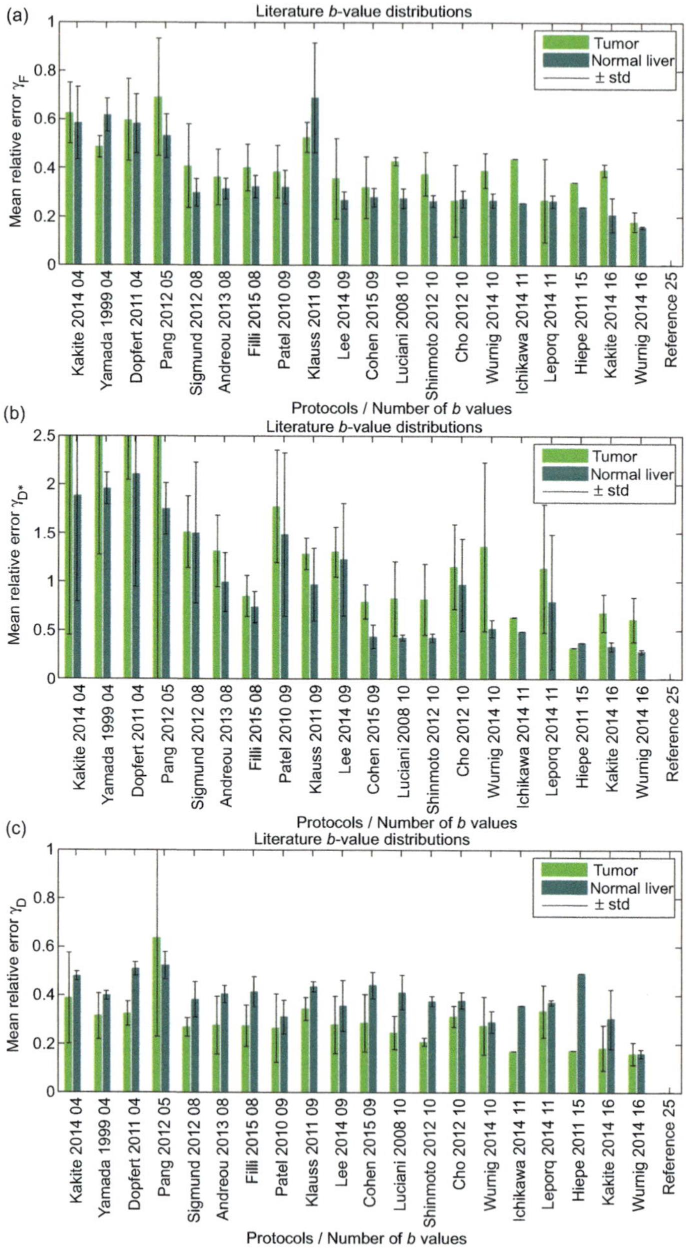

Figure 23.3 Mean relative error for *f* (a), *D** (b) and *D* (c), for various *b*-value distributions taken from the literature, relative to a reference distribution of 25 *b* values, when applied to IVIM imaging of the liver. Reprint from Ref. [54] with permission from Wolters Kluwer Health, Inc., copyright 2016.

23.4 Bayesian Inference

After nonlinear least squares and segmented fitting, Bayesian inference is the third-most-common approach to IVIM parameter estimation. Bayesian inference offers several advantages over the former two approaches:

- No initial guesses are required for any of the parameters (i.e., there is no risk of getting stuck in a local minimum).
- A measure of uncertainty is obtained for each parameter in the form of a probability distribution.
- It is possible to incorporate prior information or assumptions to influence the parameter estimation.

A possible disadvantage is the greater computational complexity in terms of both implementation and processing. Additionally, special care must be taken when specifying prior information so as not to bias the results unduly.

Bayesian inference has found application across a broad range of disciplines, and there exist many excellent textbooks devoted to the subject [55, 56]. The aim is to calculate (or sample) a joint posterior distribution, $P(\theta|\text{data})$, which gives the probability that the parameters in the set θ are "true" given the observed data. According to Bayes theorem, this posterior distribution can be expressed as follows:

$$P(\theta|\text{data}) = \frac{P(\text{data}|\theta) \times P(\theta)}{P(\text{data})}, \tag{23.1}$$

where $P(\text{data}|\theta)$ is the likelihood of observing the data given θ, $P(\theta)$ is the supplied prior distribution for θ, and $P(\text{data})$ is referred to as the evidence and acts as a normalization term (this is often ignored, and the equality in Eq. 23.1 is replaced with a proportionality).

The probability distributions for the individual parameters are obtained via a process called marginalization, whereby the joint posterior distribution in Eq. 23.1 is integrated with respect to all of the other parameters over appropriate domains. Typically, this integration must be performed numerically, and often, the distribution is sampled approximately using, for example, a Markov chain Monte Carlo approach [57]. Such marginalization may also be required for dealing with so-called nuisance parameters, such as the noise variance in the data [58].

Therefore, several choices need to be made in applying Bayesian inference to IVIM data, such as:

- The noise model used in calculating the data likelihood (e.g., Gaussian or Rician)
- The form of the prior distribution (see below)
- The central tendency measure used to provide the parameter estimates (e.g., mean, median, or mode)
- The computational process for calculating or sampling the probability distributions, for which the options may depend on the other choices above

In the following text, we summarize the various choices that have been made to date in applying Bayesian inference to IVIM data, and we refer the reader to the corresponding references for precise details on implementation.

23.4.1 Non- and Minimally Informative Priors

Perhaps the simplest choice for prior distribution is to use one that does not encode any prior information (other than constraint boundaries), such as a uniform distribution. For such a prior, the joint posterior distribution in Eq. 23.1 becomes directly proportional to the likelihood function. Under the assumption of Gaussian noise, the maximum of this likelihood function occurs at the least squares parameter estimates. However, the Bayesian approach maintains the advantage that a probability distribution is calculated, rather than iterating toward a locally optimal solution from an initial guess, and hence it may be regarded as a type of robust least squares approach.

An equally reasonable assumption may be to ascribe equal weighting to each order of magnitude for a given parameter, and one must also consider the manner in which to approach the constraint boundaries. Therefore, other choices of prior exist that are considered non- or minimally informative, such as the reciprocal distribution and the log-normal distribution [59]. These priors also encode little or no information except in cases where there is a high degree of data fitting uncertainty, which are associated with a broad likelihood function. Of course, such cases are not uncommon in IVIM data fitting, as outlined in Section 23.1, and hence these priors may still have considerable influence over the parameter estimates (see Fig. 23.4) [59].

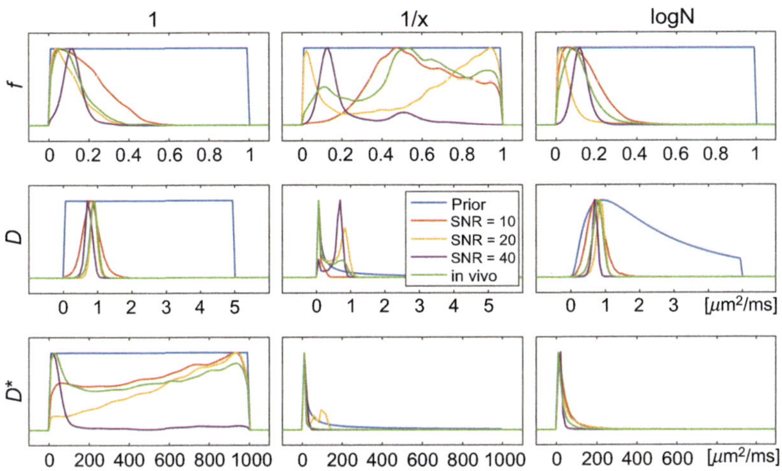

Figure 23.4 Demonstration of the impact of prior distribution (uniform, reciprocal, log-normal) and SNR on the posterior distribution (and corresponding parameter estimates) for simulated and in vivo data examples. Reprinted from Ref. [59], with permission from John Wiley and Sons, copyright 2017.

The application of Bayesian inference to IVIM data was first demonstrated by Neil and Bretthorst [8] and Neil et al. [60], who considered a Gaussian likelihood function and a prior distribution that was uniform in f and reciprocal in D and D^*. The joint posterior distribution was integrated numerically, and the maxima of the marginalized distributions were used to provide the parameter estimates. These authors used simulations and rat brain data to show that Bayesian inference provided more accurate and more precise estimates than NLLS in certain cases (e.g., for D and f at a low SNR and for D^* at a high SNR).

Variants of the approach by Neil et al. [8] using non- or minimally informative priors have been used in a range of IVIM studies assessing, for example, the impact of gradient polarity [61], techniques for dealing with respiratory motion [61–63], field strength dependence in the brain [64] and upper abdomen [65, 66], intrasite [67, 68] and intersite [66] reproducibility, correlation with dynamic contrast-enhanced magnetic resonance imaging (DCE MRI) in the kidney [69] and liver [70], and drug efficacy in terms of renal function [71].

However, despite the alleged improvement in robustness of the Bayesian approach over NLLS and segmented fitting, the parameters f and D^* still show poor repeatability and high variability in some studies [61, 63, 65–68]. Indeed Li et al. [72] presented a literature review of IVIM studies in the liver and could not conclude which approach was superior, with the parameters f and D^* estimated by the Bayesian approach displaying a higher median coefficient of variation across studies.

Nevertheless, the only two studies to date reporting direct comparisons between these approaches have both found that Bayesian inference with a non- or minimally informative prior does indeed provide IVIM parameter estimates with higher accuracy and precision than the other approaches [8, 44]. Barbieri et al. [44] compared six approaches: Levenberg–Marquardt, trust-region, fixed D^*, two versions of segmented fitting, and Bayesian inference, using both simulations and data from the upper abdomen (see Fig. 23.5). For the Bayesian inference they considered a Gaussian likelihood function, a uniform prior distribution for all parameters, slice sampling to perform the marginalization [73], and maxima to represent the parameter estimates; and they found that this approach also resulted in low inter-reader variability and the lowest intersubject variability.

Gustafsson et al. [59] presented recently a comparison of different approaches to Bayesian inference using non- or minimally informative priors for IVIM parameter estimation, using simulations and data from a mouse tumor model. These authors considered two different likelihood functions (Gaussian and Rician), three different priors (uniform, reciprocal, and log-normal), and two different measures of central tendency (mean and mode) and performed the marginalization using a Markov chain Monte Carlo approach [74]. The benefit of using a Gaussian likelihood function is that analytical marginalization is available, and indeed the results were found to be relatively invariant under this choice (in contrast to Bouhrara et al. [75]). However, the choice of prior and central tendency measure was found to be important (see Fig. 23.6), with the log-normal prior displaying the best overall performance (using either measure).

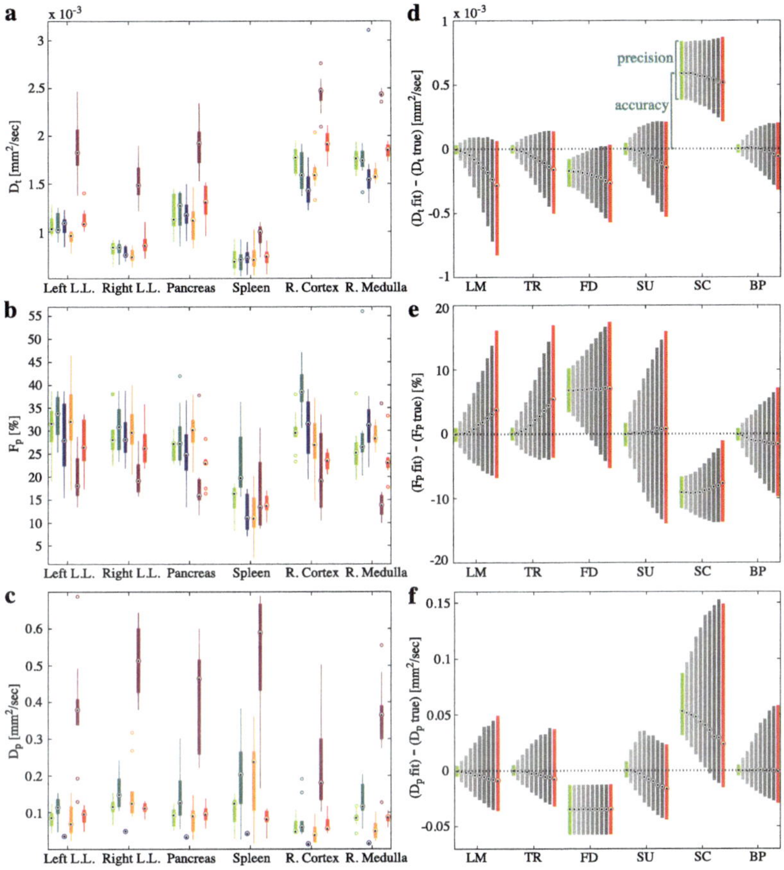

Figure 23.5 Results from experiment (a–c) and simulation (d–f) for *D* (a,d), *f* (b,e) and *D** (c,f) using: the Levenberg–Marquardt algorithm (leftmost), a trust-region algorithm, fixed *D**, two segmented approaches, and Bayesian inference with a uniform prior (rightmost). Reprinted from Ref. [44] with permission from John Wiley and Sons, copyright 2015.

23.4.2 Gaussian "Shrinkage" Prior

Orton et al. [74] considered a Gaussian prior that essentially carries the assumption that the (transformed) IVIM parameters are Gaussian distributed over a ROI, which they show to be reasonable in a practical example. Specifically, they considered a hierarchical prior structure involving a multivariate Gaussian distribution for a set of transformed parameters that had been mapped onto the entire real line. Parameter estimates and measures of uncertainty were generated using a Markov chain Monte Carlo implementation, whereby at each step the Gaussian prior was redefined using the ROI mean and covariance of the parameters from the previous step. In this way, the precise shape of the prior was driven by the data themselves, and the only assumption made was that its form was Gaussian.

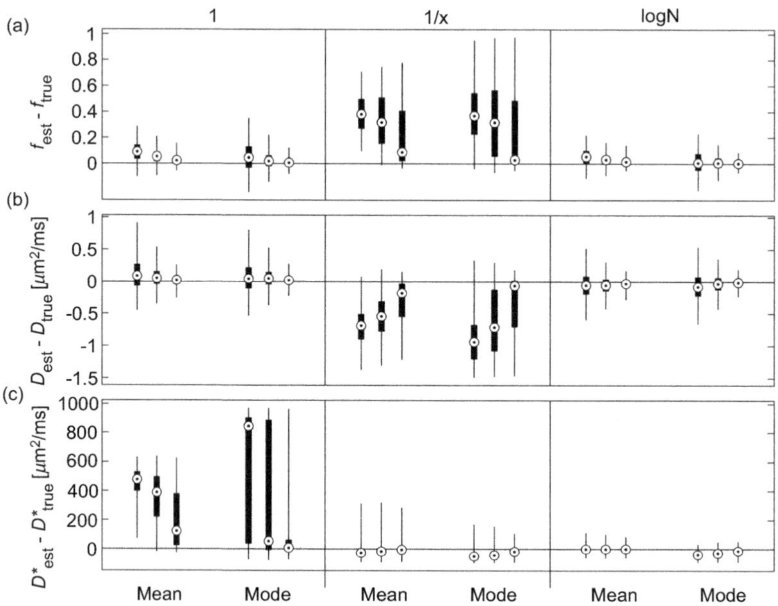

Figure 23.6 Estimation error for f (a), D (b), and D^* (c), using Bayesian inference with different priors (uniform, reciprocal, log-normal), central tendency measures (mean, mode) and synthetic data SNR (10, 20, 40). Reprinted from Ref. [59], with permission from John Wiley and Sons, copyright 2017.

Orton et al. [74] also considered a Gaussian likelihood function and a conjugate Gaussian-inverse-gamma g-prior for the nuisance parameters, such that these could be marginalized analytically. Orton et al. [74] provide a detailed explanation of this Bayesian approach, along with an appendix containing all the necessary steps for numerical implementation. These authors demonstrated the approach using liver data and compared results to those obtained using NLLS (Levenberg–Marquardt). The effect of the prior was to "shrink" parameter estimates toward the mean of the Gaussian distribution for those pixels associated with a high degree of data fitting uncertainty, and this resulted in much smoother parameter maps.

While [45] presented a simulation study (breast and liver tissue) comparing the performance of this Bayesian approach using a Gaussian shrinkage prior against the use of NLLS (trust-region) and segmented fitting. The Bayesian approach was found to produce parameter estimates with consistently higher accuracy and precision than these other methods, and cleaner parameter maps. However, a possible weakness was exposed, whereby certain tissue features corresponding to regions of high data fitting uncertainty were found to disappear completely (see Fig. 23.7). This finding suggests that the Gaussian shrinkage prior is best suited to ROIs that do not possess a substantial amount of underlying heterogeneity, or else it must be applied with caution and accompanied by rigorous uncertainty analysis.

In line with the above recommendation for the choice of ROI, Spinner et al. [76] applied this Bayesian approach to generate IVIM parameter maps of the myocardium, which displayed lower intra- and intersubject variability when compared with the maps generated by a segmented approach, with fewer outliers for f and D^*. Using simulations, these authors also showed that the Bayesian approach was associated with lower SNR requirements for the same level of bias and variation.

23.4.3 Spatial Homogeneity Prior

Freiman et al. [77, 78] introduced the concept of a spatially constrained incoherent motion (SCIM) model by using a spatial homogeneity prior within the Bayesian framework. The SCIM model is based on the assumption that parameter estimates in neighboring voxels should have a high probability of being similar in value. Freiman et al. [77, 78] reformulated the problem as the minimization of an energy functional involving a log likelihood term, which governs how well the parameters fit the data (noncentral χ distribution), plus a spatial homogeneity term that penalizes estimates that are dissimilar to those in neighboring voxels. As such, this approach uses local information to influence the parameter estimation, in contrast to the Gaussian shrinkage prior above, which uses global information, or the priors from Section 23.4.1, which treat each pixel entirely independently. Some related approaches are given in Section 23.6, on spatial smoothing.

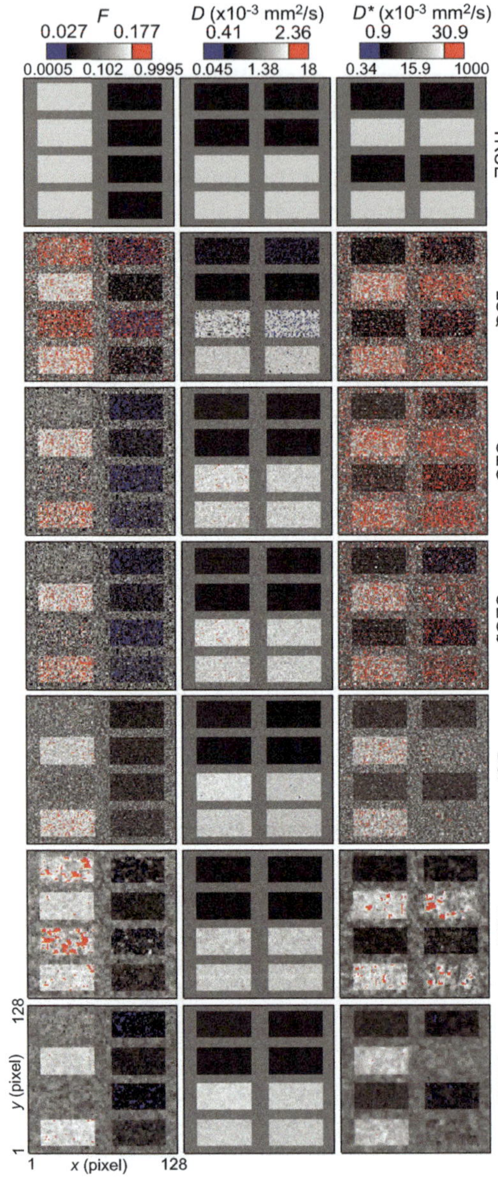

Figure 23.7 Parameter maps of *f*, *D*, and *D**, for synthetic breast data, obtained using: trust-region NLLS (LSQ), segmented fitting (SEG), and Bayesian inference with a Gaussian prior (BSP) and with a spatial homogeneity prior (FBM). Reprinted from Ref. [45] with permission from Springer Nature, copyright 2017.

Freiman et al. [77, 78] also introduced the fusion bootstrap moves algorithm for solving the optimization problem. Each iteration of the algorithm comprises two steps: firstly, a new proposal (i.e., a set of parameter maps) is generated after bootstrap resampling of the data (followed by pixel-wise NLLS fitting); secondly, this new proposal is fused with the previous iteration in an optimal way using a binary graph cut that minimizes the energy functional. That is, the parameter estimates for some of the pixels in the current solution are replaced with new parameter estimates from the proposal. Additional details and references necessary for implementing this approach were provided by While [45].

Using simulations, Freiman et al. [77, 78] demonstrated reductions in root mean square error of 80% for D^* and 50% for f and D, when compared with results from the Levenberg–Marquardt algorithm. These authors also applied the method to in vivo abdominal data and observed lower coefficients of variation and a higher contrast-to-noise ratio. Improved precision and accuracy was also observed in the simulation study reported by While [45], when compared to NLLS, segmented fitting, and, to a lesser extent, Bayesian inference with a Gaussian shrinkage prior (at the expense of a moderately higher bias). However, the approach was also shown to be susceptible to oversmoothing in regions of high data fitting uncertainty, in a manner similar to the Gaussian shrinkage prior (see Fig. 23.7). Note that the overall degree of smoothing and the relative degree of smoothing applied to each parameter are user-defined parameters.

An adaptation of the SCIM model was incorporated recently into an approach by Kurugol et al. [79] for providing simultaneous image registration and IVIM parameter estimation. That is, this extended approach accounted for motion by also solving for the optimal transformations for each individual image. These authors actually considered a probability distribution model of diffusion instead of IVIM directly but obtained IVIM parameter estimates from this model using summary statistics. The method was applied to abdominal data and resulted in significantly improved parameter estimates when compared with the results corresponding to independent image registration.

23.5 Non-negative Least Squares

While classified here as a curve-fitting method, NNLS [80], as applied to DWI data, is essentially a generalization of IVIM in that it replaces the biexponential model with a large sum of exponential decay terms. Several hundred terms may be considered, whereby each term has a different fixed diffusion constant such that in total an appropriate range of possible values is represented (typically incremented on a logscale). The optimization problem proceeds by fitting this exponential sum to the data using regularized least squares and solving for the weights. Regularization is necessary to obtain a well-conditioned system and, for example, to enforce smoothing of the resulting diffusion spectrum.

The locations of the peaks in the spectrum provide the diffusion constants, and the relative areas under the peaks provide the corresponding signal fractions—for example, f and $(1 - f)$ in the case of truly biexponential decay. NNLS has been used extensively in the study of nuclear magnetic resonance (NMR) relaxation data [81]. The advantage of NNLS with respect to IVIM is that it provides not only parameter estimates, but it also tests for the presence of additional decay terms that may be associated with other compartments within each voxel. Such additional terms would contaminate the parameter estimates from conventional biexponential fitting. Furthermore, NNLS does not require any starting guesses.

NNLS has been used to study IVIM in bone marrow [82], the prostate [83], and the brain [84] and to identify and correct for possible partial volume effects associated with large blood vessels in the liver [85]. Wurnig et al. [86] used NNLS on data obtained at as many as 68 b values to demonstrate that liver and kidney tissues are better characterized by the inclusion of a third intermediate diffusion component (see Fig. 23.8). Estimation uncertainty associated with NNLS has been compared to the Cramer–Rao lower bounds for the IVIM model using Monte Carlo simulations [87].

A related concept was presented by Kuai et al. [88] in terms of a continuous pseudodiffusion variable and perfusion fraction density function. Similarly, Kurugol et al. [89] proposed a probability distribution model of diffusion and combined it with the Bayesian approach of Freiman et al. [77, 78] involving a spatial homogeneity prior.

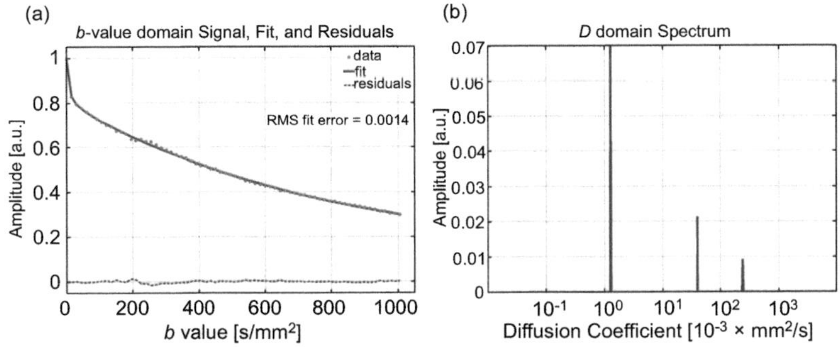

Figure 23.8 Representative data and fitted curve for liver (a), and the corresponding diffusion spectrum with three distinct peaks (b), obtained using NNLS. Reprinted from Ref. [86] with permission from John Wiley and Sons, copyright 2017.

23.6 Spatial Smoothing

A major goal of the advanced methods described in this chapter is to reduce the degree of erroneous spatial heterogeneity present in maps of the pseudodiffusion parameters. A direct approach to this problem is to enforce spatial smoothing by incorporating regularization into the data fitting, in a manner analogous to Bayesian inference involving a spatial homogeneity prior, as described in Section 23.4.3. That is, rather than estimating parameters for each voxel independently, one estimates the parameters for all voxels simultaneously by including dependency between neighboring voxels in the optimization routine.

Regularization involves the addition of a weighted penalty function to the cost function (i.e., the residual sum of squares) to be minimized. The idea is that many different sets of parameter values may satisfy the cost function to a similar degree, and one is interested in the set that also minimizes the penalty function. The weight, or regularization parameter, controls the trade-off between the two functions.

Lin et al. [90] considered a total difference (TD) penalty function and an iterative optimization routine that alternated between steps of the Levenberg–Marquardt algorithm to perform the data fitting and steps of the steepest descent technique to minimize the TD of the reconstructed parameter maps. These authors used a segmentation mask to avoid edge smoothing and demonstrated smoother parameter maps for both synthetic (lower bias and deviation) and real data in comparison with NLLS fitting, especially for data with a low SNR.

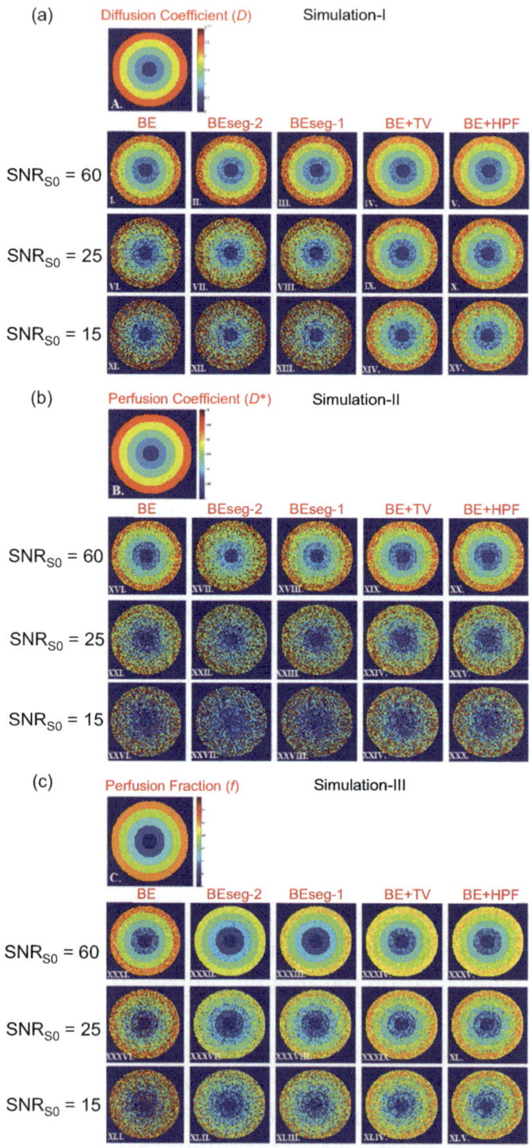

Figure 23.9 Parameter maps of D (a), D^* (b) and f (c), for synthetic bone data, obtained using NLLS, two segmented fitting approaches, and adaptive regularization using total variation and Huber penalty functions. Reprinted from Ref. [91] with permission from John Wiley and Sons, copyright 2017.

Kayal et al. [91] proposed a mask-free adaptive approach and considered both a total variation penalty function and a Huber penalty function, which essentially involved the minimization of the local gradient of the parameter maps. These authors considered synthetic and real data sets of bone and showed that the approach provided significant improvements in precision and accuracy compared to NLLS and two types of segmented fitting (see Fig. 23.9).

Perhaps a simpler approach is to apply denoising to the image data before parameter estimation. Reischauer and Gutzeit [92] used four different readily available denoising algorithms based on nonlocal means filtering, local principal component analysis, and joint rank and edge constraints, and compared their impact on parameter estimation. Using simulations and brain data (with bootstrapping) they showed that the reliability of the estimates was generally improved, both for NLLS and segmented fitting. In related work, While [45] found that rudimentary application of total variation denoising or median filtering to either the data or the parameter maps gave results inferior to those obtained using Bayesian inference with a spatial homogeneity prior.

23.7 Noise Modeling

A further limitation of conventional NLLS is that it relies on the assumption that the noise is Gaussian distributed; however, this is appropriate only for data with a sufficiently high SNR [93]. The image intensity of magnitude images is actually Rician distributed (or noncentral χ-distributed in the case of multiple receiver channels), and hence conventional NLLS introduces bias into the parameter estimates for data with a low SNR. To address this issue, several approaches have been proposed that more accurately account for various sources of noise in the data.

Lu et al. [94] used a noise-rectified least squares fitting method [95], which minimized a chi-square cost function involving the difference between the measured signal and the expected intensity calculated from the IVIM model after accounting for averaging of a Rician signal acquired at multiple channels. The optimization was performed using NLLS (trust-region) with ten random initializations. These authors used the approach to compare different diffusion models for head and neck cancer, rather than considering alternative fitting methods.

Veraart et al. [96] proposed the use of a conditional least squares estimator, which is resilient to data preprocessing steps that account for subject motion and eddy current distortions, for example. These authors considered the conditional expectation of a noncentral χ-distributed signal and minimized a weighted sum of squared deviations of the measured signal from these expectations. The estimator accounted for heteroscedasticity in the data and involved a sophisticated approach for estimating the noise [97]. The performance of the estimator on synthetic and real brain data compared favorably against a maximum likelihood estimator, NLLS, and weighted linear least squares. The approach was applied to diffusion tensor imaging (DTI) and diffusion kurtosis imaging (DKI) parameter estimation but could be extended in a straightforward manner to IVIM studies.

Dikaios et al. [98] also considered the median absolute deviation technique of Coupé et al. [97] for estimating the noise in DWI images but adapted it for the case of averaged data. This noise estimate was used to inform an approximate probability distribution function (PDF) for a Rician sum. The parameter estimation proceeded by minimizing the l_1-norm between the measured signal and either the median or the maximum (preferred) of the PDF (see Fig. 23.10). The method was shown to result in lower bias than NLLS in simulations with a low SNR, but the noise modeling did not significantly improve cancer classification in a clinical data set for neck lymph nodes.

Murphy et al. [99] proposed instead the use of a beta log-normal (BLN) error model combined with maximum likelihood estimation to account for the additional signal attenuation caused by cardiac and respiratory motion in abdominal DWI. This approach required the estimation of an extra parameter associated with the beta distribution, which governed the impact of the bulk motion, whereas D^* was held fixed. The method was tested against NLLS, and the parameter estimates were found to exhibit less dependency on gating and proximity to the heart.

Of course, one can recover a Gaussian noise distribution to good approximation by taking additional images and averaging the data, thereby increasing the SNR, but this approach is clearly limited with respect to clinically acceptable scan times. However, Zhang et al. [100] proposed that this SNR improvement might be attainable in an artificial sense, without taking additional images, using wild bootstrap resampling. These authors generated synthetic data using the residuals from a segmented fit to the original data, in a manner similar to the generation of proposals in the fusion bootstrap moves algorithm described in Section 23.4.3 [77, 78]. However, while this approach improved the precision of D^*, the uncertainty at low data SNR was shown to be less than the Cramer–Rao lower bound, suggesting that the estimation was biased. Indeed, this finding may explain the bias observed by While [45] when implementing fusion bootstrap moves.

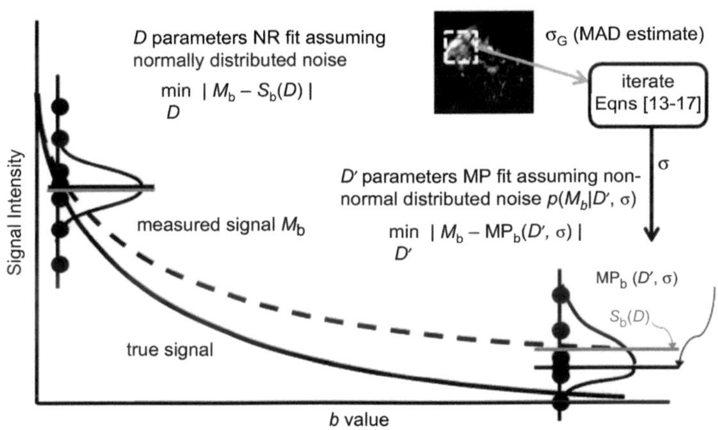

Figure 23.10 Illustration of the noise-induced bias introduced by fitting directly to the measured signal, and the closer match to the true signal that is obtained by considering instead the maximum probability (MP) of the derived PDF, where the inset illustrates the estimation of the noise variance. Reprinted from Ref. [98] with permission from John Wiley and Sons, copyright 2013.

Representing somewhat of an anomaly for this section, Huang et al. [101] proposed the use of a nonlinear mixed effects (NLME) model to account for random effects associated with the parameter estimates themselves, which are independent of the noise in the data. NLME models are typically used in longitudinal studies, but Huang et al. [101] adapted this approach to IVIM parameter estimation by considering each imaging voxel to be an independent subject. Information about the random effects associated with each voxel was obtained from sufficiently similar image data in the neighborhood of the voxel over the full set of images. These authors used simulations and brain data to demonstrate improved parameter estimation using NLME compared with estimation using NLLS on either the original or smoothed data sets.

23.8 Machine Learning

In recent years there has been increasing interest in the promise and application of machine learning in medicine [102] and medical imaging [103]. The field of machine learning encompasses a growing list of algorithms that can be trained to recognize patterns in data in order to make predictions or decisions on new data. In this way, the results are purely data driven and do not rely on any pre-existing models or assumptions.

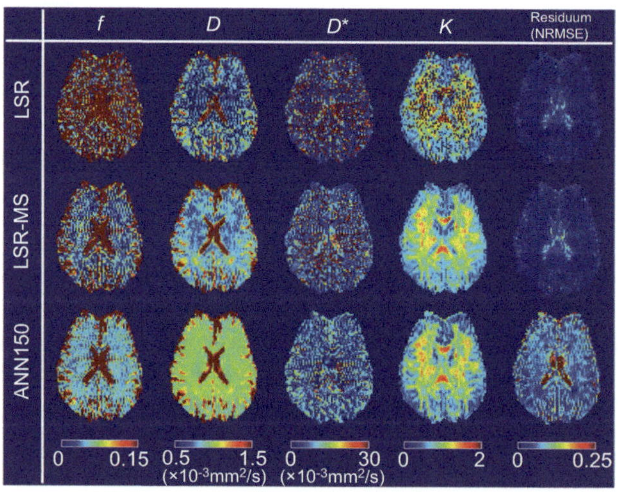

Figure 23.11 IVIM-kurtosis parameter maps (and residuals) for in vivo brain data, obtained using NLLS, segmented fitting and a machine learning artificial neural network algorithm (trained using synthetic data with SNR of 150). Reprinted from Ref. [105] with permission from John Wiley and Sons, copyright 2017.

Ciritsis et al. [104] took such a model-free approach for the purpose of tissue classification using DWI data taken at 16 *b* values appropriate to IVIM modeling [7]. These authors trained the *k*-nearest neighbors machine learning technique to distinguish abdominal organs, using only the signal intensities as learning features (from 280 ROIs of 70–200 pixels), and achieved 94.5% accuracy on new data. In addition, principal component analysis was used to find optimal subsets of *b* values, and it was found that similar accuracy could be achieved with as few as six *b* values.

Bertleff et al. [105] considered an altogether different approach by using machine learning to specifically estimate the IVIM (and kurtosis) parameters. These authors used synthetic data, appropriate to the brain, to train a machine learning artificial neural network and then tested the performance of the approach on further synthetic data, as well as on data acquired in vivo (see Fig. 23.11). The performance was found to be superior to NLLS and comparable to an extended version of segmented fitting, while generating fewer outliers, especially for D^*.

23.9 Conclusion

An abundance of methods is now available for IVIM parameter estimation in response to the rapidly growing interest over the past ten years in the potential of IVIM imaging throughout the body. Furthermore, given that the majority of the advanced methods outlined in this chapter were proposed only very recently, this number will doubtlessly continue to increase considerably over the coming years. The IVIM researcher wishing to maximize the information extracted from their data is therefore faced with a difficult choice.

Comparison between approaches is complicated. Typically, newly proposed methods are compared only against one of the conventional methods in NLLS and segmented fitting. Expository demonstrations usually target a specific body part, and results may be strongly influenced by other factors, such as imaging parameters, system and coil choice, preprocessing techniques, and especially the number and distribution of *b* values. Hence, existing presentations within the literature may be insufficient to guide the best choice of method for a given study.

Therefore, there is a great need for further comparative studies that contrast the various advanced approaches with one another over a broad range of data sets. However, unfortunately, implementation of these approaches is not always straightforward. Indeed, the increased computational complexity is generally prohibitive to the point that the majority of IVIM studies continue to use the conventional approaches and merely cite some of the advanced approaches as a possible means to improve results.

The IVIM community should therefore consider how to promote greater adoption of and comparison between the advanced approaches, whether this might be through greater availability of standardized test data sets or through an open repository of algorithms. Indeed, such an arrangement might facilitate further gains through b-value optimization or hybridization. The ideality of a new gold standard may be an unrealistic pursuit, but it should be possible to identify optimal approaches for each area of application. In this regard, there remains great potential for further substantial improvements in IVIM parameter estimation in the majority of IVIM studies.

References

1. Bromage G. E. A quantification of the hazards of fitting sums of exponentials to noisy data. *Comput. Phys. Commun.* 30(3), (1983), 229–233.
2. Shrager R. I., Hendler R. W. Some pitfalls in curve-fitting and how to avoid them: A case in point. *J. Biochem. Biophys. Methods* 36(2-3), (1998), 157–173.
3. Istratov A. A., Vyvenko O. F. Exponential analysis in physical phenomena. *Rev. Sci. Instrum.* 70(2), (1999), 1233–1257.
4. Holmstrom K., Petersson J. A review of the parameter estimation problem of fitting positive exponential sums to empirical data. *Appl. Math. Comput.* 126(1), (2002), 31–61.
5. Transtrum M. K., Machta B. B., Sethna J. P. Why are nonlinear fits to data so challenging? *Phys. Rev. Lett.* 104(6), (2010), 060201.
6. Suo S., Lin N., Wang H., Zhang L., Wang R., Zhang S., et al. Intravoxel incoherent motion diffusion-weighted MR imaging of breast cancer at 3.0 tesla: Comparison of different curve-fitting methods. *J. Magn. Reson. Imaging* 42(2), (2015), 362–370.

7. Lemke A., Stieltjes B., Schad L. R., Laun F. B. Toward an optimal distribution of *b* values for intravoxel incoherent motion imaging. *Magn. Reson. Imaging* 29, (2011), 766–776.
8. Neil J. J., Bretthorst G. L. On the use of Bayesian probability theory for analysis of exponential decay data: An example taken from intravoxel incoherent motion experiments. *Magn. Reson. Med.* 29, (1993), 642–647.
9. Levenberg K. A method for the solution of certain non-linear problems in least squares. *Q. Appl. Math.* 2, (1944), 164–168.
10. Marquardt D. An algorithm for least squares estimation of nonlinear parameters. *SIAM J. Appl. Math.* 11(2), (1963), 431–441.
11. Moré J, Sorensen D. Computing a trust region step. *SIAM J. Sci. Stat. Comput.* 3, (1983), 553–572.
12. Coleman T. F., Li Y. An interior, trust region approach for nonlinear minimization subject to bounds. *SIAM J. Optimiz.* 6, (1996), 418–445.
13. Nelder J. A., Mead R. A simplex method for function minimization. *Comput. J.* 7, (1965), 308–313.
14. Lagarias J. C., Reeds J. A., Wright M. H., Wright P. E. Convergence properties of the Nelder-Mead simplex method in low dimensions. *SIAM J. Optimiz.* 9(1), (1998), 112–147.
15. Koh D. M., Collins D. J., Orton M. R. Intravoxel incoherent motion in body diffusion-weighted MRI: Reality and challenges. *Am. J. Roentgenol.* 196, (2011), 1351–1361.
16. Andreou A., Koh D. M., Collins D. J., Blackledge M., Wallace T., Leach M. O., et al. Measurement reproducibility of perfusion fraction and pseudodiffusion coefficient derived by intravoxel incoherent motion diffusion-weighted MR imaging in normal liver and metastases. *Eur. Radiol.* 23(2), (2013), 428–434.
17. Fournet G., Li J.-R., Cerjanic A. M., Sutton B. P., Ciobanu L., Le Bihan D. A two-pool model to describe the IVIM cerebral perfusion. *J. Cereb. Blood Flow Metab.* 37(8), (2017), 2987–3000.
18. Wetscherek A., Stieltjes B., Laun F. B. Flow-compensated intravoxel incoherent motion diffusion imaging. *Magn. Reson. Med.* 74(2), (2015), 410–419.
19. Ahlgren A., Knutsson L., Wirestam R., Nilsson M., Stahlberg F., Topgaard D., et al. Quantification of microcirculatory parameters by joint analysis of flow-compensated and non-flow-compensated intravoxel incoherent motion (IVIM) data. *NMR Biomed.* 29(5), (2016), 640–649.

20. Le Bihan D., Breton E., Lallemand D., Aubin M. L., Vignaud J., Laval-Jeantet M. Separation of diffusion and perfusion in intravoxel incoherent motion MR imaging. *Radiology* 168, (1988), 497–505.

21. Penner A. H., Sprinkart A. M., Kukuk G. M., Guetgemann I., Gieseke J., Schild H. H., et al. Intravoxel incoherent motion model-based liver lesion characterisation from three *b*-value diffusion-weighted MRI. *Eur. Radiol.* 23(10), (2013), 2773–2783.

22. Concia M., Sprinkart A. M., Penner A.-H., Brossart P., Gieseke J., Schild H. H., et al. Diffusion-weighted magnetic resonance imaging of the pancreas diagnostic benefit from an intravoxel incoherent motion model-based 3 *b*-value analysis. *Invest. Radiol.* 49(2), (2014), 93–100.

23. Pieper C. C., Willinek W. A., Meyer C., Ahmadzadehfar H., Kukuk G. M., Sprinkart A. M., et al. Intravoxel incoherent motion diffusion-weighted MR imaging for prediction of early arterial blood flow stasis in radioembolization of breast cancer liver metastases. *J. Vasc. Interv. Radiol.* 27(9), (2016), 1320–1328.

24. Thoeny H. C., De Keyzer F., Vandecaveye V., Chen F., Sun X., Bosmans H., et al. Effect of vascular targeting agent in rat tumor model: Dynamic contrast-enhanced versus diffusion-weighted MR imaging. *Radiology* 237(2), (2005), 492–499.

25. Moteki T., Horikoshi H. Evaluation of hepatic lesions and hepatic parenchyma using diffusion-weighted echo-planar MR with three values of gradient *b*-factor. *J. Magn. Reson. Imaging* 24(3), (2006), 637–645.

26. Sasaki M., Sumi M., Eida S., Katayama I., Hotokezaka Y., Nakamura T. Simple and reliable determination of intravoxel incoherent motion parameters for the differential diagnosis of head and neck tumors. *PLoS One* 9(11), (2014), 1–11.

27. Teruel J. R., Goa P. E., Sjobakk T. E., Ostlie A., Fjosne H. E., Bathen T. F. A Simplified approach to measure the effect of the microvasculature in diffusion-weighted MR Imaging applied to breast tumors: Preliminary results. *Radiology* 281(2), (2016), 373–381.

28. While P. T., Teruel J. R., Vidić I, Bathen T. F., Goa P. E. Relative enhanced diffusivity: Noise sensitivity, protocol optimization, and the relation to intravoxel incoherent motion. *Magn. Reson. Mater. Phys. Biol. Med.* 31(3), (2018), 425–438.

29. Pang Y., Turkbey B., Bernardo M., Kruecker J., Kadoury S., Merino M. J., et al. Intravoxel incoherent motion MR imaging for prostate cancer: An evaluation of perfusion fraction and diffusion coefficient derived

from different *b*-value combinations. *Magn. Reson. Med.* 69(2), (2013), 553–562.

30. Iima M., Le Bihan D. Clinical intravoxel incoherent motion and diffusion MR imaging: Past, present, and future. *Radiology* 278(1), (2016), 13–32.

31. Lemke A., Laun F. B., Klauss M., Re T. J., Simon D., Delorme S., et al. Differentiation of pancreas carcinoma from healthy pancreatic tissue using multiple *b*-values comparison of apparent diffusion coefficient and intravoxel incoherent motion derived parameters. *Invest. Radiol.* 44(12), (2009), 769–775.

32. Le Bihan D., Turner R., Moonen C. T. W., Pekar J. Imaging of diffusion and microcirculation with gradient sensitization: Design, strategy, and significance. *J. Magn. Reson. Imaging* 1(1), (1991), 7–28.

33. Pekar J., Moonen C. T. W., Van Zijl P. C. M. On the precision of diffusion perfusion imaging by gradient sensitization. *Magn. Reson. Med.* 23(1), (1992), 122–129.

34. Wirestam R., Borg M., Brockstedt S., Lindgren A., Holtås S., Ståhlberg F. Perfusion-related parameters in intravoxel incoherent motion MR imaging compared with CBV and CBF measured by dynamic susceptibility-contrast MR technique. *Acta Radiol.* 42, (2001), 123–128.

35. Callot V., Bennett E., Decking U. K. M., Balaban R. S., Wen H. In Vivo study of microcirculation in canine myocardium using the IVIM method. *Magn. Reson. Med.* 50, (2003), 531–540.

36. Luciani A., Vignaud A., Cavet M., Van Nhieu J. T., Mallat A., Ruel L., et al. Liver cirrhosis: Intravoxel incoherent motion MR imaging—pilot study. *Radiology* 249(3), (2008), 891–899.

37. Patel J., Sigmund E. E., Rusinek H., Oei M., Babb J. S., Taouli B. Diagnosis of cirrhosis with intravoxel incoherent motion diffusion MRI and dynamic contrast-enhanced MRI alone and in combination: Preliminary experience. *J. Magn. Reson. Imaging* 31, (2010), 589–600.

38. Heusch P., Wittsack H.-J., Pentang G., Buchbender C., Miese F., Schek J., et al. Biexponential analysis of diffusion-weighted imaging: Comparison of three different calculation methods in transplanted kidneys. *Acta Radiol.* 54(10), (2013), 1210–1217.

39. Fujima N., Yoshida D., Sakashita T., Homma A., Tsukahara A., Tha K. K., et al. Intravoxel incoherent motion diffusion-weighted imaging in head and neck squamous cell carcinoma: Assessment of perfusion-related

parameters compared to dynamic contrast-enhanced MRI. *Magn. Reson. Imaging* 32(10), (2014), 1206–1213.

40. Cho G. Y., Moy L., Zhang J. L., Baete S., Lattanzi R., Moccaldi M., et al. Comparison of fitting methods and *b*-value sampling strategies for intravoxel incoherent motion in breast cancer. *Magn. Reson. Med.* 74, (2015), 1077–1085.

41. Lee J. H., Cheong H., Lee S. S., Lee C. K., Sung Y. S., Huh J.-W., et al. Perfusion assessment using intravoxel incoherent motion-based analysis of diffusion-weighted magnetic resonance imaging validation through phantom experiments. *Invest. Radiol.* 51(8), (2016), 520–528.

42. Meeus E. M., Novak J., Withey S. B., Zarinabad N., Dehghani H., Peet A. C. Evaluation of intravoxel incoherent motion fitting methods in low-perfused tissue. *J. Magn. Reson. Imaging* 45(5), (2017), 1325–1334.

43. Park H. J., Sung Y. S., Lee S. S., Lee Y., Cheong H., Kim Y. J., et al. Intravoxel incoherent motion diffusion-weighted MRI of the abdomen: The effect of fitting algorithms on the accuracy and reliability of the parameters. *J. Magn. Reson. Imaging* 45(6), (2017), 1637–1647.

44. Barbieri S., Donati O. F., Froehlich J. M., Thoeny H. C. Impact of the calculation algorithm on biexponential fitting of diffusion-weighted MRI in upper abdominal organs. *Magn. Reson. Med.* 75(5), (2016), 2175–2184.

45. While P. T. A comparative simulation study of Bayesian fitting approaches to intravoxel incoherent motion modeling in diffusion-weighted MRI. *Magn. Reson. Med.* 78(6), (2017), 2373–2387.

46. Wurnig M. C., Donati O. F., Ulbrich E., Filli L., Kenkel D., Thoeny H. C., et al. Systematic analysis of the intravoxel incoherent motion threshold separating perfusion and diffusion effects: Proposal of a standardized algorithm. *Magn. Reson. Med.* 74(5), (2015), 1414–1422.

47. Becker A. S., Perucho J. A., Wurnig M. C., Boss A., Ghafoor S., Khong P.-L., et al. Assessment of cervical cancer with a parameter-free intravoxel incoherent motion imaging algorithm. *Korean J. Radiol.* 18(3), (2017), 510–518.

48. Filli L., Wurnig M. C., Luechinger R., Eberhardt C., Guggenberger R., Boss A. Whole-body intravoxel incoherent motion imaging. *Eur. Radiol.* 25(7), (2015), 2049–2058.

49. Fusco R., Sansone M., Petrillo A. A comparison of fitting algorithms for diffusion-weighted MRI data analysis using an intravoxel incoherent motion model. *Magn. Reson. Mater. Phys. Biol. Med.* 30(2), (2017), 113–120.

50. Merisaari H., Jambor I. Optimization of *b*-value distribution for four mathematical models of prostate cancer diffusion-weighted imaging using *b* values up to 2000 s/mm^2: Simulation and repeatability study. *Magn. Reson. Med.* 73(5), (2015), 1954–1969.

51. Zhang J. L., Sigmund E. E., Rusinek H., Chandarana H., Storey P., Chen Q., et al. Optimization of *b*-value sampling for diffusion-weighted imaging of the kidney. *Magn. Reson. Med.* 67, (2012), 89–97.

52. Cohen A. D., Schieke M. C., Hohenwalter M. D., Schmainda K. M. The Effect of Low *b*-values on the intravoxel incoherent motion derived pseudodiffusion parameter in liver. *Magn. Reson. Med.* 73(1), (2015), 306–311.

53. Dyvorne H., Jajamovich G., Kakite S., Kuehn B., Taouli B. Intravoxel incoherent motion diffusion imaging of the liver: Optimal *b*-value subsampling and impact on parameter precision and reproducibility. *Eur. J. Radiol.* 83(12), (2014), 2109–2113.

54. Ter Voert E. E. G. W, Delso G., Porto M., Huellner M., Veit-Haibach P. Intravoxel incoherent motion protocol evaluation and data quality in normal and malignant liver tissue and comparison to the literature. *Invest. Radiol.* 51(2), (2016), 90–99.

55. Sivia D. S., Skilling J. *Data Analysis: A Bayesian Tutorial.* 2nd edn. (2006) Oxford University Press, Oxford.

56. Jaynes E. T., Bretthorst G. L. *Probability Theory: The Logic of Science.* (2003) Cambridge University Press, Cambridge.

57. Bretthorst G. L., Hutton W. C., Garbow J. R., Ackerman J. J. H. Exponential parameter estimation (in NMR) using Bayesian probability theory. *Concepts Magn. Reson. Part A* 27A (2), (2005), 55–63.

58. Bouhrara M., Spencer R. G. Improved determination of the myelin water fraction in human brain using magnetic resonance imaging through Bayesian analysis of mcDESPOT. *Neuroimage* 127, (2016), 456–471.

59. Gustafsson O., Montelius M., Starck G., Ljungberg M. Impact of prior distributions and central tendency measures on Bayesian intravoxel incoherent motion model fitting. *Magn. Reson. Med.* 79, (2018), 1674–1683.

60. Neil J. J., Bosch C. S., Ackerman J. J. H. An evaluation of the sensitivity of the intravoxel incoherent motion (IVIM) method of blood-flow measurement to changes in cerebral blood-flow. *Magn. Reson. Med.* 32(1), (1994), 60–65.

61. Dyvorne H. A., Galea N., Nevers T., Fiel M. I., Carpenter D., Wong E., et al. Diffusion-weighted imaging of the liver with multiple *b* values: Effect of diffusion gradient polarity and breathing acquisition on image quality and intravoxel incoherent motion parameters-a pilot study. *Radiology* 266(3), (2013), 920–929.

62. Jerome N. P., Orton M. R., d'Arcy J. A., Collins D. J., Koh D.-M., Leach M. O. Comparison of free-breathing with navigator-controlled acquisition regimes in abdominal diffusion-weighted magnetic resonance images: Effect on ADC and IVIM statistics. *J. Magn. Reson. Imaging* 39(1), (2014), 235–240.

63. Shan Y., Zeng M.-S., Liu K., Miao X.-Y., Lin J., Fu C. X., et al. Comparison of free-breathing with navigator-triggered technique in diffusion weighted imaging for evaluation of small hepatocellular carcinoma: Effect on image quality and intravoxel incoherent motion parameters. *J. Comput. Assist. Tomogr.* 39(5), (2015), 709–715.

64. Rydhog A. S., van Osch M. J. P., Lindgren E., Nilsson M., Latt J., Stahlberg F., et al. Intravoxel incoherent motion (IVIM) imaging at different magnetic field strengths: What is feasible? *Magn. Reson. Imaging* 32(10), (2014), 1247–1258.

65. Cui Y., Dyvorne H., Besa C., Cooper N., Taouli B. IVIM diffusion-weighted imaging of the liver at 3.0 T: Comparison with 1.5 T. *Eur. J. Radiol. Open* 2, (2015), 123–128.

66. Barbieri S., Donati O. F., Froehlich J. M., Thoeny H. C. Comparison of intravoxel incoherent motion parameters across MR imagers and field strengths: Evaluation in upper abdominal organs. *Radiology* 279(3), (2016), 784–794.

67. Kakite S., Dyvorne H., Besa C., Cooper N., Facciuto M., Donnerhack C., et al. Hepatocellular carcinoma: Short-term reproducibility of apparent diffusion coefficient and intravoxel incoherent motion parameters at 3.0T. *J. Magn. Reson. Imaging* 41(1), (2015), 149–156.

68. Lecler A., Savatovsky J., Balvay D., Zmuda M., Sadik J.-C., Galatoire O., et al. Repeatability of apparent diffusion coefficient and intravoxel incoherent motion parameters at 3.0 Tesla in orbital lesions. *Eur. Radiol.* 27(12), (2017), 5094–5103.

69. Bane O., Wagner M., Zhang J. L., Dyvorne H. A., Orton M., Rusinek H., et al. Assessment of renal function using intravoxel incoherent motion diffusion-weighted imaging and dynamic contrast-enhanced MRI. *J. Magn. Reson. Imaging* 44(2), (2016), 317–326.

70. Hectors S. J., Wagner M., Besa C., Bane O., Dyvorne H. A., Fiel M. I., et al. Intravoxel incoherent motion diffusion-weighted imaging

of hepatocellular carcinoma: Is there a correlation with flow and perfusion metrics obtained with dynamic contrast-enhanced MRI? *J. Magn. Reson. Imaging* 44(4), (2016), 856–864.

71. Jerome N. P., Boult J. K. R., Orton M. R., d'Arcy J., Collins D. J., Leach M. O., et al. Modulation of renal oxygenation and perfusion in rat kidney monitored by quantitative diffusion and blood oxygen level dependent magnetic resonance imaging on a clinical 1.5T platform. *BMC Nephrol.* 17(2016).

72. Li Y. T., Cercueil J.-P., Yuan J., Chen W., Loffroy R., Wang Y. X. J. Liver intravoxel incoherent motion (IVIM) magnetic resonance imaging: A comprehensive review of published data on normal values and applications for fibrosis and tumor evaluation. *Quant. Imaging Med. Surg.* 7(1), (2017), 59–78.

73. Neal R. M. Slice sampling. *Ann. Stat.* 31(3), (2003), 705–767.

74. Orton M. R., Collins D. J., Koh D. M., Leach M. O. Improved intravoxel incoherent motion analysis of diffusion weighted imaging by data driven Bayesian modeling. *Magn. Reson. Med.* 71, (2014), 411–420.

75. Bouhrara M., Reiter D. A., Spencer R. G. Bayesian analysis of transverse signal decay with application to human brain. *Magn. Reson. Med.* 74, (2015), 785–802.

76. Spinner G. R., von Deuster C., Tezcan K. C., Stoeck C. T., Kozerke S. Bayesian intravoxel incoherent motion parameter mapping in the human heart. *J. Cardiovasc. Magn. Reson.* 19(85), (2017), 1–14.

77. Freiman M., Voss S. D., Mulkern R. V., Perez-Rossello J. M., Callahan M. J., Warfield S. K. Reliable assessment of perfusivity and diffusivity from diffusion imaging of the body. Ayache N., Delingette H., Golland P., Mori K. (eds) *Medical Image Computing and Computer-Assisted Intervention - MICCAI* 2012, Pt 1, pp. 1–9.

78. Freiman M., Perez-Rossello J. M., Callahan M. J., Voss S. D., Ecklund K., Mulkern R. V., et al. Reliable estimation of incoherent motion parametric maps from diffusion-weighted MRI using fusion bootstrap moves. *Med. Image Anal.* 17(3), (2013), 325–336.

79. Kurugol S., Freiman M., Afacan O., Domachevsky L., Perez-Rossello J. M., Callahan M. J., et al. Motion-robust parameter estimation in abdominal diffusion-weighted MRI by simultaneous image registration and model estimation. *Med. Image Anal.* 39, (2017), 124–132.

80. Lawson C. L., Hanson R. J. *Solving Least Squares Problems.* (1974) Prentice-Hall, Englewood Cliffs, NJ.

81. Whittal K. P., Mackay A. L. Quantitative interpretation of NMR relaxation data. *J. Magn. Reson.* 84, (1989), 134–152.

82. Marchand A. J., Hitti E., Monge F., Saint-Jalmes H., Guillin R., Duvauferrier R., et al. MRI quantification of diffusion and perfusion in bone marrow by intravoxel incoherent motion (IVIM) and non-negative least square (NNLS) analysis. *Magn. Reson. Imaging* 32(9), (2014), 1091–1096.

83. Merisaari H., Movahedi P., Perez I. M., Toivonen J., Pesola M., Taimen P., et al. Fitting methods for intravoxel incoherent motion imaging of prostate cancer on region of interest level: Repeatability and Gleason score prediction. *Magn. Reson. Med.* 77(3), (2017), 1249–1264.

84. Keil V. C., Maedler B., Gielen G. H., Pintea B., Hiththetiya K., Gaspranova A. R., et al. Intravoxel incoherent motion MRI in the brain: Impact of the fitting model on perfusion fraction and lesion differentiability. *J. Magn. Reson. Imaging* 46(4), (2017), 1187–1199.

85. Gambarota G., Hitti E., Leporq B., Saint-Jalmes H., Beuf O. Eliminating the blood-flow confounding effect in intravoxel incoherent motion (IVIM) using the non-negative least square analysis in liver. *Magn. Reson. Med.* 77(1), (2017), 310–317.

86. Wurnig M. C., Germann M., Boss A. Is there evidence for more than two diffusion components in abdominal organs? – A magnetic resonance imaging study in healthy volunteers. *NMR Biomed.* 31, (2018), e3852.

87. Zhang Q., Wang Y.-X., Ma H. T., Yuan J. Cramer-Rao bound for intravoxel incoherent motion diffusion weighted imaging fitting. In: *2013 35th Annual International Conference of the IEEE Engineering in Medicine and Biology Society (EMBC)*, pp 511–514.

88. Kuai Z.-X., Liu W.-Y., Zhang Y.-L., Zhu Y.-M. Generalization of intravoxel incoherent motion model by introducing the notion of continuous pseudodiffusion variable. *Magn. Reson. Med.* 76(5), (2016), 1594–1603.

89. Kurugol S., Freiman M., Afacan O., Perez-Rossello J. M., Callahan M. J., Warfield S. K. Spatially-constrained probability distribution model of incoherent motion (SPIM) for abdominal diffusion-weighted MRI. *Med. Image Anal.* 32, (2016), 173–183.

90. Lin C., Shih Y.-Y., Huang S.-L., Huang H.-M. Total variation-based method for generation of intravoxel incoherent motion parametric images in MRI. *Magn. Reson. Med.* 78(4), (2017), 1383–1391.

91. Kayal E. B., Kandasamy D., Khare K., Alampally J. T., Bakhshi S., Sharma R., et al. Quantitative analysis of intravoxel incoherent motion (IVIM)

diffusion MRI using total variation and Huber penalty function. *Med. Phys.* 44(11), (2017), 5849–5858.

92. Reischauer C., Gutzeit A. Image denoising substantially improves accuracy and precision of intravoxel incoherent motion parameter estimates. *PLoS One* 12(4), (2017), 1–18.

93. Gudbjartsson H., Patz S. The Rician distribution of noisy MRI data. *Magn. Reson. Med.* 34(6), (1995), 910–914.

94. Lu Y., Jansen J. F. A., Mazaheri Y., Stambuk H. E., Koutcher J. A., Shukla-Dave A. Extension of the intravoxel incoherent motion model to non-Gaussian diffusion in head and neck cancer. *J. Magn. Reson. Imaging* 36(5), (2012), 1088–1096.

95. Kristoffersen A. Optimal estimation of the diffusion coefficient from non-averaged and averaged noisy magnitude data. *J. Magn. Reson.* 187, (2007), 293–305.

96. Veraart J., Rajan J., Peeters R. R., Leemans A., Sunaert S., Sijbers J. Comprehensive framework for accurate diffusion MRI parameter estimation. *Magn. Reson. Med.* 70, (2013), 972–984.

97. Coupé P, Manjón J. V., Gedamu E., Arnold D., Robles M., Collins D. L. Robust Rician noise estimation for MR images. *Med. Image Anal.* 14, (2010), 483–493.

98. Dikaios N., Punwani S., Hamy V., Purpura P., Rice S., Forster M., et al. Noise estimation from averaged diffusion weighted images: Can unbiased quantitative decay parameters assist cancer evaluation? *Magn. Reson. Med.* 71(6), (2014), 2105–2117.

99. Murphy P., Wolfson T., Gamst A., Sirlin C., Bydder M. Error model for reduction of cardiac and respiratory motion effects in quantitative liver DW-MRI. *Magn. Reson. Med.* 70(5), (2013), 1460–1469.

100. Zhang Q., King A. D., Bhatia K. S., Yeung D. K. W., Wang Y.-X., Liang D., et al. Improving intra-voxel incoherent motion MRI quantification using wild bootstrap. In: *2014 IEEE 11th International Symposium on Biomedical Imaging (ISBI)*, pp 726–729.

101. Huang H.-M., Shih Y.-Y., Lin C. Formation of parametric images using mixed-effects models: A feasibility study. *NMR Biomed.* 29(3), (2016), 239–247.

102. Deo R. C. Machine learning in medicine. *Circulation* 132, (2015) 1920–1930.

103. Parmar C., Grossmann P., Bussink J., Lambin P., Aerts H. J. W. L. Machine learning methods for quantitative radiomic biomarkers. *Sci. Rep.* 5, (2015), 13087.

104. Ciritsis A., Rossi C., Wurnig M. C., Van V. P., Boss A. Intravoxel incoherent motion model-free determination of tissue type in abdominal organs using machine learning. *Invest. Radiol.* 52(12), (2017), 747–757.

105. Bertleff M., Domsch S., Weingaertner S., Zapp J., O'Brien K., Barth M., et al. Diffusion parameter mapping with the combined intravoxel incoherent motion and kurtosis model using artificial neural networks at 3 T. *NMR Biomed.* 30(12), (2017).

Chapter 24

IVIM MRI Analysis with Low Perfusion

Emma M. Meeus[a,b,c] **and Andrew C. Peet**[b,c]
[a]*Physical Sciences of Imaging in Biomedical Sciences Doctoral Training Centre, University of Birmingham, Edgbaston, Birmingham, B15 2TT, UK*
[b]*Institute of Cancer and Genomic Sciences, University of Birmingham, Edgbaston, Birmingham, B15 2TT, UK*
[c]*Department of Oncology, Birmingham Women's and Children's Hospital Steelhouse Lane, Birmingham B4 6NH, UK*
e.m.meeus@bham.ac.uk

This chapter reviews the application of intravoxel incoherent motion (IVIM) model in low-perfused tissues. Although more commonly applied in the abdominal organs, such as liver and kidneys, IVIM can also provide valuable information in the brain. Brain and many of its related pathologies are relatively low perfused compared to the abdominal organs, but the use of a noninvasive measure of perfusion would be advantageous. However, the application of IVIM in low-perfused tissues is challenging and requires careful consideration before it can provide reliable measures for routine clinical practice and clinical decision making.

Intravoxel Incoherent Motion (IVIM) MRI: Principles and Applications
Edited by Denis Le Bihan, Mami Iima, Christian Federau, and Eric E. Sigmund

ISBN 978-981-4800-19-8 (Hardcover), 0978-0-429-42727-5 (eBook)
www.panstanford.com

24.1 Introduction

The application of IVIM model to multi-b-value diffusion-weighted magnetic resonance imaging (DWMRI) has garnered more interest in recent years. While originally applied in the brain [1], the IVIM model has been more commonly used in the abdomen, where relatively high-perfused organs, such as the liver and kidneys, have highlighted its potential [2–5]. However, the advantages of deriving quantitative parameters of both diffusion and perfusion with a single protocol are also of interest for the brain. The IVIM MRI has the potential to provide an assessment of perfusion in patients with renal failure or allergy, where administration of contrast agents is contraindicated. The recent reports of gadolinium deposits in the brain have also posed questions on the safety of gadolinium-based contrast agents, which are used in the "gold standard" perfusion MRI for the brain, the dynamic susceptibility contrast (DSC) imaging [6, 7]. In this chapter, the application of IVIM MRI in low-perfused tissues, such as those found in the brain, is reviewed.

24.2 Tissue Perfusion

This section briefly introduces the concept of tissue perfusion, why it is a valuable quantitative measure, and how it changes in pathological tissues.

Tissue perfusion, more commonly described as blood perfusion, has an important role in the delivery of oxygen and nutrients to cells in tissue [8]. The oxygenated arterial blood circulates in the microcapillary network, and it is delivered to the tissue via the blood–tissue exchange through the capillary walls. The same network is also responsible, along with lymphatics, for the transportation and removal of waste products resulting from tissue metabolism. These processes are affected by many different parameters related to the microvascular anatomy, blood circulation, and the exchange interface between blood and tissue. Therefore, a measure of perfusion can provide valuable information about the underlying microvascularity and the viability of the tissue.

The level—or degree—of tissue perfusion depends on the type of tissue and can vary to a great extent between different organs.

The most highly perfused organ is the kidney, which comprises 20%–25% of the cardiac output, that is, the blood volume pumped by the heart per minute [9]. In comparison, the cerebral blood flow in the brain is approximately 15%–20% of the cardiac output, due to the high metabolic demand and brain's inability to store energy [10]. Both of these organs are essential for life and hence sensitive to any disruptions in their respective blood supply. Autoregulation processes, which are intrinsic abilities of these organs, exist to maintain or adjust the blood flow due to any deviations. In the brain, these specialized processes manage the high metabolic demands of the brain and prevent the significant consequences that could result from cerebral ischemia [10].

24.2.1 Perfusion in Tissue Pathologies

An increase in the blood flow to specific brain regions is connected to the activation of cognitive functions [11]. This provides the link for perfusion to measure cognitive decline, for example, in diseases such as Alzheimer's [12, 13]. In general, any disruption of blood supply and hence perfusion can result in malfunction of tissue and ultimately lead to tissue death [14]. In many brain diseases, such as traumatic brain injury [15, 16], ischemic stroke [17, 18], and brain tumors [19], perfusion changes occur due to the suppression of the previously mentioned autoregulation processes. Many of these disease states also present as low-perfused tissue, although for brain tumors, this is more characteristic of low-grade gliomas [20–22].

The vasculature found in tumors is complex and is known to be unevenly distributed with irregular branching of the tumor vessels, with poorly defined hierarchy [23]. As a result, the blood flow in tumors is not constant along a single direction and may follow different paths and even change direction through the same vessel. In contrast, the vasculature in healthy tissues is arranged in a hierarchy of well-differentiated components. The tumor perfusion provides an important marker of neoangiogenesis, which is characteristic of, for example, high-grade gliomas. Previously, the histopathological assessment of gliomas has showed that the increase in the number of blood vessels progressed with the glioma grade [24]. The increase in tumor perfusion, measured with DSCMRI-derived cerebral blood volume (CBV), was also shown to be a potential biomarker for the detection of malignant progression of low-grade gliomas [25]. These studies highlight the use of perfusion in gliomas, which is also one of the applications previously studied with IVIM MRI [26, 27].

Another common pathology with characteristically low perfusion is the ischemic stroke. Multiple disease mechanisms can result in a stroke, although they all share the aspect of disruption occurring in the cerebral blood flow [10]. In an ischemic stroke, the lack of blood flow due to a narrowed or blocked artery can result in cell death. Perfusion MRI has the potential to support the rapidly required treatment decisions for acute stroke patients. However, the relative ease of applicability of DWMRI, and its extraordinary ability to confirm the diagnosis of a stroke, has meant that DWMRI has become the "gold standard" for its detection [28]. Nevertheless, the diagnosis of transient ischemic attack, where an artery is temporarily blocked, was not always detectable by DWMRI, while changes were observed in a perfusion MRI [29, 30]. This presents a favorable role for the use of IVIM MRI, which is able to derive parameters of both diffusion and perfusion in a single protocol.

Low perfusion is also presented in breast tissue and breast cancer. MRI has become an important tool in the characterization of breast cancer, and in particular the dynamic contrast-enhanced (DCE) MRI has shown promise in being highly sensitive in its detection [31, 32]. Similar to the brain gliomas, the vascularity found in the less aggressive lesions or more specifically, benign lesions, has been found to be lower compared to the malignant cases [33]. However, previous studies have shown that the use of DCE MRI can result in false positives, and DWMRI has been applied to increase the specificity [34, 35]. Once again, the combined use of diffusion and perfusion MRI provides a more beneficial scenario and a more complete investigation.

The vasculature in tumors and other diseased states provides a complicated microenvironment for investigation. The use of imaging methods, such as IVIM MRI, unique with noninvasive measures of both perfusion and diffusion, can offer invaluable information in the different steps of clinical routine, from diagnosis to the assessment of treatment response.

24.3 IVIM MRI Studies in Low-Perfused Tissues

The IVIM model has provided an alternative tool for the assessment of perfusion in tissues, while also providing a quantitative measure of diffusion [1,36]. The tissues often considered to be low perfused in "IVIM terms" have been characterized with perfusion fraction (f) values of $f \approx 0.1$ or lower. This accounts for approximately 10% of the diffusion MRI signal arising from the microvascular compartment [37]. The other perfusion parameter provided by the IVIM model is the pseudodiffusion coefficient (D^*), which describes the incoherent movement of blood in the microvascular compartment. The ratio of D^* to the tissue diffusion coefficient (D) determines the degree of the biexponential behavior in the tissue and provides an important quantity in the context of applying a biexponential fitting model to the data. Examples of IVIM parameters reported for healthy tissues of low perfusion are listed in Table 24.1, including both brain and breast tissue.

Table 24.1 Examples of previously reported IVIM parameters in low-perfused healthy tissues

Author	No. of cases	Tissue type	D	D^*	f
Wu et al. [38]	18	Gray matter	0.84 ± 0.05	8.2 ± 0.9	0.14 ±0.02
		White matter	0.77 ± 0.04	7.9 ± 0.9	0.070 ± 0.01
Grech-Sollars et al. [39]	9	Gray matter	0.75 ± 0.02	-	0.10 ± 0.002
		White matter	0.65 ± 0.01	-	0.080 ± 0.002
Chen et al. [40]	28	Breast tissue	1.84 ± 0.20	12.0 ± 7.2	0.089 ± 0.04
Liu et al. [41]	39	Breast tissue	1.96 (1.81, 2.15)	12.4 (11.3, 14.7)	0.053 (0.03, 0.59)

Note: D and D^* are in units of $\times 10^{-3}$ mm^2/s. Standard deviations (±) or quartile ranges (lower quartile, higher quartile) are reported.

The complex nature of the tissue vasculature of low-perfused tumors and other disease states has been previously investigated with the IVIM model. Some of the previous studies and the reported IVIM parameters are listed in Table 24.2. In the brain-related studies of stroke and gliomas, the IVIM parameters *D* and *f* have generally been found to be the most clinically valuable. For example, the IVIM *f* has shown value in differentiation of low- and high-grade gliomas [26, 27, 42, 43], in differentiation of recurrent tumor from treatment effects in glioblastoma, [44] and in being a prognostic biomarker in glioma patients [45]. In the detection of stroke, significantly decreased *f* values have been observed in the infarcted regions [20, 21, 46, 47], together with a decrease in the *D* parameter, which agrees with the expected pathophysiology of a stroke [21].

Table 24.2 Examples of previously reported IVIM parameters (±standard deviation) in pathological tissues of low perfusion

Author	Pathology	*D*	*D**	*f*
Suo et al. [21]	Ischemic stroke	0.42 ± 0.10	10.2 ± 4.17	0.043 ± 0.020
Bisdas et al. [26]	Low-grade glioma	0.52± 0.28	10.8 ± 7.8	0.061 ± 0.039
	High-grade glioma	0.76 ± 0.49	41.6 ± 26.1	0.107 ± 0.083
Federau et al. [27]	Low-grade glioma	-	11.4 ± 5.0	0.084 ± 0.016
	High-grade glioma	-	11.7 ± 5.8	0.127 ± 0.031
Togao et al. [41]	Low-grade glioma	1.26 ± 0.37	12.1 ± 9.7	0.058 ± 0.038
	High-grade glioma	0.94 ± 0.19	13.3 ± 9.0	0.175 ± 0.063
Meeus et al. [37]	Low-grade glioma (pediatric)	1.63 ± 0.12	7.23 ± 5.1	0.095 ± 0.032
Cho et al. [33]	Malignant breast lesion	1.32 ± 0.65†	17.7 ± 4.45†	0.091 ± 0.051†
	Benign breast lesion	1.89 ± 0.70†	18.0 ± 16.5†	0.050 ± 0.030†
Sigmund et al. [50]	Breast cancer	1.14 ± 0.32	14.9 ± 11.4	0.105 ± 0.050
Iima et al. [51]	Malignant breast lesion	1.16 ± 0.39#	24.3 ± 18.1	0.084 ± 0.023
	Benign breast lesion	2.41 ± 0.36#	68.6 ± 43.5	0.044 ± 0.043

Author	Pathology	D	D^*	f
Chen et al. [40]	Malignant breast lesion	0.81 ± 0.23	15.2 ± 12.2	0.107 ± 0.034
	Benign breast lesion	1.44 ± 0.54	12.0 ± 3.2	0.079 ± 0.037

Note: D and D^* are in units of $\times 10^{-3}$ mm^2/s.
#IVIM-D estimated using the kurtosis IVIM model.
†Deviation reported as an interquartile range.

The most common glioma type in adults is the high-grade anaplastic astrocytoma (grade III) and the glioblastoma multiforme (grade IV). However, in pediatrics the low-grade pilocytic astrocytoma (grade I) is the most common glioma type and the high-grade gliomas are much rarer [48]. This means that most of the glioma population in pediatrics is characterized by low perfusion. An example of a pediatric low-grade glioma (grade I) with IVIM D and f maps is presented in Fig. 24.1 and for a comparison, a highly perfused choroid plexus tumor is also shown. The low-grade glioma appears hypoperfused compared to the surrounding brain tissue, while the choroid plexus tumor indicates the high vascularity commonly associated with these types of tumors [49].

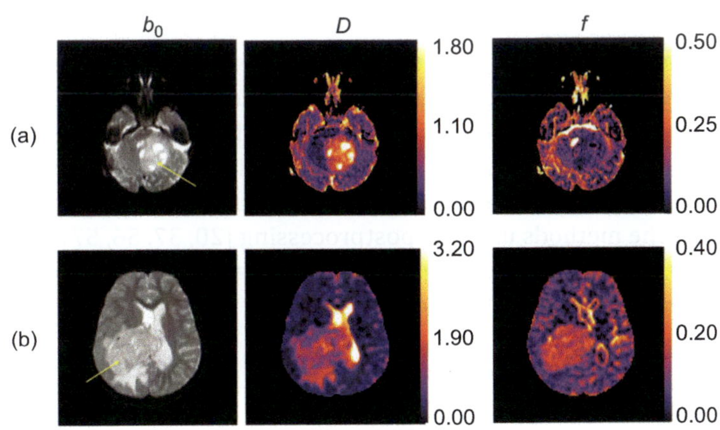

Figure 24.1 Example cases of pediatric brain tumors with low and high perfusion and the corresponding IVIM parameter maps D and f. (a) Low perfusion shown in a low-grade glioma (pilocytic astrocytoma) and (b) high perfusion in an atypical choroid plexus papilloma (grade II). The arrows indicate the location of the tumor, and the units of D are reported in $\times 10^{-3}$ mm^2/s.

In addition to brain studies, the IVIM model has also been applied in breast cancer, where the IVIM-derived perfusion fraction has indicated relatively low perfusion in some studies, particularly for benign lesions. The focus in many of these studies was the discrimination of malignant lesions from benign ones [33, 40, 52, 53], which was typically possible with the D and f parameters. However, in most cases, the D^* parameter was shown to have high variability, similarly to the previous brain studies, and was not able to discriminate between the tumors [27, 33, 37, 52]. More recently, the IVIM parameters have also shown potential as prognostic biomarkers of the treatment response to neoadjuvant treatment (NAT) [54, 55].

While the application of IVIM in clinical studies of the brain and breast has shown promise in both diagnosis and prognosis, the results have almost solely relied on the IVIM parameters D and f. In the following section, some of the challenges contributing toward the unreliability of D^* and the IVIM analysis in low-perfused tissues are discussed.

24.4 Application of IVIM MRI in Low-Perfused Tissues

The use of IVIM or any quantitative technique as a clinical application requires it to be sufficiently robust in the process of image acquisition and processing, and data fitting and analysis. Previous studies have demonstrated that the reliable derivation of IVIM parameters depends on the chosen b values and hence the DWMRI protocol, as well as the methods used for postprocessing [20, 37, 56, 57]. In this section, the IVIM analysis applied to low-perfused tissues and the technical challenges of its use are reviewed.

24.4.1 IVIM MRI Analysis

IVIM fitting is commonly performed using nonlinear least-squares approaches; and, more recently, the Bayesian probability methods have been used [56, 58, 59]. The nonlinear least-squares fitting can be constrained to different extents, and the fitting for the parameters can be performed simultaneously or in a stepwise fashion. As most of the image data is influenced by noise, the simultaneous fitting is rarely feasible due to its high degree of freedom and hence higher requirement for the signal-to-noise ratio (SNR). In previous studies focusing on the abdominal regions, the stepwise fitting, also known as the segmented approach, has been found to compute the most robust or reliable IVIM parameters [59, 60]. This was also found to be the case in a simulation study investigating low-perfused tissues of pediatric low-grade gliomas and healthy gray matter [37]. The IVIM parameters derived in this study with the segmented method were found to be significantly different to those derived with the simultaneous fitting. The segmented fitting also produced a reduced number of outliers and improved the accuracy and reproducibility of the IVIM parameters. This was particularly the case at lower SNR levels (≤ 40).

24.4.1.1 Estimation of the pseudodiffusion coefficient D^*

The low-*b*-value region is critical for the evaluation of the IVIM perfusion parameters, that is, the pseudodiffusion coefficient D^* and the perfusion fraction f. However, as indicated in many previous studies, the determination of IVIM D^* has proved challenging [37, 38, 59]. Depending on the characteristics of the signal, and in particular its degree of biexponential behavior, the IVIM D^* can be derived with some level of robustness. When $D^* \gg D$ by at least an order of magnitude, the biexponential fitting is relatively stable [61]. However, for cases where the difference between the two diffusion coefficients is smaller, the fitting scenario becomes more challenging and leads to a poor estimation of D^* [37, 38]. In the brain, a previous study by Wu et al. [38] reported the average error of estimating D^* to be 100% and 300% at an SNR = 30, for simulated tissues of gray matter and white matter, respectively [38]. In the same study, the errors were estimated to be 5% in gray matter and 10% in white matter for the perfusion fraction parameter. These results agree with other studies performed in the brain and also in previous studies of breast [60, 62]. Therefore, the overall indication is that the D^* parameter is not sufficiently robust for use in clinical practice with the current least-squares fitting approaches in low-perfused tissues.

An example of a young adult volunteer is presented in Fig. 24.2, showing the DW signal data in gray matter and white matter and the estimated IVIM parameter maps. The signal decay for the white matter shows the characteristically weak "IVIM effect" compared to that for the gray matter.

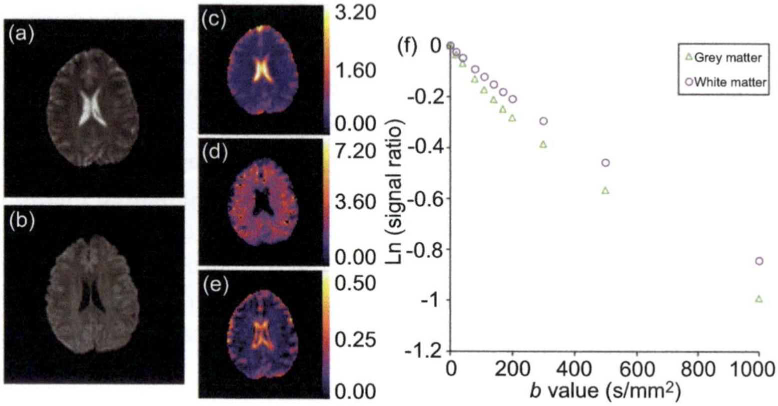

Figure 24.2 An example volunteer case analyzed with the IVIM model. The diffusion-weighted images of (a) b = 0 and (b) b = 1000 s/mm^2; the IVIM parameter maps of (c) D, (d) D^*, and (e) f; and the diffusion-weighted signal decay in (f) gray matter and white matter. The IVIM parameters maps were estimated using the segmented fitting approach with b-value distribution: 0, 20, 40, 80, 110, 140, 170, 200, 300, 500, and 1000 s/mm^2. Both D and D^* are in units of mm^2/s.

24.4.1.2 Constrained IVIM fitting approach

As discussed in the previous section, the constrained nonlinear least-squares IVIM fitting methods have provided a way to stabilize the fitting by fixing the D (and f in the segmented method) parameters for the nonlinear biexponential fitting step [37]. Although this was initially applied to increase the robustness of the estimation of D^*, the linear fitting of the log of the high b values for estimation of D and f has provided an alternative way to estimate the more robust and clinically valuable IVIM parameters in a separate fitting step. The use of this "simplified" approach has been evaluated in previous brain studies, with consideration only given to D and f, with no estimation of D^* [20, 57]. This might provide a compromise for the IVIM studies performed in the low-perfused tissues, where the D^* parameter with the current fitting approaches cannot be considered to be clinically reliable.

Separation of the "perfusion influenced" diffusion and "pure" diffusion

An important consequence of the use of segmented (or two-step [27, 46]) IVIM fitting approach is the need to estimate a *b*-value threshold that can separate the "perfusion influenced" diffusion (D^*) and the "pure" diffusion (D). In the segmented approach, the D parameter is estimated from the linear fit of the high b values and the f parameter by extrapolating the fit back to the y-intercept. The pseudodiffusion coefficient D^* is then estimated using nonlinear fitting with the other two parameters fixed. However, such an approach assumes that the high-*b*-value DW signal, above the *b*-value threshold, is unaffected by perfusion. The chosen *b*-value threshold has been previously shown to particularly affect the accurate estimation of the f parameter [40, 57, 63].

In the brain, the *b*-value threshold has been commonly set to b = 200 s/mm^2. In a previous study, the threshold for the most reliable IVIM parameters was estimated to be as high as b = 500 s/mm^2, when regions of low perfusion are considered [57]. The use of a lower *b*-value threshold was found to lead to biased estimation of both D and f parameters using simulations and also in vivo regions of gray matter (D^* was not considered in this study). The biases for D and f were the opposite, with negative and positive biases shown, respectively. In the simulated regions of higher perfusion, for example, kidney or liver, the effect of bias was considerably lower [57]. An example of segmented fitting in simulated gray matter and the use of a *b*-value threshold of 300 s/mm^2 and 500 s/mm^2 is shown in Fig 24.3. Although the linear fitting looks qualitatively similar, the error in f due to bias was −17.6% for the use of b = 300 s/mm^2 and −7.65% for the use of b = 500 s/mm^2 as the threshold. No noise was added in the presented data. These findings suggest that the use of a *b*-value threshold as low as b = 200 s/mm^2 in the brain will lead to biased results. However, the use of a higher *b*-value threshold will be more affected by noise, and therefore in some cases, the use of a lower *b*-value threshold might be more optimal [57].

Similar findings have been reported in a previous study of breast tissue. The study by Chen et al. [40] optimized the *b*-value threshold for the differentiation of malignant and benign breast lesions.

In their case, the threshold was estimated to be b = 300 s/mm^2, although for normal breast tissue, this was estimated to be b = 400 s/mm^2. The difference in the threshold was likely due to the healthy breast tissue presenting as lower perfused compared to the pathological tissues. As shown in the brain, the signal behavior with a low f and D^*/D ratio typically means that the segmented approach with a lower b-value threshold will introduce a bias in the estimated IVIM parameters.

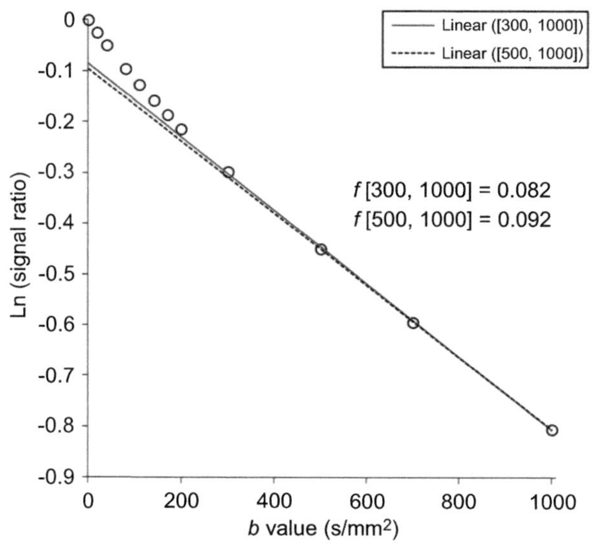

Figure 24.3 Segmented IVIM fitting approach and the use of the linear fitting to estimate D and f. The signal was simulated with values based on gray matter ($D = 0.7 \times 10^{-3}$ mm^2/s, D^* 7.0×10^{-3} mm^2/s, and $f = 0.1$), and no noise was added. The f value was estimated using b-value distributions [300, 1000] and [500, 1000], with errors of –17.6% and –7.65% to the ground truth value, respectively.

The results from these studies bring attention to the often-ignored factor of b-value threshold in the constrained IVIM fitting, which can lead to a highly biased estimation of the IVIM parameters. This seems to be especially important in the lower-perfused tissues, or in tissues where $D^*/D < 10$. Therefore, a higher threshold should be considered to reduce the systematic bias, although estimation of the SNR remains important to evaluate whether the higher b values have a sufficient SNR for a robust IVIM parameter estimation.

24.4.1.3 Data quality and SNR

Perhaps the most important consideration of IVIM analysis in any tissue type should be the data quality. Previous studies have indicated that the requirements for sufficient data quality and hence the estimation of the IVIM parameters should be stricter in the low-perfused tissues [37, 57, 61]. In a previous study with simulations of pediatric low-grade gliomas, reliable estimates of D and f parameters were computed at an SNR = 40 [37], while D^* had limited robustness. Similar findings were reported in a study by Wu et al. [38], who suggested an SNR = 30 for a healthy brain, while a study by Lemke et al. [61] reported a "critical" SNR = 50 for the reliable use of IVIM in low-perfused tissues. The "critical" SNR level for higher-perfused systems, such as kidney and liver, was as low as SNR = 8. The typical finding in the previous simulation studies of the brain was that the IVIM perfusion parameters (D^* and f) were overestimated at lower SNR levels [37, 38, 61].

Even though the IVIM analysis has been shown to be highly dependent on the data quality, most of the clinical studies reported to date have not included estimates of the image SNR levels. This provides a difficult scenario for the assessment of the reliability of the reported IVIM parameters, and in particular for the lower-perfused tissues with stricter SNR requirements. Another complication is the studies comparing IVIM parameters of two pathologies, for example, high- and low-grade gliomas. In these cases, a poorer SNR might still provide reliable results for high-grade gliomas (with higher f values and typically higher D^*/D ratio), but the estimation of IVIM parameters in the lower-perfused low-grade gliomas might be affected by noise and hence result in a less robust fitting performance and higher variability in the IVIM parameters. Therefore, in cases where the difference between two pathologies might be small, the SNR can give a good indication whether the IVIM analysis is feasible and able to estimate the parameters with sufficient accuracy and precision. Consequently, an estimate of the SNR should be of importance, in particular where IVIM parameters are used in a clinical setting as potential imaging biomarkers.

Partial volume effect in the brain

One specific challenge of IVIM analysis in the brain is the partial volume effect, which is often observed in the interfaces of cerebrospinal fluid (CSF) and the surrounding tissue. In these voxels, two components with a large difference in their diffusion signal decay result in an artificially high degree of biexponential behavior, which the IVIM model interprets as a region of high perfusion and hence as a high f value. This can also be a problem in the interfaces of low-perfused tumors and the surrounding nonpathological tissue, as shown in Fig. 24.4f. The effect has often been negated by the use of thresholding, where, for example, $f > 0.3$ has been reduced to zero [27, 46]. Either way, the IVIM parameter perfusion fraction f maps are affected by artificially high values on certain interfaces or by empty regions (pixel intensity = 0) with no quantitative values. This is problematic for the clinical use of IVIM, where interpretation of such regions is questionable. While the use of a higher resolution can help to negate such effects, this leads to a poorer SNR. A higher number of signal averages (NSA) or a higher number of signal excitations (NEX) can then be used to increase the SNR, which in turn leads to a longer acquisition time. Therefore, it is important to find a compromise between the different factors to accommodate the requirements and needs of a clinical protocol and also to ensure the appropriate data quality.

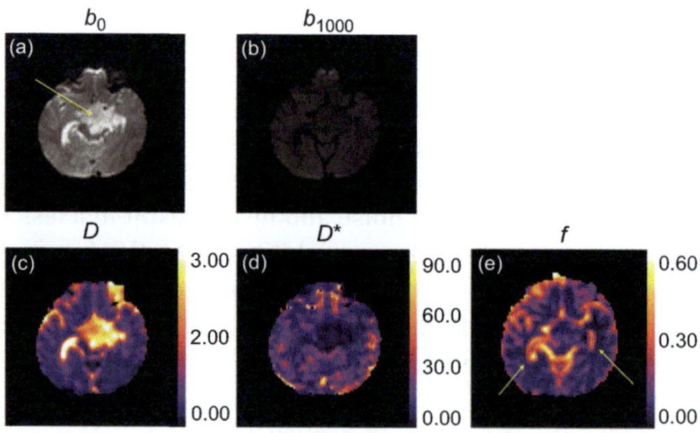

Figure 24.4 The IVIM analysis in a pediatric optic pathway glioma (low grade). Diffusion-weighted MR images of (a) $b = 0$ (arrow indicates the tumor) and (b) $b = 1000$ s/mm^2 and the IVIM parameter maps (c) D, (d) D^*, and (e) f, with arrows indicating areas with a partial volume effect (i.e., artificially high f values). The D and D^* maps are reported in units of $\times 10^{-3}$ mm^2/s.

24.5 Summary

This chapter provided an overview of the challenges related to the use of IVIM in low-perfused tissues. While most of these factors apply to IVIM analysis of any tissue type, the influence of, for example, bias from the fitting and the requirements for SNR are greater in the lower-perfused tissues. These factors also contribute to the difficulties for the robust measurement of the pseudodiffusion coefficient D^*, although the signal behavior itself (low D^*/D ratio) or the "weak IVIM effect" is likely to be the main challenge. This has meant that in the studies of the brain, the D^* parameter has been rarely reported as a potential imaging biomarker or the analysis of D^* has been completely overlooked.

Although the use of IVIM MRI analysis in low-perfused tissues remains challenging, the previous studies have shown that it can produce clinically valuable information and, in particular, provide parameters of both diffusion and perfusion in a single protocol. Therefore, the focus should now move on to the consideration of consensus of its application in tissues such as the brain and breast in order to ensure that the future clinical studies have guidance in the choice of protocols and reliable estimation of the IVIM parameters.

Acknowledgment

The data presented was acquired from the Children's Cancer and Leukaemia Group (CCLG) Functional Imaging Group e-repository. This work was funded by the Engineering and Physical Sciences Research Council (EPSRC, EP/F50053X/1) and the National Institute for Health Research (NIHR) via a research professorship (13-0053).

References

1. Le Bihan D., Breton E., Lallemand D., Grenier P., Cabanis E., Laval-Jeantet M. MR imaging of intravoxel incoherent motions: application to diffusion and perfusion in neurologic disorders. *Radiology* (1986), 161, 401–407.
2. Luciani A., Vignaud A., Cavet M., Van Nhieu J. T., Mallat A., Ruel L., et al. Liver cirrhosis: Intravoxel incoherent motion MR imaging-pilot study. *Radiology* (2008), 249, 891–899.

3. Yamada I., Aung W., Himeno Y., Nakagawa T., Shibuya H. Diffusion coefficients in abdominal organs and hepatic lesions: evaluation with intravoxel incoherent motion echo-planar MR imaging. *Radiology* (1999), 210, 617–623.
4. Chandarana H., Kang S. K., Wong S., Rusinek H., Zhang J. L., Arizono S., et al. Diffusion-weighted intravoxel incoherent motion imaging of renal tumors with histopathologic correlation. *Invest. Radiol.* (2012), 47, 688–696.
5. Gaing B., Sigmund E. E., Huang W. C., Babb J. S., Parikh N. S., Stoffel D., et al. Subtype differentiation of renal tumors using voxel-based histogram analysis of intravoxel incoherent motion parameters. *Invest. Radiol.* (2015), 50, 144–152.
6. Runge V. M. Safety of the gadolinium-based contrast agents for magnetic resonance imaging, focusing in part on their accumulation in the brain and especially the dentate nucleus. *Invest. Radiol.* (2016), 51, 273–279.
7. Stojanov D., Aracki-Trenkic A., Benedeto-Stojanov D. Gadolinium deposition within the dentate nucleus and globus pallidus after repeated administrations of gadolinium-based contrast agents-current status. *Neuroradiology* (2016), 58, 433–441.
8. Le Bihan D., Turner R. The capillary network: a link between IVIM and classical perfusion. *Magn. Reson. Med.* (1992), 27, 171–178.
9. Pinsky M. R. Functional hemodynamic monitoring: current concepts in critical care. *Curr Opin Crit Care* (2014), 20, 288–293.
10. Markus H. Cerebral perfusion and stroke. *J. Neurol. Neurosurg. Psychiatry* (2004), 75, 353–361.
11. Logothetis N. K. What we can do and what we cannot do with fMRI. *Nature* (2008), 453, 869–878.
12. Chao L. L., Buckley S. T., Kornak J., Schuff N., Madison C., Yaffe K., et al. ASL Perfusion MRI predicts cognitive decline and conversion from MCI to dementia. *Alzheimer Dis. Assoc. Disord.* (2010), 24, 19–27.
13. Johnson N. A., Jahng G. H., Weiner M. W., Miller B. L., Chui H.C., Jagust W. J., et al. Pattern of cerebral hypoperfusion in Alzheimer disease and mild cognitive impairment measured with arterial spin-labeling MR imaging: initial experience. *Radiology* (2005), 234, 851–859.
14. Calamante F. Arterial input function in perfusion MRI: a comprehensive review. *Prog. Nucl. Magn. Reson. Spectrosc,* (2013), 74, 1–32.
15. Figaji A. A., Zwane E., Fieggen A. G., Argent A. C., Le Roux P. D., Siesjo P., Peter J. C. Pressure autoregulation, intracranial pressure, and brain

tissue oxygenation in children with severe traumatic brain injury. *J. Neurosurg. Pediatr.* (2009), 4, 420–428.

16. Allen K. A. Pathophysiology and treatment of severe traumatic brain injuries in children. *J. Neurosci. Nurs.* (2016), 48, 15–27.
17. Budohoski K. P., Czosnyka M., Kirkpatrick P. J., Smielewski P., Steiner L. A., Pickard J. D. Clinical relevance of cerebral autoregulation following subarachnoid haemorrhage. *Nat. Rev. Neurol.* (2013), 9, 152–163.
18. Aries M. J., Elting J. W., De Keyser J., Kremer B. P., Vroomen P. C. Cerebral autoregulation in stroke: a review of transcranial Doppler studies. *Stroke* (2010), 41, 2697–2704.
19. Holodny A. I., Schulder M., Liu W. C., Wolko J., Maldjian J. A., Kalnin A. J. The effect of brain tumors on BOLD functional MR imaging activation in the adjacent motor cortex: implications for image-guided neurosurgery. *AJNR Am. J. Neuroradiol.* (2000), 21, 1415–1422.
20. Conklin J., Heyn C., Roux M., Cerny M., Wintermark M., Federau C. A. Simplified model for intravoxel incoherent motion perfusion imaging of the brain. *AJNR Am. J. Neuroradiol.* (2016), 37, 2251–2257.
21. Suo S., Cao M., Zhu W., Li L., Li J., Shen F., et al. Stroke assessment with intravoxel incoherent motion diffusion-weighted MRI. *NMR Biomed.* (2016), 29, 320–328.
22. Liu W., Wang B., Wolfowitz R., Yeh P. H., Nathan D. E., Graner J., et al. Perfusion deficits in patients with mild traumatic brain injury characterized by dynamic susceptibility contrast MRI. *NMR Biomed.* (2013), 26, 651–663.
23. Nagy J. A., Chang S., Dvorak A. M., Dvorak H. F. Why are tumour blood vessels abnormal and why is it important to know? *Br. J. Cancer* (2009), 100, 865–869.
24. Togao O., Hiwatashi A., Yamashita K., Kikuchi K., Mizoguchi M., Yoshimoto K., et al. Differentiation of high-grade and low-grade diffuse gliomas by intravoxel incoherent motion MR imaging. *Neuro. Oncol.* (2016), 18, 132–141.
25. Danchaivijitr N., Waldman A. D., Tozer D. J., Benton C. E., Brasil Caseiras G., Tofts P. S., et al. Low-grade gliomas: do changes in rCBV measurements at longitudinal perfusion-weighted MR imaging predict malignant transformation?. *Radiology* (2008), 247, 170–178.
26. Bisdas S., Koh T. S., Roder C., Braun C., Schittenhelm J., Ernemann U., et al. Intravoxel incoherent motion diffusion-weighted MR imaging of gliomas: feasibility of the method and initial results. *Neuroradiology* (2013), 55, 1189–1196.

27. Federau C., Meuli R., O'Brien K., Maeder P., Hagmann P. Perfusion measurement in brain gliomas with intravoxel incoherent motion MRI. *AJNR Am J Neuroradiol.* (2014), 35, 256–262.

28. Copen W. A., Schaefer P. W., Wu O. MR perfusion imaging in acute ischemic stroke. *Neuroimaging Clin. N. Am.* (2011), 21, 259–283.

29. Restrepo L., Jacobs M. A., Barker P. B., Wityk R. J. Assessment of transient ischemic attack with diffusion- and perfusion-weighted imaging. *AJNR Am. J. Neuroradiol.* (2004), 25, 1645–1652.

30. Mlynash M., Olivot J. M., Tong D. C., Lansberg M. G., Eyngorn I., Kemp S., et al. Yield of combined perfusion and diffusion MR imaging in hemispheric TIA. *Neurology* (2009), 72, 1127–1233.

31. Schnall M. D., Blume J., Bluemke D. A., DeAngelis G. A., DeBruhl N., Harms S., et al. Diagnostic architectural and dynamic features at breast MR imaging: multicenter study. *Radiology* (2006), 238, 42–53.

32. Turnbull L.W. Dynamic contrast-enhanced MRI in the diagnosis and management of breast cancer. *NMR Biomed.* (2009), 22, 28–39.

33. Cho G. Y., Moy L., Kim S. G., Baete S. H., Moccaldi M., Babb J. S., et al. Evaluation of breast cancer using intravoxel incoherent motion (IVIM) histogram analysis: comparison with malignant status, histological subtype, and molecular prognostic factors. *Eur. Radiol.* (2016), 26, 2547–2558.

34. Ei Khouli R. H., Jacobs M. A., Mezban S. D., Huang P., Kamel I. R., Macura K. J., et al. Diffusion-weighted imaging improves the diagnostic accuracy of conventional 3.0-T breast MR imaging. *Radiology* (2010), 256, 64–73.

35. Parsian S., Rahbar H., Allison K. H., Demartini W. B., Olson M. L., Lehman C. D., et al. Nonmalignant breast lesions: ADCs of benign and high-risk subtypes assessed as false-positive at dynamic enhanced MR imaging. *Radiology* (2012), 265, 696–706.

36. Le Bihan D., Breton E., Lallemand D., Aubin M. L., Vignaud J., Laval-Jeantet M. Separation of diffusion and perfusion in intravoxel incoherent motion MR imaging. *Radiology* (1988), 168, 497–505.

37. Meeus E. M., Novak J., Withey S. B., Zarinabad N., Dehghani H., Peet A. C. Evaluation of intravoxel incoherent motion fitting methods in low-perfused tissue. *J. Magn. Reson. Imaging* (2017), 45, 1325–1334.

38. Wu W. C., Chen Y. F., Tseng H. M., Yang S. C., My P. C. Caveat of measuring perfusion indexes using intravoxel incoherent motion magnetic resonance imaging in the human brain. *Eur. Radiol.* (2015), 25, 2485–2492.

39. Grech-Sollars M., Hales P. W., Miyazaki K., Raschke F., Rodriguez D., Wilson M., et al. Multi-centre reproducibility of diffusion MRI parameters for clinical sequences in the brain. *NMR Biomed.* (2015), 28, 468–485.

40. Chen W., Zhang J., Long D., Wang Z., Zhu J. M. Optimization of intra-voxel incoherent motion measurement in diffusion-weighted imaging of breast cancer. *J. Appl. Clin. Med. Phys.* (2017), 18, 191–199.

41. Liu C., Liang C., Liu Z., Zhang S., Huang B. Intravoxel incoherent motion (IVIM) in evaluation of breast lesions: comparison with conventional DWI. *Eur. J. Radiol.* (2013), 82, e782–e789.

42. Hu Y. C., Yan L. F., Wu L., Du P., Chen B. Y., Wang L., et al. Intravoxel incoherent motion diffusion-weighted MR imaging of gliomas: efficacy in preoperative grading. *Sci. Rep.* (2014), 4, 7208.

43. Lin Y. K., Li J. R., Zhang Z. Q., Xu Q., Zhou Z. Y., Zhang Z. P., et al. Comparison of intravoxel incoherent motion diffusion-weighted MR imaging and arterial spin labeling MR imaging in gliomas. *Biomed. Res. Int.* (2015), 2015, 234245.

44. Kim H. S., Suh C. H., Kim N., Choi C. G., Kim S. J. Histogram analysis of intravoxel incoherent motion for differentiating recurrent tumor from treatment effect in patients with glioblastoma: initial clinical experience. *AJNR Am. J. Neuroradiol.* (2014), 35, 490–497.

45. Federau C., Cerny M., Roux M., Mosimann P. J., Maeder P., Meuli, R, et al. IVIM perfusion fraction is prognostic for survival in brain glioma. *Clin. Neuroradiol.* (2017), 27, 485–492.

46. Federau C., O'Brien K., Meuli R., Hagmann P., Maeder P. Measuring brain perfusion with intravoxel incoherent motion (IVIM): Initial clinical experience. *J. Magn. Reson. Imaging.* (2014), 39, 624–632.

47. Wirestam R., Brockstedt S., Lindgren A., Geijer B., Thomsen C., Holtas S., et al. The perfusion fraction in volunteers and in patients with ischaemic stroke. *Acta Radiol.* (1997), 38, 961–964.

48. Sievert A. J., Fisher M. J. Pediatric low-grade gliomas. *J. Child. Neurol.* (2009), 24, 1397–1408.

49. Plaza M. J., Borja M. J., Altman N., Saigal G. Conventional and advanced MRI features of pediatric intracranial tumors: posterior fossa and suprasellar tumors. *AJR Am. J. Roentgenol.* (2013), 200, 1115–1124.

50. Sigmund E. E., Cho G. Y., Kim S., Finn M., Moccaldi M., Jensen J. H., et al. Intravoxel incoherent motion imaging of tumor microenvironment in locally advanced breast cancer. *Magn. Reson. Med.* (2011), 65, 1437–1447.

51. Iima M., Kataoka M., Kanao S., Kawai M., Onishi N., Koyasu S., et al. Variability of non-Gaussian diffusion MRI and intravoxel incoherent motion (IVIM) measurements in the breast. *PLoS One* (2018), 13, e0193444.

52. Iima M., Yano K., Kataoka M., Umehana M., Murata K., Kanao S., et al. Quantitative non-Gaussian diffusion and intravoxel incoherent motion magnetic resonance imaging: differentiation of malignant and benign breast lesions. *Invest. Radiol.* (2015), 50, 205–211.

53. Bokacheva L., Kaplan J. B., Giri D. D., Patil S., Gnanasigamani M., Nyman C. G., et al. Intravoxel incoherent motion diffusion-weighted MRI at 3.0 T differentiates malignant breast lesions from benign lesions and breast parenchyma. *J. Magn. Reson. Imaging* (2014), 40, 813–823.

54. Cho G. Y., Gennaro L., Sutton E. J., Zabor E. C., Zhang Z., Giri D., et al. Intravoxel incoherent motion (IVIM) histogram biomarkers for prediction of neoadjuvant treatment response in breast cancer patients. *Eur. J. Radiol. Open* (2017), 4, 101–107.

55. Che S., Zhao X., Ou Y., Li J., Wang M., Wu B., et al. Role of the intravoxel incoherent motion diffusion weighted imaging in the pre-treatment prediction and early response monitoring to neoadjuvant chemotherapy in locally advanced breast cancer. *Medicine (Baltimore)* (2016), 95, e2420.

56. Barbieri S., Donati O. F., Froehlich J. M., Thoeny H. C. Impact of the calculation algorithm on biexponential fitting of diffusion-weighted MRI in upper abdominal organs. *Magn. Reson. Med.* (2016), 75, 2175–2184.

57. Meeus E. M., Novak J., Dehghani H., Peet A. C. Rapid measurement of intravoxel incoherent motion (IVIM) derived perfusion fraction for clinical magnetic resonance imaging. *MAGMA*, doi: 10.1007/s10334-017-0656-6. (2017)

58. Orton M. R., Collins D. J., Koh D. M., Leach M. O. Improved intravoxel incoherent motion analysis of diffusion weighted imaging by data driven Bayesian modeling. *Magn. Reson. Med.* (2014), 71, 411–420.

59. Park H. J., Sung Y. S., Lee S. S., Lee Y., Cheong H., Kim Y. J., et al. Intravoxel incoherent motion diffusion-weighted MRI of the abdomen: The effect of fitting algorithms on the accuracy and reliability of the parameters. *J. Magn. Reson. Imaging* (2016), 45, 1637–1647.

60. Cho G. Y., Moy L., Zhang J. L., Baete S., Lattanzi R., Moccaldi M., et al. Comparison of fitting methods and b-value sampling strategies for intravoxel incoherent motion in breast cancer. *Magn. Reson. Med.* (2015), 74, 1077–1085.

61. Lemke A., Stieltjes B., Schad L. R., Laun F. B. Toward an optimal distribution of *b* values for intravoxel incoherent motion imaging. *Magn. Reson. Imaging* (2011), 29, 766–776.

62. Suo S., Lin N., Wang H., Zhang L., Wang R., Zhang S., et al. Intravoxel incoherent motion diffusion-weighted MR imaging of breast cancer at 3.0 tesla: Comparison of different curve-fitting methods. *J. Magn. Reson. Imaging* (2015), 42, 362–370.

63. Wurnig M. C., Donati O. F., Ulbrich E., Filli L., Kenkel D., Thoeny H. C., et al. Systematic analysis of the intravoxel incoherent motion threshold separating perfusion and diffusion effects: Proposal of a standardized algorithm. *Magn. Reson. Med.* (2015), 74, 1414–1422.

Chapter 25

Synthetic and Physiological IVIM Complexity

Eric E. Sigmund
Bernard and Irene Schwartz Center for Biomedical Imaging, Center for Advanced Imaging Innovation and Research (CAI²R), New York, USA
Department of Radiology, NYU Langone Health, New York, USA
eric.sigmund@nyulangone.org

Simplicity is complexity resolved.

—Constantin Brancusi

The mechanism underlying intravoxel incoherent motion (IVIM) (signal attenuation from microcirculation, in distinction from thermal Brownian motion) has been demonstrated in an increasing number of scenarios within quantitative magnetic resonance imaging (MRI). As detailed elsewhere in this volume, the combination of improved hardware, software, and anatomic accessibility has (relatively recently) led to an explosion of activity for this approach throughout the body (see Fig. 25.1).

Intravoxel Incoherent Motion (IVIM) MRI: Principles and Applications
Edited by Denis Le Bihan, Mami Iima, Christian Federau, and Eric E. Sigmund

ISBN 978-981-4800-19-8 (Hardcover), 978-0-429-42727-5 (eBook)
www.panstanford.com

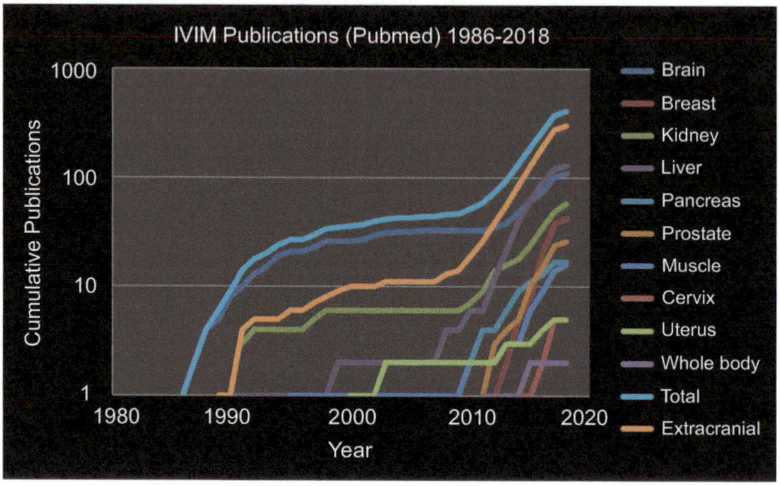

Figure 25.1 Cumulative IVIM-related publications by year overall and stratified by organ system. Three periods are evident: (i) initial discovery and investigation largely in brain tissue (1988–1998); (ii) pilot investigations in extracranial organs (1998–2008); and (iii) re-emergence and expansion of activity throughout the body (2008–present). Results were obtained via PubMed search "IVIM (or) intravoxel incoherent motion (and) (organ)." Total and extracranial categories were computed from results of the organ-specific searches.

Three periods are evident in this development: (i) an initial discovery and investigation phase, largely in brain tissue due to hardware/software availability (1988–1998), (ii) pilot investigations in extracranial organs and pathologies highly suited to vascular/microstructural decomposition, such as hepatic and renal tissue (1998–2008), and (iii) following landmark studies in several organs [1–4] and commentary [5], rapid expansion of activity throughout the body (2008–present). The rapidly growing use of IVIM has been recognized in several recent review articles [6], for example, in the body [7, 8], in the liver [9], and in the breast [10].

As the evidence base grows, however, it has become clear that the manifestations of IVIM differentiate themselves in organ- and pathology-specific ways. The tissue fraction displaying pseudodiffusion varies greatly, necessitating adaptations of acquisition and analysis. In some cases, the microcirculation is isotropic, while in others, it shows directionality in the structure and/or flow within the flow compartment. The active processes captured in the IVIM effect are also affected by such stimuli as an exercise challenge, which has motivated protocols capturing binary or dynamic changes from the baseline. In short, the occurrences of IVIM have been recognized to require treatment beyond the static isotropic model. Just as the application of structure-based diffusion-weighted imaging contrast has evolved from isotropic to anisotropic to higher and higher levels of complexity—with associated higher biological specificity—so too can we expect that a refinement of the IVIM signature to reflect more complex scenarios will amplify diagnostic potential in those situations.

For clarity, the notation of the IVIM expressions in this chapter will be

$$\frac{M}{M_0} = f_\text{p} \exp(-b \cdot D_\text{p}) + (1 - f_\text{p}) \exp(-b \cdot D_\text{t}), \tag{25.1}$$

where D_t is tissue diffusivity, f_p is perfusion fraction, and D_p is pseudodiffusivity.

25.1 Phantoms

Imitation is the sincerest of flattery.

—Charles Caleb Colton

The translational pathway of successful imaging biomarkers typically involves ongoing input from synthetic phantoms to accompany experiences in vivo. Diffusion-weighted imaging biomarkers are no exception; ice-water baths have become a very reliable diffusion phantom for static isotropic diffusion [11], and polymer mixtures/gels are also common [12–14]. A whole host of phantoms have been put forward simulating diffusion anisotropy (polymer fibers, capillaries, glass plates, and biologic phantoms) [15–22]. These systems allow controlled contrast variation, tests of reproducibility, and evaluation of new models. IVIM phantoms have also been demonstrated since the earliest uses of IVIM in clinical scanners and have grown in complexity over time (see Table 25.1 and Fig. 25.2) [23–33].

Table 25.1 Summary of IVIM phantoms employed in clinical scanners

Study	System	Flow speed	Flow fraction	Anisotropy	Fit algorithm	Flow compensation	Diffusion time	Modeling
Ahn et al. [33]	Random capillary ball	x				x		x
Le Bihan et al. [30]	Sephadex	x	x					x
Lorenz et al. [29]	Cotton; Sephadex	x		x				
Maki et al. [31]	Sephadex	x				x	x	x
Fujita et al. [32]	Single pipe	x				x		
Karampinos et al. [23]	Pipe network	x	x	x				x
Cho et al. [24]	Sponge/water	x		x	x	x		
Wetscherek et al. [28]	Single pipe	x				x	x	x
Lee et al. [25]	Sephadex	x	x		x			
Schneider et al. [27]	Sugar fibers	x						x
Ohno et al.[26]	Sponge/PPE filter	x						

Note: Different systems were employed to generate an incoherent flow. Varying amounts of quantification, encoding, analysis algorithms, and modeling have been employed to generate and understand biomimetic flow patterns to accompany the use of IVIM within in vivo scanners.

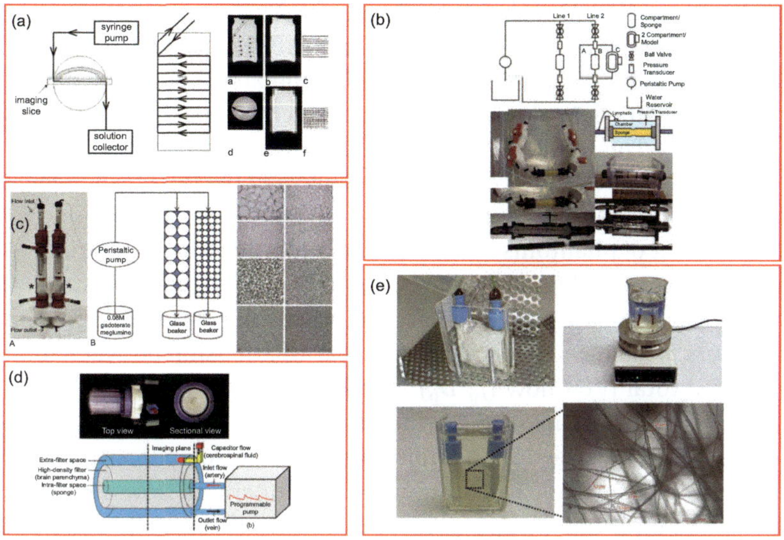

Figure 25.2 Example IVIM flow phantoms in the literature. (a) Anisotropic circumferential flow around static phantom. Reprinted from Ref. [23], with permission from John Wiley and Sons. (b) Incoherent flow through a cellulose sponge with an annular static water chamber. Reprinted from Ref. [24], with permission from John Wiley and Sons. (c) Driven flow through variable-sized Sephadex bead packs. Reprinted from Ref. [25], with permission from Wolters Kluwer Health, Inc. (d) Incoherent flow through a cellulose sponge and an annular static diffusion chamber. Reprinted from Ref. [26], with permission from John Wiley and Sons. (e) Flow through a disordered sucrose network [27].

All of these crucially employ a driven source of water motion with an incoherent flow distribution that presents a "pseudodiffusion" signal loss with diffusion-weighting magnetic field gradients. As with many fields of MRI, much inspiration for such synthetic systems was taken from nuclear magnetic resonance (NMR) research in materials science [34, 35] and adapted to the clinical MRI environment. An early synthetic IVIM phantom by Ahn et. al. [33] used a random capillary ball-shaped bundle to generate controlled incoherent flow. Another system, first demonstrated in Ref. [30] and later employed in various forms [25, 29, 31], was based on water flow through Sephadex microspheres. Alternatively, others [24, 26] employed cylindrical systems with a central flow compartment containing cellulose for flow dispersion and an annular space with water or gel. These systems allowed sampling of the flow or static spaces separately or in combination. Still other cases used single water pipes [28] or a network of water capillaries [23] to tease out higher-order features with a combination of advanced encoding and signal modeling. Another system [27] emulated microvasculature with a solidified sugarcane network of microcapillaries (diameters 2–25 μm). This system mimicked the interspersed microvascular and cellular volumes in real tissue and allowed the testing of higher-order quantification schemes.

This set of phantoms has simulated and tested the measurement of a variety of biological features (see Table 25.1). All of them allow control of flow rate with a corresponding change in pseudodiffusion markers, in some cases verifying a linear relationship between fluid flux and total IVIM flow (f_p*D_p). Another feature in some biological contexts is IVIM anisotropy, which several systems produce, given an overall flow direction in addition to transverse microcirculation [23, 24, 29]. In one case, a network of antiparallel flow segments produces clear anisotropy to test an "intravoxel partially coherent motion (IVPCM)" signal description, as might occur in muscle or renal tissue [23].

Another aspect of the IVIM analysis workflow is the choice of the fit algorithm, and synthetic phantoms allow the comparison of several methods (simultaneous fitting, segmented fitting, etc.) on the same data source [24, 25]. More generally, they allow testing of advanced encoding methods involving flow-compensated diffusion gradients [24, 27, 28, 31, 33] and diffusion time variation [27, 28, 31]. Even more broadly, complex signal models have been advanced incorporating anisotropy [36], estimating segment length or blood velocity [27, 28], or generalizing the displacement distribution [28, 37] beyond extremal cases of ballistic (short time, low velocity) and dispersive (long time, high velocity) limits.

The development of tissue-emulating ("biomimetic") systems has practical uses not only for reproducibility and translation but also for more deep understanding of tissue contrast. The original discovery of the IVIM contrast was imagined largely as an alternative measure of tissue perfusion to contrast enhancement, which is valid, although the precise expression of the microvasculature differs between IVIM and other methods (arterial spin labeling [ASL], dynamic contrast–enhanced [DCE] MRI, and dynamic susceptibility contrast [DSC] MRI). However, the application of IVIM to many organs and contexts has revealed needs for description of microcirculation beyond perfusion (such as renal tubular flow). For all of these applications, the continued refinement of synthetic systems to accompany the in vivo assay will be vital.

25.2 Anisotropy

If you're not sure where you're going, you'll probably end up somewhere else.

—Anonymous

Numerous structures in the body possess anisotropic microcirculation, and the IVIM toolbox has progressively expanded to include this feature in clinical scanner data. One example is pseudodiffusion from vascular/tubular flow in renal (kidney) tissue, particularly in the medulla (see Fig. 25.3). The "radial" pattern of tubule/duct orientation is well known in diffusion tensor imaging (DTI) [38–42], following an initial demonstration by Ries et. al. [43]. Intuitively, microscopic flow contributes to medullary anisotropy, as indirectly suggested by DTI studies showing elevated anisotropy when lower *b* values were employed [42]. Directly, several studies have now shown that the flow term shows a similar orientation pattern. One experimental demonstration employed multiple-*b*-value, multiple direction data to illustrate this collinear anisotropy of structural and pseudodiffusion tensors with projection plots ("peanut plot visualization") in a combined IVIM/DTI scheme [44]. This empirical view showed that pseudodiffusion anisotropy was comparable to that of the microstructure (see Fig. 25.3). Another approach employed an intravoxel-oriented flow (IVOF) model incorporating an apparent flow fraction tensor to capture the microcirculation and microstructural anisotropy in medullary tissue [45]. These studies have confirmed that the best representation of water transport in kidney should incorporate directionality in both flow and structural compartments. Indeed, this treatment has recently yielded diagnostic potential in the assessment of renal function in presurgical renal mass patients [46]. One of the measures most sensitive to asymmetric laterality in kidney diffusion—reflecting the compensatory redistribution of flow in response to the presence of a neoplasm and corresponding reduction in functioning nephrons—was axial medullary pseudodiffusion. This feature was only revealed in the combined IVIM-DTI analysis.

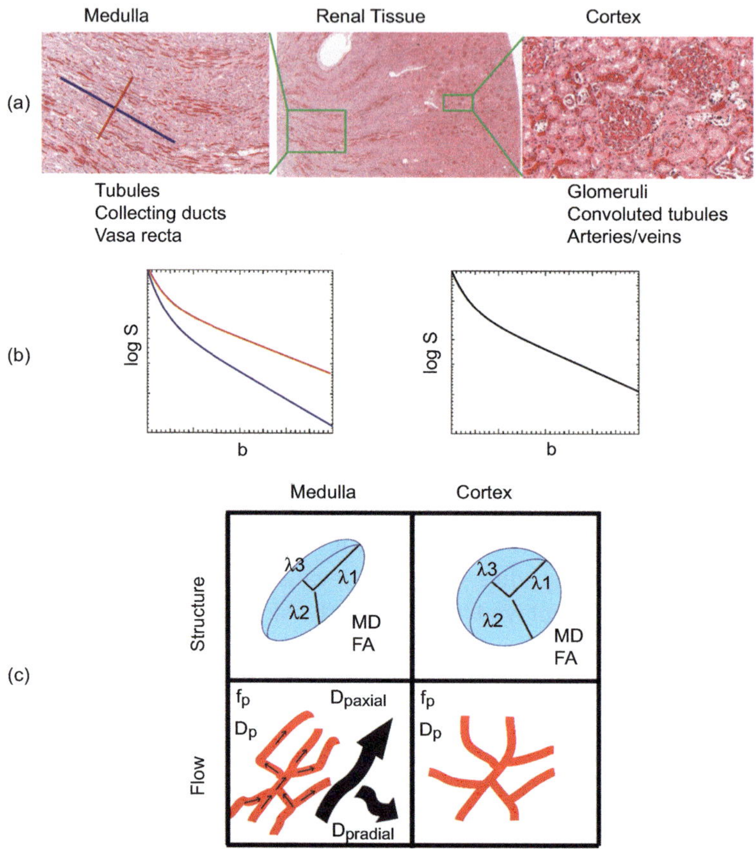

Figure 25.3 IVIM contrast in renal tissue. (a) Histological sections of the renal cortex and medulla (from Ref. [47]) show differing contributors to water transport; cortical tissue is an isotropic mixture of glomeruli, convoluted tubules, and vessels, while medullary tissue shows aligned tubules, vasculature, and ductal structures. (b) IVIM contrast as a function of *b* value shows a multicompartment response (microcirculation vs. restricted Brownian motion), with an additional component of anisotropy in medullary tissue. (c) Quantitative representations of renal DWI, with diffusion tensor indices showing structural compartments, perfusion fraction, and pseudodiffusivities (reflecting microcirculation), with the anisotropic components of D_p prominent in medullary tissue.

Skeletal muscle is another organ whose microcirculation is anisotropic. Histology confirms that a large fraction of microvasculature in skeletal muscle surrounds and is aligned with each individual myofiber (see Fig. 25.4). The IVIM signature in this organ is correspondingly anisotropic, as several studies have indicated [23, 48, 49]. One study quantified the response in an IVPCM scheme, since the perfusion component has a preferred orientation and some angular distribution around it [23]. This more complete description may aid in differentiating types of peripheral vascular disease.

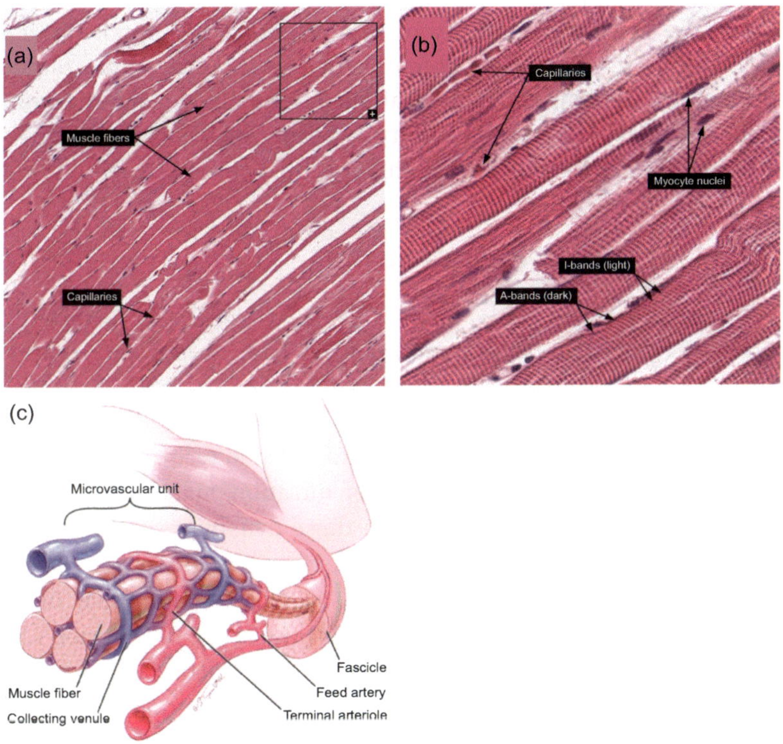

Figure 25.4 (a, b) Histologic examples from Human Protein Atlas [50] showing the alignment of capillaries with myofiber longitudinal axes in skeletal muscle. (a) https://www.proteinatlas.org/learn/dictionary/normal/skeletal+muscle/detail+1 (b) https://www.proteinatlas.org/learn/dictionary/normal/skeletal+muscle/detail+1/magnification+1 (c) Diagram of skeletal muscle microvasculature showing close alignment of microvessels with myofibers. Reprinted from Ref. [51], with permission from Elsevier.

Continuing studies in other organs have demonstrated IVIM anisotropy. Finkenstaedt et. al. [52] used a three-tensor model to describe the IVIM signature in the brain and decomposed the tensors for D_t, f_p, and D_p into planar, spherical, and linear components. Both this quantitative analysis and qualitative illustrations demonstrated deviation from spherical components in the perfusion parameters and alignment with the structural tensor. Similarly, Abdullah et. al. studied the orientation dependence of microcirculation in myocardial tissue [53]; here again pseudodiffusion showed anisotropic behavior in the same pattern as the underlying structural tensor.

These examples of anisotropy in the IVIM signal across the body signal the increased maturity of the technique and opportunities for refining its diagnostic potential by matching it to the target physiology. Ongoing technological advancements in field strength, radio frequency (RF) coil sensitivity, and especially diffusion gradient strength are expected to extend this specificity even further.

25.3 Stimulus Response

We don't grow when things are easy; we grow when we face challenges.

—Anonymous

The dynamic aspect of the IVIM pseudodiffusion term, representing processes such as perfusion or water filtration, makes another dimension of contrast available when these dynamics can be modulated by a stimulus. Examples of such stimuli might be exercise or pharmaceutical administration (such as diuretics for renal function). Federau recently summarized [54] the scope of reported observations to date of changes of IVIM perfusion fraction with a range of challenges, including muscle exercise, visual activation, hyperoxygenation, and renal pharmaceuticals (hydralazine, furosemide, etc.). In each of these cases, a comparison of IVIM contrast before and after stimulus revealed substantial changes (~30%) in the perfusion fraction; these studies exemplify the utility of combining a specific biophysical description like IVIM with a targeted challenge to distill the maximal diagnostic contrast.

Skeletal muscle water transport is transiently altered by exercise due to a combination of water exchange, myofiber swelling, and increased perfusion [55, 56]. IVIM is again a sensitive probe of this process. In forearm MRI with grip exercise by Morvan [57], response was seen in all metrics, but particularly blood volume. In a later forearm IVIM study with a high temporal resolution [58], all three parameters (but particularly f_p and D_p) were similarly elevated in the activated muscle. In calf muscle, with treadmill [49] or ergometer [59] exercise, IVIM pseudodiffusion and perfusion fraction metrics both increased. In back muscle exercise, a pre- and post-exercise protocol registered increases in tissue diffusion and perfusion fraction [60]. In a shoulder muscle study [61], selective muscle compartments targeted by a particular challenge showed significant increases in IVIM total flux $f_p{}^*D_p$. IVIM is a powerful probe of the response of microcirculation to a challenge, which is a key element in pathologies.

The kidney is another dynamic organ whose response to a challenge can be telling of its function and to which IVIM is sensitive. Renal filtration is a complex interplay of vascular flow, tubular flow, and water exchange, and pharmaceuticals can modulate individual aspects to improve diagnosis. Loop diuretics like furosemide inhibit reabsorption in the distal loop of Henle, increasing medullary tubular flow and urine output while simultaneously reducing cortical blood volume. IVIM studies have registered these changes in both preclinical studies [62] and healthy volunteers [63]. Conversely, hydralazine was observed to increase cortical perfusion fraction in a preclinical study [62]. Angiotensin II has also been observed to induce significant increases in microcirculation fractions of healthy volunteers in a triexponential signal model [64]. Here again, the pharmaceutical modulation of water transport—a crucial aspect of managing renal disease—has a corresponding noninvasive quantitative imaging measure in the IVIM approach.

25.4 Summary

Whether these are assessed by publication volume or a more focused study of individual organ-based efforts, the strength, breadth, and complexity of IVIM contrast are evidently growing within the field of quantitative MRI. While historical quandaries on whether and how IVIM signal signifies perfusion have been reasonably addressed by this progress, the increased awareness of the complexity of the IVIM signal begs focused study for the next generation of questions, researchers, and applications. Given the ubiquitous role that perfusion and microcirculation play in the body, it is surely to the benefit of MRI tissue characterization by DWI to take the IVIM contrast into account and, where appropriate, focus directly upon it. As the literature trend in Fig. 25.1 predicts, the next wave of activity will likely yield bountiful and unexpected benefits.

Acknowledgment

The author acknowledges Fred LaPolla for assistance in the literature search, Hersh Chandarana and Steven Baete for editorial review, and Margret Magid and Amy Rapkiewicz for assistance with NYU Virtual Microscope images.

References

1. Sigmund E. E., Cho G. Y., Kim S., Finn M., Moccaldi M., Jensen J. H., et al., Intravoxel incoherent motion imaging of tumor microenvironment in locally advanced breast cancer. *Magn. Reson. Med.* 2011, 65(5), 1437–1447.
2. Lemke A., Stieltjes B., Schad L. R., Laun F. B. Toward an optimal distribution of b values for intravoxel incoherent motion imaging. *Magn. Reson. Imaging* 2011, 29(6), 766–776.
3. Dopfert J., Lemke A., Weidner A., Schad L. R. Investigation of prostate cancer using diffusion-weighted intravoxel incoherent motion imaging. *Magn. Reson. Imaging* 2011, 29(8), 1053–1058.
4. Luciani A., Vignaud A., Cavet M., Van Nhieu J. T., Mallat A., Ruel L., et al. Liver cirrhosis: intravoxel incoherent motion MR imaging-pilot study. *Radiology* 2008, 249(3), 891–899.
5. Le Bihan D. Intravoxel incoherent motion perfusion MR imaging: A wake-up call. *Radiology* 2008, 249(3), 748–752.
6. Le Bihan D. What can we see with IVIM MRI? *Neuroimage* 2017, https://doi.org/10.1016/j.neuroimage.2017.12.062.
7. Koh D. M., Collins D. J., Orton M. R. Intravoxel incoherent motion in body diffusion-weighted MRI: reality and challenges. *Am. J. Roentgenol.* 2011, 196(6), 1351–1361.
8. Taouli B., Beer A. J., Chenevert T., Collins D., Lehman C., Matos C., et al. Diffusion-weighted imaging outside the brain: Consensus statement

from an ISMRM-sponsored workshop. *J. Magn. Reson. Imaging* 2016, 44(3), 521–540.

9. Li Y. T., Cercueil J-P, Yuan J., Chen W., Loffroy R., Wáng Y. X. J. Liver intravoxel incoherent motion (IVIM) magnetic resonance imaging: a comprehensive review of published data on normal values and applications for fibrosis and tumor evaluation. *Quant. Imaging Med. Surg.* 2017, 7(1), 59–78.
10. Partridge S. C., Nissan N., Rahbar H., Kitsch A. E., Sigmund E. E. Diffusion-weighted breast MRI: Clinical applications and emerging techniques. *J. Magn. Reson. Imaging* 2017, 45(2), 337–355.
11. Malyarenko D., Galban C. J., Londy F. J., Meyer C. R., Johnson T. D., Rehemtulla A., et al. Multi-system repeatability and reproducibility of apparent diffusion coefficient measurement using an ice-water phantom. *J. Magn. Reson. Imaging* 2013, 37(5), 1238–1246.
12. Wang X., Reeder S. B., Hernando D. An acetone-based phantom for quantitative diffusion MRI. *J. Magn. Reson. Imaging* 2017, 46(6), 1683–1692.
13. Pullens P., Bladt P., Sijbers J., Maas A. I., Parizel P. M. Technical Note: A safe, cheap, and easy-to-use isotropic diffusion MRI phantom for clinical and multicenter studies. *Med. Phys.* 2017, 44(3), 1063–1070.
14. McHugh D. J., Zhou F. L., Wimpenny I., Poologasundarampillai G., Naish J. H., Hubbard Cristinacce P. L., et al. A biomimetic tumor tissue phantom for validating diffusion-weighted MRI measurements. *Magn. Reson. Med.* 2018, 80(1),147–158.
15. Fieremans E., De Deene Y., Delputte S., Ozdemir M. S., D'Asseler Y., Vlassenbroeck J., et al. Simulation and experimental verification of the diffusion in an anisotropic fiber phantom. *J. Magn. Reson.* 2008, 190(2), 189–199.
16. Rydhog A., Latt J., Nilson M., Nordh E., Brockstedt S., Carlemalm E., et al. Using q-space diffusion MRI for stuctural studies of a biological phantom at 3T clinical scanner. *Proc. Int. Soc. Magn. Reson. Med.* 2007, 1534.
17. Laun F. B., Stieltjes B., Huff S., Schad L. R. Investigations of a DTI-phantom with properties similar to in vivo neuronal tissue. *Proc. Int. Soc. Magn. Reson. Med.* 2007, 1526.
18. Nilsson M., Larsson J., Lundberg D., Szczepankiewicz F., Witzel T., Westin C. F., et al. Liquid crystal phantom for validation of microscopic diffusion anisotropy measurements on clinical MRI systems. *Magn. Reson. Med.* 2018, 79(3), 1817–1828.

19. Fan Q., Nummenmaa A., Wichtmann B., Witzel T., Mekkaoui C., Schneider W., et al. Validation of diffusion MRI estimates of compartment size and volume fraction in a biomimetic brain phantom using a human MRI scanner with 300 mT/m maximum gradient strength. *Neuroimage* 2018, https://doi.org/10.1016/j.neuroimage.2018.01.004.

20. Komlosh M. E., Benjamini D., Barnett A. S., Schram V., Horkay F., Avram A. V., et al. Anisotropic phantom to calibrate high-q diffusion MRI methods. *J. Magn. Reson.* 2017, 275, 19–28.

21. Lichenstein S. D., Bishop J. H., Verstynen T. D., Yeh F. C. Diffusion capillary phantom vs. human data: outcomes for reconstruction methods depend on evaluation medium. *Front Neurosci.* 2016, 10, 407.

22. Perrin M., Poupon C., Rieul B., Leroux P., Constantinesco A., Mangin J. F., et al. Validation of q-ball imaging with a diffusion fibre-crossing phantom on a clinical scanner. *Philos. Trans. R. Soc. B* 2005, 360(1457), 881–891.

23. Karampinos D. C., King K. F., Sutton B. P., Georgiadis J. G. Intravoxel partially coherent motion technique: characterization of the anisotropy of skeletal muscle microvasculature. *J. Magn. Reson. Imaging,* 2010, 31(4), 942–953.

24. Cho G. Y., Kim S., Jensen J. H., Storey P., Sodickson D. K., Sigmund E. E. A versatile flow phantom for intravoxel incoherent motion MRI. *Magn. Reson. Med.* 2012, 67(6), 1710–1720.

25. Lee J. H., Cheong H., Lee S. S., Lee C. K., Sung Y. S., Huh J. W., et al. Perfusion assessment using intravoxel incoherent motion-based analysis of diffusion-weighted magnetic resonance imaging: Validation through phantom experiments. *Invest. Radiol.* 2016, 51(8), 520–528.

26. Ohno N., Miyati T., Chigusa T., Usui H., Ishida S., Hiramatsu Y., et al., Technical Note: Development of a cranial phantom for assessing perfusion, diffusion, and biomechanics. *Med. Phys.* 2017, 44(5), 1646–1654.

27. (a) Schneider M. J., Gaass T., Dietrich O., Ingrisch M., Reiser M. F., Dinkel J. Intravoxel incoherent motion MRI in a 3-dimensional microvascular flow phantom. *Proc. Int. Soc. Magn. Res. Med.* 2016, 920. (b) Gaass T., Schneider M.J., Dietrich O., Ingrisch M., Dinkel J. Technical Note: Quantitative dynamic contrast-enhanced MRI of a 3-dimensional artificial capillary network. Med. Phys. 2017, 44(4), 1462–1469.

28. Wetscherek A., Stieltjes B., Laun F. B. Flow-compensated intravoxel incoherent motion diffusion imaging. *Magn. Reson. Med.* 2015, 74(2), 410–419.

29. Lorenz C. H., Pickens D. R., 3rd, Puffer D. B., Price R. R. Magnetic resonance diffusion/perfusion phantom experiments. *Magn. Reson. Med.* 1991, 19(2), 254–260.

30. Le Bihan D., Breton E., Lallemand D., Aubin M. L., Vignaud J., Laval-Jeantet M. Separation of diffusion and perfusion in intravoxel incoherent motion MR imaging. *Radiology* 1988, 168(2), 497–505.

31. Maki J. H., MacFall J. R., Johnson G. A. The use of gradient flow compensation to separate diffusion and microcirculatory flow in MRI. *Magn. Reson. Med.* 1991, 17(1), 95–107.

32. Fujita N., Harada K., Sakurai K., Akai Y., Kozuka T. Separation of diffusion and slow flow effects by use of flow rephasing and dephasing. *Magn. Reson. Med.* 1992, 24(1), 109–122.

33. Ahn C. B., Lee S. Y., Nalcioglu O., Cho Z. H. The effects of random directional distributed flow in nuclear magnetic resonance imaging. *Med. Phys.* 1987, 14(1), 43–48.

34. Seymour J. D., Caprihan A., Altobelli S. A., Fukushima E. Pulsed gradient spin echo nuclear magnetic resonance imaging of diffusion in granular flow. *Phys. Rev. Lett.* 2000, 84, 266–269.

35. Seymour J. D., Callaghan P. T. Generalized approach to NMR analysis of flow and dispersion in a porous media. *AIChE J.* 1997, 43, 2096.

36. Karampinos D. C., King K. F., Sutton B. P., Georgiadis J. G. Intravoxel partially coherent motion technique: characterization of the anisotropy of skeletal muscle microvasculature. *J. Magn. Reson. Imaging* 2010, 31(4), 942–953.

37. Kennan R. P., Gao J. H., Zhong J. H., Gore J. C. A general-model of microcirculatory blood-flow effects in gradient sensitized MRI. *Med. Phys.* 1994, 21(4), 539–545.

38. Lanzman R. S., Ljimani A., Pentang G., Zgoura P., Zenginli H., Kropil P., et al. Kidney transplant: functional assessment with diffusion-tensor MR imaging at 3T. *Radiology* 2013, 266(1), 218–225.

39. Gaudiano C., Clementi V., Busato F., Corcioni B., Orrei M. G., Ferramosca E., et al. Diffusion tensor imaging and tractography of the kidneys: assessment of chronic parenchymal diseases. *Eur. Radiol.* 2013, 23(6), 1678–1685.

40. Sigmund E. E., Vivier P. H., Sui D., Lamparello N. A., Tantillo K., Mikheev A., et al. Intravoxel incoherent motion and diffusion-tensor imaging in renal tissue under hydration and furosemide flow challenges. *Radiology* 2012, 263(3), 758–769.

41. Hueper K., Gutberlet M., Rodt T., Gwinner W., Lehner F., Wacker F., et al. Diffusion tensor imaging and tractography for assessment of renal allograft dysfunction-initial results. European *Radiology* 2011, 21(11), 2427–2433.

42. Notohamiprodjo M., Glaser C., Herrmann K. A., Dietrich O., Attenberger U. I., Reiser M. F., et al. Diffusion tensor imaging of the kidney with parallel imaging: Initial clinical experience. *Invest. Radiol.* 2008, 43(10), 677–685.

43. Ries M., Jones R. A., Basseau F., Moonen C. T., Grenier N. Diffusion tensor MRI of the human kidney. *J. Magn. Reson. Imaging: JMRI* 2001, 14(1), 42–49.

44. Notohamiprodjo M., Chandarana H., Mikheev A., Rusinek H., Grinstead J., Feiweier T., et al. Combined intravoxel incoherent motion and diffusion tensor imaging of renal diffusion and flow anisotropy. *Magn. Reson. Med.* 2015, 73(4), 1526–1532.

45. Hilbert F., Bock M., Neubauer H., Veldhoen S., Wech T., Bley T. A., et al. An intravoxel oriented flow model for diffusion-weighted imaging of the kidney. *NMR Biomed.* 2016, 29(10), 1403–1413.

46. Liu A. L., Mikheev A., Rusinek H., Huang W. C., Wysock J. S., Babb J. S., et al. REnal flow and microstructure AnisotroPy (REFMAP) MRI in normal and peritumoral renal tissue. *J. Magn. Reson. Imaging* 2018, 48(1), 188–197.

47. NYU Virtual Microscope 2018.

48. Sigmund E. E., Baete S. H., Luo T., Patel K., Wang D., Rossi I., et al. MRI assessment of the thigh musculature in dermatomyositis and healthy subjects using diffusion tensor imaging, intravoxel incoherent motion, and dynamic DTI. *Eur. Radiol.* 2018, doi: 10.1007/s00330-018-5458-3.

49. Sigmund E. E., Baete S. H., Cho G. Y., Sui D., Ukpebor T., Liu K., et al. Intravoxel incoherent motion (IVIM) in healthy skeletal muscle pre- and post-exercise, *Proc. Int. Soc. Magn. Res. Med.* 2012, 4410.

50. Ponten F., Jirstrom K., Uhlen M. The Human Protein Atlas—a tool for pathology. *J. Pathol.* 2008, 216(4), 387–393.

51. Boron W. F., Boulpaep E. L. *Medical Physiology*, Elsevier, 2017.

52. Finkenstaedt T., Klarhoefer M., Eberhardt C., Becker A. S., Andreisek G., Boss A., Rossi C. The IVIM signal in the healthy cerebral gray matter: A play of spherical and non-spherical components. *Neuroimage* 2017, 152, 340–347.

53. Abdullah O. M., Gomez A. D., Merchant S., Heidinger M., Poelzing S., Hsu E. W. Orientation dependence of microcirculation-induced diffusion

signal in anisotropic tissues. *Magn. Reson. Med.* 2016, 76(4), 1252–1262.

54. Federau C. Intravoxel incoherent motion MRI as a means to measure in vivo perfusion: A review of the evidence. *NMR Biomed.* 2017, 30(11).
55. Sjogaard G., Saltin B. Extra- and intracellular water spaces in muscles of man at rest and with dynamic exercise. *Am. J. Physiol.* 1982, 243(3), R271–280.
56. Saab G., Thompson R. T., Marsh G. D. Effects of exercise on muscle transverse relaxation determined by MR imaging and in vivo relaxometry. *J. Appl. Physiol.* (1985) 2000, 88(1), 226–233.
57. Morvan D. In vivo measurement of diffusion and pseudo-diffusion in skeletal muscle at rest and after exercise. *Magn. Reson. Imaging* 1995, 13(2), 193–199.
58. Filli L., Boss A., Wurnig M. C., Kenkel D., Andreisek G., Guggenberger R. Dynamic intravoxel incoherent motion imaging of skeletal muscle at rest and after exercise. *NMR Biomed.* 2015, 28(2), 240–246.
59. Hiepe P., Reichenbach J. Functional muscle MRI in human calf muscle using IVIM. *Proc. Int. Soc. Magn. Res. Med.* 2011, p. 2013.
60. Hiepe P., Gussew A., Rzanny R., Anders C., Walther M., Scholle H. C., Reichenbach J. R. Interrelations of muscle functional MRI, diffusion-weighted MRI and (31) P-MRS in exercised lower back muscles. *NMR Biomed* 2014, 27(8), 958–970.
61. Nguyen A., Ledoux J. B., Omoumi P., Becce F., Forget J., Federau C. Application of intravoxel incoherent motion perfusion imaging to shoulder muscles after a lift-off test of varying duration. *NMR Biomed.* 2016, 29(1), 66–73.
62. Jerome N. P., Boult J. K., Orton M. R., d'Arcy J., Collins D. J., Leach M. O., et al. Modulation of renal oxygenation and perfusion in rat kidney monitored by quantitative diffusion and blood oxygen level dependent magnetic resonance imaging on a clinical 1.5T platform. *BMC Nephrol.* 2016, 17(1), 142.
63. Sigmund E. E., Vivier P-H, Sui D., Lamparello N. A., Tantillo K., Mikheev A., et al. Intravoxel incoherent motion and diffusion-tensor imaging in renal tissue under hydration and furosemide flow challenges. *Radiology* 2012, 263(3), 758–769.
64. van der Bel R., Gurney-Champion O. J., Froeling M., Stroes E. S. G., Nederveen A. J., Krediet C. T. P. A tri-exponential model for intravoxel incoherent motion analysis of the human kidney: In silico and during pharmacological renal perfusion modulation. *Eur. J. Radiol.* 2017, 91, 168–174.

Index